Ethics of Science and Technology Assessment
Volume 29

Book Series of the Europäische Akademie zur Erforschung
von Folgen wissenschaftlich-technischer Entwicklungen
Bad Neuenahr-Ahrweiler GmbH
edited by Carl Friedrich Gethmann

R. Merkel · G. Boer · J. Fegert · T. Galert ·
D. Hartmann · B. Nuttin · S. Rosahl

Intervening in the Brain

Changing Psyche and Society

With 11 Figures

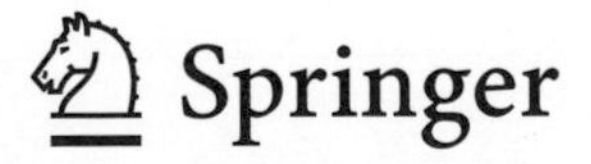

Series Editor
Professor Dr. Dr. h.c. Carl Friedrich Gethmann
Europäische Akademie GmbH
Wilhelmstr. 56, 53474 Bad Neuenahr-Ahrweiler, Germany

On Behalf of the Authors
Professor Dr. Reinhard Merkel
Universität Hamburg
Fakultät für Rechtswissenschaft
Hamburg, Germany

Desk Editor
Friederike Wütscher
Europäische Akademie GmbH
Wilhelmstr. 56, 53474 Bad Neuenahr-Ahrweiler, Germany

Library of Congress Control Number: 2007924217

ISSN 1860-4803

ISBN 978-3-540-46476-1 Springer Berlin Heidelberg New York

Springer is a part of Springer Science+Business Media
springer.com

Typesetting: Köllen-Druck+Verlag GmbH, Bonn + Berlin
Production: LE-TEX Jelonek, Schmidt & Vöckler GbR, Leipzig
Cover: eStudioCalamar S.L., F.Steinen-Broo, Girona, Spanien

Printed on acid-free paper 60/3100/YL - 5 4 3 2 1 0

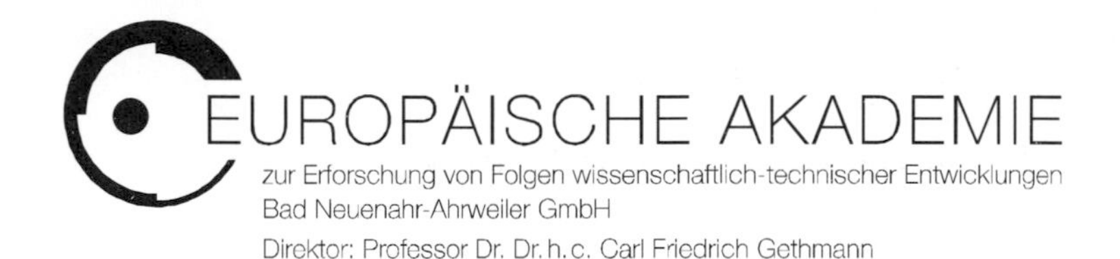

The Europäische Akademie

The *Europäische Akademie zur Erforschung von Folgen wissenschaftlich-technischer Entwicklungen GmbH* is concerned with the scientific study of consequences of scientific and technological advance for the individual and social life and for the natural environment. The Europäische Akademie intends to contribute to a rational way of society of dealing with the consequences of scientific and technological developments. This aim is mainly realised in the development of recommendations for options to act, from the point of view of long-term societal acceptance. The work of the Europäische Akademie mostly takes place in temporary interdisciplinary project groups, whose members are recognised scientists from European universities. Overarching issues, e.g. from the fields of Technology Assessment or Ethic of Science, are dealt with by the staff of the Europäische Akademie.

The Series

The series Ethics of Science and Technology Assessment *(Wissenschaftsethik und Technikfolgenbeurteilung)* serves to publish the results of the work of the Europäische Akademie. It is published by the academy's director. Besides the final results of the project groups the series includes volumes on general questions of ethics of science and technology assessment as well as other monographic studies.

Acknowledgement

The project "Intervening in the Psyche. Novel Possibilities as Social Challenges" was supported by the Federal Ministry of Education and Research (Bundesministerium für Bildung und Forschung, Förderungskennzeichen 16|1513). The authors of this study are responsible for the content.

Preface

The Europäische Akademie is concerned with the study of the consequences of scientific and technological advance both for the individual and for society at large as well as for the natural environment. One important pillar of its work is to assess the consequences of advances in medical research and technology.

In recent years, neuroscience has been a particularly prolific discipline stimulating many innovative treatment approaches in medicine. However, when it comes to the brain, new techniques of intervention do not always meet with a positive public response, in spite of promising therapeutic benefits. The reason for this caution clearly is the brain's special importance as "organ of the mind". As such it is widely held to be the origin of mankind's unique position among living beings. Likewise, on the level of the individual human being, the brain is considered the material substrate of those traits that in combination render each person unique. In view of this preeminent significance of the brain, it is understandable that, in general, interventions into the brain are considered a delicate issue and that new techniques of intervention are scrutinised with particular care. However, in doing so it is important not to go to the opposite extreme and shy away from promising new therapeutic approaches for debilitating disorders of the brain.

With respect to the new techniques of brain intervention a broad interdisciplinary perspective is required to discern irrational fear from justified concern. Hence, the Europäische Akademie established a project group consisting, on the one hand, of experts from different fields of medicine who have got first-hand experience of applying the techniques at issue and, on the other hand, of philosophers and a legal expert. The task of this team was to review the state of the art with respect to each single technique of intervening in the brain, to indicate future developments, and to address the ethical and legal issues common to all of them. The project's outcome is the book at hand.

I would like to thank the members of the project group Dr. Gerard Boer, Professor Dr. Jörg Fegert, Professor Dr. Dirk Hartmann, Professor Dr. Bart Nuttin and Professor Dr. Steffen Rosahl as well as the project's chair Professor Dr. Reinhard Merkel and its coordinator Dr. Thorsten Galert for their dedication to this project. Special thanks go to Friederike Wütscher and Katharina Mader for the editorial work in preparing the text for print.

Bad Neuenahr-Ahrweiler, January 2007 Carl Friedrich Gethmann

List of Authors

Dr. Gerard Boer, M.Sc. degree in biochemistry at the University of Amsterdam in 1970. Thereafter working at the Netherlands Central Institute for Brain Research in Amsterdam on a project investigating the role of the glial cells of the neural lobe in the hormone release process of the hypothalamo-neurohypophyseal neurosecretory system, which resulted in a Ph.D. degree in medicine at the University of Amsterdam in 1976. From 1976 onwards, the main basic research topics, first as investigator later as head of a research group, at the reorganised Netherlands Institute for Brain Research of the Royal Netherlands Academy of Arts and Science, were the neuropeptidergic and monoaminergic influences in perinatal rat brain development and the late lasting functional impairments of the brain following drug exposure in the perinatal and postnatal period (functional neuroteratology), neurotransplantation and circadian rhythm studies in rat and approaches to restore injury of the rat central and peripheral nervous system by means of cell implantation and viral vector-mediated gene transfer. Since 1990 additionally involved in discussions on the ethics of clinical neurotransplantation and other intracranial restorative surgical approaches within the Network of CNS Transplantation And Restoration (NECTAR).

Postal address: Netherlands Institute for Neuroscience, Dept. Neuroregeneration, Meibergdreef 47, 1105 BA Amsterdam ZO, The Netherlands

Professor Dr. med. Jörg M. Fegert, Professor and Chair of Child and Adolescent Psychiatry and Psychotherapy at the Universität Ulm in Germany and Medical Director of the department of Child and Adolescent Psychiatry and Psychotherapy at Ulm University Hospital. He studied medicine in Nantes, France, and Berlin, Germany, music at the Conservatoire Nationale in France and sociology at the Free University of Berlin. He got his professional training at the University Hospital of the Freie Universität Berlin. His MD thesis was published in 1987 on "Migration and psychosocial adaptation". His Habilitation/Ph.D. dealt with atopic dermatitis and child behaviour in a prospective birth cohort. From 1997 to 2001 he was Professor and Head of Department of Child and Adolescent Neurology and Psychiatry at the Universität Rostock. He was also a Visiting Professor at the Universities of Trondheim and the Franzens Universität in Innsbruck, Austria. From 1998 on he was Medical Director of the Centre of Neuropsychiatry at the Universität Rostock. In 2001 he founded the Department of Child and Adolescent Psychiatry and Psychotherapy at the Universität Ulm in Germany (http://www.uni-ulm.de/klinik/kjp). Fegert is member of different professional societies of child and adolescent psychiatry. Member of the Expert-Group Pediatric Pharmacology at the German FDA-like regulatory body, the BfArM, member of the Pediatric Psychopharmacology Initiative (PPI) of the American Academy of Child and Adolescent Psychiatry, member of the IRB/ethics committee of the Universität Ulm. Among further memberships he is member of different advisory committees and boards and member of the Federal Commission on Family Issues at the Federal Government Berlin. His main fields of interest comprise child abuse and neglect and related forensic questions, child psychopharmacology and related basic science, migration, social psychiatry and efficacy of psychosocial interventions and questions of capacity and competence in treatment decisions in child and adolescent psychiatry.

Postal address: Universitätsklinikum Ulm, Abteilung für Kinder- und Jugendpsychiatrie/Psychotherapie, Steinhövelstr. 5, 89070 Ulm, Germany

Dr. phil. Thorsten Galert, M.A. in philosophy (second subject: chemistry) at the Universität Marburg in 1997, Ph.D. in philosophy in 2004 at the same university on a thesis about animal pain, exploring fundamental problems of research in animal consciousness ("Vom Schmerz der Tiere. Grundlagenprobleme der Erforschung tierischen Bewusstseins"). Since 2004 member of the scientific staff of the Europäische Akademie GmbH and coordinator of the project that resulted in the study at hand. Since July 2006 coordinator of a project on "Potentials and Risks of Psychopharmaceutical Enhancement". Since 2006 member of the European Platform for Life Sciences, Mind Sciences, and the Humanities, a network of 60 young academics doing research at the interface between neuroscience, philosophy and psychology, funded by Volkswagen-Foundation. Research areas: applied ethics in general and neuroethics in particular; philosophy of mind; philosophy of science in general and philosophy of psychology in particular; animal consciousness in general and animal pain in particular.

Postal address: Europäische Akademie zur Erforschung von Folgen wissenschaftlich-technischer Entwicklungen Bad Neuenahr-Ahrweiler GmbH, Wilhelmstr. 56, 53474 Bad Neuenahr-Ahrweiler, Germany

Professor Dr. phil. Dirk Hartmann, Professor for theoretical philosophy at the Universität Duisburg-Essen, degree in psychology (Vordiplom) 1988, degree in philosophy and psychology (Magister Artium) 1989, Ph.D. (Dr. phil.) at the same university with a thesis on philosophy of natural sciences with special consideration of psychology 1992, habilitation with a thesis on philosophical foundations of psychology 1997 (all degrees were obtained at the Universität Marburg). In 1998 and 1999 substitute professor for philosophy at the IIWW (Interdisziplinary Institute for Philosophy of Science and History of Science) at the Universität of Erlangen-Nuremberg. In 2001 awarded Werner Heisenberg-fellowship by the DFG (Deutsche Forschungsgemeinschaft) as well as Feodor Lynen-fellowship by the Alexander von Humboldt-Stiftung. In 2001 and 2002 visiting scholar at the UC Berkeley doing research in the field of formal logic. Since 2004 full professor for theoretical philosophy at the Universität Duisburg-Essen.

Main research areas: logic, epistemology, philosophy of science, philosophy of psychology, philosophy of language.

Postal address: Universität Duisburg-Essen, Campus Essen, Department of Philosophy, Universitätsstr. 2, 45141 Essen, Germany

Professor Dr. iur. habil. Reinhard Merkel, Professor of Criminal Law and Philosophy of Law at the Universität Hamburg, Director of the Institute of Criminal Law and Penal Sciences at the same university. He studied law at the universities of Bochum and Heidelberg, and law, philosophy, and German literature at the Universität Munich; LLD at the latter university with a doctoral thesis on "Strafrecht und Satire im Werk von Karl Kraus"/"Criminal Law and Satire in the Work of Karl Kraus" which was elected "Jurisprudential Book of the Year 1995". Habilitation 1996 at the Universität Frankfurt/Main with a treatise on "Früheuthanasie – Rechtsethische und strafrechtliche Grundlagen ärztlicher Entscheidungen über Leben und Tod in der Neonatalmedizin"/"Newborn Euthanasia – Ethical and Legal Foundations of Medical Life-and-Death Decisions in Neonatology", published in 2001; venia legendi for criminal law, criminal procedural law, philosophy of law, and criminology. Member of the "Enquete Commission on Ethics and Law in Modern Medicine" of the German Parliament (Bundestag) between December 2003 and November 2005. Besides the two books mentioned, he wrote a book on the ethical and legal foundations of research on embryonic stem cells ("Forschungsobjekt Embryo", 2002), a draft legislation bill for an amendment of the German Embryo Protection Act (introduced in Parliament in January 2002), edited books on "The Debate on Euthanasia" (1990, 2nd ed. 1991), on Immanuel Kant's treatise on "Eternal Peace" (1997), and on "The Kosovo War and International Law" (2001), and published numerous essays in all major fields of bioethics and medical law, and in the areas of criminal law, philosophy of law, and international public law. He was awarded the "Jean-Amery Price for Essayistic Writing" in 1991.

Postal address: Universität Hamburg, Seminar für Strafrecht und Kriminologie, Schlüterstr. 28, 20146 Hamburg, Germany

Professor Dr. Bart Nuttin, MD, Ph.D., Professor at the Katholieke Universiteit Leuven and head of clinic in the department of neurosurgery at the University Hospitals Leuven, studied in Leuven (Belgium) and received practical training in Pretoria (South Africa) and Exeter (England). He was trained in neurosurgery in Leuven and did postgraduate courses in Cologne (Germany) and Boston (US). His Ph.D. was on "Interleukin-6 and spinal cord injury in rats" with Professor Gybels and Professor Van Damme as promoters. His clinical activity concentrates on stereotactic and functional neurosurgery. His research is now mainly focused on neurosurgery for psychiatric disorders and development of new electrodes for in vivo stimulation and recording of neurones. He developed together with his students and the psychiatry department in Antwerp electrical brain stimulation for obsessive compulsive disorder, first in animal models, and later on in patients with a treatment-resistant form of this disease. Now his group is continuing to explore this field both in animals and in humans in collaboration with the ethics committee and the advisory board for neurosurgery for psychiatric disorders in Flanders. Together with several research centers in Europe and the US he wrote guidelines on what can and should not be done in the field of neurosurgery for psychiatric disorders. He was president of the Belgian Society for Stereotactic Neurosurgery and is now president of the Benelux Neuromodulation Society and coordinator of Erasmus mundus EMMAPA.

Postal address: Department of Neurosurgery, U.Z. Gasthuisberg, Herestraat 49, B-3000 Leuven, Belgium

Professor Steffen K. Rosahl, M.D., Professor of Neurosurgery and Chairman of the Neurosurgical Clinic in Erfurt, Germany, received a MD degree from the Universität Jena in 1992. He was principle investigator in a study to develop auditory neural prostheses for electrical stimulation of the brainstem funded by the German Research Association (DFG) and conducted research on electronic interfaces to the central and peripheral nervous system funded by the German Ministry of Education and Research (BMBF) and private companies (1998–2006). As a neurophysiologist he has been working about slow brain potentials at the Department of Psychophysiology at the Universität Jena, Germany, and at the Center for Neuroscience of the University of California, Davis, USA (1990–1993). Having completed a neurosurgical residency in the program of Professor Madjid Samii in Hannover, Germany, in 1999, he developed a special interest in skull base surgery, image guidance, neural regeneration, and neural prostheses. He became an associate neurosurgeon with Professor Samii to establish the International Neuroscience Institute (INI) in Hannover in 2000. From 2003 through 2006, Rosahl held the position of Deputy Chairman at the university department of neurosurgery in Freiburg, which has become one of the largest centres for neurosurgical interventions, training, and research in Germany. He is co-author of several standardised patient consent forms in neurosurgery, a reviewer for neurosurgical journals and a member of the working group on neural prosthetics in the Initiative for Micromedicine of the German Association of Electrical Engineers (VDE). Rosahl helped to create a junior professorship for neuroelectronic systems at the Universität Freiburg in 2006. He is a member of the German Society for Neurosurgery (DGNC), the European Skull Base Society (ESBS), the German Society for Skull Base Surgery (DGSB), and the Society for Neuroscience.

Postal address: Helios Klinikum Erfurt, Abteilung für Neurochirurgie, 99089 Erfurt, Germany

Foreword

This study is the result of an extensive interdisciplinary collaboration. Regular meetings were held from the beginning of 2004 onwards. Two original members of the project unfortunately had to drop out of the group due to the burden of their other commitments. Professor Dr. K.W.M. (Bill) Fulford (University of Warwick, University of Oxford, UK) helpfully contributed to our early discussions in which we framed the contours of our subject. The team of authors is even more indebted to Dr. Anne-Catherine Bachoud-Lévi (CHU Henri Mondor, Créteil, France) who attended most of the project meetings and who contributed considerably to the chapter on "Neurotransplantation and Gene Transfer", as well as to the discussion process as a whole. The project group, in its final composition, consisted in the team of authors whose contributions are found in the present volume.

On occasion of a kick-off workshop, held in Brussels in April 2005, the project members invited a number of other experts to discuss the project's working programme and to comment on the first drafts of the chapters of the book at hand. The authors would like to thank Dr. Roger Barker, Ph.D. (University of Cambridge, Cambridge, UK), Professor Dr. phil. Michael Quante (Universität zu Köln, Cologne, Germany), Professor Dr. Barbara J. Sahakian, Ph.D., and Dr. Danielle Turner, Ph.D. (both: University of Cambridge, Cambridge, UK), and Professor Dr.-Ing. Thomas Stieglitz (Universität Freiburg, Freiburg, Germany) for their valuable contributions to the project's progress. The papers prepared and presented by these external experts were published in a special edition of the journal "Poiesis & Praxis" (Vol. 4, No. 2, 2006). A final contribution to that issue came from Professor Dr. med. Thomas Schläpfer (and his collaborators) who had been invited to share his expertise with the project group on treating depression through repetitive transcranial magnetic stimulation at a later meeting in Leuven (July 2005).

One year later, in March 2006, the project group once again invited external experts to convene in Hamburg in order to review its proceedings. By that time, detailed drafts for all the main chapters of the study were available. These drafts had been prepared by members of the project group based on their personal expertise. Consequently, these individuals should be considered the first and main authors of the respective chapters. However, even prior to the second expert workshop these papers had been extensively modified and reworked through the process of interdisciplinary discussion within the project group. Having received the comments and suggestions of their peers, the authors thoroughly revised the papers once more. Finally, after 25 days of meetings over the course of two and a half years, the project members consented to publish the results of their work as presented in this volume under common authorship.

Despite a general consensus, some controversies remain, most notably on the notion of personhood. This particular disagreement is a good example of the varying meanings which certain terms assume from different scientific and professional backgrounds. These differences in meaning, which sometimes create formidable obstacles to interdisciplinary understanding, have left their traces in several footnotes. However, we hope that it will add to the thrust of the recommendations contained in this study (Chapter 7) that we were able to jointly subscribe to them in spite of our different backgrounds and sometimes diverging perspectives.

The table below assigns the chapters of the book to their principle authors and to the external experts who reviewed them at the workshop in Hamburg. The authors are indebted to all of the reviewers for their helpful criticism and advice. Additionally, Professor Dr. med. Jörg Fegert would like

Chapter	Principle author(s)	External expert
Developmental Psychopharmacology	Professor Dr. med. Jörg M. Fegert, Universitätsklinikum Ulm, Ulm, Germany	Dr. Benedetto Vitiello, M.D., National Institute of Mental Health, Bethesda, Maryland, USA
Neurotransplantation and Gene Transfer	Dr. Gerard J. Boer, Ph.D., Netherlands Institute for Neuroscience, Amsterdam, The Netherlands	Professor Dr. Karl Kieburtz, M.D., University of Rochester, NY, USA
Central Neural Prostheses	Professor Dr. med. Steffen K. Rosahl, Helios-Klinikum Erfurt, Erfurt, Germany	Professor Dr. Eduardo Fernández, Ph.D., Universidad Miguel Hernández, Elche, Spain
Electrical Brain Stimulation for Psychiatric Disorders	Professor Dr. Bart Nuttin, M.D., Ph.D., UZ Leuven, Leuven, Belgium	Professor Dr. Alim Louis Benabid, Ph.D., Centre hospitalier universitaire, Grenoble, France
Person, Personal Identity, and Personality	Professor Dr. phil. Dirk Hartmann, Universität Duisburg-Essen, Essen, Germany Dr. phil. Thorsten Galert, Europäische Akademie gGmbH, Bad Neuenahr-Ahrweiler, Germany	Professor Dr. phil. Dieter Birnbacher, Universität Düsseldorf, Düsseldorf, Germany
Treatment – Prevention – Enhancement: Normative Foundations and Limits	Professor Dr. jur. Reinhard Merkel, Universität Hamburg, Hamburg, Germany	Professor Dr. jur. Werner Heun, Universität Göttingen, Göttingen, Germany

to thank Dr. Jacinta Tan, Ph.D. (University of Oxford, Oxford, UK), and Dr. Paul Plener (Vienna/Universitätsklinikum Ulm) for their support in drafting his chapter.

We are very grateful to Benjamin Hawkins (University of Edinburgh, Edinburgh, UK) and Dr. Bernd Seligmann (T&D Übersetzungen und technische Dokumentation, Bad Neuenahr-Ahrweiler) who undertook the difficult task of revising the English of Belgium, Dutch and German colouring with the critical eyes of native speakers. Our final thanks go to Friederike Wütscher who oversaw the whole editorial process and to Katharina Mader, Yvette Gafinen and Christian Haller for their assistance in editing this book, as well as to Katja Stoppenbrink for her effort in composing the study's glossary. Mr. Haller also helped greatly in preparing the German summary of this study.

January 2007

Reinhard Merkel
Gerard J. Boer
Jörg M. Fegert
Thorsten Galert
Dirk Hartmann
Bart Nuttin
Steffen K. Rosahl

Table of Contents

General Introduction 1

Part I
Techniques of Intervention

1 Developmental Psychopharmacology 11
1.1 Introduction 11
1.1.1 A History of Interventions in the Brain Using Psychotropic Substances 11
1.1.2 Protection of Human Research Subjects, Especially Children, and Other Related Ethical Questions 13
1.1.3 The Intervention Triad: Prevention, Treatment and Enhancement 15
1.2 History and Evolution of Child and Adolescent Psychopharmacology 18
1.3 Research Efforts and Future Perspectives 20
1.4 Interventions 21
1.4.1 Prevention 21
1.4.2 Treatment in a Developmental Perspective 24
1.4.2.1 The Example of SSRI Use in the Treatment of Childhood Depression 24
1.4.2.2 Stimulant Treatment of ADHD 30
1.4.2.3 Treating Schizophrenic Patients with Neuroleptics During Childhood and Adolescence 32
1.4.3 Enhancement 37
1.4.3.1 Stimulants 37
1.4.3.2 Emotional Enhancement 41
1.4.3.3 Ethical Concerns 42
1.4.4 Chemical Restraint 44
1.5 Ethical Problems Arising from Psychopharmacological Interventions in Children 47
1.5.1 Non-nuisance, Non-maleficence 47
1.5.2 Efficacy and Effectiveness 52

1.5.3 Autonomy 52
1.5.4 Justice 54
1.5.5 A Cultural Perspective 55
1.6 Summary 55

2 Neurotransplantation and Gene Transfer 59
2.1 Introduction 59
2.1.1 Restorative Neurosurgery by Cells and Genes 59
2.1.2 The Brain is Seat of the Human Mind 60
2.1.3 Questions to be Answered 61
2.2 Brain Structure and Capacities 62
2.2.1 Neurons Act in Networks 62
2.2.2 Networks are Formed by Genotype and Environment 63
2.3 Concepts of Cell- and Gene-based Neurosurgical Interventions 66
2.3.1 Historical Outline of Neurotransplantation in Human Beings 66
2.3.2 Several Types of Neurotransplants 67
2.3.3 The Practice of Clinical Neurotransplantation 69
2.3.4 Direct and Indirect Gene Transfer in the Brain 69
2.4 Survey of Current Experimental Human Applications of Restorative Neurosurgery 72
2.4.1 Parkinson's Disease 72
2.4.2 Huntington's Disease 74
2.4.3 Alzheimer's Disease 77
2.4.4 Amyotrophic Lateral Sclerosis 78
2.4.5 Multiple Sclerosis 79
2.4.6 Stroke 80
2.4.7 Epilepsy 82
2.5 When is Brain Disorder Eligible for Cellular or Molecular Surgery? 83
2.6 How to Design a Meaningful Experimental Human Cell or Gene Therapeutic Neurosurgical Study? 85
2.6.1 Is Sham Surgery Acceptable? 86
2.6.2 Core Assessment Protocol 89
2.7 Ethically Acceptable Retrieval and Use of Donor Material 91
2.7.1 Adult Human Cells 92
2.7.2 Human Embryo and Fetus-primary Cells 92
2.7.3 Human Embryo or Fetus-stem Cells 95
2.7.3.1 Post-implantation Embryos 95
2.7.3.2 Surplus Pre-implantation Embryos 97

2.7.3.3 Pre-implantation Embryos – Creation and Therapeutic Cloning 98
2.7.4 Animal Cells 99
2.7.5 Proportionality and Subsidiarity 100
2.8 What are the Risks of Cellular and Molecular Brain Therapeutic Interventions? 101
2.8.1 Further Aberrations in Brain Structure and Function Will Occur 102
2.8.2 Physiological Side Effects of Cellular Implants 102
2.8.3 So Far Risks of Cell Implants for the Psyche Appeared Limited or Barely Recognisable 103
2.8.4 Transfer of Personality by Neuronal Grafting is Erroneously Brought Up 104
2.8.5 Safety Aspects of Cell Implants 105
2.8.5.1 Transmissible Diseases and Tumor Formation 105
2.8.5.2 Xenografts 106
2.8.5.3 Tissue Rejection 107
2.8.6 Safety Aspects of Gene Transfer 108
2.9 Prospects 109
2.10 Summary 112

3 Central Neural Prostheses 117
3.1 Introduction 117
3.2 History of Two-way Communication Between Electrodes and the Brain 119
3.2.1 Restoration of Hearing 121
3.2.2 Visual Implants 124
3.2.3 Human-computer Interface (HCI) 126
3.2.4 Vagal Nerve Stimulation (VNS) 128
3.3 State-of-the-art & Trends 131
3.3.1 Hearing 131
3.3.2 Vision 135
3.3.3 Human-computer Interface (HCI) 136
3.3.4 Vagal Nerve Stimulation (VNS) 139
3.4 Current Limitations, Possible Solutions & Enhancement Technologies 141
3.5 Ethical Implications 149
3.5.1 Treatment 149
3.5.2 Enhancement 153
3.6 Futuristic Scenarios 156
3.7 Summary 158

4 **Electrical Brain Stimulation for Psychiatric Disorders** ... 161
4.1 Focal High Frequency Electrical Brain Stimulation ... 161
4.2 Electrical Brain Stimulation for Psychiatric Disorders ... 165
4.3 The Clinical Effects of Stimulation ... 169
4.3.1 The Effects of Acute Electrical Stimulation ... 170
4.3.2 The Effects of Chronic Electrical Stimulation ... 173
4.3.3 Side Effects and Complications ... 175
4.4 Experience of Other Research Groups ... 177
4.5 Transcranial Magnetic Stimulation ... 180
4.6 Comments on the Published Guidelines on Electrical Brain Stimulation for Psychiatric Disorders ... 181
4.7 Summary ... 185

Part II
Societal, Ethical, and Legal Challenges

5 **Person, Personal Identity, and Personality** ... 189
5.1 Preliminaries ... 189
5.2 Identity and Continuants ... 195
5.2.1 Numerical Identity ... 195
5.2.2 Identity through Change: Perdurantism ... 196
5.2.3 Material Identity and Material Continuity ... 199
5.2.4 Perdurantism Refined and Defended ... 205
5.3 Persons ... 211
5.3.1 "To Consider Oneself as Oneself" – A Transcendental Analysis of the Concept of a Person ... 212
5.3.2 "Being Capable of Having One's Actions Imputed to Oneself" – Further Cognitive, Motivational and Emotive Requirements of Personhood ... 219
5.4 Personal Identity and Personality ... 232
5.4.1 Physical Criteria of Personal Identity: Body and Brain ... 233
5.4.2 Psychological Criteria of Personal Identity I: Memory ... 235
5.4.3 Psychological Criteria of Personal Identity II: Personality/Character ... 242
5.4.4 A Narrative Approach to Personality ... 249
5.4.5 A Narrative Approach to Personal Identity ... 259
5.5 Summary and Consequences ... 272
5.5.1 Summing Up ... 272
5.5.2 Consequences ... 281

6 Treatment – Prevention – Enhancement: Normative Foundations and Limits 289
6.1 Background 289
6.2 Basic Distinctions and Affiliated Questions 293
6.3 Problems of Delineating the "Proper Limits of Medicine" by Employing the Concept of Enhancement 295
6.3.1 Preliminary Conceptual Clarifications 295
6.3.2 A Third Category: Prevention 297
6.3.3 Basic Models of Health and Disease 299
6.3.4 Deriving a Normative Standard for the Distribution of Healthcare Services 301
6.3.4.1 Three Basic Accounts of the Scope of Health Care, and the One to be Preferred 302
6.3.4.2 Limits of the Abstract Standard: "Hard Cases" and the Question of Individual Justice 306
6.4 Problems of the Treatment/Enhancement Distinction for an Ethic of Self-disposition (Self-improvement) 312
6.4.1 Enhancing One's Own Traits: Preliminary Remarks and Basic Distinctions 313
6.4.1.1 Distinguishing Law and Ethics 315
6.4.1.2 "One party" and "Two-party" Cases 316
6.4.1.3 Issues of Concern 319
6.4.2 Safety Concerns 320
6.4.2.1 Side Effects 320
6.4.2.2 Informed Consent in Cases of Enhancement 323
6.4.3 Concerns of Autonomy and Authenticity 329
6.4.3.1 Legal Considerations 330
6.4.3.2 Ethical Considerations and "Duties to Oneself" 334
6.4.4 Concerns about the Corruption of the True Nature of Human Beings 343
6.4.5 Concerns about the Corruption of the Desired Goals Themselves 348
6.4.5.1 "Win Races and Lose Racing?" – The Example of Physical Enhancements 348
6.4.5.2 Mental Performance: Output-oriented versus Engagement-oriented 350
6.4.5.3 Some Reservations 352
6.4.6 Concerns about the Expanding Medicalisation of Human Behaviour 355
6.4.7 Concerns of Justice 356

6.4.7.1 The Concept of Justice: Forms, Subjects, Objects, and Basic Distinctions ... 356
6.4.7.2 Enhancement Techniques and Distributive Justice ... 357
6.4.7.3 Mass Enhancements and Political Justice ... 364
6.5 Enhancing the Mental Features in Others ... 366
6.5.1 The Mental Enhancement of Children ... 367
6.5.1.1 Questions of Law and Legal Principles ... 368
6.5.1.2 Ethical Questions ... 374
6.5.2 The Mental Enhancement of Detainees in Prison ... 380

7 Conclusions and Recommendations ... 383
7.1 Conceptual Clarifications ... 386
7.1.1 Concerns about the Integrity of Persons ... 386
7.1.2 The Proper Limits of Medicine: Treatment – Enhancement – Prevention ... 387
7.2 Normative Foundations ... 391
7.2.1 Nonmaleficence: Avoiding Harm in Intervening in the Brain ... 391
7.2.1.1 Dealing with Side Effects in Research and Medical Practice ... 392
7.2.1.2 Minimising Harm by Careful Study Design ... 394
7.2.1.3 The Possible Harm of Enhancement ... 395
7.2.2 Beneficence: The Limits of Doing Good to Others ... 399
7.2.2.1 Treatment and Prevention ... 399
7.2.2.2 Responsibility and Liability Regarding Enhancement ... 399
7.2.2.3 Public Funding for Research ... 400
7.2.3 Autonomy: Issue of Informed Consent and Coercion ... 402
7.2.3.1 Treatment, Prevention and Research ... 402
7.2.3.2 Enhancement and the Limits of Autonomy ... 405
7.2.4 Justice: Inequality, Fair Distribution, Political Justice ... 410
7.2.4.1 Problems of Distributive Justice ... 411
7.2.4.2 Problems of Political Justice in General ... 414

Zusammenfassung ... 419
List of Abbreviations ... 475
Glossary ... 479
References ... 491

General Introduction

The aim of this study is to examine and assess a number of recently developed possibilities for intervening in the central nervous system (CNS), in particular the brain. Most of these possibilities have been opened up by innovative biomedical technologies. This is certainly true for the field of central neural prostheses covering various kinds of electronic devices which connect to the CNS in order to either influence (stimulate or inhibit) or record neural activity. The entire spectrum of technologies in this field – from electronic implants for the restoration of lost sensory function to brain-computer/machine-interfaces for the "mental" control of motor prostheses which are primarily meant to compensate for physical disabilities – is explored in Chapter 3.

The term "neural prosthetics" may generally also be applied to forms of electrical brain stimulation which are the subject of Chapter 4. This chapter focuses principally on deep brain stimulation (DBS) in which an electrical current is administered through electrodes implanted in the brain. This technique of directly interfering with endogenous neural activity can be described as "neuromodulation". It is currently used mainly on patients with otherwise untreatable central motor disturbances (e.g. pharmacologically refractory Parkinson's disease), but is also increasingly being applied to patients with mental or psychiatric disorders such as obsessive compulsive disorder or major depression. In addition to DBS, transcranial magnetic stimulation (TMS) and vagal nerve stimulation (VNS) also seem to hold new promise for the treatment of such psychiatric disorders. The potential ramifications of DBS will be discussed in Chapter 4, whilst VNS will be dealt with in Chapter 3.

Chapter 2 is devoted to neurosurgical approaches whose primary aim is the treatment of degenerative brain disorders that are sometimes accompanied by severe mental symptoms. This approach, which is currently being developed under the label of "neurotransplantation", aims principally at the replacement of lost brain cells by neural cell grafts. These implants are presently obtained from the brains of aborted foetuses, but may foreseeably be prepared from cultured and differentiated embryonic stem cells isolated from human pre-implantation embryos or from somatic stem cells present in immature and even in mature organs. Stem cells are multipotent and thus are capable of developing into neural cells and adapting to neural environments within the brain. In addition, neurotransplantation and gene transfer (or a combination of the two) are used to apply proteinous compounds locally in the brain as a substitute for neural cell malfunction, or to stimulate regeneration or inhibit degeneration of disease-related degenerating or traumatised CNS tissue.

The techniques mentioned so far all employ previously unheard of means of acting on the brain. By contrast, the subject matter of Chapter 1, psychopharmacology, is a well established method of intervening in the case of the type of brain disorders dealt with here. It was not, however, the mere novelty of certain brain interventions that motivated scientists and clinicians involved in the development and application of these techniques to share their experience and views with philosophers and a legal expert and to collaborate with them in writing this book. Rather, the driving force behind this interdisciplinary enterprise was the authors' shared interest in the controversial public debate on these new methods of intervention. For a keen observer of public and academic media it is striking that most of the concerns raised by these innovative techniques of intervening in the brain are quite well known from the longstanding debate on the use of pharmaceutical agents to influence the psyche. This is true not only of concerns about the influence of these new kinds of intervention on the individual psyche, but also for concerns regarding the possible impact of their widespread application on society in general. In view of our specific interest in scrutinising the empirical and normative soundness of these concerns, it was decided to include psychopharmacology in this study of new methods for intervening in the brain whilst leaving psychotherapy aside. We recognise the advent of major new approaches in psychotherapy, which, as we know today, also acts on the brain. However, their introduction is not accompanied by the type of concern that is regularly raised by new neurosurgical approaches.

One particular concern which has been debated most extensively in reference to pharmacological interventions relates not so much to new means, but rather to the possibility of new ends being pursued by brain interventions. This concern is provoked by an increased readiness of people not suffering from cognitive impairment or emotional disturbance in any clinical sense to consume psychoactive drugs in order to *enhance* their mood or cognitive capacities (e.g. their attention span or memory) beyond the "normal". Advances in drug development are aiding this putative tendency by providing antidepressants and psychostimulants with fewer and more tolerable immediate side effects, which lend themselves to consumption without any medical indication. For instance, if in the 1980s selective serotonin reuptake inhibitors (SSRIs) had not been considered much safer than earlier antidepressants, then Prozac® would hardly have gained fame as a "lifestyle drug" promising everyone who takes it to feel "better than well" (Kramer 1993). Methylphenidate, on the other hand, a psychostimulant better known under the brand name Ritalin®, already had a long record as a therapeutic agent before it assumed an almost emblematic role in the debate on cognitive enhancement, in the same way that Prozac® had done for mood enhancement. Its propensity to benefit healthy individuals by generally increasing cognitive functioning became apparent by the time its prescription as standard medication for the so-called attention deficit hyperactivity disorder (ADHD) in children and adolescents began to skyrocket. It is fairly obvious that, due to their growing therapeutic usage, prescription drugs containing Methylphenidate became more readily available for people seeking enhancement. Their therapeutic application thus spread the word about their applicability as "smart pills" for the cognitively "normal".

We have narrowed down the focus of Chapter 1 to *developmental* psychopharmacology since a trend currently exists towards the enhancement of minors by their parents. This raises specific additional ethical and legal issues, which are dealt with extensively in Chapter 6. Moreover, the example of psychopharmacological interventions in children and adolescents highlights issues of justice regarding the availability of treatment options with proven safety and efficacy for different population groups. Due to the fact that children do not create a large demand for psychopharmaceutical drugs, their prescription for children is usually not based on age-specific clinical trials. In addition, recent research scandals have revealed the problems of the non-publication of research results (e.g. the so-called SSRI crisis).

In addition to psychopharmacology, some of the cutting-edge biomedical technologies mentioned above, in particular the field of neural prosthetics, hold strong promises for enhancement applications. This is highlighted by the fact that the U.S. military has been funding research into "enhancing human performance" by means, for example, of brain-machine interfaces and neural implants via its Defence Advanced Research Projects Agency (DARPA) (Moreno 2006). While it is surely important to be aware of the possibility that one day soldiers may be equipped with mental control over weapons or with supernatural sight provided by retinal implants, the actual trend towards the consumption of psychopharmaceutical drugs for non-therapeutic purposes is the most useful reference point for an analysis of the normative problems associated with enhancement issues. We will see that many of the more serious challenges posed by these issues relate to the social rather than to the individual level. For example, questions of distributive justice might arise from unequal access to enhancement technologies. These would be bound to become more pressing in case the employment of particular enhancement technologies becomes more popular and widespread. Within the foreseeable future, it is highly unlikely that either neural prostheses or cell and gene therapies will surpass psychoactive substances as the primary means of enhancement for the wider public. For one thing, it is notoriously difficult to restrict access to pharmaceuticals, since professional (medical) advice and support are not necessarily required for their consumption. Furthermore, their application does not consist in a single expensive and comparatively risky surgical procedure like the intracranial implantation of electrodes, cells or genes. Finally, it adds to the consumer's feeling of safety that he can stop taking pills at any time if the desired effect turns out to be unattainable or if the effects, once attained, appear less desirable or are simply outweighed by unpleasant side effects. This may provide sufficient reason for the presumption that for quite some time to come the pharmaceutical possibilities for improving both mood and cognition will remain the standard practice against which possible further enhancement technologies need to be assessed.

The enhancement debate emerged in its present shape in the 1980s when the new molecular biological DNA techniques, and their diagnostic use in reproductive medicine, led to the possibility of enhancing one's offspring by selection. However, whilst human beings who in an early embryonic state were selected by certain genetic criteria for implantation *in utero* will later in life need to come to terms with the fact that some of their gene-based traits had been selected by others who thus set the preconditions of their continued existence, they do not experience any change from a normal to a supposedly enhanced state. By contrast, all the techniques of intervention reviewed in this study (to the extent that they suit enhancement purposes at all) will *probably* be applied only, or at least predominantly, to individuals who are able to compare a *status quo ante* with their overall situation after such an intervention. We say only "probably" because we cannot exclude with entire certainty the possibility that a type of "brave new world" may arise in which newborn babies, or even foetuses, are equipped with neuroprosthetic upgrades or fed with "soma"[1] so that eventually these children grow up without ever experiencing their "natural", unenhanced state. However, we focus our ethical and legal analysis on those cases where either people decide for themselves to undergo enhancement, or individuals get enhanced upon someone else's decision so that they can, in principle, hold the decision makers responsible for the change they experience to their way of being as a result of the intervention. This analysis, certain aspects of which we outline briefly in Chapters 1 and 3, is the main focus of Chapter 6.

The question of how individuals may come to terms with the experience of having been enhanced also relates to a second type of concern that is frequently expressed in the public debate on new biomedical interventions in the brain. It is suggested that all interventions of this kind must be treated with particular caution since they may have a particularly profound impact on the people they are applied to: The fear is often expressed that an individual may no longer be "the same person" he or she used to be prior to an intervention in the brain. In other words (i.e. philosophical terms), these interventions are said to threaten *personal identity*. No matter how we word

[1] This being the name of the "bliss" inducing drug which serves as a powerful means for the suppression of rebellion in Aldous Huxley's "Brave New World".

it, though, it is not immediately clear what precisely this concern amounts to. At this stage, we need not delve any deeper into the numerous ambiguities of these concerns about the identity of persons. They will be addressed extensively in Chapter 5.

As a group, we were engaged in intensive debates about our initially differing, and later converging, views on this subject. Therefore, we believe it to be helpful if we briefly review the main common intuition supporting the belief that interventions in the brain are particularly prone to put a person's integrity in danger, namely the basic idea that the brain is of decisive importance for who and what a person essentially is. We consider this to be true, and we would like to add that the brain assumes this special importance *by virtue of* being the organ that physiologically sustains all mental processes. We state in Chapter 5 that an important element of a person's identity is her own conception of who she is. This self-concept is constituted by memories; self related beliefs, thoughts and emotions; concerns, hopes and ambitions for the future, all of which represent mental states or processes. We do not presuppose that these mental phenomena are nothing but brain states or processes. However, we subscribe to the less controversial view that there can be no change in the mind without a concurrent change in the brain.[2] Therefore, it makes sense to assume that all mental states and functions pertinent to personal identity can be interfered with by either deliberately introducing, or inadvertently causing, changes in the cellular and molecular networks of the CNS.

While this reasoning is in accord with the empirical findings of neuroscience, it seems nevertheless premature to maintain that the mind-brain relation outlined here must also hold the other way around, i.e. that each and every change of the brain would need to go along with some change in the mind. It must be conceded that such a position can hardly be refuted on empirical grounds. Its protagonist can always defend his view against apparent counter-examples by claiming that the relevant difference (to be couched in psychological terms) has not been described appropriately or is yet to be detected. However, given the available data, it seems that sometimes even extensive structural changes in a person's brain – whether they are induced by trauma or, for that matter, by neurosurgical procedures – are not associated with any noticeable impact on a patient's behavioural dispositions, cognitive capacities and emotional condition in normal daily life. Nor, for that matter, do they appear to impact on his own, or anyone else's, understanding of who he is (as a person or in any other relevant way).

Unfortunately, in spite of several decades of ground-breaking advances in neuroscience, our knowledge of the physical realisation of mental phenomena does not allow us to reliably predict just which particular inter-

[2] This comparatively parsimonious view is sometimes expressed by stating that processes of the mind *supervene* on brain processes.

ventions in the brain will leave mental processes unaffected. On the contrary, sometimes even minute modifications of brain processes produce unexpectedly grave changes in behaviour, and thus also in the underlying mental condition of the respective individual. Given all this, it makes good sense to adopt the cautionary approach set out above, according to which all interventions in the brain deserve to be handled with particular care. Practically no intervention in the structure or functioning of the human brain can be undertaken in complete certainty that it will not affect mental processes, some of which may eventually come to play a key role in a person's self-concept. We hope that this preliminary clarification of the relationship between brain and mind will help to prevent this justified caution from being taken to an unreasonable extreme. Such an approach might hold that, since intervening in a person's brain is ultimately tantamount to interfering with his or her identity, it would be best to declare all interventions in the brain taboo. Considering the numerous well established methods of therapeutic intervention, this seems to be a hopelessly misguided stance on the matter.

By the time the authors of this book decided to join forces in exploring this subject, it emerged as a basic consensus that there are no grounds for establishing any such taboo. This, of course, goes without saying for those of us who have been, or are still, working with the intervention techniques scrutinised in this study. However, the philosophers and legal experts participating in this project equally agree that we should not regard the brain as an organ better left completely untouched. Nevertheless, specific dangers may well be associated with novel techniques of intervening in the brain as a result of their potential to affect the psyche. The overarching goal of our joint venture was, therefore, to clarify the scope of this potential danger by exploring, as far as we are able to tell, a heretofore unparalleled multiplicity of factual and normative aspects related to this subject.

We do, of course, gratefully acknowledge the valuable work that has already been done on many of the topics we investigate in this study. In recent years, numerous workshops and conferences took place, gathering experts from different disciplines who have explored the ethical, social and legal issues surrounding brain science and the emergent neurotechnologies. The proceedings of those meetings (e.g. Marcus 2002; Garland 2004; Raeymaekers et al. 2004) usually make do with presenting a multitude of different disciplinary perspectives, however. In writing this book we, by contrast, were aiming at a more integrated, interdisciplinary result by repeatedly discussing every draft until everyone was ready to subscribe to the joint outcome. There have been but a few previous projects on the topics of this study which pursued a similar approach. Two of them are worthy of particular mention here. The debate on biotechnological possibilities of enhancing various kinds of human traits has been stimulated by the influential report of the U.S. President's Council on Bioethics titled "Beyond

Therapy" (President's Council on Bioethics 2003).[3] Within the European Union, the ethical aspects of so-called "Information and Communication Technologies implants" (ICT implants, dealt with in this study under the heading of "Central Neural Prostheses") have been addressed by the European Group on Ethics in Science and New Technologies (Hermerén et al. 2005). The present study is not only comparable to these two reports in being the outcome of an interdisciplinary and consensus-oriented approach, but it also shares their mission to provide decision-makers in science and politics with advice. Therefore, the final chapter (Chapter 7) of this book contains a concise summary of its most important results and, wherever possible, recommendations for future action. It is our hope that in this way we succeeded in providing a useful contribution to the ongoing international debate which is still in its infancy but which needs to be developed at an appropriate pace to meet the challenges raised by new possibilities for intervening in the brain.

[3] The "ENHANCE Project" with a similar thematic scope has been launched only recently (in October 2005) funded by the European Commission's Sixth Framework Programme. For details see the project's website at http://www.enhance-project.org/index.html, accessed on December 15th, 2006.

Part I
Techniques of Intervention

1 Developmental Psychopharmacology

1.1 Introduction

1.1.1 A History of Interventions in the Brain Using Psychotropic Substances

Fantasies of intervening in the psyche and the use of psychotropic agents have a venerable history in mankind. Even in prehistoric times, substances like opium, cannabis, coca, peyote and alcohol were used, especially in the context of religious and magic rituals and other cultural practices. In ancient Greece, for example in the Hippocratic writings and the writings of Dioscourides and Galen, the use of opium was recommended for the treatment of pain and sleep disorders, particularly in women. Helleborus was the treatment of choice in psychiatric diseases. The Greek authors distinguished the black helleborus, a purgative, from the white helleborus, a substance which induced vomiting. Ancient Greek medical writings show that doctors believed psychiatric illnesses to have somatic foundations. They therefore tried to heal through the extraction of illness-inducing substances using emetics or purgatives. As can be seen, the concept of the so-called "biological psychiatry", meaning physical interventions in the psyche through somatic changes by means of pharmaceutical agents or other manipulations with an impact on the human brain, is a very old one. In the Middle Ages in Europe, cathartic methods using purgatives, emetics or phlebotomy retained some of their importance whilst different herbal extracts of plants with greater or lesser toxicity gained ascendance in the monastic medicine. Women collecting these plants and having some knowledge about their therapeutic effects often risked to be accused of witchcraft. The word "psycho-pharmacon" was introduced in 1584 by Reinhardus Lorichius of Hadarmar in the title of a book of prayers: "Medication for the soul".

The precursors of psychotherapy in the religious and monastic context became increasingly important in the conception of interventions in the psyche. Even as late as the 19th century, crude interventions such as cold baths or various mechanical machines, wheels and coercive chairs were recommended as treatment for psychiatric disorders (Schneider 1824). At the same time, the first chemical discoveries of psychotropic agents were being made, with the first descriptions of the active components of herbal plants like Morphine and Scopolamine. In 1826, sedation by bromides started the first era of modern sedatives. In the middle of the 19th century, Paraldehyde and Chloralhydrate (sedatives still currently in use) were developed. The famous psychiatric textbooks of Kraepelin in 1899 and Bleuler in 1916 showed a hapless polypharmacy in the pharmacological treatment of psychiatric diseases with a central concept of *sedation*. In 1903, the synthesis of the first barbituric acid (barbital) introduced a new era in psychopharmacology. Klaesi published his famous sleeping cures in 1920. The main focus of psychotropic intervention in these times was the treatment of agitation and aggression in severely disturbed psychiatric patients. No pharmacological treatment of mood disorders or other psychiatric symptoms such as hallucinations was as yet possible. Therefore other interventions based on Cardiazol, insulin shocks or induced fever constituted the main focus of interest in somatic interventions in the psyche in the first half of the 20th century, until the effects of Lithium in the treatment of mania were discovered in 1949.

The idea of enhancing cognitive functioning also dates back far in ancient times. The stimulating plant Ephedra vulgaris was used by Chinese physicians such as Ma Huang over 500 years ago. The use of the Khat shrub Catha edulis in East Africa and the Middle East is relatively unchanged to the present day, where the custom of chewing leaves of the plant has been widespread for at least 700 years. Cathinone, the active ingredient, was only isolated in 1970.

It was not before 1880 that the active ingredient Ephedrine was isolated, finally leading to its characterisation in 1920. Ephedrine was widely used in the treatment of asthma. Increased efforts to search for a synthetic substitute led to the rediscovery of amphetamine that was synthesised 40 years before. Since then, many analogues of amphetamine have been developed and characterised, including the popular street drug, Methamphetamine, which was synthesised in 1912 in Darmstadt by Merck. During World War II, amphetamines came into use in the military as a means to keep pilots awake and vigilant during long flight hours. The first condition amphetamine was clinically used for was narcolepsy. Although not curative, it revolutionised therapy for this condition by making the patients relatively symptom free.

The use of stimulants in children dates back to 1937 when Bradley first used Benzedrine® and noted "a spectacular change in behaviour" along with "remarkably improved school performance". Ritalin®, which is used so often now, was first synthesised by L. Panizzon and named after his wife Marguerite (nicknamed "Rita"), who occasionally used it to improve her tennis performance. It was patented in 1950 and advertised by Ciba-Geigy thus: "it acts more carefully and longer than caffeine and amphetamines and does not involve habituation."

The story of the Coca plant Erythroxylon, which was used in South America 2000 years ago, seems comparable. The active ingredient Cocaine was first isolated in 1800, rapidly gaining popularity as an ingredient in tonic drinks such as Coca Cola and remaining popular until recent times. Its pharmacological use shifted from application as a local anaesthetic or a cure for a range of physical and psychological maladies (depression, indigestion, asthma, neurosis, syphilis and drug and alcohol addiction) to current practice of abuse as one of the most popular illicit street drugs in its various forms of powder, freebase and crack.

1.1.2 Protection of Human Research Subjects, Especially Children, and Other Related Ethical Questions

One of the consequences of the Nazi medical crimes on psychiatric patients, mentally retarded people and sick children was the Nuremberg Code. Following this tradition, the Helsinki Declaration and the Convention on Human Rights and Biomedicine of the European Council have also been enacted. Protection of human research subjects has become imperative, especially for interventions in children and the human psyche. In this chapter, therefore, we will focus on the developmental aspect of intervening in critical phases of development in the discussion of psychopharmacotherapy.

While psychopharmacotherapy is widely used especially in most First and Second World countries where there are high levels of prescription, there is still a lack of research on the developmental aspects of psychopharmaceutical interventions in the developing brain. Children who are treated with psychotropic agents often show age-specific reactions and side effects. Efficacy and safety issues are not the same over the age span. The earlier in a child's life a therapeutic intervention starts, the more likely it will be to influence brain development and modify plasticity and capacity (Carlezon and Konradi 2004) and therefore the more likely long-term consequences might be. These long-term consequences may be beneficial, but they could also consist of late onset side effects leading to drug dependencies or late impairments such as tardive dyskinesia, which is related to neuroleptic treatment, especially with the classical neuroleptics. By focusing on developmental aspects of psychopharmacology, we will describe in this chapter the use of pharmaceutical agents in different developmental stages to *prevent* or *treat* psychiatric illness, and to *enhance* cognitive and/or emotional functioning in human beings, particularly in children and adolescents but also during the life span. Some classes of substances will be used to illustrate the classic questions as well as conflicts that might arise in the future, related with the introduction of new possibilities of intervening in the brain dealt with in the other chapters like deep brain simulation. These general questions of ethical importance are the standard questions of *efficacy* and *effectiveness* as well as the combination of different forms of interventions and *safety issues.* The use of an intervention against a patient's will is also taken into consideration with the example of chemical restraint.

These days, questions of health resource *allocation*, determining who gets access to what form of treatment, are relevant to the ethical discussion on medical innovations. If we refer here to the principles which have been introduced into medical ethics by Beauchamp and Childress (2001)[4], ques-

[4] The first edition of their "Principles of Biomedical Ethics" dates back to 1977. In 1979 a similar set of principles formed the basis of the so-called "Belmont Report" issued by the National Commission for the Protection of Human Subjects of Biomedical Research.

tions of justice and autonomy should be of prime importance in ethical discussion of psychopharmacology. In contrast, however, it is the primary questions of nonmaleficence *(primum non nocere)* and beneficence which seem to be the aspects which are particularly well studied in psychopharmacological interventions.

One might presume that ethical debates on novel interventions in the brain would focus first on the dangers to the first research subjects and patients (nonmaleficence), before focusing on the question whether there are scientific proofs of an overall beneficence and a positive cost benefit relationship of a new intervention. Questions of justice like access to care, access to new interventions are usually discussed later in the development of novel and often very expensive technologies – unfortunately, the differences of medical development in different regions of the world mean that only a small group of patients in first world countries obtains access to new forms of intervention.

The developmental focus underlines the importance of the concept of *autonomy* and the difficulties associated with this. In the treatment of children, but in a different way also in the treatment of mentally retarded people or people suffering from dementia, questions of patients' rights will become increasingly important. Who can and should consent to treatment? How important is the assent of the person who has to tolerate the treatment? Can parents decide on preventive interventions or enhancement in children whilst the children are too young to articulate their will or do not recognise the problems the parents have with their behaviour? Who defines the problems? Who decides about the cure and who has to take the pill? These are the standard questions in the triangle of parent, child and doctor or legal guardian, patient and doctor.

Regarding autonomy, another dimension is quite important: that of society. One of the historical tasks of psychiatry has always been the *restraint* of aggressive or dangerous psychiatrically ill patients. From the beginning of modern psychiatry in the 19th century this aspect was regulated in police law. In the context of intervening in the psyche, the interests of society can conflict with the personal interests of a subject. For example: is so-called "chemical restraint" acceptable to avoid harm to self or others? Individual rights of freedom and autonomy are sometimes overruled by mechanical or chemical interventions in psychiatrically ill patients. These classic ethical questions will be discussed in this chapter against the background of some examples from different classes of psychopharmacological agents. This will lay the groundwork of possible future discussions that will accompany the introductions of new forms of interventions in the psyche.

1.1.3 The Intervention Triad: Prevention, Treatment and Enhancement

This chapter on interventions in developmental psychopharmacotherapy will be subdivided into *preventative interventions, treatment in a developmental perspective, and enhancement (and restraint).* These three forms of intervention have to be distinguished. Treatment and enhancement are currently discussed for many new interventions in the brain represented in this book.

Preventative interventions or interventions at an early state of development influencing brain development and therefore future personality traits are little discussed. However, as the example of novel antipsychotics in the prevention of schizophrenia shows, the question of preventative intervention in the brain raises many ethical considerations. The same is true for the debate on the potential use of interventions for restraint.

Experts in neurosciences are increasingly speculating about issues of prevention and neuroprotection. If, in a few years' time, we are able to define specific targets in order to enable us to offer protection to the neural system, some parents would certainly wish to use these techniques for the benefit of their children. The wish to have a healthy and well born (eugenic) child is a very natural and ancient one. But this possibility raises troubling questions. Who will defend the children's rights in these decisions? What are the ethical questions arising from clinical trials aimed at preventing potential neuropsychiatric illnesses in seemingly healthy children, especially when the risk of morbidity is a relative risk, depending on multiple factors in the environment? What justifies interventions in nature, where nurture can also be protective and when there is only a risk rather than the certainty of developing a severe psychiatric disease?

Enhancement of sensory functions is well accepted because we usually presume that prosthetic interventions only improve natural functions or replace impaired functions without changing the personality. What about psychopharmacological agents changing attention and behaviour in school, school success etc.? The use of stimulants in children and adolescents not only for the treatment of ADHD but also for cognitive enhancement during examination periods appears to be growing, especially in the United States (Fegert et al. 2002; McCabe et al. 2005). The President's Council on Bioethics in its study "Beyond Therapy – Biotechnology and the Pursuit of Happiness" summarises:

> It is precisely the effectiveness in improving attentiveness, focus, and steady conduct – coupled with the absence of serious side effects, when they are properly administered in small doses – that makes these drugs attractive also for the treatment of inattention, distractibility, and impulsivity in children who do not manifest the full disorder. Indeed, these drugs have the capacity to enhance alertness and concentration in children without any symptoms whatsoever. All these reasons conspire to make the use of stimulants to control behaviour a fascinating and important case study for the pursuit of 'better children' through psychopharmacology. (President's Council on Bioethics 2003:74)

Emotional enhancement is another issue of intervening in the psyche and the personality in the so-called "Prozac® Generation". Isn't it justified that even normal individuals want to escape from natural mood changes by using for example SSRIs to improve their emotional stability in a society where good mood and optimism is a real need for success in the work place?

Another ethical debate concerns the potential for abuse of psychopharmacological substances as means of chemical restraint. Interventions in the brain can also limit the autonomy of people especially if they could harm themselves or others. The debate about restraint is somewhat similar to the ethical debate about enhancement but reflects the other side of the coin with regard to intervening in the brain to reduce potential risks even against the will of a person.

In the psychopharmacotherapy of psychiatric disorders, neurotransmitters, receptors, signal transduction and so-called second messengers all play an important role. A *neurotransmitter* is a substance synthesised and released from neurons. It is released from nerve terminals in a chemically or pharmacologically identifiable form and interacts with postsynaptic receptors, causing the same effects as are seen with stimulation of the pre-synaptic neuron. Cell surface receptors have two major functions: They have to identify specific molecules (neurotransmitters, hormones, growth factors and sensory signals) and they have to activate a response via effectors. Among the different neurotransmitter and neuropeptide systems we can describe the serotonergic system, the dopaminergic system, the noradrenergic system, the glutamatergic system and the GABAergic system. For this context, the monoaminergic systems are the best studied, because most current effective antidepressants and antipsychotics target these systems. Generally we distinguish different substance classes:

- *Antidepressants and anxiolytics* including tricyclic and tetracyclic drugs, selective serotonin reuptake inhibitors (SSRIs), monoamine oxidase inhibitors (MAOIs) and other mostly combined reuptake inhibitors such as Venlafaxine, Duloxetine and so on. These substances are usually used for the treatment of (major) depression, anxiety disorders and obsessional compulsive disorders.
- *Other anxiolytics:* Benzodiazepines are used for the treatment of anxiety disorders and acute states of agitation or panic.
- *Antipsychotics.* Classic antipsychotic medications are the phenothiazines, Butyrophenone, neuroleptics such as Haloperidol, and different derivatives. These classic conventional antipsychotic drugs have a multitude of well known effects and side effects. They are used for the treatment of schizophrenia and schizoaffective disorder, substance induced psychosis, mania, personality disorders, Tourette's syndrome and different states of aggression or self-injurious behaviour. The so-called atypical novel antipsychotics are Clozapine, Olanzapine, Quetiapine, Risperidone, Arip-

iprazole, Ziprasidone and others. All these antipsychotic substances can also be used for the acute treatment of mania but there is another substance group for the treatment of bipolar disorders, the "mood stabilisers".

- *Mood stabilisers and drugs for the treatment of bipolar disorder.* Lithium is the oldest and best studied substance that can prevent relapse in bipolar affective disorders. It is effective in reducing suicide rates in this population, but feared for its narrow therapeutic window (the effective versus toxic plasma levels) in treatment. It can be also used for the treatment of aggressive behaviours in children and adolescents, if other interventions have failed (Gerlach et al. 2006). Antiepileptic drugs like Valproate, Carbamazepine, Lamotrigine and Topiramate are also used as mood stabilisers.
- *Sedatives-hypnotics.* Barbiturates can be used as sedatives, for example in order to induce sleep.
- *Psychostimulants* like Methylphenidate, Amphetamine and Modafinil are used for the treatment of children with attention deficit hyperactivity disorder.

We will limit our discussions of interventions in a developmental perspective to a few practical examples of ethical problems and debates in the use of psychopharmacological substances in childhood and adolescence. We will focus on the three most commonly used substance classes in this age group: stimulants, antidepressants and antipsychotics. Therefore, we will deliberately omit other important substance classes such as mood stabilisers and/or antiepileptic drugs, anxiolytic drugs and sedatives. The example of the abuse of anxiolytic drugs and the tragedy of a generation of women dependant on prescription drugs is well known and does not need to be illustrated in this chapter. Before starting with the main chapter on interventions we will give a short overview of the history of developmental psychopharmacology. At the end of this chapter we will focus on aspects of the different roles of doctors, researchers, the industry and the state in medical innovations. This chapter is not intended to be an exact or detailed history of child psychopharmacology, nor is it meant to detail the neurobiological foundations of treatment. Instead, it will offer some insights into future perspectives of drug development and an overview of the different conflicts of interests influencing medical progress. *The main aim of this chapter is to use well-known examples of conflicts and problems in developmental psychopharmacology in children and adolescents to highlight future perspectives in the ethical debate on novel techniques and medical innovations.*

1.2 History and Evolution of Child and Adolescent Psychopharmacology

Child and adolescent psychopharmacology had an early start in 1937 when Bradley reported that some children with disruptive behaviours showed a seemingly paradoxical improvement when treated with racemic amphetamine (Benzedrine®). His first publication describes the exploratory use in thirty, mostly preadolescent, children in a residential treatment facility. He cited one of the children in his report: "I start to make my bed and before I know it, it is done." Finally he established that "Fourteen out of thirty responded in a spectacular fashion." In the same issue of the American Journal of Psychiatry, Molitch and colleagues (Molitch and Eccles 1937; Molitch and Sullivan 1937) reported that this drug also improved cognitive functioning in children and adolescents. This was the first observation on the possible enhancement effects of stimulants. Cutts and Jasper (1939) reported age- and disorder-specific paradoxical side effects: an excitation due to phenobarbital in children with behavioural disorders. Bradley and his co-workers published more case reports throughout the 1940s (Bradley and Bowen 1940; Bradley and Green 1940; Bradley and Bowen 1941). Independently from this group Bender (Bender and Cottington 1942) also communicated her experiences with the use of psychostimulants. By 1950 Bradley had treated 350 preadolescent children with psychostimulants. The early studies on stimulant treatment focused on institutionalised hyperactive children, often with brain damage, cerebral dysfunction and developmental disorders, and the body of literature gradually increased. Between the 1960s and the 1990s, over 250 reviews on stimulant treatment and over 3,000 articles were published on stimulant effects (Swanson 1993). By 1996, 161 randomised controlled trials had been published, including five studies on preschool children, 150 studies on school aged children, seven studies on adolescents and nine studies in adults (Spencer et al. 1996). 133 trials studied Methylphenidate, Dextroamphetamine was used in 22 trials, and Pemoline in 6 trials. Improvement occurred in 65% to 75% of all children randomised to stimulants in these studies. This is confirmed by different reviews of the trial literature (Dulcan 1997; DuPaul and Barkley 1994; Greenhill et al. 1999). Paul Wender (1971) postulated in his book "Minimal brain dysfunction", that therapeutic effects of stimulants in ADHD are based on alterations of the neurotransmission of catecholamines in the brain. He was the first researcher who explicitly discussed the dopaminergic neurotransmitter hypothesis with respect to stimulant use in children. The previous idea of a paradoxical effect expressed by Bradley was finally laid to rest by Rapoport's seminal NIMH study published in "Science" in 1978, showing that normal children and normal adults as well as children with ADHD all react with better concentration and reduction of impulsivity and hyperactivity under stimulant exposure. Since that time the hypothesis of a disorder-specific medication effect has been much criticised and general questions of enhancement have arisen again. In contrast to this early start of child neuropsychopharmacology with discovery of the effects of stimulants in following decades, child psychopharmacological research has remained focused on stimulant effects and alternative treatments in ADHD and the replication of adult psychopharmacology findings in children and adolescents.

The so-called biological revolution in adult psychiatry began with some accidental findings in the 1940s and 1950s. In 1949 J. Kay discovered the anti-manic effects of Lithium. In 1955, Delay and Deniker described the antipsychotic properties in adults of Chlorpromazine (initially synthesised in 1950). This was the first modern antipsychotic agent and the precursor of all phenothiazine neuroleptics. The first anecdotal description of its use in children was published by Heuyer et al. in 1953. The authors prescribed doses up to two milligram per kilogram to 6 children and adolescents aged 5 to 14 that they had diagnosed with psychosis and agitation. It is important to state that at that time the concept of early or infantile psychosis in French psychiatry was very broad. As early as in 1955, Freedman et al. conducted a placebo controlled study of 159 hospitalised children with mixed diagnoses treated with doses of 30–100 mg of Chlorpromazine. Iproniazid, the first monoamine oxidase inhibitor (MAOI), was developed as a therapeutic drug for tuberculosis but showed psychotropic properties during its development for clinical use. Friedman described in 1955 an increase of awareness and language production in children with autistic disorders who had been treated with MAOIs. In 1957 R. Kuhn described the antidepressant activity of Imipramine, and the era of pharmaceutical treatment of depression truly began. In child and adolescent psychopharmacy, the tricyclic antidepressants (TCAs) were first reported to be useful in treating enuresis (McLean 1960; Poussaint and Ditman 1965), and ADHD (Krakowski 1965 and Rapoport 1965). The first descriptions of the clinical effects of TCAs in childhood depression (Lucas et al. 1965; Frommer 1972) appeared and the same clinicians (Frommer 1967) had the impression that MAOIs were helpful in treating children with depression. Today we have to come to the conclusion that no proof exists of any superiority of TCAs over placebo in children with depression (Fegert and Herpertz-Dahlmann 2005).

In 1958 Paul Janssen developed Haloperidol, the first butyrophenon neuroleptic. Neuroleptics were quickly described as useful agents, not only in psychotic disorders in children but also in hospitalised children with autistic disorders (Fish 1960a,b) and Tourette's disorder (Challas and Brauer 1963, Chapel et al. 1964). In 1960 Chlordiazepoxide (Librium®) was the first of the benzodiazepines introduced by Sternbach. As early as in 1961 Chlordiazepoxide was also used clinically in children. Kraft et al. (1965) published observations in 130 children with mixed psychiatric diagnoses treated with Chlordiazepoxide. In the 1970s and 1980s, drug development was increasingly standardised, with placebo controlled trials becoming the established method of proving the efficacy and describing the side effect profile of a new drug.

Over the decades, the phases of drug development have become more and more rigorously implemented in adult psychopharmacology. The first important discoveries had been accidental clinical observations, heroic single case studies or clinical observations. No pharmacological knowledge about the pharmacokinetics or pharmacodynamics of a substance and no animal observations had to be collected prior to clinical use in humans at that time. With the evolution of drug development methodology, patient safety has acquired increasing protection in the standardised stages of drug development. This is not true for advances in child and adolescent psychopharmacology, which still consists of open clinical experiments, which entails experimenting with substances, previously described as effective in adults, in several children with psychiatric disorders. Until now, most of the psychopharmacological agents used in children have been administered "off label", in which the prescribing physician takes responsibility for prescription of a drug beyond the remit of its licence. Following changes in the legislation in the last ten years, pharmaceutical companies have begun to consider the potential use of new psychopharmacological agents in children in their drug development plans. This is in response to requests from regulatory agencies, and we still do not know whether this will influence the future of child psychopharmacology so that interventions in the developing brain will be based upon more scientific evidence, which would make the prescription of psychopharmacological agents to children and adolescents less fraught with risk.

The molecular mechanisms of drug action will have to be unravelled before scientifically-founded interventional choices can be made in the future. Up to now, physicians and child psychiatrists have used observation from adult work to guide child psychopharmacology, and we have not completely understood the underlying molecular mechanisms in a developmental perspective. There is a wealth of literature from animal work on the effect of early exposure to drug leading to lasting modifications of brain function both physiologically and behaviourally. Human observations of developmental effects of drug use during pregnancy and in developmental periods after birth are of course less direct and less common (Swaab and Boer 2001). Until now, the clinical use of psychopharmacological drugs in children and adolescents has been insufficiently based on animal work modelling the impact of an intervention at different developmental stages. We often even lack age-specific data on the pharmacokinetics and -dynamics of substances used in children and adolescents.

1.3 Research Efforts and Future Perspectives

There is a clear correlation of the influence of expected market size with research efforts in industry (Entorf et al. 2004). Changes in the market with more common use of pharmacological interventions in children during the

1990s (Zito et al. 1999, Austin et al. 2002) and regulatory changes in the United States granting additional months of patent exclusivity in exchange for research in children (Food and Drug Administration Modernization Act, Best Pharmaceuticals for Children Act) with similar impending regulations in the EU, have stimulated more psychopharmacological studies in children. Until early 2004, 36 pediatric psychopharmacological studies had been requested by the U.S. Food and Drug Administration (FDA), the American regulatory agency (this corresponds to 13% of all studies requested in pediatric drugs). Ten pediatric psychopharmacological drugs had been granted a six-month additional exclusivity by the FDA. This shows that without regulatory interventions the market alone cannot improve the situation of safety and efficacy of psychopharmacological treatments in children. Expected market size determines what compound will be tested in a given population. Therefore patients with rare diseases or age groups that usually do not get ill are at risk. We speak of "orphan drugs" in the context of drug treatment of rare diseases; and children may be considered "therapeutic orphans".

1.4 Interventions

1.4.1 Prevention

In a consensus statement on prevention the World Psychiatric Association (WPA) defined three major aims of prevention (WPA December 2003). *Primary prevention:* The identification of, and interventions with, high risk groups was recommended, for example prenatal care, healthy start to life programmes, good parenting, collaborative multi agency programmes. *Secondary prevention:* Pre-morbid intervention in mental illness such as depression, post-traumatic stress disorder, substance abuse or psychosis was recommended. *Tertiary prevention:* This was defined as early intervention in mental illness, for example in community-based treatment and rehabilitation programmes. The World Psychiatric Association also defined goals in educating the community about mental illness (secondary prevention) and stigma reduction (tertiary prevention).

In this chapter we will focus on pre-morbid pharmacological interventions in mental illness or early intervention in mental illness, and we will take the unique example of novel antipsychotics and schizophrenia prevention. We would have liked to focus on so-called "neuroprotection" in cases of early child abuse and neglect, but the literature on the neuro-protective effects of some antiepileptic drugs also known as mood stabilisers is insufficiently researched and documented to enable this, consisting only of some clinical observations and interpretation of animal data. An overview of well-researched prevention programmes in child and adolescent mental health or adult mental health (Fegert 2004b; Warner 2004) shows that the most effective prevention programmes in child psychiatry and adult psychiatry may not require a psychiatric or psychopharmacological intervention, but rather a medical or psychosocial intervention. Home visiting and nursing programmes, early infancy projects and similar interventions were effective in reducing child abuse, conduct disorder, substance abuse, adult depression, etc. Even in schizophrenia, improved obstetric care for women with schizophrenia and first degree relatives of people with schizophrenia proved to be effective. In this context, the pre-morbid detection and early intervention for the prevention of schizophrenia with atypical neuroleptics will be an interesting example of a pharmacological intervention in the developing brain.

In 1996 Yung and McGorry defined the so-called "schizophrenia prodrome", characterised by sleep disturbance, depressed mood, social withdrawal, suspiciousness, perplexity, change in sense of self or others, poor appetite, raising thoughts, impulsivity or disinhibition, memory problems, anxiety, anger, irritability, deterioration of functioning, poor concentration, loss of motivation, fatigue perceptual changes, somatic complaints, thought blocking, odd behaviour and elevated mood. Although this is a very unspecific list of symptoms, with some of these being quite common in adolescents in puberty, the American Psychiatric Association defined "prodromal schizophrenia" in DSM III, the diagnostic and statistical manual for the classification of psychiatric diseases in the United States. Here we find in the definition such unspecific behaviour as social isolation and withdrawal, impairment in role functioning, peculiar behaviour, impairment of personal hygiene, blunted or inappropriate affect, digressive speech or poverty of ideas, odd beliefs or magical thinking, unusual perceptual experiences (illusions), and lack of initiative, interests or energy. 10–50% of Australian 16-year olds reported having at least two of these non-specific symptoms. McGorry stated that these symptoms of schizophrenia prodrome are a mixture of assimilated psychotic symptoms, neurotic and mood related symptoms and various changes in behaviour. In his research, based on these symptoms McGorry and his co-workers found that 41% of all individuals meeting various criteria for prodrome would go on to develop first episode schizophrenia within one year, and a further 15% would develop it within two years. In an interventional study of 522 patients referred to the PACE Clinic, 135 met study criteria and 59 were finally randomised into two treatment groups. The first group received individual and family support and SSRI treatment, if indicated, for six months (n = 28). The other intervention group received the same support and open label Risperidone therapy (1–2 mg per day) plus cognitive therapy for six months (n = 31). At six months, 35.7% (10 out of 28) of those receiving supportive care had developed first episode psychosis. In the other group of those receiving low dose Risperidone and cognitive intervention, 3 out of 31 (9.7%) had developed first episode psychosis during six months, and 3 more had a first episode during the subsequent six months (Philipps et al. 2000). The onset of psychosis was therefore possibly delayed in about 7 of the early interventional or Risperidone prevention group. Philipps concludes that in subjects manifesting symptoms of the "schizophrenia prodrome", the transition to frank psychosis appears to be less frequent in those given drug treatment and cognitive therapy than in those not given such treatment. But is this perilous intervention with a strong atypical neuroleptic justified? This positive outcome seems to be very striking. In 7 out of 31 subjects the onset of illness was delayed or prevented but at the same time out of 31 early intervention subjects, 21 had been told that they were at risk for schizophrenia but in fact did not develop it; thus they would have been taking Risperidone unnecessarily. Furthermore, three patients developed early Schizophrenia despite taking Risperidone. So they, too, had taken the preventive Risperidone therapy without benefit. A German group (Klosterkötter et al. 2001) developed the Bonn Scale for Assessment of Basic Symptoms, a 66 item measure of prodromal disturbance in thought, language, perception and affect. In their 10-year follow up of clinic outpatients they found that 49% of their outpatients developed schizophrenia as compared with 70% of those with an identified risk by the Bonn Scale for Assessment of Basic Symptoms developed schizophrenia (positive predictive value). The authors reported a low false negative rate that means the sensitivity was high at 0.98 and a moderate false positive rate with specificity being at 0.59. They concluded that their screening instrument is applicable to a broad identification of at-risk persons in a general population. But this might be a dangerous conclusion, because their study was conducted in a highly selected population where 49% of all referred outpatients developed schizophrenia. In the general population the base rate with risk of developing psychosis is at about 1%. According to Bayes' theorem, the positive predictive value of 70% in this special outpatient population drops to 2% in the general population. Therefore one might understand why in Germany many people had objections when this group wanted to leave the outpatient setting and go to schools with their screening instrument in a research project, in order to identify at-risk patients qualifying for an early pharmacological preventive intervention. Given the results of McGorry, also in a highly selected population with a number needed to treat of about four for preventative effects of psychotropic medication in at-risk subjects, the number needed to treat in general population based sample would be very high, whilst the risk to harm by the side effects of the medication without any preventive benefit would also be high. Preventative medication in the schizophrenia prodrome may not work because the screening and selection of cases might be inadequate. The symptoms are very unspecific, and psychosis in childhood is an extremely rare condition. Less than 1% of all schizophrenic disorders start before the age of 10, less than 4% before the age of 14; as a result, very early onset psychosis before the age of 11 or early onset psychosis are low frequency disorders that are difficult to detect in the general population, for example through school based programmes. It is for this reason that the Australian Intervention Program was criticised by European authors (Fegert 2003). Even if the intervention is effective for some of the identified individuals, intervention might be harmful to those individuals with false positives on screening. Finally, there may be much better ways to identify the target group by training the general population to recognise symptoms of schizophrenia and thus reduce the duration of untreated psychosis that is related with negative outcome of schizophrenia in many studies.

1.4.2 Treatment in a Developmental Perspective

1.4.2.1 The Example of SSRI Use in the Treatment of Childhood Depression

A scandal highlighting the problem of off-label use. In paediatrics and child psychiatry, "off-label" use and unlicensed use, are very common. Most of the medicines used to treat children are not approved by the regulatory agencies for an indication in this age group. Child psychiatrists usually rely on results found in adults and then try to adapt dosages and treatment strategies to the needs of the paediatric age group. There is often no research on age-dependent pharmacokinetics, which means that dosing is a risky single-case based strategy. Children are not small adults; this is well known, but there is inadequate research on psychotropic medication in children. Written requests by the American regulatory agency FDA did stimulate research on antidepressants in children and adolescents. In order to get patent extension, several pharmaceutical companies studied their products in this age group and submitted the results to the agencies. Unfortunately, they did not usually publish unfavourable results. Therefore clinical recommendations which relied on published literature, for example in treatment parameters or clinical guidelines, recommended the use of SSRIs in children and adolescents for the treatment of depression. The so-called SSRI debacle, which we will describe below, illustrates the risk of publishing seemingly positive case series without control groups. Many novel interventions in the brain are first published in the same way for example as case reports or case series without any blinded controls or other controlled design. There might be a natural tendency to underreport negative observations and overestimate positive effects.

Since the first airing of the BBC Film "The Secret of Seroxat®" on the 13th of October 2002 in Europe as well as in the United States, an increasing amount of publications and contradictory information has caused a vivid debate about risks and benefits of SSRI treatment in depressed youth. Many parents and depressed children are alarmed and their spontaneous reactions to reports in the media are increasingly posing a further risk in the treatment of depression in child and adolescent psychiatry. The general acceptance of the use of psychotropic agents in the treatment of children and adolescents, which had grown in the last decade (Zito et al. 2000), is now declining. There is an ongoing discussion on publication bias and the need of transparent information for the public, prescribers and patients. The fact that the new European Clinical Trials Data Base (EUDRACT) will not be publicly accessible raises questions of the importance of transparency and treatment safety on the one hand and patent holder propriety issues on the other. Well founded critical reviews (Angell 2004) as well as conspiracy theories on the cooperation of doctors and industry (Healy 2004) and personal reports of families who lost a child under SSRI treatment (with many other factors not taken into consideration) have spread, causing concern and controversy.

Many clinicians now avoid the off-label prescription of SSRIs and have returned to tricyclic antidepressants. In some countries, for example in Germany, a majority of physicians had never given up using tricylics, because of a conservatism reinforced by the labelling situation – due to historical labelling procedures some tricyclics are labelled in some European countries for the use in childhood depression, despite the absence of proof of their efficacy for this indication in this age group in a clinical trial or a meta-analysis (Greenhill and Waslick 2004).

Of the remaining clinicians who are still prescribing SSRIs, some tend to use low dosages to avoid harm, ignoring the fact that children and adolescents generally metabolise antidepressants more rapidly than adults (Brent 2004; Findling 2004). Some refrain from prescribing SSRIs even in situations where we can find promising results (such as posttraumatic stress disorder [PTSD] and anxiety) and have established indications with childhood labelling of different substances in different countries, as in SSRIs for obsessive-compulsive disorder.

The European Medicines Agency (EMEA) has reinforced these attitudes by issuing a general warning against SSRIs on April 25th 2005, recommending strong warnings across the European Union to doctors and parents about risks of suicide-related behaviour. The EMEA's Committee for Medicinal Products for Human Use (CHMP) concluded that "these products should not be used in children and adolescents, except in their approved indications" (Doc. Ref. EMEA/CHMP/128918/2005 corr).

Development of the SSRI controversy. In January 2003 the FDA approved Fluoxetine for paediatric use in major depressive disorder (MDD) and obsessive compulsive disorder (OCD). The British Modern Humanities Research Association (MHRA) issued a warning about Paroxetine in children and adolescents based on a confidential report concerning 3 studies with Paroxetine including 748 children and adolescents. Events possibly related to suicide occurred in 3.7% in the treatment group and 2.5% in the placebo group. This means that there was a non significant ($p = 0.50$) increase of relative risk (1.5, 95%CI: 0.6, 3.4). Even though during the 30 day follow up period event rates in the Paroxetine group were further elevated to 5.3% vs. 2.8%, the increase of relative risk still remained non significant ($p = 0.12$).

Adding the data from the other trials including children with OCD, possibly suicide-related events went down to 2.4% in the therapy group vs. 1.1% in the placebo condition ($p = 0.07$) and to 3.4% vs. 1.2% if the 30 day follow-up period was included ($p = 0.01$). The authors of the report conclude: "This means that any possibility of a protective effect is minimal, but the excess risk could be over 5-fold".

From this time on the public discussion mainly focussed on risks in treatment with SSRI, avoiding the issue of poor treatment outcome and lack of proof of efficacy. Clinicians, in contrast, stressed the clinical effectiveness and importance of SSRIs based on their personal impressions. Some epidemiologists started to discuss the general decrease of suicide rates since the introduction of these medications in search of a proof of their general benefit (Olfson et al. 2003).

In July 2003 the FDA addressed a request for paediatric suicidality summary data to the patent holders of 8 other antidepressant products. Wagner et al. published their study on the efficacy of Sertraline in August 2003. At the same time Wyeth issued a warning to doctors concerning Venlafaxine and pro-actively obtained a label upgrade in the United States while the MHRA issued a warning on Venlafaxine. The FDA sought external review to reclassify possible suicide-related events at Columbia University.

At the end of 2003 the British agency's warning regarding antidepressants was extended to a contraindication of all SSRIs except Fluoxetine, followed by a FDA general warning in March 2004 after a first FDA public hearing in February and a warning by Health Canada (http://www.fda.gov/cder/drug/antidepressants/default.htm, accessed on December 14th, 2006). Whittington et al. (2004) published in the Lancet the first systematic review of published vs. unpublished data and concluded:

> Data for two published trials suggests that Fluoxetine has a favourable risk-benefit profile, and unpublished data lend support to this finding. Published results from one trial of Paroxetine and two trials of Sertraline suggest equivocal or weak risk-benefit profiles. However in both cases, addition of unpublished data indicates that risks outweigh benefits. Data from unpublished trials of Citalopram and Venlafaxine show unfavourable risk-benefit profiles.

Different papers claimed that we need full access to data of positive and negative trials (3, 4, 14). In June 2004, New York state attorney Eliot Spitzer filed a law suit charging United Kingdom-based drug company Glaxo Smith Kline with "repeated and persistent fraud alleging that it only published positive results of its Paroxetine trials". In summer 2004 the case was settled with the payment of more than two million US dollars. Since the FDA hearing there had been rumours that the FDA had suppressed a critical report by the FDA's child psychiatrist Andy Mosholder stating that there is a two-fold risk of suicide-related behaviour in the use of SSRIs compared to placebo. The United States' Congress started an investigation against FDA. Finally in August 2004 the British Medical Journal and the

New York Times gained access to Dr. Mosholder's 33-page memorandum and the FDA launched a criminal investigation to find out who leaked the report. The results of the reclassification analysis by the Columbia team were published on the internet by the FDA in August. In mid-August 2004 the Treatment for Adolescents with Depression Study (TADS – a publicly-funded randomised controlled clinical trial done by a research team) was published in the Journal of the American Medical Association. This was the first study comparing medication against psychotherapy and the combination of both to placebo. The combination of Fluoxetine with cognitive behaviour therapy (CBT) offered the most favourable statistically significant results over placebo and showed a response rate of 71%. Fluoxetine alone (with a response rate of 60.6%) was statistically superior to CBT alone (43%, the response at of placebo being 34.8%). With respect to suicide risk, the authors found that clinically relevant suicidal thoughts were present in 29% of the sample at baseline and improved significantly in all four treatment groups, with the combination therapy showing the greatest reduction. In that sample of 439 youths suffering from moderate to moderately severe MDD (CDRS-R t score average was 76 at the beginning of treatment, with current major depressive episode duration median being 48 weeks) seven patients (1.6%) attempted suicide. As in the other studies, there was no completed suicide. CBT had a specific beneficial effect on suicidal ideation.

The TADS Fluoxetine and placebo data have been included in the FDA risk analysis, and were presented in September 2004 at a second public hearing. The members of the two advisory committees concerned (the Psychopharmacologic Drugs Committee and the Paediatric Advisory Committee) concluded that the finding of an increased risk of suicidality in clinical trials was a group effect and recommended that a trials warning related to an increased risk should be applied to all antidepressant drugs whether previously studied or not, and a patient information should be provided to children and their caregivers with every prescription. They reached a split decision (15 for and 8 against) recommending a so-called "black box warning" but were unanimous that these drugs should not be contraindicated because the access to these therapies was important for those who could benefit. The controversy over the pros and cons of a black box warning was made public by the New England Journal of Medicine, which asked to committee members to comment on this issue (Newmann 2004; Brent 2004).

On Friday, October 15th, 2004, the FDA launched a strategy, including a black box warning, to strengthen safeguards for children and adolescents treated with antidepressant medications.

On April 25th, 2005, the CHMP of the EMEA concluded that these substances "should not be used in children or adolescents except in their approved indications".

Table 1.1: Black Box Warning Issued By the FDA October 2004

Suicidality in Children and Adolescents

Antidepressants increase the risk of suicidal thinking and behavior (suicidality) in children and adolescents with major depressive disorder (MDD) and other psychiatric disorders. Anyone considering the use of [Drug Name] or any other antidepressant in a child or adolescent must balance this risk with the clinical need. Patients who are started on therapy should be observed closely for clinical worsening, suicidality, or unusual changes in behavior. Families and caregivers should be advised of the need for close observation and communication with the prescriber. [Drug Name] is not approved for use in pediatric patients except for patients with [Any approved pediatric claims here]. (See Warnings and Precautions: Pediatric Use)
Pooled analyses of short-term (4 to 16 weeks) placebo-controlled trials of nine antidepressant drugs (SSRIs and others) in children and adolescents with MDD, obsessive compulsive disorder (OCD), or other psychiatric disorders (a total of 24 trials involving over 4,400 patients) have revealed a greater risk of adverse events representing suicidal thinking or behavior (suicidality) during the first few months of treatment in those receiving antidepressants. The average risk of such events on drug was 4%, twice the placebo risk of 2%. No suicides occurred in these trials.

Access to care and national differences in treatment approaches. Access to care and the possibilities of surveillance of side effects are different across European countries. In some countries a majority of depressed patients are seen by general practitioners or paediatricians, whereas in other countries child psychiatry is well developed as a speciality and there are sufficient treatment facilities for both inpatient and outpatient psychiatric treatment of childhood depression. In an analysis (Fegert et al. 2004; Zito et al. 2004) based on a Dutch cohort of 72,570 enrollees, a German cohort of 480,680 enrollees and a Mid-Atlantic State Children's Health Insurance Program (SCHIP) cohort (comparable to the others in its middle class composition) of 125,157 enrollees, a wide disparity across systems has been found. Antidepressant prescriptions were 15 times greater in the United States middle class sample than in the German, and 3 times greater than in the Dutch cohort despite a similar theoretical approach to child psychiatry. Older girls were most common recipients of prescriptions in Dutch and German cohorts, whereas 5–14 year olds were more prominent in the United States cohort. Sub-class analysis showed that tricyclic antidepressants are still the most prescribed antidepressant drugs for young people in Germany, whereas in the United States and Dutch population SSRIs were the most commonly prescribed drugs. Table 1.2 gives an overview of antidepressant prescriptions. Paroxetine (27% Netherlands, 24% United States) accounted for a quarter of all antidepressant prescriptions in the Dutch and United States cohort, while Imipramine and Amitriptyline constituted 45% of the prescriptions in Germany (Fegert et al. 2004).

Table 1.2: Leading Antidepressants as a Proportion of All Antidepressant Users

Leading antidepressants as a proportion of all antidepressant users						
	Dutch n=390	%	German * n=522	%	US-SCHIP n=2067	%
Drug 1	Paroxetine	27	Imipramine	32	Paroxetine	24
Drug 2	Amitriptyline	16	Amitriptyline	13	Sertraline	23
Drug 3	Fluoxetine	14	Opipramol	12	Fluoxetine	18
Drug 4	Imipramine	14	Doxepine	11	Bupropion	18
Drug 5	Fluvoxamine	9	Fluoxetine	7	Trazodone	7
> 1 drug	5.9%		5.4%		21.3%	

* Excluding herbal medicines
Source: Fegert et al. 2004

Fluoxetine prescriptions ranked at a middle level of 7% in Germany, 14% in the Netherlands and 18% in the United States population. Co-medication was common in the American population (21.3%) while in the Dutch and German cohort the rates were much lower (5.9% and 5.4% respectively). Herbal medicines such as Hypericum (St. John's Wort) were not included in this comparison, but another study in a German sample (Kölch et al. 2004; Fegert et al. 2006) has found Hypericum to be the predominant drug prescribed for childhood and adolescent depression in Germany. The data shows that the prescriptions of Paroxetine or Venlafaxine may be an important health issue in United States-populations and in the Netherlands or the United Kingdom but are not such an issue in Germany where ineffective medications for the treatment of depression, such as TCAs with their high risk profile (Amitai and Frischer 2006), are more widely prescribed.

Consequences. The discussion on contraindications, black box warning, different warnings and prescription restrictions has caused considerable political fallout and confused many patients, parents and doctors. There is a situation of relatively low risk but unclear benefit in the treatment of depression with most of the known SSRIs except Fluoxetine. There has been no pooling of efficacy data with the same methods at the FDA, so we only have information of the risk of the drug class but not whether there is an overall positive trend for efficacy. Many patients have been alarmed about these warnings and do not understand the notion of a statistically significant but clinically small risk signal. This makes sudden withdrawal from a clinically effective medication a high risk associated with this type of situation where information is skewed.

The non-transparency of research results caused a major *credibility problem* for doctors and industry. As in the United States, it will be important in the future in Europe to have sponsors of clinical research other than industry. Because of their vested interests, combined trials with psychotherapy or psychosocial intervention and medication or trials with psychotherapy alone will never be sponsored by the industry (Vitiello et al. 2004). We need a better understanding of the interface between publicly-funded and industry-funded research and better opportunities for integration and collaboration in paediatric psychopharmacology and treatment research. According to European regulations and national law in many European countries, *group benefit* is the only ethical principle that legitimises clinical trials in children. Therefore research data must be made fully available to the public. Research physicians should not sign trial contracts which give the sponsor an absolute or relative right to veto publication. More research on the long-term effectiveness and long-term safety of psychopharmacological treatments in children and adolescents is needed. We need better information for patients and parents, general practitioners, paediatricians, child and adolescent psychiatrists and the media.

There are no simple answers to complex situations. Banning an entire group of medications involves a higher risk for patients and doctors and takes us back to a situation that we had in the 80s and the early 90s of the last century in most of the countries in Europe, where long-term non-evidence-based treatments or insufficient access to treatment were common for children in need of child psychiatric interventions. The SSRI crisis dramatically illustrates the fact that we do not need any more ideological controversies and conspiracy theories on child psychopharmacology, but that instead we need more evidence and more, better research for the benefit of children in order to have balanced treatment strategies founded on a sufficient scientific evidence base.

1.4.2.2 Stimulant Treatment of ADHD

According to Schwabe and Paffrath (2005), there has been a 40-fold increase of Methylphenidate prescriptions in Germany over the last ten years. Elliger (1991) estimated, based on a supposed daily dose of 30 mg and a mean treatment duration of 150 days, that about 2,500 children were treated with Methylphenidate in Germany at the beginning of the 1990s. Ten years later it was found that 68,000 children were treated with Methylphenidate (Fegert et al. 2002). Safer et al. (1996) found a 2.5-fold increase of prescriptions in the United States from 1990 to 1995. The overall treatment prevalence he found was 2.8% in children aged 5–18. Angold et al. (2000) found, in their great Rocky Mountains study, a treatment prevalence of 7.3% of all children, but only 34% of these children treated with stimulants fulfilled all diagnostic criteria for ADHD. Different study groups have described important regional differences (Rappley et al. 1995; LeFever et al. 1999; Fegert et al. 2002). In the above mentioned study, Fegert et al. found that the stimulant prevalence was the highest in the age group between 9 and 15 years, at 2.5%. Boys were more frequently treated than girls (2.5–3.1 times more often). 90% of all prescriptions concerned Methylphenidate, and less than 10% of the boys treated with stimulant medication had been co-medicated. Co-medication included many irrational combinations with phytopharmaca, benzodiazepines and other non-phytosedatives. These combination therapies were mostly prescribed by general practitioners and paediatricians whilst the combination with atypical neuroleptics apparently was more favoured by child psychiatrists. There is still an ongoing debate on the long-term effects of Methylphenidate treatment especially with respect to the development of substance abuse disorders. Most of the published studies described an even lower risk in patients that had been treated for ADHD (Biederman et al. 1999; Molina et al. 1999; Paternite et al. 1999; Levin and Kleber 1995), and others found no influence at all (Barkley et al. 2003; Weiss and Hechtmann 1993; Chilcoat and Breslau 1999; Burke et al. 2002). Only Lambert and Hartsough (1998) found an increased risk. Different regulatory agencies have issued warnings or conducted hearings on other different possible long-term effects or serious side effects of stimulant treatment, such as possible cardiac problems or hallucinations. New formulations with slow release, imitating a twice daily or thrice daily Methylphenidate dosing regime have entered the market, reducing the stigmatisation of children who previously had to take their medication in school. New classes of so-called non-stimulant interventions such as Atomoxetine have also found a place in the market for the treatment of children suffering from ADHD. So, at the end of 2005 the number of children treated with a stimulant or non-stimulant medication for ADHD is the highest ever seen in the United States and in many countries in Europe.

There is good evidence for this approach. The Multimodal Treatment Study of Children with ADHD (MTA) and the MMT (Hechtman et al. 2004) both showed that pharmacological treatment with a sophisticated titration technique is comparable or superior to any other approach. In general there is no additional benefit to be expected from combined pharmacological and psychotherapy. It is only in cases with co-morbidities that combined treatment strategies may be superior to pharmacotherapy alone. Based on these multimodal treatment studies, pharmacoeconomic discussions have arisen about the general usefulness of psychotherapy in this field. While the European standpoint is still that psychosocial interventions and medication should be combined and in less severe cases psychosocial interventions should be tried first, in the United States medication is usually the first approach in trying to address the problem of ADHD.

Because stimulants were introduced in child psychiatric therapy so early, there is a lack of sound pre-clinical studies that are now usually conducted in early phases of drug development. Still, very little is known about the exact pathogenesis of ADHD at the molecular level. There seems to be good evidence for a genetically inherited vulnerability, as Biederman and Faraone

(2005) reported that most studies with focus on the dopamine D4 receptor "have assayed a variant known as the exon III 7-repeat allele, which produces an in-vitro blunted response to dopamine." There are other possibilities, for example of the dopamine 5 receptor and the 148-bp allele, which have been reported as well. The genetic factors are amplified through different influencing factors throughout child development, such as pregnancy and delivery complications, neglect, abuse, hours of television viewing, etc., thus presenting a broad but also "fuzzy" range of influences or underlying mechanisms. This seems to result in a dysregulation of frontal-subcortical circuits. When confronted with cognitive tasks, differential activation of neural systems can be assessed using neuroimaging studies of ADHD patients as compared to healthy subjects. For example, Durston et al. (2003) reported that children with ADHD activated frontostriatal regions ineffectively when compared to healthy controls, and also activated a network of regions (including more posterior and dorsolateral prefrontal regions). In addition to this complex mosaic of possible triggers, the cellular mechanisms of functioning of Methylphenidate (about sixty years after it was first synthesised) and other stimulants remain unknown.

Evidence from neuropharmacological studies seems to confirm the hypothesis that ADHD is founded on a disequilibrium of catecholaminergic neurotransmission, especially within the dopaminergic system (Solanto 2002). Neuroimaging studies show an increased density of dopaminergic transporters in the striatum of adult ADHD patients (Dougherty et al. 1999) which can be altered (decreased) through administration of Methylphenidate (Krause et al. 2000). There seems to be sound evidence that Methylphenidate binds to the dopaminergic transporter on the neural cellular membrane, thus blocking the reuptake of dopamine from the synaptic cleft back into the presynaptic neuron, which in turn increases the concentration of dopamine within the synaptic cleft (Solanto 1998; Volkow et al. 2005; Chen et al. 2005). In addition to the abovementioned reuptake blockade there seem to be other mechanisms of Methylphenidate action, as behavioural alterations after administration of Methylphenidate have been observed in mice lacking dopamine transporters (Trinh et al. 2003).

1.4.2.3 Treating Schizophrenic Patients with Neuroleptics During Childhood and Adolescence

In surveys of the current state of research, the lack of controlled studies of atypical neuroleptics has been criticised. Findings concerning the adult age group are generally assumed to be applicable to adolescents. Currently there is insufficient data available which is specific to the adolescent age group. The general reason for this lack is the worldwide problem of "off-label use" of substances legally permitted for use in adulthood with children and adolescents, which has been previously discussed. Currently in the Federal Republic of Germany, as in most countries of Europe, no atypical neuroleptics are licensed for the treatment of schizophrenia in childhood and adolescence (as at the end of 2005). Since autumn 2001, *Risperidone* has been labelled from age five for another indication (disruptive behaviour), because sufficient data on effectiveness, and above all on therapeutic safety, are available for this (Findling et al. 2001; Croonenberghs et al. 2005; Fegert and Herpertz-Dahlmann 2005). Gillberg's survey (2000) shows that even for the "old", typical neuroleptics few studies exist, most of them open studies. Here Gillberg cites fewer than 10 noteworthy studies, and in a survey of the last 35 years he is able to point to another 50 studies that contain case reports of one to six patients treated. Truly controlled studies, namely those able to present a genuine basis of evidence, are extremely rare; thus, among the studies he mentions there are still those that make reference to the treatment of autism and other behavioural abnormalities. Thus, according to the criteria of the international psychopharmacological algorithm project (Jobson and Potter 1995), high standards of evidence and verification are missing.

This persistent situation has led us to question whether protective regulations might not generally lead to psychopharmacological advances being withheld from adolescents. Largely due to the terrible medical crimes of the Nazi era, ethical standards and protective regulations ranging from the Nuremberg Code to the Declaration of Helsinki, adopted by the World Medical Association, were developed to protect those considered "incapable of consent". Indeed, a primary problem in child and adolescent psychiatry is the fact that in many discussions children and adolescents are seen as generally incapable of consent. Rothärmel (1999), together with Rothärmel et al. (1999), have suggested that in such contexts "informed consent" can become a construct that is opposed to the real interests of children, because in the consultation parents act as proxies on behalf of the children, though the children are expected to cooperate in the treatment. Thus, in places where American English is spoken a distinction is made between "assent" and "consent". "Assent" indicates the adolescent's willingness to undergo treatment, which though it does not have the status of legal consent is still a prerequisite for clinical research.

Patient information, informed consent and assent in off-label treatment. The current practice in the treatment of adolescent patients with schizophrenia in Europe is to conduct an individual clinical trial using an atypical neuroleptic. However, this treatment is adopted exclusively in the interest of healing the patient, as an individual decision. Adolescents generally seem to show considerable psychological maturity, and many adolescents are perfectly able to understand issues concerning medication. Nevertheless, especially in the acute stage of a first schizophrenic illness, prescribers should proceed with caution and on the assumption of a limited capacity for consent because of the impact of psychopathology. This means that the physician should assume that acutely ill patients cannot sufficiently evaluate the nature, meaning, or scope of the administration of medicines, and that therefore, in addition to the patient's consent, the consent of the person with custody is absolutely necessary. Thus the consultation in a situation of off-label use (described in German law as "an individual clinical trial") must be rather more thorough, in many respects, than for a treatment in the context of authorisation, that is, of specialised research. On the basis of therapeutic freedom, the doctor can opt for a treatment that is not yet labelled in this form, but must consult about the matter with the individuals concerned and also explain the legal alternatives. The advantages of the drugs to be taken, their digestibility, side effects, onset of effects, duration of effects, and target dosage must all be discussed. Placing such considerable demands on the consultation discussion entails legal risks, for the doctor will be held responsible for any lack of thoroughness in the consultation or, in reality, for insufficient documentation of the consultation process. Therefore, what distinguishes the competent consultation is the designation, at the beginning of treatment, of a significant measure indicating the quality of the process. It must be borne in mind, particularly in the treatment of adolescent patients with schizophrenia, that patients' understanding of treatment efforts in consultation will change with the increasing success of the treatment. Consequently, some consultation discussions must be repeated, i.e. followed through in a broader context. Consultation with adolescents is more of a continuous process than a one-time task completed at the beginning of treatment. For instance, if the doctor records specific follow-up questions with the documentation from the consultation, then it will be easy to present proof, in the event of any subsequent legal-medical dispute, that an appropriate consultation discussion has taken place.

Empirical impressions on the questions of participation of children in treatment decision. In conducting a broader investigation of the rights of children and adolescents to information and participation in psychiatric treatment, Rothärmel et al. (2005) investigated, with the support of the Volkswagen Stiftung, a random sample of consecutive admissions to child and adolescent psychiatric treatment in Rostock and Ravensburg. In total, all consecutive inpatient admissions to both support clinics were included in the sample, with 296 cases in the age range of seven to seventeen years. Through factor analysis, different scales were obtained from a questionnaire. Relevant here is the "Participation Scale"; it consists of eight items and indicates a significant internal consistency (Cronbach's Alpha 0.87). Participation at the beginning of treatment had significant effects on motivation measured at the first and fifth week of treatment and also on the evaluation of the quality of treatment at the end of treatment (Beta coefficient 0.518***, 0.245*, 0.183*). Particularly for the beginning of treatment, the considerable participation of the patients through sufficient consultation accounted for 25% of the total variance with regard to motivation. Since, in child and adolescent psychiatry, schizophrenic illnesses usually make their first appearance in adolescence, we are considering in this context only the partial random samples of the over-14 year old patients (n = 161). Nineteen of these patients had a schizophrenic illness; an additional nineteen had the diagnosis of borderline personality disorders (F 21/DSM IV 301.22) and thus belonged to the treatment group for which the use of atypical neuroleptics is considered. For the patients of this diagnostic group, decisions concerning treatment were made by others far more frequently than was the case with other over-14 year-old child and adolescent patients (with reference to the diagnosis group ICD-10, F 2/DSM IV 295x-298x, chi2 = 7.504, p = 0.23). Because these patients were asked at the same time to what extent they would want to have the option to be the sole decision-makers for their own treatment, it was possible to establish the astonishing fact that these significantly impaired patients reflected in a fully realistic manner on the greater necessity of decision-making by others given their illness. The patients with schizophrenia, personality disorders, and eating disorders had the least desire (meaning not at all) to be entitled to make determinations about important questions of treatment (such as the admittance to treatment, medicinal dosages, eating guidelines, etc.) for themselves, as compared with the other patients of the same age. The relationship between autonomy, participation, and heteronomy is thus a highly sensitive matter that must be treated with a view to the patient's well being and the individual patient's situation. It must, however, be said by way of qualification that, in the context of acute schizophrenic symptoms, among the criteria for exempting a patient from completing an interview was "danger of doing substantial harm," and thus the most seriously affected patients could not be included in these interviews.

The adolescents under treatment for schizophrenia were directly questioned in interviews as to how they had understood the consultation on medication. Here are a few quotes from their responses: "So I can get a little more rest from the voices in my head"; "For my head, so I can be normal again"; "...to repress the visions, I had and to be more calm"; "Don't know – actually things should be better for me then." 57.1% of the patients were, by their own account, informed of side effects and long-term consequences. Only 14.3% of this patient group were consulted concerning alternative medications. However, in the overall random sample, one third of the patients were consulted concerning alternatives for treatment. This proportion of one third indicates far from optimal provision of information of all patients, but is nevertheless much better than in this specific group of very dependent patients with schizophrenia. To the interview question of how the decision was first made to prescribe medication, patients responded: "The doctors decided on the first day"; "It was determined by the doctor at the ward"; "I got something else from my doctor but it was switched at the clinic"; "They just said I should take some of them. That's what the doctors told me"; "I was asked, with my parents." These results show that the general concept of increasing the autonomy of the patient may not be acceptable or appropriate for all patients, depending on their developmental age and specific conditions.

Evidence base as a prerequisite for the formulation of treatment standards. The question of whether a certain form of therapy can be designated as standard has played a critical role since the Aciclovir decision of OLG (Higher Regional Court) Cologne (05/30/1990 – see Fegert et al. 1999). In that case, doctors were criminally convicted for failing to apply an off-label medication for a given diagnostic indication, even though it was regarded as standard practice in international literature in the field. The effort to establish quality and a greater evidence base has led professional organisations to set up guidelines to diagnostics and therapy. In the German guidelines for "Schizophrenia, schizoid-type and delusional disturbances," the argument is made that typical and atypical antipsychotics are (with the exception of Clozapine) the psychopharmaceuticals of first choice. This conclusion agrees with the current guidelines of German and American adult psychiatric professional groups, in particular for the treatment of schizophrenic patients with so-called negative symptoms. However, no adequate evidence base currently exists on effectiveness for this recommendation in childhood and adolescence. At the time of the review of these guidelines, three studies (Mandoki 1997; Kumra et al. 1998; Krishnamoorthy and King 1998) were available on Olanzapine, with a total sample size of 21 patients. These pertained to un-controlled, open observations. With regard to the use of Risperidone in treating childhood and adolescent schizophrenia, the authors of the German guidelines at that time were only able to make reference to Quintana and Keshavan (1995), Groevich et al. (1996), and Armenteros et al. (1997), who collectively made observations of a total of thirty patients in open trials. It can certainly be said that results from six short observations of open treatment describing altogether the effects of two different substances with approximately 50 adolescent schizophrenic patients cannot be considered an adequate evidence base for such a recommendation. This recommendation was, however, correct in other qualitative aspects and was even elaborated in a consensus process by the three professional societies of child and adolescent psychiatry in Germany.

In their survey of neuroleptic efficacy, which covered five placebo-controlled studies, twenty-four open studies and three case studies, Toren et al. (1998) arrived at the conclusion that the most convincing empirically obtained evidence of effects available are for Clozapine. Meanwhile, there are certainly other open studies on newer substances as well, such as Quetiapine (McConville et al. 1999; Shaw et al. 2001). However, even today no general designation for the highest standard of evidence can be made, the prerequisite being two or more controlled studies for a substance not a substance group.

The current, problematic, state of affairs with respect to available data and the law leads to a heterogeneous practice of making and writing prescriptions, compounded by the changes in care that occur as patients move between different practitioners at the clinics. Because of the deficient state of studies on childhood and adolescence, practitioner prescribing is driven by practical experience and experience gained from adolescent psychiatry concerning effectiveness. As a result, structural deficits should not be conceived so much in terms of their relation to proven effectiveness as to therapeutic safety. In any case, data concerning the effectiveness of antidepressants shows that even with respect to the effectiveness of substances, manifestly age-specific variations can arise. Some key questions remain: questions concerning specific age-appropriate dosages; questions concerning the particularly pronounced, age-dependent side effects such as elevated Prolactin-levels (e.g. Turrone et al. 2002) with and without clinical consequences; questions concerning the long-term implications of medically "trivial" physical side effects such as weight-gain, and so on. The process of treatment can be substantially hindered by the fact that, for example with an already paranoid patient and his greatly worried parents, a discussion must take place concerning off-label use, which then appears to be something seemingly forbidden or a mere experimentation. Thus many patients in the clinic wonder if they will be treated as guinea pigs. It is often possible to defuse these fears in discussion and move towards a genuine informed consent. Occasionally this difficult beginning can itself lead to a greater level of compliance because, in contrast to those on conventional treatment, patients receiving off-label treatment are better informed and consulted. In planning the course of treatment, it is necessary to ensure that consultation discussions are designed such that they are adequately documented and that the persons who are in fact entitled to give consent are involved in making the decision. This means obtaining consent from those having responsibility of a child or adolescent, and any adolescent who is able to grasp the scope of the decision. With treatment of children with atypical neuroleptics, consultation on dietetic measures is mandatory for children and those looking after them, particularly for younger children, as past experience shows they tend to have even greater weight gain.

1.4.3 Enhancement

Conceptual issues related to "enhancement" will be addressed in Chapter 6. In the present context, suffice it to say that we would like to focus on "neuroenhancement", defined by Hall as "the use of drugs and other interventions to modify brain processes with the aim of enhancing memory, mood and attention in people who are not impaired by illness or disorder." (Hall 2004)

1.4.3.1 Stimulants

Stimulants could be called universal enhancers because they are capable of modifying the behaviour and improving the performance of any person who takes them. Specific enhancers in contrast are only effective for a specific handicap and bring people with that specific handicap back to normal functioning, for instance eyeglasses, and hearing devices (according to the above definition one might even not call them enhancers at all). The United States President's Council imagined a situation where the tolerance with respect to the diversity of behaviour would decrease, and expressed concern that eventually "using psychotropic drugs might become, for an increasing number of children, a social necessity or expectation – merely to keep up." (President's Council on Bioethics 2003:90)

Fegert (1999) has pointed out that with current demographic trends of less children being born in developed states, the pressure for children to fulfil the expectations of parents is increasing, so conformity to standards and norms will reduce diversity in future generations. In a similar vein, the President's Council maintains:

> This enhanced ability to make children conform to conventional standards could also diminish our openness to the diversity of human temperaments. As we will find with other biotechnologies with a potential for use beyond therapy, behavior-modifying drugs offer us an unprecedented power to enforce our standards of normality. Human societies have always had such standards, but most societies (and certainly our own [the United States]) have in practice tolerated fairly significant deviations from them, and have greatly benefited from such tolerance. (President's Council on Bioethics 2003:88)

Another concern that the President's Council raises with respect to universal enhancement by stimulants is a moral concern.

> By medicalizing key elements of our life through biotechnical interventions, we may weaken our sense of responsibility and agency. And, technologies aside, merely regarding ourselves and our activities in largely genetic or neurochemical terms may diminish our sense of ourselves as moral actors faced with genuine choices and options in life. These concerns are especially serious with regard to children, where those who are treated are not the ones making the choice to seek treatment. (ibid.:92)

As Steven Hyman put it in his presentation to the Council: "There are symbolic messages to children about self-efficacy. Behavioral control comes from a bottle. We have the problem of anabolic steroids for the soul." (cited in President's Council on Bioethics 2003:92) Another moral argument is the matter of "brain doping":

> Artificial enhancement can certainly improve a child's abilities and performance (at least of specific tasks, over the short run), but it does so in a way that separates at least some element of that achievement from the effort of achieving. (ibid.:93)

Finally, consistent with its overall conservative attitude the Council argues that enhancers might just threaten "the innocence and the simple joys of childhood." (ibid.:94) A special protected phase of development such as childhood (Ariès 1960; deMause 1974) is a very late notion in human development and only common in our literature from about the time of the French Revolution. Conservative writers such as Postman (1982) have suggested that the modern media reduce this time of innocence. More and more features of adolescent behaviour seem to be embraced by adults, and the fading away of childhood seems to be one of the symptoms of our society. The President's Council concludes with respect to stimulants:

> It would be paradoxical, not to say perverse, if the desire to produce 'better children,' armed with the best that biotechnology has to offer, were to succeed in its goal by pulling down the curtain on the 'childishness' of childhood. And it would be paradoxical, not to say perverse, if the desire to improve our children's behavior or performance inculcated short-term and shallow notions of success at the expense of those loftier goals and finer sensibilities that might make their adult lives truly better. (President's Council on Bioethics 2003:94)

Stimulating agents have been utilised for ages to stay vigilant and the practice of using performance enhancing substances such as nicotine and caffeine (Koelega 1993) are a widespread custom in our days. As mentioned in earlier chapters, the idea of using psychopharmacological medication to enhance cognitive performance is as old as their use in clinically disturbed children and adolescents itself (Bradley 1937; Molitch and Eccles 1937). The next subsection will give an overview on the commonly widely used substances.

Methylphenidate and Amphetamines (Ritalin®, Medikinet®, Medikinet retard®, Concerta®, Equasym®, Adderall®). Even though the idea of augmenting one's performance using psychopharmacology is about 70 years old, nowadays an increasing number of college students use stimulants to perform better in their exams (see table 1.3 Potential use, misuse and abuse of stimulants).

Table 1.3: Potential Use, Misuse and Abuse of Stimulants

Potential Use, Misuse and Abuse of Stimulants	
Full ADHD criteria	Proper use
Some ADHD symptoms	Improper use
No diagnostic criteria met at all	Iatrogenic false use
Non-ADHD-symptoms or use in adults	Off-label therapeutic use
To enhance performance	Non-therapeutic use
To elicit euphoria	Abuse

McCabe et al. (2005) showed in their current survey a 6.9 % life prevalence of non-medical stimulant abuse among college students in the United States. This issue was covered by the New York Times and television reports as well. It seems safe to say that Methylphenidate and Amphetamines have moved beyond the paediatrician's and psychiatrist's office into the everyday's life of a growing number of young adults. As little data exists on possible effects of their usage in healthy subjects, we need to rely on our knowledge of their effects on people suffering from ADHD. Methylphenidate (MPH) and the related Amphetamines appear to influence dopaminergic pathways. While Amphetamines increase the output of dopamine, MPH seems to work by influencing the DAT – a dopamine transporter in the neuron's membrane. Amphetamines were used as early as World War II (where it was employed to keep pilots awake and alert during long flight hours) to enhance attention, but MPH's effects appear to extend far beyond that. It seems to calm the hyperactive child down, improve the accuracy on memory tasks in intellectually sub-average children (Aman et al. 1991), lead to a gain in academic performance (Schmidt et al. 1984), have beneficial effects on working memory (especially in subjects with lower baseline capacity) (Mehta et al. 2000) and even seems to make mathematical tasks more interesting (Volkow et al. 2004). But as Rapoport pointed out in 1980, MPH does not only increase the cognitive performance of these who suffer from ADHD – it is a "universal enhancer" which also seems to work in the healthy user, and is, as pointed out in the report of the President's Council, "capable of modifying the behavior and improving the performance of anyone who takes them." (2003)

The effects of MPH and d-Amphetamine in children with ADHD have been studied using multiple approaches, and are still under constant evaluation. Although little is known about possible long term effects of Methylphenidate and Amphetamine consumption (and there are still ongoing discussions about genotropic effects and the influence on later drug abuse), the volume of prescribed stimulants continues to rise, both within the United States (which consumes 80 % of the world's MPH production) and Europe. The prescription of MPH early in life (the stimulant is approved by the FDA for the use in children from six years of age but is, in spite of that, fairly often prescribed even to preschoolers, see Zito et al. 2000) raises particular concerns about possible impact of long-term stimulant medication on the developing child (Carlezon and Konradi 2004).

Modafinil (Provigil®). This relatively new non-amphetamine stimulant can be found in the recent literature as newest model of a psychopharmacological "Swiss Army knife". It seems to increase the vigilance of people working night shifts (Walsh et al. 2004) (and was even endorsed for this indication by an FDA group in 2003), improves the cognition in adults with ADHD (Turner et al. 2004), enhances learning processes in mice (Beracochea et al. 2003) and seems to possess antidepressant potential as well (Ferraro et al. 2002).

The role of Modafinil as a potential universal enhancer is supported by a long list of possible indications:

> [...] treatment of Alzheimer's disease, depression, attention-deficit disorder (ADHD), myotonic dystrophy, multiple sclerosis-induced fatigue, post-anaesthesia grogginess, cognitive impairment in schizophrenia, spasticity associated with cerebral

> palsy, age related memory decline, idiopathic hypersomnia, methamphetamine ('Ice') abuse, jet-lag, fatigue in Charcot-Marie-Tooth Disease (CMT), and everyday cat-napping. (http://www.modafinil.com, accessed on December 14th, 2006)

Whether or not this psychopharmacological agent will match the wide distribution of MPH remains to be seen.

Selective memory enhancement. Memory is, as the report of the President's Council points out, "important also for allowing and enabling us to 'know' [...] *who we are.*" (President's Council on Bioethics 2003:214) Although most of the recent scientific efforts to enhance memory concern treatment of the symptoms of Alzheimer's disease and dementia, it can be easily seen that the prospect of an improved memory is tantalising for the healthy as well.

While there have been some publications (with contradictory results) about phytopharmacological alterations of memory (Wesnes et al. 2000; Solomon et al. 2002; Persson et al. 2004) there are recent efforts to identify new promising substances. In her review of possible ways to manipulate human working memory Barch (2004) emphasised the importance of dopaminergic and cholinergic pathways for enhancing working memory, while only mixed results were available for noradrenergic and serotonergic pathways. Methylphenidate appears to increase spatial working memory in novel situations, but impair previously established performance due to a decrease in accuracy (Elliott et al. 1997). Mattay found an increase in working memory with Dextroamphetamine, but only in subjects with a low baseline capacity (Mattay et al. 2000).

1.4.3.2 Emotional Enhancement

> *Why don't you take some SOMA when you have these dreadful ideas of yours, You'd forget all about them. And instead of feeling miserable, you'd be jolly. So jolly.*
>
> *Aldous Huxley (1932) Brave New World*

The idea of "Feeling 'better than well'" (Hall 2004) which was addressed in Huxley's classic novel "Brave New World" is as old as mankind, but never before have we possessed such powerful means to accomplish that goal without having to risk too much in the process. The selective serotonin reuptake inhibitors (SSRIs) such as Prozac®, Paxil®, Zoloft®, Celexa®, Lexapro® and Effexor®, which have been extensively discussed earlier in this chapter, were originally developed to battle depressive symptoms (and also found to be useful in OCDs). They do, however, seem to have the additional potential to alter moods in the mentally undisturbed as well, hence their reputation as "happy pills" which could be used – as the President's Council points out – "to ease the soul and enhance the mood of nearly anyone." (President's Council on Bioethics 2003:207)

The widespread use of and increasing numbers of prescriptions (Zito et al. 2003) for SSRIs should be critically questioned, not just because of latest concerns regarding a possible influence on suicidality in adolescents, but also because these substances seem to have the potential to alter personality traits as well along with their mood altering effects. As Knutson et al. (1998) made clear, the administration of SSRIs has significant effects on negative affect and affiliative behaviour, even in subjects who do not suffer from depression or other psychopathology. SSRI administration reduced assaultativeness and negative affect and enhanced indices of social affiliation in a cooperative task in a placebo-controlled study of 51 healthy volunteers (Knutson et al. 1998). Comparable effects on social intervention were also reported for the use of the SSRI Citalopram by Tse and Bond (2001).

The effects of SSRIs on personality traits are described by the President's Council as follows:

> Loss, disappointment, and rejection still sting, but not as much or as long, and one can cope with them with less disturbance of mind. Sensitivity also declines, along with obsession, compulsion, and anxiety, while self-esteem and confidence rise. Fear, too, is reduced, and one is more easily able to experience pleasure and accept risk. Mental agility, energy, sleep, and appetite become more regular, typically increasing. And mood brightens – though not to the point of perpetual bliss or anywhere near it. People do indeed feel better. (President's Council on Bioethics 2003:245)

The question, however, still remains: "Can we become numb to life's sharpest sorrows without also becoming numb to its greatest joys?" (ibid.:229)

While SSRIs enable people with mental illnesses to experience a life which would be out of reach because of, for example, their genetic predisposition, one has to wonder if "feeling good" is the ultimate goal to be reached for the healthy or whether suffering, sorrow, longing and hunger for improvement in fact "make for a fuller and more flourishing life." (ibid.:258)

1.4.3.3 Ethical Concerns

> *"I'd rather be myself," he said.*
> *"Myself and nasty. Not somebody else, however jolly."*
> *Aldous Huxley (1932) Brave New World*

Multiple ethical concerns have been raised during the ongoing debate about neuroenhancement. With respect to MPH, the President's Council emphasised the problem of social conformity and raised the question of whether we would be tempted to "treat difficult or non-conforming children as problems" (President's Council on Bioethics 2003:89), thus diminishing human diversity. The Council also expressed its concerns about using the direct influence of a substance to the brain to change a child's behaviour without the child having to learn to "behave appropriately" (ibid.:91) for itself. Additionally Nylund (2000) pointed out that ADHD questionnaires and rating scales are based on norms from a white middle class population, leading to a possible overrepresentation of poor, non-white racial and ethnic groups diagnosed with ADHD, because different sociocultural backgrounds can contribute to behaviours that are interpreted as "restless" or "fidgety".

This discussion could be summed up by this question: whether a life without any effort, pain, difficulties and experiences is worth living; or, in plain words: "no pain, no gain?". Although experts agree upon the fact that people in need of psychopharmacological intervention (for example the mentally disturbed) need to have access to the psychopharmacological armamentarium, it is not so evident that drugs should be used to sanitise the experiences of normal life. Thus the President's Council in his chapter on "Better children" came to the conclusion: "Life is not just behaving, performing, achieving. It is also about being, beholding, savoring." (President's Council on Bioethics 2003:94)

In addition to issues of the diminution of experience through psychopharmacology, there are issues about distributive justice to be considered. Butcher (2003), Farah (2002) and Hall (2004) raised fundamental questions concerning the use of enhancing drugs in our society: What would happen if only the wealthy gain access to enhancing substances? Although from our viewpoint a two class society seems far fetched at the moment, the possibility does nevertheless exist, and in the United States, the managed care system has effectively created a two-tier system of those able and unable to access healthcare respectively. Cognitive resources for the healthy, being expensive, can result in a modern caste system, with cognitive resources only being available to those with enough money to hand. There would be no need for the wealthy to achieve academic excellence through hard work as pharmaceutical shortcuts enter the scene. If, on the other hand, enhancing drugs would be available for everybody, the question remains, would this disadvantage those who deliberately refuse to take drugs in a society in which cognitive enhancement is a standard procedure and performance levels are consequently artificially raised? It remains unclear whether the level of cognitive performance for the whole human species could be raised by using enhancing pharmaceuticals in large quantities. Refusing to be part of an "enhanced society" (and thus staying "natural") would mean to intentionally choosing to live one's life at a lower baseline of functioning than the average.

Finally, there is no evidence whether psychopharmacological substances do alter personality in one way or the other on the long run. It is intriguing to speculate, however, whether an individual who has become used to an enhanced, perhaps more positive functioning would remain so after the medication is discontinued or revert to a now unfamiliar and dimly remembered baseline personality.

So far these questions must remain unanswered, as we are on the edge of a new development, where we cannot see the future. It would appear necessary to stay cautious and keep vigilant watch on this development, as there are at the moment no definite results concerning long term safety and ethical implications available to us.

1.4.4 Chemical Restraint

In the treatment of children, and in a different way also in the treatment of mentally retarded people or people suffering from dementia, questions of patient choice will become increasingly important as already discussed in the example of atypical neuroleptics. Who can, and should, consent to treatment? How important is the assent of the person who has to tolerate the treatment? Can parents decide on preventative interventions or on enhancement in children whilst the children are still too young to articulate their wishes or recognise the problems the parents have with their behaviour? Who defines the problems? Who decides about the cure and who has to take the pill? These are the standard questions in the triangle of parent, child and doctor or legal guardian, patient and doctor. Where autonomy is concerned, an additional dimension is important: that of society. *Restraint* of aggressive or dangerous psychiatrically ill patients has always been one of the historical tasks of psychiatry. In the context of intervening in the psyche, the interests of the society may conflict with the personal interests of a subject. For example: is so-called "chemical restraint" acceptable to avoid harm to self or others? Individual rights of freedom and autonomy are sometimes overruled by mechanical or chemical interventions in psychiatrically ill patients, in the interests of protecting either themselves or others. These classical ethical questions will be discussed in this chapter against the background of examples from different substance classes. This will provide a framework for possible future discussions that will accompany the introduction of new forms of interventions in the brain.

The term "chemical restraint" in itself bears some potential for dispute (Crumley 1990) and is still not accepted by the American Psychiatric Association (APA), which considers this term imprecise, inaccurate and pejorative, and prefers to use the phrase "drug used as restraint" (Riordan 1999). Nevertheless, this term is widely used within the literature concerning restraint of children and adolescents and is well defined in the "Practice parameters" of the American Academy of Child and Adolescent Psychiatry (AACAP):

> A drug used as a restraint is a medication used to control behavior or to restrict a patient's freedom of movement and is not standard treatment for the patient's medical or psychiatric condition. Chemical restraint is different from the ongoing use of medication for the treatment of symptoms of underlying illness. (Masters et al. 2002)

Similar definitions can be found in the existing literature (Sorrentino 2004; Wynn 2002) and in the definition of the Health Care Financing Administration (Department of Health and Human Services 1999).

Discussion of different types of restraint (including mechanical, physical and chemical) and seclusion began about 200 years ago and led to dispute between European and American psychiatrists (or "alienists" as they were called at that time) throughout the 18th century, with a British group led by

John Conolly opposing mechanical restraint on the one side, and American alienists emphasising the need for mechanical control as the only means of controlling the "liberty-loving American" (Deutsch 1949) on the other.

The synthesis of chloralhydrate (which entered the American market in 1870) by a German pharmaceutical company, along with the use of opiates, bromides, alcohol and (later on) barbiturates, opened new possibilities in the management of agitated and psychotic patients by the turn of the century (Colaizzi 2005), thus ending the debate about the pros and cons of mechanical restraint.

Nowadays, different (psycho)pharmacological substances are used to control problematic behaviour and restrain patients. They include antihistamines (e.g. Diphenhydramine and Hydroxyzine), benzodiazepines (e.g. Diazepam, Lorazepam, Midazolam), opiates (e.g. Fentanyl), barbiturates (e.g. Pentobarbital), beta blockers (e.g. Propanolol), Lithium, Carbamazepine, atypical antipsychotics (e.g. Olanzapine, Ziprasidone, Quetiapine) and typical antipsychotics (e.g. Chlorpromazine, Fluphenazine, Haloperidol, Perphenazine, Thiothixene, Trifluorperazine; the butyrophenone Droperidol received a black box warning from the FDA due to its QT-prolongation and torsades de pointes dysrhythmias). Combinations, for example Haloperidol with Lorazepam (Battaglia et al. 1997; Bieniek et al. 1998), have also been tried.

Dorfman and Kastner (2004) evaluated the use of both mechanical and chemical restraint in paediatric psychiatric patients within an emergency medicine residencies and paediatric emergency medicine fellowships setting. They found that the most commonly drugs recently used to restrain children and adolescents were benzodiazepines, butyrophenones and antihistamines, followed by phenothiazines, opiates, barbiturates and others. Vitiello et al. (1991) found no significant difference in the efficacy of pro re nata (PRN, meaning according to need) medication when compared to placebo in a study of 21 boys between 5 and 13 years to whom medication was administered for the control of physical aggression, disruptive behaviour and temper tantrums.

According to Sorrentino (2004), an ideal drug for chemical restraint would have 1) efficacy in children; 2) multiple routes of administration; 3) non-addictive properties and no induction of tolerance; 4) minimal side effects with a good safety record and 5) cost-effectiveness. So far, such a drug does not exist. When it comes to indications for the use of seclusion and restraint, the "Practice parameters" of the AACAP (Masters et al. 2002; Barnett et al. 2002) points out that the application of these methods is only indicated "to prevent dangerous behavior to self or others and to prevent disorganisation or serious disruption of the treatment programme including serious damage to property". This, unfortunately, leaves considerable room for personal interpretation. Possible goals of chemical restraint suggested by Sorrentino (2004) are:

1. Decreasing the patient's anxiety and discomfort
2. Minimising disruptive behaviour
3. Preventing escalation of behaviour
4. Reversing the underlying cause, if identifiable

It is crucial that chemical restraints should always be offered first to the patient as voluntary treatment before involuntary measures are instituted, in order to emphasise the self-directedness of the applied pharmaceutical measures (Sorrentino 2004). Pharmacological substances often seem to be used as an aid where seclusion is not feasible. Sufficient data exists that an "unlocked seclusion policy" leads to an increased use of "as needed" tranquilising medications (Antoinette et al. 1990).

When we start to discuss chemical restraint and its potential impact on children, we always need to consider the possible alternatives in managing aggressive behaviour. "Time-out" is often used at psychiatric wards as a means of giving a child the opportunity to "cool down" by him- or herself. It is defined by the AACAP as "a process in which a child or adolescent can calm down usually by being quiet and disengaging from current stressors. The time-out may be conducted without removing a child from peers (inclusionary) or with the child's removal (exclusionary). It may be staff-directed or at the child's request (self-directed)" (Masters et al. 2002). It has been shown that seclusion in a time-out room can be problematic for children and adolescents with a history of physical or sexual abuse, as it has potential for re-traumatisation (Barnett et al. 2002). We need to know how patients themselves feel about different treatment modalities offered in an "out of control" situation. Miller (1985) showed within a sample of 40 children, that young patients perceived time-out as a punishment and not as a self-regulated aid to lower their aggression level. Kazdin (1984) found that although mothers of hospitalised children found time-out to be the most acceptable method, children in fact preferred medication. In adults, Wynn (2002) noted that different studies suggest that both patients and staff prefer the use of pharmacological restraint to the use of physical restraint and seclusion, as the first is perceived more as "treatment" whereas the latter more as some sort of "punishment".

When we look at this topic from an ethical viewpoint, we should ask whether the child who presents with acute aggressive problems that clearly require management either physically or pharmaceutically has had comparable difficulties in his former (which in this context is understood as "pre-hospital") life, indicating an inherent need; or whether the behavioural problems stem from the surrounding environment at a psychiatric ward. It is well known in the literature that aggression among children at psychiatric wards peaks during unstructured times (Measham 1995) and Wynn (1996) described a peak in the afternoon and early evening for aggression at an adult psychiatric ward.

There is a probable lack of recognition of the need to change staffing factors associated with an increase of violence in psychiatric units, such as inappropriate nursing staff-to-patient ratios, too many non-nursing staff on planned leave, staff becoming involved in cycles of aggression and coercion, staff sadism, staff conflicts, lack of boundary-setting by staff in response to patient limit-testing and emotions amongst staff of fear and anger. Finally, staff must demonstrate competent therapeutic approaches (Masters 2002). In a nutshell: we must always ask whether pharmaceutical control of behaviour is necessary in itself, or in order to compensate for deficits within a hospital or parental or school environment which promote "artificial" aggressive behaviour.

To sum up, the possible conclusions that can be drawn include the following three points:

- First, the administration of chemical restraints must always be questioned in terms of necessity, and possible amelioration which can be achieved by changing the hospital environment.
- Second, (psycho)pharmaceutical substances should only be used after several attempts to offer the aggressive child support in controlling their violent behaviour have failed.
- Third, and most important, a distinction between a child's behaviour problems and himself/herself (Masters 2002) should be made by the staff, in order to use chemical restraint not as some sort of punishment, but as an appropriate step to help the patient regain self-control.

1.5 Ethical Problems Arising from Psychopharmacological Interventions in Children

1.5.1 Non-nuisance, Non-maleficence

Primum non nocere ("First, do no harm"), one of the oldest principles of medical ethics, is the plea that medical interventions should not do damage to patients. Novel interventions are often associated with burgeoning hope in severely affected patient groups. Pharmaceutical marketing adds to this general expectancy and therefore many parents and children are prepared to take the risk of new interventions in order to gain relief from a serious and chronic condition. Patients as well as parents in controlled clinical trials usually say that despite the increased risks, if they had the choice they would prefer to be in the drug arm compared to the placebo arm of the study. Harm avoidance and risk reduction does not seem to be the first aim of either doctors or patients. From an ethical point of view, as long as the effects of a certain intervention are not well established by sound scientific studies, the first consideration should not be whether it works but whether it harms. It has only been possible to discuss some of the substance classes currently used in child psychopharmacology here. With respect to all interventions mentioned in this chapter, there remain *open questions of drug safety.* Stimulants, for example, have now been used for more than half a century, but fundamental questions of preclinical mechanisms and long-term safety remain unanswered and even unasked. This demonstrates that once a drug is widely accepted due to its high efficacy in short-term trials, long-term safety questions in general will not be addressed because there are no research sponsors interested in long-term safety studies and a correspondingly low public interest in these questions. It is only in the last few years that long-term safety has become a political issue and some funding has been provided to create clinical networks for pharmacovigilance and pharmacoepidemiological procedures, in order to establish and monitor safety in everyday practice. The standard voluntary reporting systems currently in place are not reliable because they depend on the patients' and doctors' willingness to report side effects, and are skewed by a tendency to report exotic rather than common side effects. Furthermore, patients often have no access to side effect reporting systems whilst doctors often shy away from reporting because this is associated with considerable paperwork. When the FDA invited The Paediatric Expert Panel in summer 2005 to comment on possible serious side effects like hallucinations and cardiac side effects of stimulant treatment, the only indications the agency could refer to were sporadic spontaneous reports. There is no way of quantifying the relationship between these spontaneous reports and the prescriptions, so relative risk cannot be calculated, and the magnitude of the serious side effects of a widely-used drug remains unknown. This is an example of how interventions that could have an impact on the developing organism and the maturating brain need careful long-term follow up, and not only of patients in clinical trials.

There are inherent problems associated with extrapolating interventional trial study results to the clinical setting. Study patients are usually a highly select population with lower co-morbidity and profiles of symptomatology that are easier to treat as compared to clinic patients. Co-morbidity and co-medication are much more frequent in real life situations than in trials. That leads to a general underestimation of risks due to the combination of different interventions. Research programmes are usually targeted at the detection of an effective intervention, while documenting possible risks at the same time. This has nothing to do with safety in clinic situations, where patients are treated for months or even years not only with one drug, but with combinations of drugs or different drugs in turn. These patients are not usually followed up. This lack of studies leads to ever more debates on the safety of stimulant treatments, often sponsored by lobby groups like the Scientologists who have vested interests, and many obscure theories have even found their way into scientific journals, causing additional harm and anxiety to families and patients. Only the scientific investigation of the long-term consequences of a medical intervention in the maturating brain, not only in animal models but in real life situations, can answer these questions and provide a reliable evidence base for treatment decisions. In contrast, the current discussions of evidence based treatments centre on pharmaco-economic considerations with respect to effectiveness rather than to safety and not at all on long-term safety. It is clear that the industry has no direct motivation for studying the long-term safety of their compounds (Vitiello et al. 2004), particularly if they are being widely used. When drugs manufactured by different patent holders are combined, there are no commercial sponsors willing to study the consequences of the combinations. It is clear that the state or health insurance systems must sponsor research in this field in order to protect patients from risks of novel interventions. Another question that is related to the potential harm of stimulants is the question of whether the burden of illness justifies any pharmacological intervention. Comparing the diagnostic manuals in the United States and the rest of the world (DSM-IV vs. ICD-10) one can easily see that the American criteria allow for the inclusion of many more children under the diagnosis of ADHD than the much stricter ICD-10 criteria. Santosh applied an ICD-10 diagnostic algorithm to the well-known MTA sample and found that only about a third of the patients fulfilled ICD-10 criteria. In this subgroup with more clearcut symptoms, the effects of medication were even more convincing than in the DSM-IV sample. So we can ask the question whether early intervention with a drug is justified in the mild cases. This question is particularly pertinent to treatment in the very young. In Europe the stimulant treatment of preschoolers is still rare. In contrast, Zito and Safer (2005) showed that in the United States a considerable proportion of children in the preschool age range is treated with stimulants, and there are even children under the age of 3 treated for ADHD. There must be concern with respect to long-term consequences because these interventions in preschoolers occur in a phase of massive brain development. All the animal literature leads us to suspect long lasting effects of these interventions. This must not mean that these interventions will be harmful; it is conceivable that they are even curative at this age whilst they can induce only symptomatic changes in older children. However, who studies this question, and is it ethically permissible to conduct prospective trials on this in humans? In any case, in the interests of safety, we should follow up the children treated very early with stimulants as a naturalistic study of a high risk cohort.

Turning to SSRIs, the SSRI debate demonstrates that medications generally thought to be safe, and demonstrated to be safe in adults, can nevertheless carry specific risks to other age groups. The side effect of "activation" is well known in adults but its significance as a signal of behavioural activation and suicidal thinking is only found in children and adolescents. There is even a different side effect profile of SSRIs, with most side effects appearing in smaller children (Safer and Zito 2006). What the SSRI debacle underscores is the importance of age-specific safety considerations. It is worth noting that at the same time there is no debate about the older antidepressants, which have well-known but much higher safety risks. It is difficult to kill oneself with overdoses of SSRIs, but this can easily be done with a tricyclic antidepressant. Obviously these debates on safety also are connected with marketing of the drugs and the stockholder interests involved. One does not have to wholly subscribe to the provocative conspiracy theories of David Healy (2004), expounded in a polemic written by the British psychopharmacologist, physician and medical historian ("Let Them Eat Prozac"), to accept that there was a clear publication bias (Whittington et al. 2003) that resulted in prescribers only being aware of the positive studies of efficacy. In the United States, John March is now setting up a nationwide psychopharmacology pharmacovigilance network, sponsored by the NIMH (March 2005 and March et al. 2004). One can conclude that the SSRI debacle shows that the political rules of the game (that is, the current drug regulatory environment) need to change in order to prioritise the public health value of clinical trials above their profitability for the pharmaceutical industry and academic medical centres (March 2005).

In general, the methods of collecting data on side effects have to be improved, validated and standardised. It is incredible that up to now, in general verbatim reports of patients are "translated" by agencies not involved in clinical care, resulting in verbatim references such as "hung", "hang", "cut", "self-harm" and so on being translated into sweeping, inaccurate labels such as "emotional lability".

For every new intervention in the brain, there should not only be a debate about the secure way of scientifically measuring the effects of the treatment but also a scientifically sound measure of expected and unexpected side effects, such as in the Columbia recording system of suicidal behaviour and thinking. Inter-rater reliability for different criteria must be established if we wish to collect reliable data concerning potential harm of interventions in the brain.

A last example in our plea for a stronger emphasis in safety is the use of atypical neuroleptics and the recent discussion of the appropriateness of their use in general in adults and in comparison to older drugs (Lieberman et al. 2005). Atypical neuroleptics are a new substance class of medication with potential use for children and adolescents that has been introduced to the market without any relevant studies in adolescents suffering from schizophrenia. Children and adolescents tolerate typical antipsychotics less well than adults and often react with early-onset dyskinesia. As a result, the new alternatives are widely used in the treatment of childhood schizophrenia. In a preventive study, Risperidone has even been used in adolescents to prevent schizophrenia; but there is no labelling of any of these substances for the use in children or adolescents for the indication of schizophrenia due to the lack of clinical trials in this age group. Some studies, especially with Risperidone, address the problem of disruptive behaviour (Findling et al. 2001; Fegert

2003; Croonenberghs et al. 2005). From these studies we have learned that children have a different side effect profile with atypical neuroleptics as compared to adults, with more weight gain in smaller children and some adverse events related to high prolactin levels. In general the problem of weight gain for some of these second generation antipsychotic drugs increasingly seems to be a limiting factor of their use. The Clinical Antipsychotic Trials of Intervention Effectiveness (CATIE) study in adult patients with chronic schizophrenia (Lieberman et al. 2005) showed that treatment with Olanzapine was particularly associated with more discontinuation for weight gain or metabolic effects, whilst the use of first generation antipsychotics was associated with more discontinuation due to extra-pyramidal side effects. Olanzapine was superior to the other drugs with respect to treatment adherence. At present, there is controversy about the possible safety of atypical drugs because of their propensity to induce weight gain and alter glucose and/or lipid metabolism in the young, with possible longer-term consequences for physical health. Given the higher proportions of extra-pyramidal reactions in adolescents and the higher importance of hormonal changes in a developing metabolism there is no sound database for a cost-benefit evaluation of novel antipsychotics in the treatment of schizophrenia in children and adolescents. This situation will change in the next few years because the FDA has issued a written request to all the pharmaceutical companies marketing atypical antipsychotics, requiring studies for the indication of schizophrenia and/or hypomania/mania in children and adolescents. These studies have start in 2006, be conducted on a worldwide base and take into account gender differences and national differences. Up to now, most of the studies have addressed a small number of mostly male and predominantly Caucasian children. The study of girls and children from ethnic minority backgrounds, who might have a different reaction with respect to the side effect profile, is still rare.

With respect to the three most important psychopharmacological substance classes used in children and adolescents, we have to conclude that most of the safety issues remain unaddressed. There is sensible change in progress with respect to study policies and the acceptance of the risks related to off-label use, but these changes will take a long time. With respect to novel interventions in the brain, one can draw the general conclusion that there is also an initial focus on their therapeutic effects in adult patients with severe diseases. Clinical trials tend to be performed in highly selected monosymptomatic populations to prove the effectiveness of the compound; side effects are only observed opportunistically but there is often no standardised way of studying potential side effects. Questions of long-term safety and long-term vigilance of the consequences of the intervention, especially in the developing brain, are usually not addressed. This constitutes a remarkable risk in the treatment of children and adolescents, that we would find intolerable in adult medicine.

1.5.2 Efficacy and Effectiveness

In contrast to safety issues, there is an overwhelming body of data proving the efficacy and even long-term effectiveness of stimulant use in ADHD. The effect sizes of stimulants for ADHD are high (larger than one) the numbers needed to treat are small, and placebo effects are also small for this indication. On the other hand, SSRIs are not only a problem because of the safety issues but especially because of a lack of superiority over placebo in many trials. Only Fluoxetine has proven consistently superior to placebo in all trials amongst children and adolescents with depression. Placebo rates are high in children with mild depression, which depression trials tend to study. That means that these children respond very well just to the attention of a study doctor and that sometimes the addition of medication may bring little benefit in comparison to this psychosocial effect. The lesson to learn from the SSRI debacle is that positive effects are usually over-reported and overestimated from highly selected clinical case series. The scientific community must ensure that in the future negative research results are equally accessible for meta-analyses and clinical recommendations.

With respect to new interventions in the brain, we should distrust single case reports or small case series even if they report fantastic results in extremely complicated and previously therapy-resistant cases. Only a statistically sound controlled study and its replication in another study context can give us certainty about efficacy questions. The recent controversy of the atypical neuroleptics shows that new treatments are not always superior to the old ones. Therefore designs with active comparators are needed for clinical treatment decisions (Freedmann 2005) and for pharmacoeconomic considerations. New interventions in the brain should have to prove that they are superior or at least equal in their results compared to a predefined gold standard of current treatment before they can gain general acceptance.

1.5.3 Autonomy

Treatment decisions in children are always difficult because the standard dyadic relationship in the informed consent contract between patient (who gives informed consent) and physician (who provides information and offers the medication) is replaced by a triangulated relationship between parent(s), doctor, and child. This can lead to some complications. For example, in the case of stimulant treatment of preschool or primary school children with ADHD, the child does not usually see a problem from his or her perspective, but the parents and teachers do. They want the child's behaviour to change. Parents may decide that the child should take pills to reduce educational conflicts. At the same time it is these parents who both define the problem and give consent on their child's behalf. Could they really represent the child's wishes and his or her best interests in that case? Classically, many patients with ADHD stop medication when they reach the age of puberty because they cannot understand why they should take this medication and the parents no longer have the power or control to force them to do so.

From this dilemma there arises a general question: Should a person or the community be allowed to define a problem and at the same time consent on behalf of the person that has to undergo the intervention? Our interviews with young inpatients in a child psychiatric setting have shown that particularly adolescents suffering from (mostly first episode) schizophrenia do not wish to make their own decisions about their medication. Somehow, these young people know that they have to take this medication, but they do not want to take the responsibility for doing so. So they seem to accept parents and doctors taking important treatment decisions on their behalves. There is no simple rule how to deal with the dilemmas that result from conflicts of respecting the will of a patient and respecting their needs or best interests.

In the case of severely mentally retarded individuals with auto-aggressive (self-harming) behaviour, it has been shown that respecting a patient's wishes to refuse medication can be harmful to them and the need of 24 hour supervision for many weeks or months. In some published cases (Häßler and Fegert 1999) it has been demonstrated that Risperidone treatment, given with the permission of court orders in these cases, could paradoxically lead to much more autonomy for these patients. Instead of being confined to and observed in their beds all day and night, medication enabled these patients to take part in normal group activities.

So if there could be a new intervention in the brain that would allow us to "heal" paedophilic sex offenders, would it be ethically acceptable for a court or a state administration to force sex offenders to undergo this new intervention even against their will? What about decisions concerning preventative interventions in very young children? Is it justifiable for parents, out of their understandable fears of a future relative risk of a certain disease, to treat their children with so-called neuro-protective substances? Would it even be ethical to carry out research studies with children who cannot give their own consent, in order to study the preventative potential of a drug in a new intervention? In the case of vaccinations the consent of parents is usually accepted, and numerous vaccination studies had been performed with children who cannot consent. However, is the model of vaccination really instructive when it comes to very early interventions in the developing brain? Isn't there a risk that the fears of parents will translate into interventions that might change the developing personality of their offspring?

Another series of questions pertains to the field of *chemical restraint.* Is it ethical to use interventions in the brain to calm people down? Restraint is not only used to dominate aggressive children. Psychopharmacotherapy of institutionalised mentally retarded people or seniors is quite common. A distinction must be made between the more or less articulated will of the patient, their assent or consent or dissent, and their best interests with respect to a given intervention in the brain. This is because psychiatric disorders can cause patients to act against their best interests. This gives rise to the possibility that a judge or another person, such as a guardian, may take the treatment decisions by proxy for the patient. But can a guardian consent to interventional research in a person who does not want the intervention? If this is not the case, how can safe and effective interventions, including chemical restraint, be developed for those high-risk patients in forced treatment conditions?

1.5.4 Justice

The three examples from the field of child psychopharmacotherapy have shown that, in general, the treatment of children today cannot be based on the same level of safety data as the treatment of adults. Consequently, a highly vulnerable subgroup of our population that should be particularly well protected ironically suffers from an unacceptable lack of data concerning age specific dosages and effects as well as side effects, even for the most commonly used drugs in child and adolescent psychopharmacotherapy. Children can therefore be described as *therapeutic orphans*. The health and economy discussion about justice of distribution of healthcare interventions is increasingly dominated by allocation issues. Will it be possible for everybody in a given society to be granted the same access to new intervention techniques? Even now there are dramatic differences with respect to the use of new pharmacological agents between the United States, some countries of Europe and, especially, countries in the Third World. Will new interventions only be accessible to rich, well insured citizens of wealthy countries? Do the patients with the most severe symptomatology get the best treatment? Even our current pharmacoepidemiological comparisons between the United States and Europe show wide differences. In Germany, for example, fixed budgets in outpatient care lead to a very conservative prescription pattern concerning psychopharmacological drugs in children and adolescents. The first generation neuroleptics and the old tricyclic antidepressants still dominate the German market, whereas in the United States more than 90% of the prescriptions to children and adolescents are for new and much more expensive drugs. As a new drug is not always the better or even safer option, there is no simple answer to the question whether a restrictive system with fixed budgets that stimulates the prescription of old and cheap generic drugs or a system that encourages innovations is more conducive to general mental health. In Germany there is a risk that patients may not profit from the advances of interventions, but at the same time German patients are less at risk from aggressive marketing strategies for novel interventions. The National Health Service in Britain, for example, has not adopted slow release stimulants for free-of-charge treatment because there is no proof of superiority with respect to the therapeutic effects of the slow-release medication over repeated administration of a regular pill. Still, is a more convenient regime of drug intake and the reduction of stigma at school just a cosmetic effect, or should such aspects be taken into consideration? At present in the UK, well-off parents can always buy long-acting stimulants for their children, whereas poorer families have to rely on the National Health Service. In the future, pharmacoeconomic studies that take into account quality-of-life measures and calculate the benefit of novel interventions in the brain in terms of quality-adjusted life years will be very important in the process of making available alternative treatments or new interventions in the brain.

1.5.5 A Cultural Perspective

Disease concepts may vary between cultures. The perception of whether a small boy is hyperactive or not differs considerably between e.g. China, Mediterranean countries like Greece, Italy or Spain, and countries like the United States, Germany or the Netherlands. Many cultural differences are reflected even in the diagnostic systems used in the United States and Europe. This variation of diagnostic systems leads to an enormous difference in drug consumption between European countries and the United States (the lack of access to psychosocial interventions in the U.S. may be an exacerbating factor). Many of our study results are based on definitions of psychiatric diseases in that particular society.

The concept of the importance of a child's or an adolescent's individual will might appear very strange in the Japanese culture, for example, where the family usually decides the measures to be taken for a sick family member, even an adult. So, many ethical questions concerning novel interventions in the brain must be answered in different ways with respect to different cultural backgrounds. If we want to rely on the public control of forced interventions in the best interest of the patient, we have to make sure that the culture that defines this best interest subscribes to universal humanitarian principles and is ready to accept that every human being has fundamental rights. So if, according to some philosophical definitions, a small child is not yet a person, and if this human being with all the potential of personhood undergoes a preventive intervention in his brain, will this affect his future personality? Would this constitute an attack on his rights as a human being? These days there is widespread enthusiasm for the future possibilities of neuroprotection, once we can define molecular targets. But who can consent to neuroprotective interventions in the most needy, for example in children neglected and traumatised in infancy by their natural parents?

1.6 Summary

In this study of novel interventions in the brain, psychopharmacology is, historically, the oldest and currently best known technique of biological intervention in the brain to change psychical states such as mood and psychiatric disorders. This chapter focussed on developmental psychopharmacology in particular because this field allows bringing out a number of critical issues which also pertain to those novel types of interventions in the brain that will be explored in the following chapters. First of all we provided an overview of the current psychopharmacological substance classes used in the treatment of children and adolescents with psychiatric problems. Three major substance groups were chosen to introduce the reader to current ethical conflicts and technical problems of treatment and research in the field of developmental psychopharmacology:

1. The case of treating childhood depression with selective serotonin reuptake inhibitors exemplified the manifold problems of off-label use. Generally, more than 75% of all medications prescribed to children in psychiatric hospitals are used off-label, that is without empirical evidence from age-specific safety and efficacy studies. The mere possibility of SSRIs increasing the risk of suicidality in children and adolescents highlights the necessity of adequate safety testing for different age groups. In general, it is reasonable to assume that the earlier a therapeutic intervention in the brain starts the more likely it may influence the plasticity frame development and therefore lead to long-term consequences. These consequences could be beneficial, but they also could consist of late-onset side effects. Furthermore, the SSRI debacle substantiated the risk of publication bias resulting from conflicts of interests between researchers and pharmaceutical companies.
2. The example of stimulant treatment of attention deficit hyperactivity disorder and the possible use of stimulants for enhancement served to underline that psychopharmacological interventions can be applied not only for treatment but also for enhancement purposes. Reliable diagnostic instruments are urgently needed to distinguish between healthy people, who want to enhance their normal cognitive functions, and people suffering from a cognitive deficit or, more general, from a condition that can be regarded a psychiatric disease or disorder.
3. The last case from developmental psychopharmacology, the example of atypical or novel neuroleptics, illustrated the special importance of issues of capacity and informed consent in the case of young patients with severe psychiatric illnesses. The debate on schizophrenia prodrom and the studies on prevention of schizophrenia by treating prodromal adolescents has been critically reviewed, first from a consequentialist stance employing a utilitarian analysis of the risks and benefits of preventative psychopharmacological interventions, and then from the point of view of respect for persons elucidating possible conflicts between parental decisions and young patients' wish of autonomy.

The findings from these case studies were subsequently reviewed against the background of the so-called Belmont Principles, which are widely recognised in the medical world. In the context of developmental psychopharmacology, the principle of nonmaleficence urges greater efforts to establish the long-term safety of psychopharmacological interventions in children and adolescents. The principle of beneficence, on the other hand, calls for more empirically sound data on the efficacy and effectiveness of such interventions. The principle of respect for persons and the related issue of autonomy have to be considered not only for the relationship of doctor and patient but rather with respect to a triangle of possibly conflicting interests between parents, children and doctors. The informed consent paradigm with its usual exchange of medical information against consent does not easily apply to that context. Children have their own informational needs and should assent to psychiatric interventions even if their consent is not legally sufficient to legitimise them. Another issue of autonomy discussed in this chapter relates to the usage of chemical restraint in psychiatry. Finally, psychopharmacological interventions in children and adolescents raise major concerns with respect to the principle of justice. Due to the fact that many medications approved for adults have not been studied in children, they are sometimes called "therapeutic orphans". Regulatory mechanisms should be introduced to ensure adequate testing for drugs tailored to the needs of small groups of the population that do not offer profitable markets.

The "orphan" situation now so typical for child and adolescent psychiatry may in the future become a common situation for many other patient subgroups. The better we understand the underlying molecular and genetic mechanisms of some psychiatric diseases, the more we recognise that seemingly similar symptomatologies can be caused by completely different pathways. Thus, we will have to deal with smaller groups of patients to whom a certain therapeutic approach might apply. As a consequence, questions of protection of special populations like children, elderly or demented people, mentally retarded people etc. will become increasingly important. In the long run, the development towards specialised treatments for different genotypes is likely to reframe the medical legal and ethical debate on (distributive) justice.

Presently most new interventions in the brain concern adult patients with severe diseases and pessimistic prognoses. In the future we might have the capacity to intervene in the development of children by neuroprotective interventions leading to a higher resilience to risks of developing psychiatric disorders in the first place. However, the ethical and legal preconditions of research into neuroprotection still remain unstudied and poorly discussed.

2 Neurotransplantation and Gene Transfer

2.1 Introduction

Research on the nervous system has been intensified over the last decades and still is booming. Basic neuroscience has dramatically increased the knowledge of cellular and molecular mechanisms of brain functioning. As a result cellular and molecular disarrangements that go with the variety of neurological, neurodegenerative and psychiatric disorders have been identified, although the primary causes of these disorders remain largely unknown. In cases of acquired or degenerative loss of nervous functions, pharmacological treatments are still mainly directed towards the amelioration of symptoms and the limitation of secondary tissue damage. This clinical problem together with the development of new potential therapeutic techniques such as cell grafting or implantation and gene transfer, have led to the exploration of interventions in the nervous system that can tentatively be called "restorative neurosurgery". A shift from animal experimentation to clinical trials occurred rapidly and experimental neurotransplantation surgery in patients with neurological and neurodegenerative disorders has taken place over several decades. Neuroscience, however, is just beginning to explore cellular and molecular interventions in diseased, degenerating or traumatised human nervous systems. Are we approaching an era of interventions in the brain that will revolutionise treatment of thus far untreatable brain disorders? And if so, how do we ensure that these interventions will be performed in a safe, adequate and acceptable way? How do we judge and prevent the risks of unwanted changes in brain function and in the human psyche?

2.1.1 Restorative Neurosurgery by Cells and Genes

In particular, neural tissue grafting has attracted great interest for its potential as a treatment for human neurodegenerative diseases. The basis for this was the discovery that immature nerve cells (neurons) can survive implantation in the brain of laboratory animals, something which adult neurons are unable to do. Immature nervous tissue taken from unborn foetuses can develop normal neuronal properties in the adult nervous system. Immature neurons grow and differentiate and form functional contacts with host brain neurons. The grafting of human embryonic nerve cells would therefore allow replacement of lost neurons in the case of a disease like Parkinson's disease in which the loss of so-called nigro-striatal dopaminergic nerve cells seems to be a primary cause. They might also allow reconstruction of a brain circuit like that of the striato-frontal system, effected by Huntington's disease, through the supplementation of the atrophic striatal spiny neurons.

However, the neuronal loss in such neurodegenerative diseases may also be ameliorated or even stopped by the implantation of cells that provide trophic support in order to keep the neurons at risk alive. These cell implants should do so by the release of neuro protective or neuralgrowth-stimulatory proteineous compounds. Such factors can not be applied systemically due to a short half life in vivo and the need to apply them locally to prevent any negative side effects on nearby intact systems. The genetic modification of the affected cells, or their neighbouring cells to let them locally produce such factors has also been proposed as a possibility. This does not involve a cell implantation but treatment involving a "gene transfer by injection". Cell implantation and genetic modification may even be combined when the implanted cells are modified to express a therapeutic gene. Cell and gene therapy for the diseased or traumatised brain, however, are both invasive interventions in the human brain, the organic basis of our personhood. Such interventions cannot be reversed or halted in the way that a patient is able to stop taking a drug. Even if the treatment has a built-in termination process that can kill the implanted or genetically modified cells in case of unwanted side effects arising, or when the prescribed period of therapy should end, the organisation of the brain at the point of termination is never the same as that prior to intervention.

2.1.2 The Brain is Seat of the Human Mind

There is no doubt that the central nervous system (CNS), and in particular the brain, is the "seat" of the biological processes that underlie human identity and personality, and thus a person's character and mental capacities. It is of central importance for our behaviour, perceptions, thoughts and feelings and regulates body functions such as heart rate, muscle responses and control of our immune system. It works in conjunction with both our bodies and the outside world. It is *the* organ of our personhood and, in this respect, it is a unique and indispensable organ for human self-consciousness.[5] Alternatively, one can say that our mind is our brain in action. Without this action the human mind is gone.

Small differences in the structure and organisation of the brain lead to different functional capacities and, therefore, to differences in mental and physiological processes directed by and derived from the brain. Such differences underlie differences in personality between individuals. These differences are only partially determined by the genotype as even identical twins differ in functional capacities and personality. Neurodegenerative and traumatic disorders obviously alter the organisation of the nervous system and,

[5] This uniqueness is further explained by the (albeit fictional) thought experiment of human brain transplantation. The result will be that the brain donor will see him-/herself as having received a new body. On the other hand, the recipient 'person' will cease to exist. Brain transplantation, therefore, does not exist or should be defined as body transplantation.

therefore, the functioning of the brain. Cell implantations in the brain and gene transfer to brain cells which aim to restore brain functions will never be able to restore the structure and organisation of the brain prior to the impact of the disease or trauma. Therefore, unwanted physiological and mental side effects will occur on the recipient of any form of intervention. However, these side effects may be very subtle and will not necessarily be obvious in normal daily life.

This chapter will focus on interventions in the brain in the field of restorative neurosurgery. The goal of these interventions is tissue repair or the introduction of physical changes in brain chemistry in order to relieve the symptoms of certain diseases. Neurodegenerative diseases like Parkinson's disease (PD), Huntington's disease (HD), Alzheimer's disease (AD), amyotrophic lateral sclerosis (ALS) and multiple sclerosis (MS), as well as acquired nervous trauma as the result of a stroke or spinal cord injury, are the first candidate diseases for such approaches. The neural grafting of fetal brain cells (neurotransplantation) in PD and HD patients was the first experimental clinical treatment explored because precise aims could be formulated for these interventions (implanting nerve cells to deliver dopamine and supplementing interneurons in the striatum of the brain in the respective cases). Clinical research is less advanced for other neurodegenerative diseases and in the field of brain trauma, where the target for restoration is larger or less well-known. In these cases, the potential target for intervention in the CNS is largely unknown and this is crucial knowledge for any restorative neurosurgery. In principle, if a brain disorder can be pinpointed to a particular (local) cellular or molecular origin, or a target site for regeneration can be identified, then cell or gene therapy may be possible. For psychiatric disorders incompatible with normal life, which are potentially caused by a multiplicity of interrelated factors, cellular and molecular interventions in the brain may not be feasible unless one finds a specific target which can be reached through the efficient treatment of a particular sub-symptom. This may not be unrealistic as nowadays the deletion of single genes in transgenic animals can show dramatic behavioural effects in areas such as drug dependency, anxiety, depression and fear conditioning, indicating the possibility of existing primary targets.

2.1.3 Questions to be Answered

Several interconnected ethical and normative questions arise from clinical neurotransplantation and gene transfer. When and how should a brain disorder be subject to (safe) cellular or molecular intervention? How can we design meaningful and morally acceptable experimental studies of the effects of these procedures on human beings? What criteria should be employed to evaluate the outcome of experimental restorative neurosurgery? What should be the correct procedures for the retrieval and use of embryonic tissue from aborted fetuses or collected from organ donor?

What criteria should govern the use of human stem cells when derived from in vitro human blastocysts (their stem cells are nowadays seen as a very potent source of cells for tissue repair of all organs thereby providing a future solution for many life-threatening organ failures, including brain failures)? Should we permit the use of cells from prenatal animal sources in order to circumvent the ethical problems surrounding the use of human fetuses? Can genetic modification be safely established? Finally, given the view that the CNS will be altered by an intervention, how do we weigh up the benefits and the risks of any such procedure for the patient? Before discussing these points, it seems appropriate to shortly outline the organisation of the brain and its principle functional processes as well as the current status of experimental neurotransplantation and gene transfer in human patients.

2.2 Brain Structure and Capacities

The nervous system consists of a central part and a peripheral part. The nerves arising from the spinal cord and the nodes of certain neurons in the body (ganglia, retina, and olfactory epithelium), serve to innervate the organs, muscles and skin and comprise the peripheral nervous system (PNS). The brain and the spinal cord are referred to as the central nervous system (CNS), whereby the spinal cord is the means through which the CNS is able to communicate with the PNS. The CNS receives input from the body and from the environment through sensory, auditory and visual organs as well as chemicals (including hormones). This information is processed and either generates an output in the form of bodily, emotional, cognitive and anticipatory reactions or is kept and stored as memory for future challenges. The individual brain acquires and accommodates these mechanisms in its developmental period, but these mechanisms remain subject to active self-organising and reorganising changes throughout life.

2.2.1 Neurons Act in Networks

The basic units of the nervous system are the neurons. These cells have a cell body and many cell processes (neurites), one of which is the axon that transfers a pulse to other neurons or to non-neuronal targets outside the nervous system. The message to other neurons is carried in chemical compounds – neurotransmitters – that are released at the contact zone of the axon, the synapse. Examples of neurons having a peripheral target rather than other neurons are motoneurons (innervate the muscles) and neurosecretory neurons (releasing hormones into the circulation). The release of the emitted messenger is always evoked by so-called action potentials, a moving change in electric membrane potential arising at the cell body and traveling along the axon. The sum of these action potentials of individual neurons as well as the continuous changes in the membrane potential of the neurons, make up the electro-encephalogram (EEG) which can be measured by placing electrodes on the surface of the skull. The human brain contains about 10^{11} neurons (about 20 times the world population of humans). Each neuron receives the input of an average of 1,000 synapses on their neurites (having an estimated total length of 100,000 km in the human brain). This is an amazing number of nodes per cell and within the CNS for internal brain communication. Neurons by themselves are functionless units. However grouped, either in nuclei or in layer structures, neurons make up networks that mutually interact to form information-processing units. Within a substructure of the brain, different types of neurons have different connections and use different chemical compounds for signal transfer. These neurotransmitters reach different types and quantities of receptors on the target site of the synapse, thereby affecting intracellular molecular machinery in the receiving cells. For a single neuron, the mix of incoming signals will be integrated, and will lead either to the adaptation of cell functions or to an action potential via its axon, i.e., a message to its target (after a change of its membrane potential above a certain threshold). In addition, the human brain contains glial cells. There are around ten times as many of these than the total number of neurons in the brain. These cells are involved in the regulation of signal transduction. Various subtypes of glial cells have different functions among which the electric isolation of axons is but one. The result of all the interactions of neurons in the human brain steers or directs both body functions and the psyche.

2.2.2 Networks are Formed by Genotype and Environment

Different groups of neurons are incorporated into different networks of functional activities in the brain known as neuronal systems. If parts of these systems or their connections are lost (as in the case of degeneration or trauma) or are not properly working (as the result of toxins or the transient overexposure to neuro-active compounds), the functional capacity of the system is affected. The neuronal cell acquisition of the human nervous system takes place both before and after birth, and continues in young children up to approximately three years of age. Neuronal networks are formed throughout this period too but continue to be formed up to approximately 18 years of age, i.e. until after puberty, when the nervous system is said to be fully matured. Brain development is an orchestrated process whereby the "birth" of neurons during fetal life is genetically defined, but the differentiation, maturation and organisation of neurons depends on the appearance of other groups of neurons and on molecular signals from non-neuronal cells. Thus, the connectivity of neurons depends on the temporal profile of particular signals. During development, neurons are often born in excess and compete for survival by establishing connections with their targets (see figure 2.1).

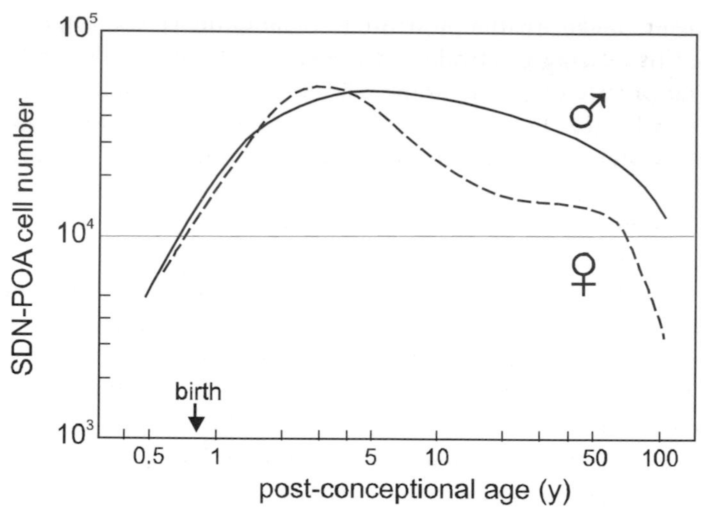

Figure 2.1: Prenatal and Life-time Changes of Neuronal Cell Number in the Sexual Dimorphic Nucleus of the Preoptic Area in Male and Female Humans

The curves show the fast acquisition of cells in the perinatal period reaching maximal levels only at the age of three to four years for both sexes, and a maturational period with (normal) cell loss until puberty significantly higher in girls than in boys, leading to an average 5-fold difference (note the logarithmic scale). It is just a single example of the long lasting brain developmental period in humans and the influence – in this case sexual hormones – of factors outside of the CNS.

Adapted from Swaab et al. (1992)

The early period of development of the brain is very sensitive to the external factors that may interfere with brain cell activity. It is claimed that any circumstance known to interfere with the functioning of the adult nervous system, when imposed on the developing brain, will (or at least could) alter the functional capacities of the brain permanently (Swaab and Boer 2001). In other words, the regulatory systems of neuronal circuits in the mature brain, the blueprint of which is determined by the genotype, are "set" differently by external factors and experiences during the maturing period. The lasting effects that occur following exposure to neuro-active chemicals present in food, the environment or in medicines and drugs, as well as to external factors like stress, which act on the developing nervous system via endogenous hormonal and neurotransmitter responses, are the result of changes in the cellular make-up, organisation and the synaptic strength of neuronal systems. Pre- and postnatal estrogen exposure modifies later psychosexual capacities and gender identity, corticosteroids affect psychomotor behaviour, maternal smoking enhances the incidence of homosexuality amongst female offspring and could be correlated with aggressive behaviour in children of both sexes, neuroleptics impair later learning ability, cocaine impairs later vigilance (detection of actions), and there are more examples to illustrate this interaction (Swaab and Boer 2001). In humans it is difficult to isolate the precise cause of certain characteristics amongst the myriad of stimuli to which a child is exposed. However, as shown above, individual experiences organise the functional capacity of the brain. The knowledge that small changes in the nervous system induced during the perinatal period of brain developmental result in lasting changes to physiology and behaviour, was previously described as behavioural teratology or functional neuroteratology[6]. Nowadays, this topic also attracts attention in studies on gene-environment interactions as the role of external influences on brain development may be identifiable in the gene expression profiles of nervous structures and may underlie the occurrence or onset of neurological and psychiatric disorders in later life. Above myriad of influences stresses the fact that each brain develops uniquely in its own particular environment, i.e. to its own phenotype. Therefore, the moulding of the nervous system during the development of the brain strongly contributes to the identity and personality of the individual including their capacity to adapt to, or cope with, external challenges.

The influence of external factors on the organisation of the nervous system continues throughout life through self-reorganisation and changes in number and strength of synaptic connections. This process is called brain plasticity. The window of opportunities for these self-adaptive changes of the nervous system is also set during the period of brain development. For instance, the cognitive abilities of humans depend on the level of plasticity in the nervous systems. A professional activity, for example playing music or learning a second language, will modify the organisation of the brain for the performance of these tasks in everyday life. However, not every nervous system has the same capabilities in this respect.

The lesson to learn from all this is that intervention in the brain by cell implantation or the genetic modification of cells will modify the organisation of the brain. Therefore, besides the intended therapeutic effects of an intervention on the neural disorder, lasting collateral functional effects cannot be excluded, and must, perhaps, even be expected. This, however, does not mean that restorative neurosurgery should be ruled out completely, although we must consider these factors when assessing the risks and benefits of a particular treatment. Ideally, any side effects occurring in patients will be very subtle and will not be obvious in normal daily life.

---

6 This has to be distinguished from classical teratology, i.e., when gross malformations are visible.

2.3 Concepts of Cell- and Gene-based Neurosurgical Interventions

2.3.1 Historical Outline of Neurotransplantation in Human Beings

The loss of neurons in the CNS as the result of degeneration or trauma following an accident does not initiate a process of self-repair. Though neurogenesis takes place at low levels in the adult CNS, the loss of neurons in the above cases is definitive. In addition, in the situation of cell damage, when for instance processes of neurons are transected, neuronal connections cannot autonomically be repaired. The replacement of damaged or degenerated neurons with new ones that will integrate into the broken neuronal system or circuit was successfully undertaken in animals and so became a possibility for human beings too. Immature neurons appeared capable of integrating into the nervous system after implantation, which is not the case for adult neurons. Moreover, damaged neurons that do not restore their connections spontaneously, often maintain the intrinsic capacity to regenerate. Thus, the challenge is to find the conditions to evoke and guide regenerative fiber growth in the damaged brain.

The history of neurotransplantation goes back to 1890, when Thompson attempted to transplant neocortical brain tissue taken from a cat into the brain of dogs. His experiment largely failed, and it took until the 1970s for the work of Das and Altman (1971) and Björklund and Stenevi (1979) to show that only fetal neurons survived brain tissue grafting and that these cells are also able to reconstitute neural circuitry. Thereafter, the grafting of fetal nervous tissue was widely used in animal studies to investigate the processes of brain development. It was also applied as a possible repair strategy in a variety of animals to repair brain damage and neurological disorders.

Development towards a human application of these techniques accelerated after the observation of Perlow et al. in 1979 that grafting fetal nigral cells into the striatum of substantia nigra-lesioned rats reversed the motor disturbances. These rats were regarded as a partial model for Parkinson's disease since the gradual loss of dopaminergic neurons of the substantia nigra was seen as the origin of the movement disorders. Models of the disease were developed in primates that better represented the complexity of the disease in humans, with symptoms like tremor, rigidity and bradykinesia (Björklund 1992). Subsequent transplantation studies strongly validated the work undertaken in rats (Bakay et al. 1987; Fine et al. 1988; Bankiewicz et al. 1990). These results led to the first clinical studies in 1987, in which human fetal substantia nigra-containing tissue was placed in the dopamine-poor striatum of late stage PD patients (Lindvall et al. 1989; Madrazo et al. 1991). Hundreds of patients world-wide have received this experimental treatment since then. The first results were variable and were far from a complete and persistent recovery from the disease (e.g., Lindvall et al. 1989, Lindvall 1997; Madrazo et al. 1991; Olanow et al. 1996; Mehta et al. 1997).

The history of neural grafting in human PD can be seen as the test bed for neuron supplementation techniques as a therapeutic intervention in the human brain. It showed cell implantation deep inside the brain to be surgically feasible and proved that restorative neurosurgery using immature neurons is possible, at least in principle.

2.3.2 Several Types of Neurotransplants

The above-mentioned application of neural grafts in PD is meant to supplement the function of the lost nigro-striatal neurons and to restore the dopaminergic input in the striatum. Neuronal grafting is currently also clinically studied in HD patients. In HD it aims at rebuilding the defective stri ato-frontal pathway.

Immature neurons can either be obtained in one of three ways: i) directly from aborted human embryos and fetuses, ii) indirectly by in vitro proliferation and/or differentiation of stem or germ cells towards the neuronal phenotype, or iii) through the differentiation of the cell lines of neural precursor cells ("brain-committed cells"). Genuine stem cells, with the potential to differentiate into neuronal cells (and other organ-specific cell types), can also be collected in three different ways: i) as embryonic stem cells (ESCs) from the blastocyst (pre-implantation embryo), ii) as embryonic germ cells from post-implantation embryos, or as ii) somatic stem cells (SSCs) from organs in late embryonic, fetal, neonatal and adult stages. They can also be obtained from umbilical cord blood. The presence of SSCs in adult organs (often also called adult stem cells) introduces, in principle, the possibility for neural autografts or for the patient to act as their own donor. Brain-committed cells are, for instance, the LBS-neurons (neurons by Layton BioScience Inc.) that originate from a human teratocarcinoma. Teratocarcinomas are tumors of the reproductive organs that are composed of embryonic-like cells that were transformed in the laboratory into fully differentiated, non-dividing neurons (Borlongan et al. 1998). Finally, as neurons of non-human mammals can match the functional capabilities of human cells (Isacson and Deacon 1997), implants taken from the brains of pig fetuses are thought to be applicable as well.

However, therapeutic approaches that involve something other than "simply" supplementing neurons are needed when the neuronal functioning of the anomaly within the brain has an indirect effect on neurons such as in AD or MS. These other therapeutic techniques include the implantation of a particular type of glial cells and the implantation of cells that release chemical compounds to substitute the function of lost neurons (molecular versus cellular replacement), or release compounds that can stop, prevent or counteract the degeneration or malfunction of diseased neurons (molecular treatment) (see figure 2.2). Such cells do not need to be neural cells but can

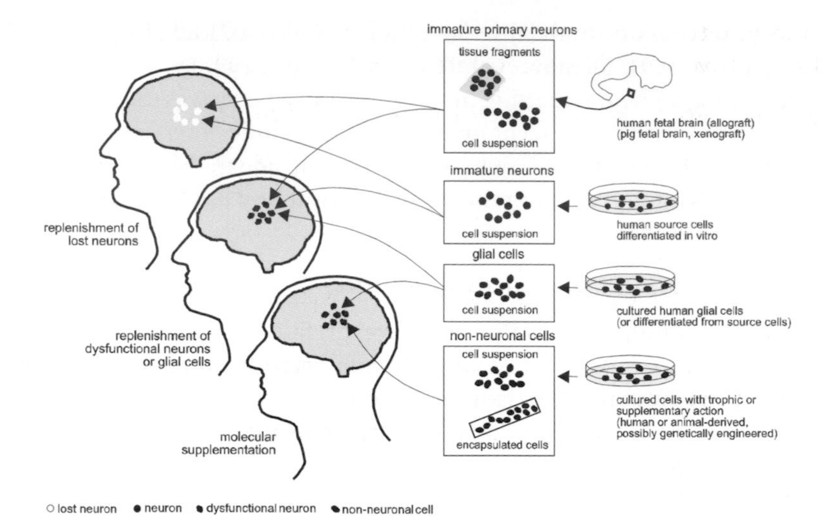

Figure 2.2: Neurotransplantaion as a Kind of Restorative Neurosurgery Comes with a Variety of Possibilities for Various Types of Defects in the CNS

When neurons are lost in neurodegenerative diseases, or following a brain trauma, immature neurons, either dissected from young stages of the human (or pig) brain or manifactured in the laboratory from relevant sources (e.g stem cells, certain teratotomas, germline cells, etc.), can, upon grafting, replace the loss through a process of maturation and integration in the affected host nervous circuit over a period of several months. Embryonic and fetal brain tissue can either be placed as tissue fragments or as cell suspensions, but have to be dissected at the proper immature stage of donor development for the neurons to be replenished. Similarly, immature neurons can replenish dys- or malfunctioning neurons, whereas glial cell loss in the nervous system ("supporting" brain cells present 10-fold the number of neurons) can also be supplemented after these cells are proliferated in the laboratory to the volume needed. However, instead of cell replenishment, cells can also be implanted for their specific action on damaged, degenerating or dysfunctioning brain areas by releasing supporting or growth-stimulating proteins (molecular supplementation; cells as chronic proteineous drug delivery preparations). These cells do not necessarily have to be neural cells. They can even be animal-derived cells, especially when encapsulated by semi-permeable membranes that avoid tissue immunorejection. The growth of cells in the laboratory is often accompanied with genetic modification either to direct proper neuronal differentiation or to equip them with a gene for the overexpression of a therapeutic compound prior neurotransplantation.

The use of cultured cells allows auto-transplantation as well. Cells withdrawn or dissected from the patient him-/herself are used for laboratory growth, thereby again preventing the need for immune-suppression therapy when grafted.

also be non-neural cells isolated from other human organs, like fibroblast taken from the skin. Some of these approaches are already in the first phase of clinical evaluation. In the case of MS, for instance, glial cells of the oligodendocytic type are the cells to be supplemented and only implants with cells that have been grown and purified in vitro are used.

2.3.3 The Practice of Clinical Neurotransplantation

The survival and integration of transplanted nerve cells depends on their plastic growth capacities at the stage of maturation in which they have not yet fully developed their complex neurite connections and bio-electrical interactions. In the brain developmental period each type of nerve cells has its own time window of "birth" and its own pace of maturation. The transplantation of entire brain sub-regions might thus easily result in one cell type surviving and another, more mature, cell type failing to do so. Consequently, a large brain part may survive transplantation as a tissue mass, but it can or will not easily develop its normal organisation in the recipient brain, nor develop the proper connections with, or within, the damaged neuronal systems of the brain. In other words, neurotransplantation strategies in human patients add new cells of particular types (cell suspensions), or place fragments of immature brain structures (minced tissue) but cannot aim to replace entire brain structures that are lost due to severe damage or trauma, as occurs, for example, in the case of heart and kidney transplantation. Nothing will be removed from the CNS for replacement, and parts cannot be replaced like a module of a defective computer. Neurotransplantation should therefore not be described as brain transplantation, but only as brain cell or brain tissue grafting.

In practice, neurotransplantation in defective areas of the human brain consists in the precisely directed injection of microliter quantities of suspensions of nerve cells or tissue fragments prepared from defined areas of fetal brain known to contain the needed cell type in an immature state or prepared from cells specially cultured and modified for it in the laboratory. The injected mass is about 100,000 times smaller than the volume of the adult brain (approximately 1.5 liter). This type of intervention requires surgical precision and accuracy, but it is not an extremely severe, physically invasive operation on the patient. Transplanted nerve cells have to mature and integrate for proper restoration of the lost brain function to occur. The possible therapeutic effects of neurotransplantation are, therefore, never immediate, but develop over a period of several months, not unlike the time frame of brain cell maturation in the intrauterine fetal stages (Isacson and Deacon 1997).

2.3.4 Direct and Indirect Gene Transfer in the Brain

Modification of the gene expression of cells in a living organ became possible with the development of viral vectors – genetically modified viruses that infect a cell, but cannot replicate nor evoke its disease effects – that can deliver a therapeutic gene in a target cell. This form of gene transfer aims to i) restore protein expression in a hereditary failing molecular or cellular process, ii) compensate for the loss of particular protein expression (in degenerative diseases) or iii) (over)express proteins that have symptom-relieving or restorative effects as a locally delivered drug (as externally delivered non-proteineous drug can have). Gene transfer can additionally be used to iv) block the endogenous expression of proteins which cause the symptoms of a disease or v) frustrate tissue self-repair following trauma making use of siRNA (small interfering RNA) technology[7]. In the nervous system two approaches can be distinguished for the (over)expression of proteins: in vivo (direct) and ex vivo (indirect) gene transfer (Kaplitt and During 2006). The first approach involves the injection of viral vectors carrying the gene of interest directly into the brain tissue of the patient. In the second approach the cells to be implanted are genetically modified in vitro, and then harvested for implantation surgery (figure 2.3). For the latter case also non-viral vector transduction methods are available in which the cells can be cultured as single cells.

The potential applications of gene transfer in restorative neurosurgery are manifold. In vivo transduction could equip degenerating neuronal or glial cells with properties to survive damage, to restore a lost function, or to release compounds that serve these purposes in adjacent cells. In vivo gene transfer for neurotrophic factors like nerve growth factor (NGF), brain-derived neurotrophic factor (BDNF), glial cell-derived neurotrophic factor (GDNF), ciliary neurotrophic factor (CNTF) and neurotrophin-3 (NT-3) in animal models for neurodegenerative diseases and neurotrauma have shown themselves to be very potent in increasing cell survival and/or promoting axon sprouting. Viral vector-mediated gene transfer has been applied experimentally in human beings for diseases outside the nervous system and, recently in the CNS as a myriad of neurological disorders may also be treatable according to the results of animal experimentation (Tuszynski 2002; Kaplitt and During 2006). Viral vectors not only need to be able to infect a post-mitotic neuron, but it should also have no toxic or immunological effects on CNS tissues and should provide long term, and preferably controllable, gene expression of the therapeutic protein that should be locally effective without affecting intact neighbouring neural systems too much.

Currently lentiviral (LV) vectors and adeno-associated viral (AAV) vectors are vectors that efficaciously and directly transduce the CNS tissue without direct or short term toxicity for neuronal cells. Whether it is safe for use in the human brain in the long term still has to be established. Clinical trials with both ex vivo gene transfer and direct gene transfer are currently being performed in PD and AD patients (see below).

---

[7] Small interfering RNAs (siRNAs; also called "short interfering RNAs") are a class of 20–25 nucleotide-long RNA molecules that interfere with gene expression. They are naturally produced as part of the RNA interference (RNAi) pathway, but can be designed and artifically applied to inhibit endogenous expression of proteins from a particular gene.

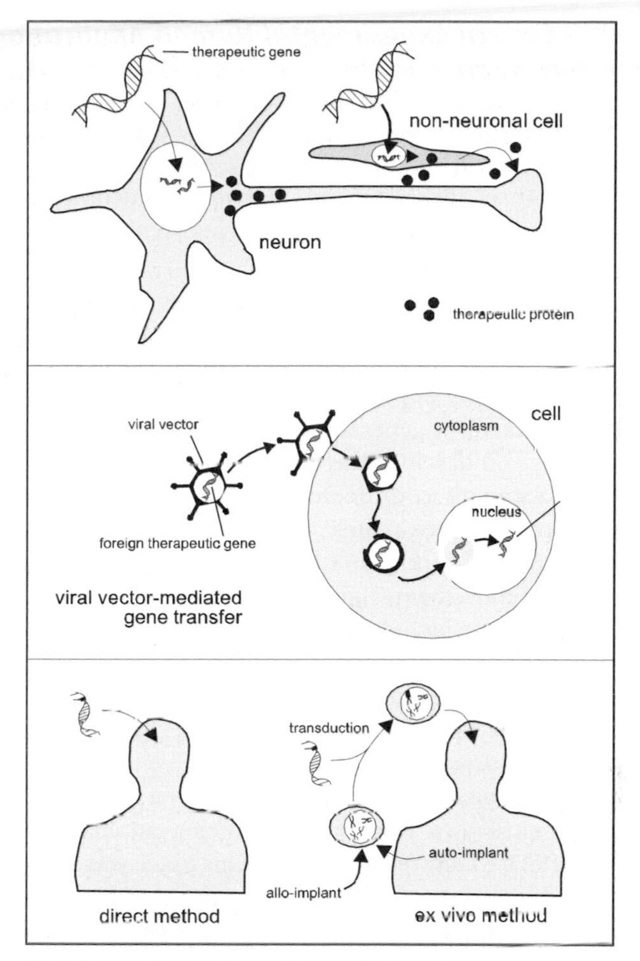

Figure 2.3: The Principles of Gene Transfer for therapy

Either a neuron or a non-neuronal cell can be modified by the insertion of a gene (transduction) for the production of survival-enhancing and growth-stimulating factors or of factors that mimic or enhance neuronal functions in the impaired or damaged CNS. Nowadays, the most efficient and safest way to modify neurons is the use of viral vectors. Viral vectors are viruses that are (re)constructed so that they can infect a cell but do not have the capacity to multiply following infection. This is achieved by creating viruses that do not contain the DNA for their reproduction but instead contain the DNA of the therapeutic gene, which can be delivered to the target cell nucleus to initiate the transcriptional and translational machinery for the synthesis of the therapeutic protein.

Viral vector-mediated transduction can be applied by direct injection into the CNS or it can be used in combination with neurotransplantation (ex vivo transduction). When the source cells used to grow transplants are obtained from the patient her-/himself, auto-implantation is also possible in order to prevent the immune-suppression treatment required following the allografting of cells from human donors or animal sources.

2.4 Survey of Current Experimental Human Applications of Restorative Neurosurgery

Clinical application of cell implantation and gene transfer in human brain disorders has not reached the level of therapy. All treatments still are in the experimental phase as the beneficial functional outcomes are variable, unpredictable or not present at all. The following section surveys briefly the achievements in this area to date.

2.4.1 Parkinson's Disease

PD is primarily caused by the slow loss of dopaminergic neurons in the substantia nigra so that their dopamine transmitter function in the striatum eventually disappears. PD is generally age-specific: approximately 1% of the population over age 60 develops the disease. An appropriate dopaminergic signal is vital for a smooth, coordinated function of the body's muscles and movement. As soon as approximately 80% of the dopamine-producing cells are lost, the symptoms of Parkinson's disease appear. The key signs of PD are tremor, slowness of movement, rigidity and loss of balance. Other signs of Parkinson's disease may include small, cramped handwriting, stiff facial expression, a shuffling walk, muffled speech and depression. Current pharmacological treatments with dopamine agonists and dopamine precursors reduce the symptoms in the early stages of the disease. However, with progress of the nigral degeneration, these drugs cease to be effective.

Dopamine cell supplementation began with open trials of striatal placement of the patient's own dopamine-producing adrenal medulla tissue (Backlund et al. 1985; Madrazo et al. 1987). This tissue was used experimentally as an alternative source of dopamine in order to circumvent the ethical problems following the use of human fetal brain tissue obtained from elective abortions (Boer 1996). The outcomes of this and later studies by other groups were disappointing and must be considered to have largely failed: not enough of the transplanted tissue survived, amelioration of the motor disturbances was absent or minor, and no relationship existed between dopaminergic cell survival and behavioural response. Other approaches of bypassing the use of human embryonic tissue have been tried, including cells obtained from the patient's own stellate ganglion but only modest antiparkinsonian effects are reported in a small number of patients (Itakura et al. 1997). As a corollary of the above clinical results, as well as the significantly better functional effects of immature tissue transplants in the case of parkinsonian rats and monkeys, a move towards the use of human fetal dopaminergic neurons in patients was inevitable (Boer 1999).

Intracerebral transplantation of human fetal dopaminergic neuron-containing mesencephalic tissue fragments, or cell suspensions thereof, obtained from the remains of legally induced abortions, were placed in the dopamine-depleted caudate-putamen complex of late stage PD patients. So far, more than 300 patients with PD have undergone this allograft surgery, but under different conditions of donor tissue treatment, graft placement, surgical approach and pre- and post-grafting treatment and symptom evaluation. Months after the implantation surgery several clinical centres observed consistent and clinically meaningful benefits in small groups of patients in open trials using a relatively strict common protocol of pre- and post-surgery evaluation of graft survival and disease symptoms (Peschanski et al. 1994; Defer et al. 1996; Levivier et al. 1997; Mendez et al. 2002). Others, however, reported more variable or negative results (Freed et al. 1992; Lopez-Lozano et al. 1997). The benefits on the Unified Parkinson's Disease Rating Scale (UPDRS) often go hand in hand with dopaminergic cell survival as measured by fluoro-dopa PET scanning, which indicates graft survival.

Recently, the results of randomised double-blind sham surgery-controlled neurotransplantation studies in PD were published (sham surgery performed as a hole drilled in the outer layer of the skull bone but without penetration of a canula into the brain) (Freed et al. 2001, Olanow et al. 2003). At the outset, the design of such studies was criticised with respect to the fact that this large-scale study, including ~20 patients in each group, was performed at too early a stage, i.e., when optimal methods for tissue procurement, graft preparation and implantation had not yet been established (Widner 1994). The studies did, however, demonstrate that there was no lasting placebo effect, and that anti-parkinson effects were found primarily in the younger group of patients (Freed et al. 2001). Moreover, several patients in the treatment group developed abnormal involuntary movements and these movements were regarded as major side effects of this study. The modest improvement in neurological rating scores, only partly comparable with other studies (Isacson et al. 2001), and the occurrence of dyskinesias aroused widespread scientific interest and debate about the future of cell replacement therapies in PD (Brundin et al. 2001; Dunnett et al. 2001; Isacson et al. 2001). The fact that the study was double-blind and sham-controlled eased the initial methodological criticism and led the media to take these results as sound evidence that the technique of neural tissue transplantation in general was faulty and ineffective (Vogel 2001). This interpretation, however, is erroneous, as the net effects are dependent on the particular technique used (Björklund 2005). What was predicted by Widner and Defer (1999) became true: the results of a suboptimal grafting procedure challenged the therapeutic value of cell therapy in PD. Journalists called the results a failure, thereby harming the field that tries to develop novel cell replacement therapies in brain diseases (Dunnett et al. 2001). However, the field of experimental clinical neurotransplantation agreed that dopaminergic cell implantation in PD cannot be recommended as, or even be called, a therapy (Polgar et al. 2003). Further improvement of the technique is needed and the cause of the dopaminergic graft-related dyskinesias needs to be unraveled.

In addition to cellular therapies in PD, phase I studies are currently also being performed with AAV vector-mediated gene transfer, based on a series of successful studies with in vivo and ex vivo AAV and LV vector-mediated gene transfer in PD animal models (Raymon et al. 1997; Freese 1999; Kordower et al. 2000; Shen et al. 2000; Le and Frim 2002). One trial tries to mimic the results of deep brain stimulation (DBS) in the subthalamic nucleus (STN) of the brain. DBS is shown to be an effective method to treat many PD patients in the late stages of the disease when L-dopa medication starts to fail. The application of AAV-GAD vectors (containing the gene for glutamic acid decarboxylase [GAD], the enzyme synthesising the major inhibitory neurotransmitter gamma amino butyric acid [GABA] and upon overexpression causing a chronic release of GABA) in the animal STN results in similar result as electrical stimulation (During et al. 1998; 2001). According to the interim clinical findings (Feigin et al. 2005), AAV-GAD treatment in the STN appears to be safe and well-tolerated in advanced Parkinson's disease, with no evidence of adverse effects or immunologic reaction. One year after treatment, patients exhibited a 27% statistically significant improvement in motor function on the side of their body corresponding to the treated part of the brain, with no improvement for the untreated side. A second phase I clinical study uses AAV-AADC, a vector that introduces the gene for L-amino acid decarboxylase (AADC) in the striatum of PD patients (http://www.avigen.com, accessed on December 7th, 2006). This enzyme catalyses the synthesis of dopamine, and is known to decrease with progression of PD. In parkinsonian monkeys, the vector has been effectively applied (Bankiewicz et al. 2000; Sanftner et al. 2005) and may be of continuing clinical benefit (Bankiewicz et al. 2006).

2.4.2 Huntington's Disease

HD is a rare autosomal dominant neurodegenerative disease that causes devastating disorders. It affects principally people above the age of forty. The disease inalterably proceeds towards a multi-faceted cognitive deterioration, motor disorder-associated chorea and bradykinesia as well as psychiatric disturbances such as depression and irritability. The clinical symptoms – at least in the early stages of the disease – are related primarily with a hypofunctioning and a degeneration of the medium spiny GABAergic neurons in the striatum. In the later stages of the disease, cortical and sub-cortical structures, anatomically connected with the striatum, become affected too. The disease is fatal within 15 to 20 years of its onset in most patients (Bird and Coyle 1986) and has no cure or any effective treatment. Besides the search for therapeutic agents like neurotrophic factors which act against the molecular mechanisms of neurodegeneration in HD, therapeutic research also focuses on GABAergic nerve cell supplementation therapy.

Intrastriatal implantation of (striatal) fetal ganglionic eminence tissue was able to reverse a large number of the motor and cognitive deficits brought about by striatal lesions of various kinds in animal affected by HD (cf. Peschanski et al. 1995). Several indicators suggest that implanted neurons do mature normally, are mainly GABAergic and express both the expected corresponding neuropeptides (substance P, met-enkephalin, somatostatin or neuropeptide Y) and the dopaminergic and muscarinic receptors. Host afferent axons both grow into the grafts and connect to grafted neurons (cf. Wictorin 1992), and functional reconnection of grafted GABAergic cells to the experimentally denervated target neurons of the globus pallidus also develops. Grafted neurons do not reach more remote projection zones such as the substantia nigra, pars reticulata, but the globus pallidus is by far the most important projection zone of striatal neurons in primates and in humans. Behavioural analysis of grafted animals to a large extent confirms the rewiring of cortical output circuits in which striatal neurons normally act as first relay cells (Dunnett et al. 1988; Kendall et al. 1998; Palfi et al. 1998; Hantraye et al. 1990).

The converging evidence in animal studies, outlined above, has led to trials of intracerebral grafting in patients with HD. Except for the study carried out by Hauser et al. (2002), all studies involved patients at an early stage of the disease. The safety and feasibility of the grafting procedures appeared almost unquestioned in all studies (Kopyov et al. 1998; Bachoud-Lévi et al. 2000b; Fink et al. 2000; Rosser et al. 2002) except in the Hauser et al. (2002) study where patients at a more advanced stage of the disease, and patients with a history of neurological problems, were included and some subjects developed subdural hemorrhages or required surgical drainage. The latter may indicate that patients at an advanced stage of the disease are particularly sensitive to medical interventions. No noticeable side effects were reported in the other studies except for difficulties encountered in obtaining a good compliance of patients for drug treatment and, in particular, for immunosuppressive drugs (Bachoud-Lévi et al. 2000b; Rosser et al. 2002). An autopsy in one patient, who died of causes unrelated to the transplant 18 months after surgery, revealed the presence of a large graft that contained a large number of neurons phenotypically similar to GABAergic medium-spiny striatal neurons (Freeman et al. 2000). Moreover, the grafted cells did not exhibit any signs of the disease, e.g. nuclear inclusions, in contrast with the host neurons in the surrounding striatum.

Conclusive clinical benefits so far have only been shown in the Créteil clinical trial by Bachoud-Lévi et al. (2000b; 2002). The other study, whose clinical data has now been published (Tampa trial; Hauser et al. 2002), was inconclusive. This was possibly due to the type of patients included or the fact that it allowed too short a follow-up time (Peschanski and Dunnett 2002). In Créteil, an improvement in motor, cognitive and functional abilities became apparent only at about twelve months in three of five HD patients, and remained so in the subsequent two years (Bachoud-Lévi et al. 2000b). These clinical results matched with the reduction of both the striatal and the frontal hypometabolism as measured by positron emission tomography using ^{18}F-fluorodeoxyglucose (Gaura et al. 2004). In a fourth patient, this improvement was transient, starting around nine to ten months after a first right-side unilateral graft, and lasted up to five months after a second left-sided graft. In this patient, the secondary loss of all improvements coincided with the disappearance of the grafted tissue as evaluated with MRI (Bachoud-Lévi et al. 2002), indicating a link between graft survival and clinical benefits. In the fifth patient, the graft was never active for reasons that remain unknown, and MRI scans still shows declining signals for the striatal metabolic activity (Bachoud-Lévi et al. 2002). Therefore, despite the absence of a control group, the coincidence of results acquired in various domains (clinical, images, electrophysiology) and analysed blindly, strongly point to the efficacy of neurografting. The positive treatment result in a very small population of HD patients obtained in a single centre trial initiated in 2001, initiated a large, controlled randomised trial on 60 patients at the early stages of HD in France and Belgium (Multicenter Intracerebral Grafting in HD, MIG-HD). For control purposes, and to avoid the use of sham surgery, 30 patients randomly received transplants either after 13–14 months or after 33–34 months, with a follow-up of all patients towards 52 months. Currently, this strategy is being replicated in a separate study in which the results of grafts conducted in Belgium, Germany, Switzerland and Italy will be compared with a large cohort of non-treated patients in the UK. Therefore, the efficacy of fetal neural grafts as putative therapy for HD will be fully known in the next three to five years.

The sustainability of the positive effect resulting from grafts is currently being assessed in the patients from the Créteil's pilot study (Bachoud-Lévi et al. 2006). The gene defect is still present and the patients' condition is expected to deteriorate at some point in the future. This secondary deterioration has appeared heterogeneous so far, starting at 4–5 years in the case of motor symptoms and after 6 years in the case of cognitive functions. Thus, the potential therapeutic effects of fetal striatal grafts possibly fade away due to a process of remission. This indicates that a neuroprotective treatment of the graft is needed as an unavoidable complement to the initial surgery. However, the graft will remain the only therapy able to restore lost functions and, therefore, will be indicated in patients exhibiting the symptoms of HD.

A number of experimental studies conducted on animals affected by HD striatal lesions have demonstrated that various neurotrophic factors can provide neuroprotection. Among these factors CNTF appeared to offer the most effective protection. However, the short half life of the CNTF in plasma, its inability to cross the blood brain barrier and its severe side effects (inflammation, cachexia) in a phase I/III clinical trial in patients with ALS (Cedarbaum et al. 1995), precludes its systemic administration. Following the positive results of striatal protection in rats and non-human primates using CNTF-delivering mini-pumps (Anderson et al. 1996) or gene therapy approaches (Emerich et al. 1996; 1997; Mittoux et al. 2000; 2002), an intraventricular implant of encapsulated CNTF-producing cells was chosen for a phase I trial (Bachoud-Lévi et al. 2000a). Cells were taken from a baby hamster cell line engineered to synthesise and release large amounts of CNTF which were subsequently introduced into semi-permeable tubes with pores i) permitting CNTF and all nutrients to cross the membrane, and ii) excluding larger proteins (e.g. antibodies) and cell processes to traverse. The cell encapsulation method has the advantage that in the clinical situation it immuno-isolates the cells, whereas removal of the device can stop the treatment whenever needed. The capsule was inserted into the lateral ventricle of six HD patients using stereotactic neurosurgery and was retrieved and exchanged every six months during a two year period. Little, if any, ^{18}F-fluordeoxyglucose-determined metabolic change was observed in the ipsilateral striatum, but significant recovery of normal electrophysiological values was associated with active CNTF-releasing tubes in three patients (Bloch et al. 2004). There were no adverse effects related to the procedure. However, secondary adverse effects (mainly depression) related to the interruption of the procedure were observed a few months after the extraction of the last tube, showing the symbolic and emotional aspect of such therapy.

2.4.3 Alzheimer's Disease

AD is a neurodegenerative disease associated with the formation of tangles and plaques in the brain, resulting in neuronal atrophy leading first to mild forgetfulness (which can be confused with age-related memory change) and an inability to solve simple mathematical problems and followed later by severe cognitive deficits and problems in speaking, understanding, reading and writing. In the final stages of the disease, patients often exhibit anxiousness or aggressiveness and become in need of total care. The precise cellular or molecular origin of the disease is not known, so that there is no clearly definable "point of attack" at which to fight the cause of the disease nor its progress. Yet certain symptoms can be traced back to changes in particular brain nuclei. For instance, cholinergic neurons of the basal forebrain atrophy and die in the brains of those affected with AD. This process has been correlated with attention deficits and an overall cognitive decline. As the application of NGF in this area has shown to protect cholinergic cell loss following their axotomy (cf. Lad et al. 2003), the chronic delivery of NGF in the human basal forebrain to reduce, or prevent, the loss of cholinergic nerve cells could possibly result in the relief of these symptoms (Tuszynski 2002).

In order to investigate the effect of NGF in AD patients, local application is needed as infusion of NGF in the ventricles of the brain results in intolerable side effects. For instance, rats and monkeys undergoing cholinergic cell rescue procedures using NGF lost their appetite leading to severe weight losses, and this was also observed in a clinical trial of NGF infusion involving three AD patients (which had to be stopped because of painful side effects were experienced by the patients; Eriksdotter Jonhagen et al. [1998]). These negative effects were not observed in subsequent studies in which autologous NGF-secreting cells were implanted into the cholinergic basal forebrain of aged monkeys in which a substantial reversal of age-related neuronal atrophy was achieved (Tuszynski et al. 1998; Tuszynski and Blesch 2004). This had led to a phase I clinical trial of ex vivo NGF gene delivery through the implantation of transduced fibroblasts isolated from the skin of the AD patient, grown and transduced ex vivo (Tuszynski et al. 2005). In this study, after a mean follow-up of 22 months in six AD subjects, no long-term adverse effects resulting from the NGF occurred. Preliminary outcomes showed the Mini-Mental Status Examination and Alzheimer Disease Assessment Scale-Cognitive subcomponent to be improved suggesting cognitive decline have decelerated. Serial PET scans showed significant increases in cortical ^{18}F-fluorodeoxyglucose after treatment, indicating a return of brain activity at pre-disease stages. The brain autopsy from one subject suggested robust neurite growth responses to NGF.

2.4.4 Amyotrophic Lateral Sclerosis

Amyotrophic lateral sclerosis (ALS) causes the progressive degeneration of motoneurons of the CNS. If the motor neurons die, the ability of the brain to initiate and control muscle movement is lost. The course of the symptoms starts with muscle weakness in one or more muscles of the hands, arms, legs or of the muscles involved in speech, swallowing or breathing. This then develops into twitching and a cramping of muscles, impairment in the use of the arms and legs (paralysis), "thick speech" and, in advanced stages, difficulty in breathing and swallowing, eventually leading to death. Yet, for the vast majority of ALS patients, their minds remain unaffected throughout. Currently there is no treatment for this disorder starting with loss of function of the motoneurons in the spinal cord.

Ciliary neurotrophic factor (CNTF) has been shown to protect motoneurons from deterioration. Thus, subsequent patient studies with this peptide were initiated. Systemic delivery of hCNTF in ALS patients, however, had no beneficial effect on the primary (limb strength and pulmonary function) or secondary end points (individual function tests and activities-of-daily-living outcome measures and survival; Miller et al. 1996), but has been frustrated by peripheral side effects, as well as the molecule's short half life, and its inability to cross the blood-brain barrier. Aebischer and his collaborators (Sagot et al. 1995; Tan et al. 1996) have conducted experiments in mice with symptoms of ALS which showed that encapsulated baby hamster kidney cells, genetically engineered to make CNTF and placed intracerebroventrically or intrathecally, also reduced the degeneration of these neurons. Trials in human ALS patients in 1996, using the same procedure described above in the treatment of HD but involving the implantation of the CNTF-releasing tube intrathecally in the lumbar CNS (Aebischer et al. 1996; Zurn et al.

2000), showed no evidence that the CNTF alleviated motor neuron deterioration (P. Aebischer, personal communication). One of the reasons for this could be that insufficient amounts of CNTF were released or that the intervention was too late to be of use (Schorr et al. 1996).

Huang et al. reported significant improvements in ALS patients after the implantation of human fetal olfactory ensheathing glia cells in the motor cortex of the brain at an international conference in 2004. However, the rationale of this surgery, advertised as a therapy to both prolong the life span and improve the quality of life of patients, is not based on animal experimentation, and the study has still not been published in a peer-reviewed journal in which the methods they employed would be evaluated in detail.

2.4.5 Multiple Sclerosis

Multiple sclerosis (MS) is an unpredictable, chronic disease of the CNS, whose symptoms can range from the relatively benign to the somewhat and potentially devastating. Pathologically, MS is characterised by the presence of areas of demyelination and predominant T-cell perivascular inflammation in the brain white matter, which disrupts efficient communication between the brain and other parts of the body. MS is believed to be an autoimmune disease that attacks the nerve-insulating myelin. Common symptoms of MS include fatigue, weakness, spasticity, balance problems, bladder and bowel problems, numbness, loss of vision, tremors and depression. Symptoms are determined by the location of the lesion and thus not all symptoms affect all MS patients. Symptoms may be continuous or may be sporadic. These periods of remission may be complete, leaving no residual damage or leaving only partial permanent impairment. A variety of medication can be used to treat the disease symptomatically, but there is, as yet, no cure for the demyelination in MS. New therapies, therefore, need to aim at reducing specific autoimmune responses and to assist in remyelination. It is the latter goal in which neurotransplantation may have potential.

Animal studies have shown remyelination processes following cellular therapies in experimental demyelination (Kocsis et al. 2002). The use of Schwann cells, glial cells that normally insulate axons in the PNS, were found to remyelinate fibers in the CNS of rats and reinstate message transmission (Kohama et al. 2001; Bachelin et al. 2005). In a 2001 pilot study Tomothy Vollmer and co-workers (http://www.myelin.org/schwannupdate.htm, accessed on December 7th, 2006) transplanted autologous Schwann cells in three patients with MS and found that the technique was safe. Further studies are needed to determine whether the cells can also repair myelin and aid functional improvement in patients. Other cells for remyelination are olfactory ensheathing cells that inhabit the nose but can also make myelin (Franklin et al. 1996; Lakatos et al. 2003) and neural stem cells, which assist to stimulate remyelination by endogenous oligodendrocyte precursor cells or mature themselves into oligodendrocytes and subsequently produce myelin in the CNS (Totoiu et al. 2004; Copray et al. 2006). In one recent study scientists found that in mice with an MS-like disease, transplants of stem cells travelled to multiple areas of damage and matured into myelin-forming cells. Animals undergoing such transplantation showed a decrease in myelin damage and nerve fiber destruction. Some animals also regained lost movement in their legs or tails (Pluchino et al. 2003; Pluchino and Matino 2005).

A large clinical trial using autologous SSCs from bone marrow or blood as peripheral implants not as brain implants, combined with high-dose immunosuppression, revealed slight neurological improvements in 21% of the MS patients and a stabilisation of the clinical condition in approximately 70% of the patients trialed by completely abrogating the inflammatory process in the brain as evidenced in magnetic resonance imaging (Fassas et al. 2002). However, the procedure is associated with a transplant-related mortality risk of around 3% to 8%. Therefore, it cannot be recommended for the treatment of a chronic, non-lethal disease like MS. However, the systemic or peripheral approach of cellular treatment has the advantage that the skull need not be opened up for surgery. On the other hand, a direct approach of the MS lesion area for any type of therapy may be more effective and reduce the chances of side effects due to maladaptive myelination in uninjured parts of the brain.

2.4.6 Stroke

Brain stroke occurs when blood supply to, or within, the brain region stops. A stroke can occur anywhere in the CNS and is caused either by a cerebral infarction, as a result of a blocked artery (ischemic stroke) or by an intracranial or cerebral haemorrhage as a result of weak arteries or an aneurism in the brain that ruptures (haemorrhagic stroke). The symptoms a stroke victim experiences depend on which areas of the brain are involved and can include, amongst other symptoms, an abrupt loss of vision, coordination, sensation, speech, paralysis and loss of consciousness. Brain stem strokes are especially devastating and life threatening because they can disrupt the involuntary vegetative functions essential to life. When blood supply is blocked, brain cells die as they are deprived from oxygen (ischemia), and they start to release toxic chemicals that threaten surrounding tissue (the ischemic penumbra). In ischemic stroke, the acute goal is to restore blood flow to the area and to prevent cell death in the penumbra. Thrombolytic drugs are nowadays applied as a "blood clot-buster" to restore blood flow (Pulsinelli et al. 1997). A variety of cytoprotective agents can be used in the post-acute phase for up to six hours (Endres et al. 1998), but their effectiveness is poor and the treatment window limits its application to only a small number of patients. In hemorrhagic stroke, however, thrombolytic drugs would actually have a detremental affect (Schellinger et al. 1997). If spontaneous clotting does not occur and hematoma increases in size, a rapid neurosurgical intervention may be needed to stop bleeding. Depending on the site, the duration and the severity of the blocked or hampered blood supply, the patient usually recovers, but often a lasting defect remains due to a loss of brain tissue, which is also visible in brain scans. The brain can compensate for this damage to some extent. Some neurons may only have been temporarily damaged, not killed, and the plasticity of the brain allows it to reorganise neuronal networks so that other parallel brain areas can take over functions stimulated by physical, occupational, and speech and audiology rehabilitation programmes. However, large infarctions or chronic cases of small strokes require tissue repair. The ischemic penumbra is the target area for both restoration and the prevention of further neuronal degeneration.

The possibilities of neurotransplantation guided experimental studies in rodent early stroke models to either replace the lost neurons or place cells as a source of trophic factors to enhance plasticity phenomena for recovery of function. It proved to be effective in many studies (cf. Abe 2000; Nishino and Borlongan 2000). Fetal neurons (Netto et al. 1993) and cultured LBS neurons, grown and differentiated from a malignant human testicular carcinoma (Borlongan et al. 1998) were found to integrate with existing neurons in the stroke affected area in rats and to correct cognitive and motor skill problems. In addition, human neuroprogenitor cells (Kelly et al. 2004), human bone marrow stem cells (Zhao et al. 2002) appear to exhibit a similar effect, and these cells differentiate themselves to resemble the neighbouring cells in the site of the lesion. However, the observed functional improvements are possibly mediated more by proteins secreted from the implanted cells than by cell supplementation since the integration of implanted cells in the host brain is limited. Thus, an upregulated host brain plasticity may be the underlying mechanism. This trophic mechanism is also assumed to take place following implantation of human umbilical cord blood cells (Vendrame et al. 2005) or porcine choroid plexus tissue (Borlongan et al. 2004), but concurrent angiogenesis may occur as well (Jiang et al. 2005).

The early positive and encouraging results with the LBS neurons in rat stroke models has led to clinical trials in patients with chronic motor defects resulting from an ischemic stroke. The cells were implanted with multiple injections around the area of the brain lesion in patients whose stroke occurred six months to six years previously and who had a fixed motor deficit that had remained stable for at least two months in order to evaluate any possible improvements resulting from the procedure. This phase I trial, including twelve patients, showed no adverse cell-related serologic or imaging-defined effects up to 18 months after surgery. There was also evidence of improved metabolism at the implant site in seven patients and some improvement on the European stroke scale score in six patients (Kondziolka et al. 2000). A positive correlation was found between glucose metabolic activity in the stroke area and motor performance (Meltzer et al. 2001) and cognitive function improved for those patients treated for basal ganglia stroke after six months (Stilley et al. 2004). The subsequent phase II trial with LBS neurons using pre- and postoperative, observer-blind evaluations and control patients for comparison, revealed no significant benefit in motor function, although several patients noted measurable improvements of their functional defects in daily life compared to pre-surgery state (Kondziolka et al. 2005). So again neuron implantation is feasible in patients with motor area infarction, but a genuine and reproducable therapy was not reached. Other types of transplants, such as fetal porcine cells (Savitz et al. 2005) and cell suspensions from immature human nervous and hemopoietic tissues (Rabinovich et al. 2005), were also applied in small pilot studies with partial success. However, these studies were not based on any preclinical animal studies.

2.4.7 Epilepsy

The hallmark of epilepsy is the occurrence of usually unpredictable, spontaneous seizures in the brain. These seizures are an event with a particular focus in the CNS; the cause is not precisely understood. It is either a symptom of specific congenital diseases or acquired following injury to the brain from sclerosis, tumors, abscesses, strokes or gliosis. Focal epilepsies can often be controlled by drugs that favour inhibitory over excitatory neurotransmission. Seizure activity, however, persists in approximately 35% of the patients taking these anti-epileptic drugs (Devinsky 1999). Medically intractable epilepsy, in cases of an identifiable epileptic focus, may be treatable through lesion surgery. Even so, in a number of patients surgery fails to control the seizures, and many patients cannot be surgically helped because of the (often extremely high) risk of losing important brain functions such as speech and motor control. Among the various new treatment techniques under investigation (Rosenfeld 2002), neurotransplantation and gene transfer were recently proposed after breakthroughs in the treatment of epileptic animal models (Freeman 2000).

Cells engineered to release GABA, the major inhibitory transmitter, or adenosine, known to suppress seizure activity, have been applied successfully as anticonvulsant treatments in rats experiencing chronic seizures (Löscher et al. 1998; Gernert et al. 2002). GABA-releasing cells are conditionally immortalised neurons genetically modified to over-express the GABA-synthetising enzyme GAD under the control of tetracycline. These cells, when placed intraparenchymally in the brain of animals experiencing spontaneous seizures, brought about a reduction in the number of spontaneous seizures (Thompson and Suchomelova 2004; Thompson 2005). The adenosine-releasing cells were modified by the genetic inactivation of adenosine kinase or aminase enzymes that normally break down adenosine. Encapsulated in semi-permeable membranes (see above in the section on HD), these cells prevent kindling-induced epilepsy in rats when placed intracerebroventricularly (Huber et al. 2001; Guttinger et al. 2005a).

The first human pilot study of the implantation of GABA-producing cells was performed in epilepsy patients who failed to respond to conventional epilepsy medication, and who are candidates for the surgical removal of a portion of the brain in order to control seizures (D. Schomer et al.; communicated at the 58th Annual meeting of the American Epilepsy Society, New Orleans 2004). These cells were fetal porcine neurons and the study aimed primarily to look at cell survival, host reaction, and clinical side effects. An ability to control seizures was reported in two out of three patients in this unblinded study. However, during the subsequent epilepsy lesion surgery, no implanted tissue was detected. The study was stopped as a result of this and also because of the concern about safety of porcine xenografting (see below). Currently, fundamental research is moving towards the option of using (human) neural stem cells as they differentiate into GABAergic neurons (Chu et al. 2004) following brain implantation. Moreover, they can be genetically modified so that they release seizure-reducing molecules (Guttinger et al. 2005b).

If cell implants can have an anti-epileptic effect through the release of seizure-reducing compounds, direct genetic modification of the cells in or around the epileptic focus would be an obvious alternative. The generation of AAV and LV viral vectors, which are capable of stable transduction of neurons, is an example of this type of strategy. Indeed, animal studies showed that an overexpression of galanin (Haberman et al. 2003; Lin et al. 2003) and neuropeptide Y (NPY) (Richichi et al. 2004; Noe et al. 2005) revealed significant anticonvulsant and anti-epileptic effects. Phase I studies with AAV-NPY treatment in intractable epilepsy are reported to be on the way (Neurologix; http://www.neurologix.net, accessed on December 7th, 2006).

2.5 When is a Brain Disorder Eligible for Cellular or Molecular Surgery?

The history of cellular intervention in the human brain started with the autologous implantation of adrenal medulla tissue fragments in the striatum of the PD patient. The first presentation of these studies immediately provoked the question whether enough basic studies had been performed to justify such an experimental clinical treatment. Adrenal implantation in rat models for the parkinsonian dopaminergic failure of the brain have shown reversal of the motor symptoms, but is it enough evidence to justify a clinical trial? One of the fundamental requirements in clinical research is that a sufficient body of animal studies, in particular those carried out in non-human primates, be reported before trials on human beings can be performed. It will, however, always be difficult to determine what volume of animal results justifies the intracranial application of cells or genes in the human CNS. This will remain an area of ethical controversy, but the safety of the procedures and the possibility of beneficial effects on a neurological or neurodegenerative disease, which cannot be treated adequately in any other way, must prevail (Sladek and Shoulson 1988; Hoffer and Olson 1991). Several factors must be taken into consideration: i) the risk-benefit ratio for the patient; ii) the need for treatment in the light of the severity of the disease; iii) the time and money required and iv) the effects of trials on the experimental animals involved and, in particular, on non-human primates. Animal "models" for brain diseases however will never completely match with the symptomatology and prognoses in the case of human patients. This is also true for the various rodent and monkey models of neurodegenerative diseases like PD, HD, ALS, etc. Thus, the final efficacy of any intervention in the brain will require trials in human beings that carry some risk of negative effects. These considerations should be made separately for every disease in which cellular or molecular neurosurgery could conceivably have a beneficial effect, independently of similar considerations for other diseases, before clinical trials can be morally justified. As explained above, the brain is a very heterogeneous organ and both the type, and the site, of intervention will differ in every disease, and thus the possible risks will also vary.

The team that performed the first stereotactic neurotransplantation of autologous adrenal medulla tissue argued that the frustrating lack of treatment for the advanced PD patients had weighed heavily in their considerations, and that the respective national and university-based ethical committees agreed to start this enterprise (discussions at the Eric K. Fernstrom Foundation Symposium on "Neural grafting in the human CNS", Lund, Sweden, June 18th–22nd 1984). Hundreds of patients world-wide were subjected to this auto-transplant surgery after very positive results were presented by Madrazo et al. (1987). Many teams offered it as a therapy, but in the end the field had to conclude that cell survival and recovery effects were both negative. This history of adrenal medulla auto-implants in the brain of PD patients illustrates the difficulty of determining what level of prior animal experimentation is required to establish the efficacy and safety of a new clinical treatment. It also illustrates that a move towards the first clinical trial is often prompted by the absence of any effective existing treatment (Boer 1996, 1999, 2006).

A basic requirement, however, is obviously that any brain disorder elected for cell or gene transfer must have a defined target for the intervention, determined by the results of animal experiments. A new trial without such a background can not be accepted because of unknown risks for human brain functions.

2.6 How to Design a Meaningful Experimental Human Cell or Gene Therapeutic Neurosurgical Study?

Facing a future with various types of therapeutic cell and gene trials in various human brain diseases, strategies on how to control efficacy of these new treatments needs to be discussed. Human experiments that are methodologically bound to give non-interpretable results are unethical (Felten 1994). However, this is also true of unnecessary control treatments in human beings. Randomised blind evaluation clinical trial methodology has been the gold standard for establishing the effectiveness of medicines for the last 50 years. The standard trial must show that a particular drug treatment correlates with a hypothesised outcome and that no other factors are responsible for this correlation (Kenny 1979). In the case of individual human subject, one cannot simultaneously both give and withhold a treatment. The comparison of patients pre- and post-treatment is hard to measure accurately and can easily be biased by artifacts (Kraemer 2004). It is, therefore, regarded as inferior to a comparison between an experimental and placebo group. For pharmacological trials, extensive guidelines have been published to reach this goal of strict control. Nowadays the randomised double-blind, placebo-controlled design, with an expectation of clinical relevant outcomes, is often the legally required standard (CPMP Working Party on Efficacy of Medicinal Products 1990). However, surgical implantation of cells or gene transfer in the brain cannot simply be compared with pharmacological treatment as one would not implant non-therapeutic cells or genes in the brain for control. Such a control in itself, even if not harmful for the patient, will make it difficult, or even impossible, to provide the "real" treatment if it appeared to be truly beneficial in the end. For experimental neurosurgery, and thus also for neurotransplantation and gene therapy surgery, legal guidance is largely lacking. Thus, there is a new need to establish what controls can, or should, be included to obtain meaningful results.

Experimental human studies on cell and gene therapy differ from drug therapy trials in that the former are invasive treatments with irreversible effects, even in those cases in which the activity of the implanted cells or inserted genes is "silenced" through either a process of cell killing[8] or the transcription of inactivating systems[9]. The guidelines for experimental

---

[8] Before implantation cells can be equipped with the herpes simplex virus thymidine kinase gene (HSV-tk), rendering them susceptible to the cytotoxic effects of ganciclovir which subsequently will kill the cells that were implanted. An inflammatory response to remove the debris is the consequence.

[9] In the case of gene therapy one can stop gene expression when the Tet-Off and Tet-On expression systems (Baron and Bujard 2000) are applied in the recombinant transgene. The expression of a putative therapeutic transgene will then be dependent on the activity of the inducible transcriptional activator doxycycline. In Tet-Off, doxycycline in the drinking water will block expression, in the Tet-On system expression will be on in the presence of this tetracycline derivative, and blocked when it is left out the drinking water.

(neuro)surgery are, of course, the general ones given by the WHA Declaration in Helsinki (2000), and by the Council of Europe Convention on Human Rights and Biomedicine (1997). Ad hoc groups of international scientists have formulated core assessment protocols for the process of neural grafting in PD (CAPIT-PD) (Langston et al. 1992; Defer et al. 1999; Widner and Defer 1999) and HD (CAPIT-HD) (Quinn et al. 1996) that recommend stringent pre- and post-surgical evaluation to determine recovery from the disease symptoms. However, any further guidance is lacking. Nevertheless, the field of experimental clinical restorative neurosurgery moves fast and guidance is urgently needed.

Due to the invasiveness of cell-based therapeutic trials, they have seldom been placebo-controlled, but this type of trial has been applied in the case of implants in peripheral organs like muscles (Tremblay et al. 1993). A true control treatment in neurotransplantation, equivalent to the use of non-efficacious dummy pills in gold standard pharmacological studies, would involve the irreversible implantation of non-functional fetal nerve cells. For the brain, however, this type of placebo surgery is problematic as its invasive character is more of a risk since nervous tissues self-repair is virtually absent. The "gold standard" approach of (normally reversible) pharmacological studies in humans cannot be applied (similarly, heart transplantation has never been placebo-controlled in human beings). But is this enough reason to also ban sham-controlled trials (surgery without placement of cells or genes) in which neither patient, nor evaluator, knows whether the brain has been touched or not? Sham-controlled, or imitation, surgery trials include a placebo for the expectations of the surgery, not for the result of the cellular or molecular intervention. If sham-controlled studies are also not acceptable, is there an alternative study design that can provide meaningful and interpretable data as ethically required for clinical trials?

2.6.1 Is Sham Surgery Acceptable?

Sham surgery is a completely new aspect in neurotransplantation research that had never received a critical evaluation in the scientific literature until Freeman et al. (1999) published a plea in favour of this approach in PD grafting studies. Until that time, the clinical trials with grafting in PD patients had always been open trials and were performed under different conditions in terms of the donor tissue treatment, the graft placement, the surgical approach used, the pre- and post-grafting treatment and the symptom evaluation. Due, or partially due, to these differences, surgical outcomes were variable from trial to trial, leading to the criticism that a credible body of evidence on the efficacy of the treatment had not been obtained since both investigator bias and placebo effects on the patient side could have affected the results of the open trials (Felten 1994; Freeman et al. 1997, 1999). Thus double blind placebo-controlled studies were needed. The central question raised by Freeman et al. (1999) was: "Under what circumstances are the risks to subjects assigned to the placebo group in a medical or surgical trial justified, and what risks are reasonable in order to determine the benefits and adverse effects of a given intervention?" Three criteria were listed that must be met before randomised double blind placebo-controlled trials could be carried out: i) the study should address an important research question that cannot be answered by a study with an alternative design that poses a lower risk to the subjects, ii) there must be preliminary but not conclusive evidence that the intervention is effective, and iii) the treatment should be sufficiently developed so that it is unlikely that it will become obsolete before the study has been completed. For neurotransplantation in PD, the case discussed by Freeman et al. (1999), the latter two criteria pose no problems as it was, at that time, generally acceptable to assume that the treatment could be effective, even though it still needed to be perfected, and that adverse effects had not been prominent (Brundin et al. 2000; Dunnett et al. 2001). The criterion for discussion is, therefore, the first one, which is a general point for all clinical trials involving invasive experimental restorative neurosurgery. The sham surgery in PD patients justified by Freeman et al. (1999), and applied in the studies of Freed et al. (2001), Watts et al. (2001), Olanow et al. (2003), does not control for placebo clinical changes due to the implantation surgery itself as no cells are implanted in the sham group (see before). The justification is therefore only defendable on the basis of control for investigator bias or placebo effects for the perception, or expectation, of the patient. Freeman et al. (1999) stated that the risks of participating in the study are "reasonable" in relation to the possible benefits (sham patients undergo one imitation surgery and will then wait one year to obtain the "real" treatment if the benefits of the procedure has been shown). Frank et al. (2005) recently reviewed the adverse effects reported in the double-blind sham surgery-controlled trials for PD, and concluded that i) it was generally safe and well tolerated, ii) effects were not attributed to the placebo surgery and iii) de facto harm occurred more frequently in subjects with the "true" intervention. However, the risks of surgery were not zero and they must be regarded as being as serious as risks arising from a placebo drug treatment. There are the medical risks of local or general anesthesia (six to eight hours) during the surgery itself as well as of the immune suppression therapy (cyclosporin for at least six months) and of the risks related to the significant exposure to radiation during the repeated PET scans possibly needed in the evaluation period (Boer and Widner 2002). These procedures were thus enforced on control PD patients at a moment when i) the neurografting technique remained suboptimal in terms of neuronal survival and striatal reinnervation, ii) a significant number of PD patients worldwide had cell implants without evidence of a long-lasting therapeutic effect, and iii) compelling evidence had been presented that the clinical course of the engrafted PD patients parallels the development of the dopaminergic graft measured with the surrogate marker F-dopa uptake in PET scans (as animal studies

embryos (blastocysts), as well as from adult organs and umbilical cord blood. However, stem cells from the human blastocysts are, at present, the best pluripotent source material. The process of characterisation, isolation, purification, laboratory growth and differentiation of early and late age retrieved stem cells differs and is not completely understood even under "harnessed" laboratory control. Thus, one cannot claim that adult rather than early embryonic tissue has to be used as source for stem cells as opponents of the use of human prenatal stem cells do. Each source of tissue or cell retrieval must remain open for appropriate use for therapeutic purposes as each source of cells has its own particular set of ethical problems.

2.7.1 Adult Human Cells

When it became obvious that adrenal implants had failed in the case of PD, the idea of autologous transplants did not vanish, because of the advantage of avoiding immunological problems and the absence of the need for a donor. Combined adrenal chromaffin/peripheral nerve tissue (Date et al. 1997) or chromaffin/Sertoli cell implants (Date et al. 1997; Sanberg et al. 1997), stellate ganglion or globoid bodies (Itakura et al. 1997; Nakao et al. 2001; Arjona et al. 2003) were used in small cohorts of PD patient as a corollary of successful studies in rat and/or monkey models. The ethical evaluation in these cases concerns the possible loss of function due to the removal of (dopamine-producing) cells elsewhere in the body. This aspect is a minor one if cells for transplantation originate from e.g. a skin biopsy, as in the studies in AD patients with genetically modified NGF-producing fibroblasts (Tuszynski et al. 2005). An obvious exclusion criterion will be the autologous cellular treatment in cases of an inherited disease like HD in which the implanted cells would then have the same disease-related genotype.

Yet another process of autologous transplantation is the collection of the patient's own SSCs in order to grow and differentiate them into the cell type needed for restorative neurosurgery. Currently somatic stem cells are primarily obtained through tissue punction of bone marrow of the patient. This procedure is also used in the area of cancer treatment and, in particular, Hodgkin's disease and non-Hodgkin's lymphomas, where it is collected prior chemotherapy and given back to the patient afterwards in order to safeguard bone marrow function (Hahn et al. 2001). Again, there seem to be no ethical objections against bone marrow retrieval as long as the isolation of these cells presents a minimal burden for a patient who can benefit from subsequent treatment or an amelioration of his/her disease symptoms.

2.7.2 Human Embryo and Fetus-primary Cells

The grafting of embryonic neurons in the case of PD, in particular, opened the way for discussion of the ethical acceptability of the use of human abortion remains in the clinic and laboratory. For decades, research on pre-viable and non-viable fetuses and their tissues has been carried out by embryologists and physiologists. These data can be found in handbooks on embryology and intrauterine development (Falkner and Tanner 1978; O'Rahilly and Müller 1987) and have contributed to measures that have helped to safeguard early prenatal human life. Thus, in itself, the use of prenatal tissues has not been seen as ethically objectionable (Gareth Jones 1991). However, the notion that the use of embryonic and fetal cells would become of therapeutic value for large groups of patients (not only patients with brain diseases, but also patients with hematological, liver, thymic and pancreatic disorders; McCullagh 1987), and might be in great demand, was said to encourage induced abortions that would otherwise not have occurred (as it would be seen as a form of donation and, therefore, as a noble and selfless act for the benefit of humanity). The issue can, therefore, not be completely separated from the ethical aspects of the decision on elective abortion (Boer 1994, 1999).

The moral basis of the current legal practice of elective abortion in many countries is that the interest of the woman's physical and social health can be balanced against the interests and viability of the embryo or fetus *in utero* as a human being-to-be. Many national and international organisations, national institutes of ethics as well as, for instance, the Parliamentary Assembly of the Council of Europe and a Working Group of the European Commission, and scientists working in the field themselves have provided ethical guidelines for the use of body remains for experimental and clinical research (Peel Report 1972; CNESVS 1984, 1990; BMA 1988; Boer 1994; De Wert 2002). Despite marked differences, they all aim to solve the above-mentioned ethical problem by trying to achieve a complete separation between the decision about abortion and the possible donation of the remains (the so-called *separation principle;* Boer 1999; De Wert 2002). It would then be similar to the generally accepted use of organs or tissue from deceased babies, children or adults (cf. table 2.1). Leaving aside the fact that some people give the embryo and fetus an absolute right to the protection of life, which makes the use of the resultant material a crime of "complicity after the fact" (Bopp and Burtchaell 1988), even if induced abortion is regarded as unethical, it cannot be concluded that it is inherently wrong to save lives with donated abortion remains (Robertson 1988; Boer 1994).

Of course, informed consent should be obtained for the donation. The main additional requirements should be that the timing and method of tissue retrieval should not inhibit efficient medical care in the interest of the woman and the unborn child. Similarly, no financial remuneration should be involved for the woman undergoing the abortion. The consent procedure and the extent to which one can deviate from standard abortion procedures in order to obtain useful tissue, without violating principles of efficient handling, remain open to differences in opinion (De Wert et al. 2002). In none of the informed consent procedures of any of the guidelines has a role been set aside for the begetter of the unborn child. In view of the equal legal posi-

Table 2.1: Example of guidelines for the use of human embryonic or fetal tissue for experimental and clinical neurotransplantation and research (as formulated by the Network of European CNS Transplantation And Restoration, NECTAR) that also fulfil the requirement for the separation principle of decisions on the termination of pregnancy and the subsequent donation of the tissue remains from the abortion.

1. Tissue for transplantation or research may be obtained from dead embryos or fetuses whose death resulted from legally induced or spontaneous abortion. The death of an intact embryo is defined as the absence of respiration and heart beat.
2. Intact embryos or fetuses should not be kept alive artificially for the purpose of removing usable material.
3. The decision to terminate a pregnancy must, under no circumstances, be influenced by the possible, or desired, subsequent use of the embryo or fetus and must, therefore, precede any introduction of the possibility of donation. There should be no link between the donor and the recipient, nor designation of the recipient by the donor.
4. Neither the procedure nor the timing of abortion must be influenced by the requirements of the transplantation activity when this would be in conflict with the woman's interest or would increase embryonic or fetal distress.
5. No material can be used without informed consent of the woman involved. This informed consent should, whenever possible, be obtained prior to the abortion.
6. Screening of the woman for transmissible diseases requires informed consent.
7. Nervous tissue may be used for transplantation as suspended cell preparations or tissue fragments.
8. All members of the hospital or research staff directly involved in any of the procedures, must be fully informed.
9. The procurement of embryos, fetuses or their tissue must not involve any form of profit or remuneration.
10. Every transplantation, or research project involving the use of embryonic or fetal tissue, must be approved by the local ethical committee.

Published on behalf of NECTAR by Boer (1994)

tions of men and women (in Western societies), fathers may have legal rights in making this decision as well, similar those in the case of the donation of organs from a deceased child. On the other hand, some women do not want (for personal reasons) to involve the biological father in the process of terminating the pregnancy. In other cases, the identity of the father is unknown at the time of abortion. These are practical arguments for not routinely seeking consent of fathers and seeking only the consent of the mother (Boer 1994). In the case of a good parental relationship, the father's view will be taken into account by the woman. If father's consent were a requirement for donation, the ultimate consequence would be that no donation would be possible where the man cannot be consulted as well, regardless of the mother's opinion.

Modifications of the method of abortion for the purpose of getting suitable material for transplantation could involve an additional burden on the women involved, and thus conflict with the best interests of her health. This objection vanishes for modifications that impose little or no additional risk to the woman. However, postponement of the abortion may be emotionally burdensome for women as well as not being in agreement with the above-mentioned separation principle (Boer 1999; De Wert et al. 2002). Adhering to this separation principle has a strategic function, as it conceives of the abortion and the use of the remains as separate practices, thereby circumventing any of the accusations of complicity or questions of morality as mentioned above. A change in the method of abortion employed does not jeopardise the procedure of the separation of decisions. In practice a planned implantation surgery infrequently is not cancelled for the simple reason that no, or not enough, donor tissue is available.

2.7.3 Human Embryo or Fetus-stem Cells

The finding that the ESCs from the inner cell mass (ICM) of the human pre-implantation embryo at the blastocyst stage can be isolated, propagated and differentiated into many different types of cells in vitro, including neurons, raised the possibility of growing transplants for engraftment in patients with neurodegenerative diseases or neurotrauma. Theoretically, as these totipotent ESCs can multiply indefinitely, the ICM of a single human pre-implantation embryo would be sufficient to treat large cohorts of patients (Palacios et al. 1995; Rohwedel et al. 1998; Thomson et al. 1998). However, the precise conditions for achieving and harnessing cell lines for neural cell supplementation are far from established (Deacon et al. 1998) and research using human pre-implantation embryos remains necessary. Human cells with the pluripotency of ESCs can be found also as embryonic carcinoma cells (ECCs) and as embryonic germ cells (EGCs) from the germinal primordium of the post-implantation embryo (Shamblott et al. 2001). Furthermore, neuroprogenitor cells from the embryonic or fetal brain can be used as source cells to grow neural cell grafts. Finally, the somatic stem cells (SSCs) and/or progenitor cells from the embryonic or fetal organs, or from umbilical cord blood, appeared to have the ability to form neural cells. Ethically speaking, the source or donor situation is quite different (figure 2.4) and needs separate discussion.

2.7.3.1 Post-implantation Embryos

When stem cells or progenitor cells are retrieved from post-implantation human embryos, the situation is similar to when primary neurons are retrieved and used for immediate grafting. The guidelines for donation following elective abortion thus also hold for the use of the remains for isolation and proliferation of neuroprogenitor cells, SSCs, or EGCs. Two main aspects are, however, different. Informed consent must, of course, be obtained for different research goals such as the establishment of a cell line for research or possible cell therapy. Secondly, screening of the woman for transmissible diseases can be omitted as safety tests can be performed on the cultured cells.

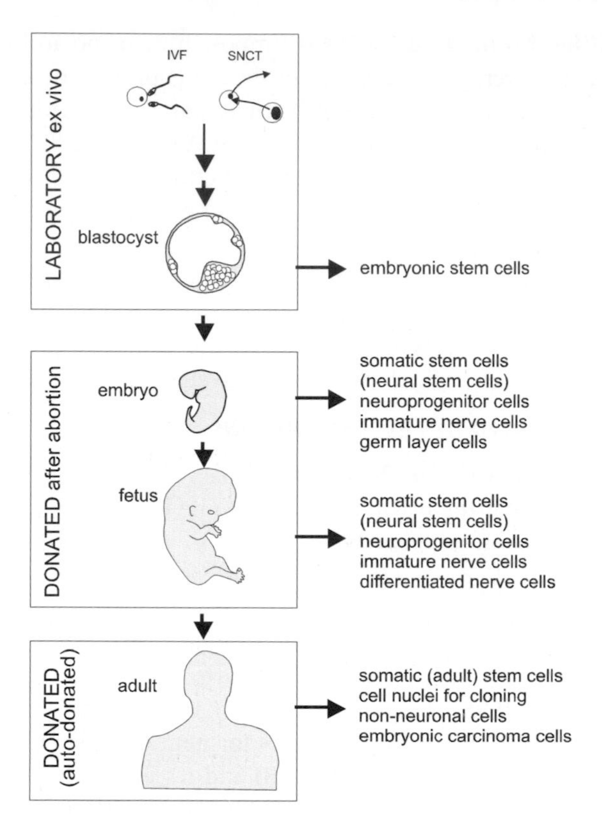

Figure 2.4: Present and possible future sources of obtaining or growing cell transplants for human restorative neurosurgery

The first steps in experimental neurotransplantation were based on the use of mesencephalic tissue retrieved from human embryos and fetuses containing immature but differentiated dopaminergic nerve cells from the substantia nigra. Meanwhile, several new developments have taken place or are foreseeable. First, the embryonic or fetal remains of human abortion could also be the source of neural stem cells and neuroprogenitor cells (stem cells that passed the first stages of differentiation), which can be proliferated in a laboratory culture and differentiated for neurotransplantation. Neural stem cells also appear to be present in the adult brain, but it is unclear whether this can be a source of cells to grow neurografts. Stem cells are also present in many other organs in the embryonic, fetal and adult stages of human development. These SSCs (somatic stem cells) appeared multipotent as well and may also be a potential source for the growth of neurografts. ESCs (embryonic stem cells) present in the inner cell mass of the pre-implantation embryo (blastocyst stage) are easier to expand than SSCs. Their potential as source cells for the preparation of differentiated cells of various organs, including the brain, is great. The pre-implantation embryos could come from the donation of spare embryos from a parents' in vitro fertilisation (IVF) programme or be created for the purpose of obtaining these ESCs from donated sperm and egg cells from adults (egg cells could perhaps also come from the remains of aborted female fetuses). Finally, an in vitro pre-implantation embryo as a source of stem cells could also be obtained through somatic cell nucleus transfer (SCNT, also called "therapeutic cloning"). The DNA of the patient is then placed in an enucleated donated egg cell, which would provide a method of solving the problems related with the immunological rejection of transplants.

For a more detailed explanation see the main text that refers to the present diagram.

2.7.3.2 Surplus Pre-implantation Embryos

So far, the potency of mammalian ESCs for expansion and differentiation appears to be superior to that of SSCs and other types of pluripotent or multipotent cells. There is thus a strong scientific wish as well as a need to explore ESCs from human blastocysts as source cells in order to grow transplants. The creation of human blastocysts is a current practice in in vitro fertilisation (IVF) programmes that help to fulfill the desire of couples with particular reproduction problems to have children. In the research preceding this now common treatment, human blastocysts were created as a means of developing the methods now employed in this procedure. The in vitro creation and sacrifice of human pre-implantation embryos is still mainly limited to research in the field reproductive medicine (infertility treatment, causes of congenital diseases and miscarriage, and improvement of the techniques and quality of IVF treatment). It is licensed under the strict control of regulatory bodies in some countries, whilst in others it is completely forbidden. This is indicative of the differences in moral views in different societies on the human value of the in vitro pre-implantation embryo.

Due to the burden of the necessary hormonal treatment, current practice in IVF protocols is that the collection of egg cells is performed once. After IVF, and some days of growth and quality control in the dish, blastocysts are then implanted in the uterus for pregnancy, or deep frozen for a second attempt or for subsequent pregnancies. At some point, the frozen embryos are no longer needed and are regarded as "surplus" embryos (also called rest, residual, spare or supernumerary embryos). Although extreme pro-life activists claim that these human beings-to-be must not be destroyed and can only be thawed for implantation in the womb, pragmatism leads to destruction. If the use of the remains of an aborted post-implantation embryo can be justified ethically, the use of "surplus" embryos cannot be rejected. The protection of the *in vitro* human blastocyst, a liquid-filled tissue sphere with undifferentiated cells (Scothorne 1968; Singer 1990), should not be held in higher esteem than that of an intrauterine human embryo in which organogenesis into a visible human being-to-be has taken shape. This reflects the principle of relative worthiness of protection of an embryo, which gives increasing protection as intrauterine development progresses (HER 1994). However, the relative simplicity of the procedure might explain the fear of some people in society that there may be a temptation to use the human pre-implantation embryos for commercial purposes.

Many, but not all, of the guidelines developed for the retrieval and donation of the embryonic or fetal remains after elective abortions are also of value for the donation of "surplus" embryos. The decision not to implant opens the door to the possibility of donation. The removal and cultivation of cells from pre-implantation embryos that would otherwise be destroyed could be regarded as analogous to the practice of tissue donation. In both

this was a failure because of limited graft survival (Fink et al. 2000; Larsson and Widner 2000).

The ethical discussion in xenografting covers the concept, welfare and choice of animals as a source of transplants as well as the dangers of infection, the need for long-term immunosuppressive treatment of the patient, and the psychological acceptance by the recipient. Many of these points have also been discussed in view of the shortage of organs for patients suffering from end-stage organ failure (Nuffield Council on Bioethics 1996). Animal protectionists challenge and oppose the use of specially bred animals as a source of transplants, since the special breeding conditions – necessary to control the pathogen status of the source animals – would introduce yet another violation of animal integrity and would hamper animal welfare through a new type of factory farming. Ethically speaking, there should be no difference between breeding animals for food or breeding them to harvest cells or organs for transplantation (Daar 1998), providing that suffering can be kept to a minimum. With all due respect for the life of animals, the integrity and autonomy of a pig should not be viewed as comparable to that of a human being. One might even say that breeding for transplants serves a higher goal than food production. Any validation of animal welfare should, however, be weighed against the potential benefit to patients, and animals used for animal-to-human transplants are to be protected by laws specifically designed to protect animal.

The greatest concern connected with xenotransplantation is that of the possibility of pathogens, specifically viruses and prions, jumping the species gap (Butler 1998) and the need for this procedure to be accompanied by lifelong immunosuppression treatment. These problems are absent when genetically modified animal cell lines are used, encapsulated in semi-permeable polymers for the local release of neuroregenerative or neuroprotective proteins in the nervous system (Aebischer et al. 1996). Cells from lower animals or even invertebrates can even be applied.

2.7.5 Proportionality and Subsidiarity

Possible objections against the use of human embryos for research and therapy are also connected to the ethical principles of proportionality and subsidiarity. The *principle of proportionality* states that the use of embryos in this way must serve an important goal in the interest of human health. It is difficult to claim that isolating cells from human abortion remains, or from "surplus" or created pre-implantation embryos, is disproportional if tissue is discarded anyhow. In many societies, elective abortion is legally accepted and research on pre-implantation embryos has been, and continues to be, used for research into the causes and treatment of infertility. It would be inconsistent to reject the research on cell replacement therapies in human beings that may lead to the effective treatment of yet untreatable neurodegenerative diseases and neurotraumas.

The *principle of subsidiarity* in restorative surgery with human cell implants would imply that the goals of research or experimental clinical application should neither be achievable using cell sources other than the human blastocyst, embryo and fetus, nor by methods other than cell therapy itself. First of all, one has to realise that research on cellular replacement therapy is presently focusing on the establishment of cell lines for transplantation. An endlessly cultured cell line with the capacity to form e.g. dopaminergic or GABAergic neurons would theoretically eliminate the need to obtain new material for new patients ("dopaminergic and GABAergic neuronal transplants from the shelf"). This may be reached with human ESCs from blastocysts but also with human EGCs and the multipotent neuroprogenitor cells from human embryos and fetuses. Calling a halt to this research would obstruct important developments that may in the end avoid the need for human embryo tissues and that could, moreover, be applied in large cohorts of patients from large scale laboratory cell cultures. However, the finding that stem cells are everywhere in the human body, even in adulthood, challenged the principle of subsidiarity and gave rise to new criticisms from people who do not accept the use of human embryonic and fetal remains (Oduncu 2003). These SSCs have now been isolated from bone marrow, liver, skin, fat tissue as well as the CNS. Their capabilities seem remarkable and are described as "blood into brain, brain into blood cells" (Bjornson et al. 1999; Brazelton et al. 2000; Mezey et al. 2000; Toma et al. 2001). At this very moment, however, the capacity for proliferation and differentiation of ESCs are superior to those of SSCs. Limiting the field to the use of SSCs would delay research in clinically operational and efficacious cellular treatments in many diseases causing organ failure, including those of the nervous system. Thus, although the principle of subsidiarity is meant to express concern for the moral value of the embryo, it is a sign of ethical one-dimensionality to present every alternative which does not use early human embryos as being morally superior a priori (De Wert 2002). Xenografting, as an alternative for the use of allografts, is at present no alternative either. From the perspective of animal ethics, one may question whether it is reasonable to breed and kill animals in order to obtain transplants when, e.g., residual human IVF embryos can be used that would otherwise be discarded.

2.8 What are the Risks of Cellular and Molecular Brain Therapeutic Interventions?

Ideally, cell and gene restorative therapy in brain disorders should be able to completely reverse the disability without affecting the psyche of the patient compared to its status prior to the disease. Changes in personality undoubtedly occur in all brain diseases but also in normal life in relation to changes in circumstances and new experiences (see before). Changes are either directly or indirectly related to the disease. They are directly related when particular nervous functions are affected and indirectly related if the physical, psychological and social situation of patients is altered by the burden of the symptoms, limited potential of daily autonomous handling, fear, depression, stress, uncertainty about the future and a possible loss of self-respect and self-confidence. If the burden of the disease's symptoms can be eliminated, or alleviated, by neurorestorative interventions, many of these personality aspects will subsequently improve, simply because the patient feels better and healthier. These are welcome effects on their personality and not unwanted side effects. In this respect, these brain interventions are not different from a pharmaceutical therapy that aims to treat the origin of a disease. Neuro-active medication is often also prescribed to treat the symptoms of personality changes observed in psychiatric and neurological diseases the origin of which in the central nervous system cannot be precisely identified and localised. The possible negative consequences of the latter treatments, however, are largely reversible when medication is stopped. The question, therefore, remains whether cell or gene transfer will affect the neural regulatory body functions and the psyche in an unwanted and irreversible way.

2.8.1 Further Aberrations in Brain Structure and Function will Occur

Would it be possible to have a cell or gene therapeutic treatment that is beneficial without introducing any type of mental change not related to, or induced by, the disease? It is clear that any restorative intervention in the brain will never totally bring about the "old structural and organisational situation". The therapeutic effect will be reached with nervous circuits that deviate and differ in structure and capacity from the pre-disease situation. This is particularly the case as plasticity phenomena will also have occurred during the progress or course of the disease. Slight changes in the cellular make-up or molecular functioning of the brain and its nervous pathways and circuitries *will* have physiological and behavioural consequences. Thus, surgical brain interventions *must* have side effects! All effective interventions will, in fact, have some side effects no matter how temporary or unrecognisable they seem to be. The ideal treatment – one that is effective and has no side effects – remains nothing more than a utopian ideal. Side effects must be accepted, but are they identifiable? If so they should, of course, be outweighed by the clinical improvement of the disease symptoms.

2.8.2 Physiological Side Effects of Cellular Implants

Besides possible recognisable side effects on the psyche, the newly structured organisation of the brain by neurotransplantation may also result in unwanted physiological effects. Neurotransplantation in the intact brain of rodents has been shown to alter physiology. Three examples from the literature on transplantation in animals illustrate this: i) the increase in cognitive capacities of aged rats following implantation of fetal septal brain grafts in the hippocampus (Gage et al. 1984), ii) the increase in masculine and feminine sexual behaviour of female rats following neonatal implantation of male preoptic brain tissue (Arendash and Gorski 1982) and iii) the change in circadian rhythm by rat inter-species grafting of the fetal suprachiasmatic nucleus (the biological clock of the brain; Ralph et al. 1990).

The recent notion that in PD patients who received an intrastriatal human fetal mesencephalic graft dyskinesias occurred more frequently than in sham-controlled subjects (Olanow et al. 2003; Freed et al. 2003) indicates that the grafted dopaminergic cells or the other nerve cells in the graft also have such physiological effects other than those wanted to restore the symptoms. The grafted tissues have re-arranged or re-structured the neuronal circuitries of the striatum so that control of motor functions is set differently and steering of body movements deviates from the intact situation of non-PD persons. This side effect, only recognised after a long history of dopaminergic cell grafting in PD patient (Hagell et al. 2002; Freeman et al. 2001) indicate once more that negative symptoms are sometimes hidden. It also re-emphasised that findings in animal models can never completely predict the results of the same approach in the diseased human and that unexpected side effects may show up in the clinical trial. Such an observation clearly sends the clinical neuroscientist back to their animal experiments to find out the cause of this side effect and to design new strategies for improved experimentation in human beings, if at all feasible. Meanwhile, some studies seem to indicate that the uneven distribution of reinnervation of the stratum in dopaminergic cell engrafted PD patients may be the cause of the disturbing dyskinesias (Maries et al. 2006).

2.8.3 So Far Risks of Cell Implants for the Psyche Appeared Limited or Barely Recognisable

Neurotransplantation adds small neural cell masses to the recipient brain, either as cell replacement therapy or as a source for substances that are beneficial to dysfunctional or damaged neurons. It does not, and cannot, replace large parts of the CNS with similar parts from donor brains and cannot replace entire neuronal circuits. It is unlikely that the micro-implants which are currently applied experimentally in patients would create a complete new brain with a new set of neuronal circuits, bringing about a different personal identity or, in the case of nervous xenografts, a non-human identity. Identity is not linked to a single, clearly defined, brain structure. Identity, as a reflection of declarative information on self, others, time and the environment, is stored in the entire brain and its networks in a dynamic fashion. The brain is not static but continuously changing and adapting its neuronal cell function and sensitivity and its cellular connectivities. However, as indicated above, small changes in the nervous system can definitely reflect personality changes from functional neuroteratology studies as well as neurografting studies in intact animals. When personality changes occur as the result of neurological and psychiatric diseases, particular brain surgical interventions may bring about additional changes beyond the ones that had to be cured and thus should be called side effects. The altered regional cellular and molecular make-up will change neural functioning of a particular neuronal network or of a series of networks in the CNS which then become active at a different level of homeostasis and, therefore, result in altered behavioural performance in daily life. Such personality changes are almost always subtle in the few studies on personality changes in programmes of experimental restorative neurosurgery with fetal dopaminergic neurons in PD, the test bed disease for many types of interventions (Sass et al. 1995; Diederich and Goetz 2000; McRae et al. 2003). Thus, no major complications for the psyche of a patient are reported that would balance out the gains in terms of therapeutic effects. However, one has the problem to distinguish the alterations due to the progress of PD itself, the changes induced by ongoing drug intake, those of the mechanical lesion from the surgery (penetration of a grafting cannula) as well as of the implanted dopaminergic cells. Though little research has been reported, Diederich and Goetz (2000) concluded, on the basis of various available neurophysiological and behavioural studies in PD patients subjected to with various treatments that fetal tissue, that transplantation does not induce significant cognitive changes or long term psychiatric complications. Unwanted side effects such as major contraindicative changes in personality or altered identity have so far not appeared to be major risks when the brain is locally treated with cell supplementation.

2.8.4 Transfer of Personality by Neuronal Grafting is Erroneously Brought Up

The transfer of personality has been put forward as a possible, unwanted side effect of neurotransplantation of human or pig fetal brain tissue (Walters 1988; Polkinghorne 1989; Linke 1993). Personality, as stated above, is not located in a single neuronal cell type or in a small brain area, but comes to expression from the activity of the neuronal networks of the brain, with all their inputs and outputs from and to other networks in the brain and elsewhere in the body. Personality is acquired and based on the formation and strength of these networks, the backbone of which is established by the genetic programme of human nuclear DNA during early and late (up to puberty) brain development in interference with external conditions, but which remain adaptable throughout someone's life (through mechanisms of neural plasticity, see before). Thus, transfer of personality from (minced or suspended) fetal donor tissue to the host brain is erroneously put forward as a possible drawback in neurotransplantation. The maturing and functional integration of the implanted fetal neurons will, moreover, be directed by the adult conditions of the site of implantation in the host, which are totally different from those in the fetal and immature brain.

2.8.5 Safety Aspects of Cell Implants

Cellular and gene therapeutic interventions in the brain of course also have several safety implications that need intensive control.

2.8.5.1 Transmissible Diseases and Tumor Formation

Before implantation of cells from human sources, the presence of transmissible diseases should be checked. In case of a short time interval between the retrieval of the tissue from human abortion remains and the actual surgery, this requires informed consent of the woman involved, as (time-consuming and blood-based) tests have to be performed on her bodily fluids prior to donation and use of the aborted fetal tissue. This is routine procedure in all existing protocols of neurotransplantation involving embryonic mesencephalic tissues. The EC Directive of the European Parliament and Council on setting standards of quality and safety for the donation, procurement, testing, processing, storage and distribution of human tissues and cells (2003), requires serology tests for HIV 1 and 2, hepatitis B and C, Treponema pallidum and HTLV-I and II. Contaminations preclude the direct use of these tissues for implantation. More tests are sometimes added to these standard procedures. For example, in France the law requires additional tests for toxoplasmosis, EBV, CMV, VZV together with a risk-benefit assessment by the doctor (it is also mandatory that blood samples, taken from the patient before and after grafting surgery, are stored for checking the serology of immunological status of the host. Similarly, seroconversion had to be checked for EBV, CMV and VZV). Storage and hibernation of the abortion remains would make it possible to carry out these tests without blood sampling from the woman. However, in the case of primary neural cells, this is done at the expense of neuronal cell survival following grafting (Frodl et al. 1994).

The tests described above are, of course, also necessary when allogeneic ESCs, EGCs, fetal neuroprogenitor cells or SSCs are to be used as implants, or when cell lines from human embryonic teratocarcinoma are to be applied. Cell cultures can be tested for pathogens during the proliferation, differentiation and storage phase before final use. Control for the presence of infectious organisms will then be part of the "good laboratory practice" (GLP) of the cell line production facility. Cell lines derived from human ESCs appeared to be sensitive to mutations (Maitra et al. 2005), which may perhaps make them unusable for therapeutic purposes such as late-passage cell lines and highlights the need for periodic monitoring for genetic and epigenetic alterations. A major problem, however, is the frequent occurrence of brain tumors in animal studies when ESCs, either undifferentiated or differentiated into neuronal phenotypes, are used as neurografts. Causing a tumor is in fact the most feared complication of any stem cell-based therapy. ESCs injected in an undifferentiated state and not given proper guidance, can form a tumor in virtually any location (Asano et al. 2006). Experimental human application should therefore not be started until this event is better understood and can be controlled. Further research is needed on this. As i) there is no evidence to date that cancer is caused by bone marrow-derived SSCs, whereas ii) it can be used as autograft and iii) it is not ethically controversial, research in this field of stem cell therapies focuses more and more on the use of SSCs. However, as claimed above, the ESC may, in the end, be the cell that is needed because of its genuine totipotent character.

2.8.5.2 Xenografts

For pig xenografts, proposed as an alternative for human allografts as pig nerve cells (as well as those from other mammals) can integrate and function perfectly to repair the injured brain in other mammals (Huffaker et al. 1989; Isacson et al. 1995; Galpern et al. 1996; Belkadi et al. 1997), screening is needed not only for animal-to-human transmissible diseases but the chances of zoonosis occurring must also be considered. This is a great concern as world wide attention is given nowadays to the fact that not only viruses, but also prions, may jump the species gap (Butler 1998). Large disease outbreaks in humans of the Ebola and Marburg monkey viruses, of the simian-derived HIV AIDS virus and, more recently, of bird flu seem to ward against any use of xenografts in human. Barker et al. (2000) still formulated a series of criteria that should be fulfilled in case pig xenografts are to be used in humans: i) microbiological specification of the pig strain, ii) biosecurity of animal production, iii) sterile tissue collection, iv) creation of a tissue archive and safety database, and v) an investigation of porcine endogenous retroviruses (PERVs). Even assuming that the use of domestic pigs – which have been in contact with humans for long periods of time – as source animals for cells will be less dangerous, the potential occurrence of zoonosis cannot be completely avoided by pathogen-free breeding. PERVs are integrated into the genome, as are retroviral DNA sequences in the human genome, and other mammalian species (Weiss 1998). Zoonosis could, therefore, also be a result of DNA recombination and adaptation, leading to the expression of known, or newly formed, retroviruses. Though not directly pathogenic for humans, pathogenicity of porcine viruses can change unpredictably when they cross species. The chance of cross-species infection (Patience et al. 1997) increases with the closeness of contact of grafted and host cells following neurotransplantation, and the reduced competence of the immune system in patients taking immunosuppressant drugs following grafting surgery. In a worst-case scenario, xenotransplants could introduce a highly infectious, or possibly lethal, pathogenic virus that would not only affect the graft recipient but could also (through human-to-human contacts) lay humanity open to a new plague (the "Trojan xenotransplant") (Butler 1998; Bach et al. 1998).

To the xenograft recipient, the benefit of a successful transplant will certainly outweigh the risk of any subsequent, unwanted effect of infection by a pig virus. To society in general, however, the possibility of setting off a new human epidemic requires fundamental virology studies before any ethical judgments are passed.

So far, patients who have received pig organ or tissue transplants (Nasto 1997; Stoye et al. 1998; Heneine et al. 1998) or who have undergone dialysis using pig kidneys (Patience et al. 1998) have shown no signs of porcine virus-induced pathogenesis. Clinical studies with porcine embryonic mesencephalic dopaminergic grafts in the brain should always include long-term, post-operative screening on the expression of PERVs in serum samples (Isacson and Breakefield 1997). Possible consequences for the patient when hazardous viruses do show up have hardly been considered in the neuro transplantation field. If it affects just the patient, it is to be regarded simply as a side effect. If it becomes a highly transmittable, life-threatening disease, it could require, in extreme cases, the isolation of the person receiving the xenotransplant.

2.8.5.3 Tissue Rejection

The brain is regarded as an immunological privileged organ in which tissue rejection is mild or absent. This knowledge stems from intra-species neurografting (allografting) in mammals, including non-human primates. The immune system reaches the brain without hesitations if interspecies neurografting is applied (xenografting), indicating that foreign body rejection can act in the CNS, as it can when bacterial or viral infections occur. Clinical trials with allografts are performed with or without immune suppression treatments. The disadvantages of life-long term immune suppression are known from organ transplantation surgery. Omitting immune suppression following neural grafting remains a subject of controversy, as do the results. Claims of long term dopaminergic cell survival in PD patients following neurotransplantation were presented, but a good correlation between cell survival and functional motor recovery was only reached in patients that had an ongoing immunosuppressive treatment.

Immunological responses can be prevented when the cells for implantation are encapsulated in semi-permeable membranes. Then, even cells from non-human species can be used as implants (Aebischer et al. 1996). However, the implant is then, and will only be, useful as an intracranial or subarachnoidal biological drug delivery device generating a missing compound in the brain and releasing a trophic protein following genetic modification of the encapsulated cells to fight or ameliorate neurodegeneration (the use of artificial cells as a vector for gene therapy). Supplementation of lost neurons or glial cells to reconstruct neuronal pathways in neurodegenerative diseases is impossible with such an approach.

2.8.6 Safety Aspects of Gene Transfer

Gene transfer inserts a copy of the particular gene into the nuclear DNA. It could potentially revolutionise medicine, as a working copy of a defective gene could be inserted to treat genetic metabolic disorders, such as lysosomal storage diseases that account for mental retardation and affects the CNS in young children. Nowadays inserting genes into brain cells may also offer ways to slow down, or even reverse the damage from neurological disorders and stimulate brain reconstruction upon cellular therapy. Gene transfer to post-mitotic neurons (and other neural cells) has been achieved by several classes of viral vectors (Hermens and Verhaagen 1998). Herpes simplex viral and adenoviral vectors for gene transfer into brain cells must be banned for clinical trials (except perhaps for the killing of a brain tumor), because of the toxicity for several neuronal cell types. However, the use of AAV and LV vectors may be feasible in patients as absence of toxicity and destructive immunological responses (though immune responses are induced against the virus components) as well as long-term expression of the transgene are hallmarks for these vectors (Kordower et al. 1999; Tenenbaum et al. 2003). However, due to the death of patients in clinical trials outside the field of neural deficiencies, gene transfer has come under a cloud (Gansbacher 2003). Thus, even more than in cell therapy research, safety aspects are an important focus in the field of experimental gene transfer in the brain.

Aberrant insertion of the transgene in the genome of the host (i), the occurrence of integration of virus sequences at uncharacterised integration sites (insertional mutagenesis) (ii), as well as the insertion of the transcriptional active sequences that could result in activation of otherwise silent genes (iii), may have devastating effects or may perhaps even lead to disorganisation or tumor formation in the CNS. Furthermore, this cannot be corrected afterwards. Even the application of co-transduction with killer genes could have traumatic effects due to the inflammatory and immunogenic responses that will occur when activation of this safety system is indicated. Insertional mutagenesis by random gene addition has, so far, not been observed. Moreover the spread of viral vectors in the CNS is very limited so that the chance of major transduction of cells outside the area of injection is minimal (this is also of importance to ascertain absence of genetic alterations in germ line cells). Biosafety of AAV vectors is especially accepted, and the use of (Parvovirus family) AAV subtype 2 vector has been cleared for phase I studies in humans, also because the wild type AAV2 is not known to be an etiological agent in any disease in human beings (Tenenbaum et al. 2003). Therefore, safety aspects then mainly have to deal with side effects of the over-expression of the gene of expected therapeutic value.

Gene transfer by viral vectors in the brain has some specificity as not all vector types transduce all cell types of the brain, and not all AAV vector types have the same efficiency in transducing cells. The main side effect of a therapeutic gene may be the constitutive over-expression of the synthesised protein, its effect for the transduced cell and, if released, for cells that do not need the treatment. In other words, an uncontrollable, long term local effect that changes the functional balance of nervous pathways and circuits not affected by the disease, which may lead to unwanted structural or molecular alterations and thus to unwanted activities in the CNS. The application of NGF, for instance, has been shown to induce neuropathic pain in human patients (Pezet and McMahon 2006). This quite likely results from the neurite growth-stimulatory potency of this protein, which could have led to an abnormal pattern of synaptic connectivity between nerve cells or its modulatory role on the action of BDNF also involved in pain. However, as the brain is a very heterogeneous structure each substructure of which is acting in many physiological and mental functions, one cannot say that gene therapy with, for example, the gene for NGF expression in one area of the brain will have the same side effect when applied in another area. Other side effects on the basis of (newly) established, but misdirected, neuronal contacts will affect different functions. Considering aspects mentioned above, any new clinical trial of gene transfer for molecular neurosurgery of the diseased or traumatised brain should not be limited to tests of the primary outcome for the disease parameters but always include safety issues and tests on personality.

2.9 Prospects

It is not unlikely that clinical neuroscience is rapidly entering an era of experimental cellular and molecular neurosurgery. In particular, stem cell and gene technology are rapidly progressing fields in medical science, which are likely to make restorative interventions possible and will, therefore, also be embraced quickly for the development of new therapeutic strategies in human brain dysfunctions. Newspapers and broadcast media frequently report on these developments and the use of human ESCs for organ repair is presently a topic of worldwide debate as well as of ethical concern on the political agendas[11,12]. The CNS, however, is a structurally

[11] The case of fraud of the South Korean researcher Hwang Woo-suk in the report on the first establishment of therapeutic cloning of human embryonic stem cells must be seen as a shadow cast over all purported breakthroughs in cloning and stem-cell technology and a grave act that damages the very foundations of science. However, it should not be viewed as an argument to stop research in this field that had raised hopes of new cures for hard-to-treat diseases.

[12] Both in Europe and the USA politicians play a role in societal debates. In 2006 both the European Commission and the Bush government in the US banned the financing of any ESC research. In Europe, however, many national governments, as well as many other national governments world-wide, do permit state money to be used for ESC research (UK, Netherlands, Belgium, France) under strict conditions and surveillance by the competent authorities.

heterogeneous organ, in which, unlike in other organs such as liver, heart or skin, each substructure acts within a different set of physical and mental functions and is directly or indirectly connected to other substructures in neuronal networks and whose output systems are connected to other organs. Neurons, and the quality of their connections to other neurons and non-neuronal cells, are the basic elements for these functions. Moreover, if one realises that the brain is the organ delivering the human mind, one can imagine that surgical intervention by implanting nerve cells, or genetically modifying their functions for the restoration of defects in nervous functioning, should be considered with caution and must strive not to disturb intact physiological functions and cognitive, emotional and motivational aspects of personhood. One, therefore, has to find the sole, or primary, disease-causing target for any intervention and perform cellular/molecular surgery in such a way that only that target is modified for its beneficial effects.

Current experimental interventions are mainly researched to solving the problem of a neurodegenerative disease or a brain trauma. Targets nowadays can be defined in these cases, and animal models have been developed in which restorative cell and gene therapeutic interventions are shown to be of some efficacy. Definitive breakthroughs, however, have not been made in patient studies, though solid claims of beneficial effects in the absence of maleficence are definitively reported in the case of grafting immature fetal neurons in the brain of PD and HD patients. The variability of therapeutic outcome in patients and the logistical and technical problems of obtaining enough appropriate donor material, though, cannot "stamp" this intervention as a therapy. If at some point in the future, human stem cells can be harnessed in the culture laboratory to develop into any kind of neural cell in specified, ready-to-integrate states, transplants better able to survive and integrate themselves in the host brain may be achieved. Moreover, cells can then be grown easily in greater numbers and can be obtained as autologous cells, preventing immunological rejection following implantation in the CNS (Armstrong and Svendsen 2000; Roybon et al. 2004).

Whereas cellular and molecular surgical interventions are developed and experimentally investigated in clinical trials for the cure of neurodegenerative conditions and the effects of trauma in the human brain, they are also often discussed as interventions for psychiatric disorders. In particular, gene transfer has been proposed as a potentially viable future strategy for the clinical treatment of behavioural and psychiatric disorders (depression, anxiety, schizophrenia and cognitive disorders). Fundamental research in animal models of these diseases of the brain revealed significant effects following genetic manipulation of synapse functioning and strength (see reviews Dunning 2006; Green and Nestler 2006). Whereas initially this was investigated in transgenic animals[13], nowadays the potency of viral vector-mediated gene transfer is more and more appreciated for more precise and direct molecular or cellular intervention in very local brain areas. Through this technique, insight is gained into the basic and local mechanisms of motivational, emotional and cognitive (as well as physiological) capacities of the CNS. Many aspects of behaviour and cognition have, moreover, been compartmentalised in the CNS, so that selective and discrete interventions may indeed be possible to correct existing anomalies or acquired pathologies. Current psychopharmacotherapy – which doubtless has advanced treatment in psychiatric disorders – do not have this advance of selectivity as drugs reach not only the target for intervention and, therefore, always result in side effects with the risks of non-compliance for the treatment. Even though the exact mechanisms and the pathologies are still hardly understood, psychopharmacotherapy has its effects on synaptic transmissions. So, will it then soon be possible to improve the mental capacities of the psychiatrically or psychologically diseased persons by viral vector-mediated gene therapeutic intervention on defined aspects of neurotransmission in the CNS? The answer is no, as one still is not able to define the exact targets for interventions well enough and since animal models are usually poor models for the complexity of human psychic anomalies. Moreover, the obstacle of finding the proper target is not the only problem as viral vector type, control of "therapeutic" transgene expression (Baron and Bujard 2000) and safety aspects must also be resolved (see above). In particular, in vivo regulatable gene expression may tune a local effect in the brain to correct specific abnormal behaviour.

Like cell transplants in neurodegenerative diseases, the effects of gene transfers will not be instantaneous as gene expression first has to be translated in molecular changes at the cellular level which takes more than a few days. One may also ask the question whether a single primary target can be defined for therapy. Behavioural and psychiatric diseases may relate more to limitations in the function of neuronal systems either by aberrancy of connectivity or by limitations in potency to adapt to the

---

[13] In transgenic animals, the genome, the nuclear DNA of all cells of the organism, has been modified through ex vivo insertion, deletion or mutation of a gene in the fertilised egg cell prior implantation. This technique is used in life science to determine the importance and specific task of the protein transcribed and translated from a particular gene for the organism, its development and its adult functioning, and to investigate its involvement in particular molecular and cellular processes. As all cells of the body are genetically modified from early prenatal development onwards, compensating growth mechanisms may occur – and certainly will occur during the formation of neuronal networks in the CNS – so that in behavioural studies the precise function of the gene is obscured. Viral vector-mediated gene transfer permits to genetically modify cells in adulthood and can, moreover, be applied locally by a single injection. The genetic modification can thus be targetted.

Both cell and gene therapy for the diseased or traumatised brain are invasive interventions in the human brain, the organic basis of our personhood. Contrary to medication, whose intake can simply be stopped, these invasive interventions are either irreversible or only partially reversible. Moreover, they will never be able to restore the condition of the brain prior to the onset of the disorder in terms of morphology and the quality and extent of neuronal circuits. Unwanted physiological and mental side effects related to interventions can, therefore, occur in the recipient, although they will not necessarily be recognised in normal daily life. It is argued that, if a brain disorder can be pinned down to a particular (local) cellular or molecular origin, then cell or gene therapy with minimal side effects may be foreseeable. It is, therefore, most important to evaluate experimental interventions in the brain in carefully designed clinical trials where patient selection and outcome measures – on the disease symptoms and on side effects – are part of a core assessment protocol (CAP) dedicated to the particular brain disease targetted by the intervention. Only in this way can the results of various types of intervention be compared for genuine efficacy, and the disputable, but currently performed, control of treatments through sham surgery will be rendered unnecessary.

Ethical guidelines on the retrieval and use of human embryonic cells for transplantation have been established by several international research organisations, as well as by national authorities. However, the irresolvable controversies about elective abortion and, to an even greater extent, the logistical demands for large quantities of "cells from the shelf", has led to the search for other neural cell graft sources. The discovery of the potencies of embryonic stem cells, cells able to clone themselves indefinitely and to grow and differentiate in any type of cell in the body, could make the latter possible. However, this has re-opened debates on ethical guidance. The in vitro creation and sacrifice of human pre-implantation embryos is still mainly limited to research in the field of reproductive medicine. It is licensed under the strict control of regulatory bodies in some countries, and completely forbidden in others (which shows the different views of different societies on the human value of in vitro pre-implantation embryos). It is argued that the use of embryonic stem cells from surplus pre-implantation embryos from an IVF programme (supernumerous blastocysts) must be permitted and could, in principle, be an endless source of stem cells as cell lines. In addition, cells from animal sources are regarded as an alternative for grafting (and applied in PD and HD patients without therapeutic effect). However, ethical discussions on xenografting cover not only the welfare and choice of animals as a source of transplantation material, but also the dangers of animal infections (zoonosis) and the need for long-term immunosuppressive treatment of the patient. In addition, there are concerns about the psychological acceptance by the recipient of this kind of treatment. Finally, there is the possibility that neural grafts will be developed from somatic (adult) stem cells that are present in many organs of the body. In principle (i.e. not for a genetic brain disorder) the patient could then be his own donor. Cell therapies based on self-donation have the advantage of circumventing any type of immune rejection following implantation but, so far, somatic stem cells cultured in the laboratory differentiate in a less potent way than embryonic stem cells.

The risks of cellular and molecular brain therapeutic interventions have frequently been described as the fear that one's personal identity will change or that a transfer of personality traits might take place. However, identity is not linked to a particular brain structure. Biologically speaking, this is the result of the activity of the brain as an entity with neuronal networks that interact dynamically with the environment (plasticity). The minute amounts of cells used for transplantation cannot induce the transfer of personality traits. Moreover, it is unlikely that this procedure could cause changes in the entire brain sufficiently significant to bring about a change in personal identity. Major cognitive changes or long term psychiatric complications will not occur either, but it is quite reasonable to expect subtle personality changes. This may not necessarily show up in routine daily life, but it may well show up in the case of extreme challenges for the individual in society. However, the benefit/risk ratio will veer towards the positive. A safety risk with grafts developed from embryonic and somatic stem cells is the development of tumours. Currently, fundamental studies are underway to harness these stem cells during differentiation into pure populations of neural cell types. The experimental human application of stem cell-derived grafts should, therefore, not start until differentiation is better understood and can be better controlled.

It is not unlikely that clinical neuroscience is fast entering an era of experimental cellular and molecular neurosurgery. Cell transplantation and gene transfer could potentially revolutionise brain restorative medicine, that is to say the treatment of brain defects or prevention of brain degeneration. Recently, gene transfer has also been proposed as a viable future strategy for clinical treatment of behavioural and psychiatric disorders such as depression, anxiety, schizophrenia and cognitive disorders.

3 Central Neural Prostheses

3.1 Introduction

Everyone takes the limits of his own vision for the limits of the world.

Arthur Schopenhauer

The nervous system is one of the most influential human physiological systems. Virtually every organ in the human body is contacted by a nerve. Most bodily functions are under neural control or modulated by neural activity. This is the reason why any loss of neural function may cause deleterious impairment of health.

The major constituents of the nervous system are neurons. The human brain roughly contains about 10^{12} of these nerve cells (Poliakov 1972; Nicholls 2001). The neurons contact each other, and some of them receive contacts from up to 25,000 others forming about one hundred trillion interneuronal connections in the brain. In these so-called synaptic connections, neurons receive excitatory and inhibitory signals that modulate the electrical potential on its cell membranes. These incoming electrical potentials can add up to lower the membrane potential of the neuron until it passes a threshold of self-excitation. Subsequently the neuron's membrane becomes completely depolarised within a millisecond, leading to an electrical impulse that is mediated to the target connections of this neuron. The neuron is equipped with fibre extensions for these actions: "neurites" to receive signals, "axons" to transmit them. If a neuron in a compound functional system is damaged, it ceases to send electrical impulses to its partner or target neurons in the neural network or to target cells in peripheral organs. If the neuron is a receiving station for peripheral events, then the message cannot be transferred to the nervous system.

Excitation of a neuron can be forced or mimicked by direct external electrical stimuli. Theoretically it would be possible to replace the damaged nerve cell by an electrical stimulator that connects to the target. However, since the damaged neuron is a terminal of thousands of biochemical contacts (synapses) and thus receives input from many other neurons, it is hard to see, in view of current technology, how an artificial stimulator could be designed to replace a single neuron in practice. On the other hand, in some instances it may also be hard to limit the effects of electrical stimulation to a specific target pathway. Due to the multitude of synaptic contacts and also due to the nature of signal propagation involving neurotransmitters, hormones, ion channels, and changes in the chemical milieu of the brain tissue, excitation or inhibition may spread to other functional systems (also see Section 3.5.1). Still, even with today's technology, we are already capable to partially restore a damaged neural pathway by an electrical stimulator with just one or two contact sites. To understand this apparent paradox, one has to explore a basic principle of neuronal activity – the "all-or-nothing" rule.

It basically says that a neuron generates an explosive action potential of maximal voltage ("all") whenever its membrane potential exceeds a certain threshold. When electrical stimulation is applied through nerves, this action potential travels to all the partner neurons with fibre extensions present in this nerve. Viewed from the perspective of its partners, the neuron remains "silent" as long as the threshold is not exceeded. The threshold can be reached either by spatial and temporal summation of incoming information from the neuronal network or artificially – by an electrical stimulus or "electric shock".

Electrical stimulation takes advantage of the fact that only the first group of neurons in a neural network is excited in such a crude artificial way. The next members of the chain receive a "natural" input through the anatomically formed interneural connections. The whole artificial setup works like an electrical switch that can turn on a complete neural pathway by only a few electrodes that contact neural tissue. Until now, neuroscientists have managed to place electrode arrays with a maximum number of a few hundred contacts in the central nervous system and only a fraction of these microelectrode-neural tissue interfaces becomes functional. Of course, the electrodes may also be used the other way around – to pick up electrical activity generated by the neurons in order to operate a computer or other machines (see Chapter 2.1).

Technology is just beginning to exploit the possibilities of such electrical stimulation and detection systems. Until the 1960s, it was impossible – if not unthinkable in scientific terms – to restore a lost neural function by connecting electric circuits to the human nervous system. 45 years later, 200,000 profoundly deaf people use cochlear implants in daily life, and 80–90% of them can understand speech (Illg et al. 1999).

Just as with the PC revolution and the Internet, prominent specialists in the field failed to foresee this development. As an example, Merle Lawrence, then director of the Kresge Hearing Research Institute Michigan, summarised the concerns among scientists at the beginning of the evolution of cochlear implants, stating that "independent of the number of electrodes one implanted in the inner ear, a frequency representation will never be reached (Merzenich 1974).

The development of neuroelectronic devices as an ongoing process has been gathering pace in recent years. Having entered into medical practice for the treatment of neurological disease, it is now speculated on their possible role in enhancing the capabilities in healthy human beings.

To assess the potential benefits, risks, and limitations of connecting such devices to the central nervous system, a closer look from a historical perspective would seem recommendable. From there we will move on to the current state of the art of neuroelectronic interfaces, their limitations and possible ways to overcome them in the future. Finally, we will deal with ethical implications of this technology and their possible impact on society. To separate fiction from science, a short section on futuristic scenarios will be added. However, as truth is the daughter of time, the story of central neural prosthesis as well as our judgements about this technology will have to be reconsidered with every new development.

3.2 History of Two-way Communication between Electrodes and the Brain

The further backward you look, the further forward you can see.

Winston Churchill

After the pioneering experiments of Luigi Galvani in the 1790s, it was the primary discoverer of bioelectricity, Alessandro Volta himself, who first experienced auditory sensations evoked by electrical stimulation when he placed two wires at his water-filled outer ear canal in the beginning of the 19th century (Volta 1800).

In 1870, two German researchers (Eduard Hitzig and Gustav Fritsch) electrically stimulated the brains of dogs. They found that areas in the cerebral cortex were related to motor function. Another German, Fedor Krause, one of the fathers of modern neurosurgery, systematically mapped the human brain in conscious patients undergoing brain surgery by the turn of the last century (Morgan 1982; Zimmermann 1982).

The neurosurgeon Wilder Penfield took up this line of research and extensively studied the localisation of several brain functions in the 1940s and 1950s (Penfield 1950a; Penfield 1950b). He also noted that electrical stimulation of the temporal region of the brain in alert patients could stimulate the recall of past events.

In 1956, the Canadian neurologist James Olds reported on research in which he had electrically stimulated the "pleasure centre" in the brains of rats. After implanting electrodes in the rats' hypothalamus, he attached a device that allowed the rats to activate the electrical impulse. He found that the rats would become so obsessed with self-stimulation that they would literally starve themselves to death (Olds 1958a; Olds 1963).

José Delgado coined the term "stimoceiver" – a composite of "stimulator" and "receiver" for an electronic device that is partially implanted into the brain, and allows for both electrical stimulation and detection of electrical brain activity (Delgado 1969; Delgado et al. 1976).

Delgado showed that many behavioural patterns could be evoked or interrupted by electrical brain stimulation. In one of his most controversial experiments he implanted electrodes in the skull of a bull. By waving a red cape, Delgado provoked the animal to charge. Then, with a signal emitted from a hand-held radio transmitter, he made the beast stop in mid-lunge and trot away.

The publication of Delgado's book "Physical Control of the Mind" met with a decidedly cool reception, mostly because it implied wider application of these techniques in humans. By 1975, Delgado had linked the brain electrodes with computers, creating both the first BCI and a method of "two-way transdermal communication with the brain" at the same time:

> The most interesting aspect of the transdermal stimoceivers is the ability to perform simultaneous recording and stimulation of brain functions, thereby permitting the establishment of feedbacks and 'on-demand' programs of excitation with the aid of the computer. With the increasing sophistication and miniaturization of electronics, it may be possible to compress the necessary circuitry for a small computer into a chip that is implantable subcutaneously. In this way, a new self-contained instrument could be devised, capable of receiving, analysing, and sending back information to the brain, establishing artificial links between unrelated cerebral areas, functional feedbacks, and programs of stimulation contingent on the appearance of pre-determined patterns. (Delgado et al. 1976)

While Delgado's work may have appeared dubious with respect to funding, intent and scientific methodology, other researchers gained considerable insights from his experimentation with two-way communication between the central nervous system and electronic devices.

With a much clearer stress on therapeutic intention, medical professionals teamed up with bioelectrical engineers to create a whole new field for the treatment of patients who had lost neural control of sensory or motor functions. As a result, "neural prostheses" for the deaf and the blind demonstrated the technical feasibility of bridging damaged sensory receptors by direct electrical stimulation of the nervous system by the end of the 1960s.

The term "neural prosthetics" summarises technologies aimed at the restitution or bridging of lost or disturbed neural function (e.g. sensory or motor deficits), while "neuromodulation" refers to technologies that are aimed at influencing erroneous function in neuronal networks, either by blocking abnormal excessive endogenous electrical spike activity or by stimulating impaired activation of it within relevant neuronal circuits in various diseases (e.g. Parkinsonism, pain, mood disorders; see Chapter 4). Sometimes, both fields are subsumed under the more general term, "neuroprosthetics" (Hoffmann and Dehm 2005). The disorder to be treated by either of the two may be caused by degeneration, a localised lesion (like a tumour) or a trauma.

Neural prostheses have been developed for the central and for the peripheral nervous system. Central neural prostheses in the sense of the present topic are electronic devices that connect to the brain for the purpose of stimulation or detection of activity of the human brain. For obvious reasons, restorative medicine has taken the lead in human electronic implantation. The complete loss of motor function or a sensory channel (e.g. hearing, vision) is a terrible disaster for the individual patient and the bridging of the gap, even if only partial, is not only a very rewarding method of treatment for such cases, it is also considered a highly prestigious, at times heroic endeavour (House and Urban 1973; Schindler 1999).

Until now, most central neural prostheses involve electronic devices or micro-electro-mechanical systems (MEMS) that operate with potentials and currents communicated between the brain and the electronic device via various electrode-tissue interfaces.

The European Group on Ethics in Science and New Technologies (EGE) has recently tried to categorise two groups of electronic implants for the human body: those that permit an intake of information from the environment – *internalising implants* – and others that convey information from the body to the outside world – *externalising implants* (Hermerén et al. 2005). This classification can be applied to central neural prosthesis as well, since there are devices that generate input into the brain's sensory pathways and those that operate electronic actuators or MEMS controlled by brain activity. The common ground for the two-way interaction between the brain and the implants is electricity – either produced by an electrical stimulator or by the biological tissue itself.

Apart from "deep brain stimulation" (DBS, e.g. electrical stimulation to inhibit the activity of the subthalamic nucleus in Parkinson patients – see Chapter 4 –, the most advanced central neural prostheses today comprise the auditory implant, the visual implant, and the human-computer interface (HCI). All three still are unidirectional devices at present, but Delgado's studies, existing implants for motor cortex stimulation to relief patients from chronic pain (Gharabaghi et al. 2005), and experimental work considering a sensory prosthesis (Morris 2002) indicate that the HCI principle of detecting brain electrical activity at the level of the cortex may also work in the reverse direction, so that these implants may soon advance to become a bidirectional interface. In the next chapter we will summarise the history and present technological basis of the major central neural prostheses as a premise for the discussion of their social and ethical impact.

3.2.1 Restoration of Hearing

Hearing implants, which are now worn by more than 200,000 people worldwide, certainly constitute the most successful human sensory artificial devices at present (Pfingst 2001; Rauschecker and Shannon 2002). The Volta effect of hearing by electrical stimulation (see previous section) was rediscovered by American radio engineers in 1925, who then called it "electrophonic hearing" (Steven and Jones 1939).

Extensive research on the auditory system was really sparked by an incidental discovery in 1930. A group of researchers led by the physiologists Wever and Brey had been performing an experiment that involved direct electrical recording from a cat's hearing nerve (Wever and Bray

1930). The animal was placed in a sound-shielded room with two of the investigators talking to each other. The electrode attached to the hearing nerve was connected to a loudspeaker in the adjacent room to make the electric discharge of the nerve audible. This loudspeaker was suddenly noticed to transmit what sounded like human speech to the experimenter next room. It turned out that the peripheral auditory system can partially transform an auditory stimulus analogously into electrical signals that travel along the hearing nerve. The characteristics of the electrical signals ("cochlear microphonics") closely followed the physical properties of the sound input – like in a telephone. At that time, the telephone had already penetrated major areas of social life, so the – however wrong – conception that human hearing might be founded on the same principles, with the cochlea working just like a microphone, came as a boost to auditory research.

From that time on there have been attempts to transfer sound information directly to the auditory nerve or to the brainstem – bypassing the middle ear and even the cochlea as the physiological receivers and transmitters that are damaged in a variety of pathological conditions leading to profound deafness. The result of these endeavours was a device that could receive sound stimuli via a microphone and transform the acoustic characteristics into a series of time-distributed and intensity-modulated electrical impulses. With multiple electrodes on silicone carriers passed into the cochlea to contact the remaining nerve fibres (neurites) replacing the biological receptor cells (less refined than in nature, with a maximum of 23 electrodes today) in a frequency-specific order from the basal to the apical turns (cochlear implant) or onto the cochlear nucleus at the brainstem when the auditory nerve too was destroyed, these impulses were conveyed to the auditory pathway which ultimately terminates in the temporal cerebral cortex. In later years the implants advanced to multi-electrode arrays with each electrode docking to a specific frequency channel, and the speech encoding strategies for the sound processor have been considerably improved to provide speech comprehension for the patients (see below).

In 1957, the French otologist Djourno and physicist Eyries eventually published the first scientific report on direct electrical stimulation of the hearing nerve in a human, based on a solid amount of data. Following a radical removal of a cholesteatoma in the mastoid bone of a patient, they placed an electrode on the nerve and connected it to a primitive speech processor – a principle of sensory implantation that, basically, is still applied today (Djourno and Eyries 1957). The French patient could hear sounds and even understand a few words for more than a year by use of the implant. Later in this chapter it will be shown that a learning process is involved in speech comprehension with an auditory implant.

The work of Djourno and Eyries was taken up by American surgeons. The first series of single-channel human cochlear implants (CI), published in 1961, was rather unsuccessful due to toxic and infectious complications (Doyle et al. 1964). Researchers in Germany were more reluctant to transfer their ideas to the operating theatre, but in 1963, Zöllner and Keidel already conceived what was to become known as the multi-channel CI some 20 years later (Zöllner and Keidel 1963).

Prompted by the early complications and the fact that the patients could not understand speech, a period of great scepticism followed, even though there was another successful implantation in a congenitally deaf patient at Stanford University in 1966 (Simmons 1966). To a majority of experts it seemed obvious at that time that these implants could not reproduce the complexity of the human inner ear with respect to speech processing. The pioneers in the field suddenly found themselves branded as scientific pariah (Schindler 1999).

This situation changed significantly when the first successful clinical series with four patients was published in 1971 (Michelson 1971) and even more so after several hundred patients had been implanted with a CI described by William House in 1973 (House and Urban 1973).

Boosted by the newly aroused commercial interest, multi-electrode implants were advanced faster than expected even by enthusiasts and, despite all doubts, the first recipients were reported to be able to understand speech in 1981 (Clark et al. 1981; Michelson and Schindler 1981). In the meantime, and almost unnoticed at first, the head and neck surgeon William House, together with his neurosurgeon colleague William Hitselberger in Los Angeles, had once more boldly advanced the limits of neural interfacing in humans. On May 24, 1979 they pushed an electrode directly into the brain stem at the level of the hearing nucleus in a profoundly deaf patient suffering from destruction of both hearing nerves (Edgerton et al. 1982). The electrode was connected to an external speech processor that transformed the sound from a small microphone into electrical impulses just like the cochlear implant did. Against many odds, the patient could hear as well as most of the recipients of single-channel cochlear implants. What is more, after the auditory brainstem implant (ABI) was exchanged two years later due to malfunction, she is still using that same replacement implant to the present day.

The safety of both CI and ABI was improved by transcutaneous transmission with magnetic coils in the mid 1980, almost excluding former complications such as infections and plug malfunction. Psychophysiological research involving gap detection, recovery functions, and conceived frequency of amplitude modulation proved that the patients could process the temporal information contained in the electroacoustic signals in almost the same way as normal hearing listeners. It was concluded that a properly designed speech processor could preserve the important temporal features of speech for these patients (Shannon and Otto 1990).

versity – Cyberkinetics, Inc. – is planning to develop a commercially available system ("BrainGate") in the near future. With the cooperation of a German company, active implants are being developed that are supposed to allow wireless transmission of signals, so the implanted subjects could be free of external wires and move around while they turn their thoughts into mechanical actions.

Another U.S. company (Neural Signals, Inc.), together with a research group from Atlanta, follows a "semi-invasive" strategy based on cone-shaped glass electrodes that are coated with biochemicals extracted from the patient's knees to stimulate nerve growth with gold wire electrode leads. These electrodes are placed on the surface of the brain, but neural processes (axons) can grow into the cones to form connections with the gold wires. This BCI has also been applied to patients who were able to control computer cursors by electrical brain activity generated during imagined movements (Friehs et al. 2004).

Medical indications for therapeutic application of a motor BMI include movement disorders, more specifically brain or spinal cord injury, cerebral palsy, stroke, and the degenerative disorders amyotrophic lateral sclerosis, multiple sclerosis, muscular dystrophy – generally disorders, where patients have lost the ability to perform motor tasks due to loss of function either after brain lesions or lesions to spinal motor neurons (Friehs et al. 2004).

A brain-machine interface could help these patients – after a period of training – to move artificial limbs by thinking about moving them or even to regain (limited) control of there own muscles. The number of patients who might benefit from such a device is hard to estimate. Just for spinal cord injuries, there is a population of about 30,000 patients in Germany alone for whom a BMI could be a therapeutic option. This figure would translate into more than 100,000 patients in the United States. Market interests may soon become a factor that could propel research just as effectively as it has in cochlear implantation for the restoration of hearing.

Now that there are a number of reliable interfaces between neural tissue and electrodes in both clinical routine (see Chapter 4) and research, naturally there are also efforts to take up Delgado's early experiments from the 1960s and 1970s and to develop devices for electrical stimulation of very specific areas in the brain. While these experiments continue to cause public concern because of their potential for abuse (see discussion on ethical issues below), practical considerations come into play from very different directions:

Rats guided by electrical stimulation can already be made to run, climb, jump or turn left and right through microprobes the width of a hair, implanted in their brains. Stimuli are transmitted from a computer to the rat's brain via a radio receiver strapped to its back. One electrode stimulates the "feelgood" centre of the rat's brain, two other electrodes activate the cerebral regions which process signals from its left and right whiskers (Talwar et al. 2002). Those remote-controlled "robot rats" (Nicolelis 2002) could perhaps help to find earthquake victims.

3.3.4 Vagal Nerve Stimulation (VNS)

Compared to the latest anti-epileptic drugs, VNS therapy in epileptic patients has shown similar efficacy in clinical trials and the long-term results are even more positive, with continued improvement in seizure reduction for up to two years (Ben Menachem 2002; Ben Menachem and French 2005).

Still, VNS has not been generally accepted for use as a first line or even second line therapy because it is a surgical procedure. Moreover, the safety of MRI examinations, especially in 3Tesla scanners which may be needed in these patients in the course of the disease has not yet been established.

The side effects of VNS are totally different from those seen with antiepileptic medication. There have been no pharmacological interactions, cognitive or sedative side effects reported in any age group. Side effects are restricted to local irritation, hoarseness, coughing and, in a small number of patients, swallowing difficulties when the stimulator is on. The latter complication tends to disappear over time. Since stimulation is delivered automatically, patient compliance is guaranteed. The cost of the currently available "VNS Therapy System" (Cyberonics Inc.), when spread out over an average battery life of eight years, is reported to be less than the cost of using a new anti-epileptic drug over an eight-year period, and if frequent hospital stays due to seizures can be avoided, there might even be real cost savings with the system (Ben Menachem and French 2005).

With respect to the treatment of depression, Nemeroff et al. recently commented on the current situation in anti-depressant treatment:

> Considerable strides have been made over the past 2 decades in the development of safe and efficacious antidepressants. Although truly novel therapies with mechanisms other than monoamine neurotransmitter reuptake inhibition represent an active area of investigation, they are years away from being clinically available. Unfortunately, up to 50% of patients with depression do not achieve remission with currently available treatments in short-term (i.e., 6–8 weeks), double-blind, clinical trials. (Nemeroff et al. 2006)

In this situation, new treatment methods were desperately needed for a disorder as common as depression. In Section 2.4 we have already sketched the rationale for including vagus nerve stimulation in the treatment plan. The first clinical trial, an acute (3-months period) open-label study with patients resistant to usual treatment, started at Baylor College (North Carolina, USA) in 1998, showed promising results (Rush et al. 2000; Nahas et al. 2005). A naturalistic follow-up study carried out by the same group with prolonged stimulation for one year confirmed these results, showing a (not statistically significant!) sustained response rate of 40% (12 of 30 patients) to 46% (13/28) and a significantly increased remission rate over the acute trial of 17% (5/30) to 29% (8/28). Moreover, significant improvements in function between acute study exit and the 1-year follow-up assessment as measured by the Medical Outcomes Study Short Form-36 were observed (Rush et al. 2005b).

Other studies, also combining VNS and treatment as usual (TAU), confirmed an improved long-term outcome of this combination over the usual treatment alone (George et al. 2005; Nahas et al. 2005). It was concluded that longer-term vagus nerve stimulation treatment was associated with sustained symptomatic benefit and sustained or enhanced functional status.

However, a 10-week acute, randomised, controlled, masked trial comparing adjunctive VNS with sham treatment in 235 outpatients with nonpsychotic major depressive disorder (n = 210) or nonpsychotic, depressed phase, bipolar disorder (n = 25) at Baylor College failed to yield definitive evidence of short-term efficacy for adjunctive VNS in treatment-resistant depression. Effects of VNS + TAU were compared to Sham + TAU. In this study, medication was kept stable.

Response rates (>/=50% reduction from baseline) on a 24-item rating scale (Hamilton Rating Scale for Depression) were 15.2% for the active (n = 112) and 10.0% for the sham (n = 110) group. With a secondary outcome scale, based on self-report of the patients (Inventory of Depressive Symptomatology, IDS), response rates were 17.0% for active VNS and 7.3% for sham. VNS was well tolerated: Only 1% of the patients (3/235) left the study because of adverse events (Rush et al. 2005a). These ambiguous results show that there is a definite need for further research in this field – especially with respect to the mode and mechanisms of vagal nerve electrical stimulation.

At present, the delivery of VNS involves a surgical procedure that includes exposure of the carotid artery. Apart from cosmetic issues, MRI scanning options are restricted. In both epilepsy and depression, some patients will receive little to no benefit, despite having had surgery.

If ways were found to deliver VNS less invasively, or if it could be predicted which patients will benefit of the clinical applications, VNS would probably be used more widely. Preliminary attempts at stimulating the vagus nerve using a transcranial magnetic stimulator (TMS) have not been successful, partly because it the difficulty of finding reliable indicators to confirm that the TMS has activated the vagus (George et al. 2000). Another possibility might be to develop a temporary percutaneous method of stimulation (George et al. 2000) to test in advance whether a patient would benefit from an implant.

A PET study with epilepsy patients found that increased blood flow in the right and left thalamus during the initial VNS stimulation correlated with decreased seizures over the next few weeks (Henry 2002). This suggests that, if ways can be found for the transcutaneous stimulation of the vagus, functional imaging may help to select the patients most likely to benefit from this therapy.

It is also not clear yet if different fibre systems are involved in the different effects of VNS. Stimulation can be delivered at different amplitudes, frequencies and with different pulse widths, and at various duty cycles (ON/OFF time). It would appear that if stimulation parameters are varied from those commonly used for epilepsy (or depression), VNS might produce different CNS effects (George et al. 2000).

Apart from epilepsy and depression, ongoing research indicates that clinical indications may broaden in the future. Potential application of VNS for anxiety, cognitive enhancement in neurodegenerative diseases like Alzheimer's, migraines (Groves and Brown 2005), and the mediation of high blood pressure (Rosahl 2006) are currently under investigation.

3.4 Current Limitations, Possible Solutions and Enhancement Technologies

> *Linking the human nervous system and brain directly to a computer opens up innumerable possibilities, not only in the future world of medicine, but also as a potential way of technically evolving all humans. This, however, presents something of an ethical problem. Nevertheless, the only way to actually find out what is realistically possible and what is not is to carry out practical experimentation using implant technology and to witness the results.*
>
> *Ken Warwick (Warwick 2005)*

Implants have a general disadvantage over other methods employed to restore or even enhance neural function: they involve a more or less invasive surgical procedure. Still, their development has been pursued with considerable perseverance for a number of important reasons, which we have to keep in mind when wondering why anybody would seriously consider surgical connection of artificial devices to the human brain: Neural implants

- can restore neural function where all other methods fail (e.g. CI, ABI, retinal implant),
- can function continuously without the implantee having to pay any attention to them or having to interrupt or alter his or her normal behaviour,
- can be completely hidden under the skin, invisible to others,
- can be turned off easily,
- can be recharged without having to remove the implant.

To judge the actual weight of these advantages, we ought to take a closer look at the current limitations in the field of central neural implants. While auditory implants have been improved considerable over the last 40 years, and visual implants appear on the clinical horizon, there are still no prostheses for the restoration of the sense of taste, smell and touch yet. The latter has already been addressed (Sampaio et al. 2001, Tyler et al. 2003; Krupa et al.

2004, Rita 2004) and – in combination with motor prosthesis – the bionic arm is no longer pure fiction as encountered in Schwarzenegger movies.

The first limitation affecting all sensory implants today is that they contact the neural tissue with a relatively small number of electrodes as compared to the multitude of neurons involved in the sensory pathways. Larger electrode arrays are currently under investigation for implantation in the visual cortex (Normann et al. 2001; Fernandez et al. 2005). However, the more electrodes become available on a small space, the more cross channel interaction is to be expected, possibly leading to a deterioration of the performance of the implant.

Second, implants today are placed in sensory pathways that have been severed before. With a lesion in the central nervous system there usually is little chance of natural regeneration. To the contrary, other elements in the severed pathway degenerate, too, when not in use. An early station in the auditory pathway for instance, the spiral ganglion, may lose as many as 75% of its cells when the hearing nerve is severed. The same is true for the peripheral sensory and motor elements one a peripheral nerve is cut off. Degeneration may be delayed by delivering protective substances or continuous electrical stimulation to the structures at risk of degeneration. There are also attempts to place implants at a higher level in the sensory pathway (e.g. the colliculus inferior or the hearing cortex in the auditory path) where degeneration after nerve injury is minimal.

Third, the electrodes contacting the neural tissue are prone to rejection and degradation. They may also damage the neural tissue they are supposed to stimulate. Therefore, researchers are looking into ways of coating of the materials in vitro, either with epithelial cell layers or with non-degradable surface layers.

Fourth, the neural interfacing of electrodes is still far from mimicking the anatomical and physiological connections in a neural network. To improve the performance of auditory brainstem implants, for instance, it may be of advantage to place the electrodes as close to their neural target structures.

This is the principle behind current research with penetrating brainstem electrodes for the cochlear nucleus (Schindler 1999; McCreery et al. 2000; Rosahl et al. 2001; Rosahl 2004).

From the perspective of today's technology, however, it is hard to see how the electrochemical basis of thousands of synapses can be replaced by an electronic system. It might not be reasonable at this point even to try to "rebuild", completely, a synaptic network. To restore sensory pathways, "bioinspired" systems in hearing and visual prostheses (Fernandez 2000; Fernandez 2002, Fernandez et al. 2005) partially mimic the function of biological receptors and sensor cells by "translating" signal received from the environment into physiologically "acceptable" electrical stimulation patterns that can be relayed to neurons in the remaining intact part of sensory pathway information via electrode arrays. At that point the intact portion of the central nervous system takes over to process this information further in its usual way. To improve the performance of a sensory implant, one therefore has to improve the way the information is delivered to the first intact neurons. Ideally, the implant would have to excite and inhibit these neurons in a pattern identical to the physiological paragon. This would involve several thousand electrode contacts in a volume of a few cubic millimeters – a setup that is unlikely ever to be realised. Alternatively, the (electrical) input/output functions of a group of neurons may be simulated, so that an array of electrodes connected to neuronal tissue on one side and a signal processor on the other would just have to deliver stimuli in a charge pattern that equals the one that is present in a given group of neurons at a given time in response to a given environmental stimulus. This is, basically, where research and clinical application stands today. It remains to be seen to what extent it will be possible with these systems to completely restore normal sensory pathways by neuroelectronic interfaces. However, the better these interfaces become, the more one could imagine that electronic connections to the brain that allow contacting biological structures involved in memory formation and higher cortical functions can be established one day – be it merely by modulating the amount of neurotransmitters in a specific area of the cerebral cortex or in a functionally specific neuronal network. Improvement of these functions would be particularly welcome for patients with neurodegenerative disorders like Alzheimer's disease – but if there were ever a very low-risk way to extend human memory capacity by directly connecting it to artificial devices with a, it is hard to see how healthy people too would not want to take advantage of such a possibility (see section on possible solutions below).

As of today, technology has not advanced that far and there are no such devices on the horizon yet. In a functional retina implant, for instance, colour vision would not be possible since all visual information is converted into a grey scale. Also, the understanding of speech and the perception of music with any multi-channel implant of today's technological generation connecting to a secondary or tertiary neuron of the auditory pathway will probably remain rudimentary, as has already been demonstrated in auditory brainstem implants.

Stimulation that is purely based on electrical impulses is further limited by the refractory properties of neurons, which respond only to a limited number of impulses per time interval. Perhaps one of the most important limitations in research on sensory implants is, however, that their efficacy can ultimately only be tested in humans. On the other hand, it is exactly this consideration that also poses a temptation that researchers could not always resist in the past. As soon as commercial interests will be involved, ethical dams may well be in danger of breaking (see discussion on ethical issues below). Such interests may arise in particular with the development of devices that could not only *restore* severed sensory function, but *computer-enhance* human capabilities.

For Human Machine Interfaces, particularly for the control of artificial limbs, crucial limiting factors are the spatial and temporal resolution of the electrical brain activity that reflects the ongoing neuronal activity, as well as the speed and accuracy of three-dimensional movements to be performed in response to these brain signals. Also, sensory (haptic) feedback from prosthetic arms can not be provided yet, and motor functions are restricted to very basic movements so far.

Size, biocompatibility, durability, and energy supply are basic problems for all neuroelectronic implants, but considering recent developments, these do not appear to remain critical in the long run. It is still not possible to connect more complex brain structures such as the hippocampus – a formation of neural tissue in the temporal lobe involved in memory formation and retrieval – or speech centres with electronic circuitry, although research studies in that direction are currently under way (Iatrou et al. 1999; Alataris et al. 2000; Gholmieh et al. 2002; Gholmieh et al. 2004) and will be dealt with later in this section.

Scientists have adopted several strategies to overcome these present limitations. Some of such strategies will be summarised briefly in the next section to provide an understanding of current top-of-the-line research in this field.

Possible solutions. Speed as a limiting factor in the performance of BCIs can be increased even without manipulating the interface itself, just by "tuning" the output functions on the technical part. For instance, with a pointing device or a virtual keyboard connected to a BCI, it may be possible to predict an intended target from an early anticipated trajectory and to place the cursor or pointer at the predicted endpoint. Recent research has indicated that with such a higher performance 96-electrode BCI it is possible to design a fast and accurate key selection system with a speed of 6.5 bits per second or approximately 15 words per minute(Santhanam et al. 2006).

When considering improvement of the quality of complete neural-electronic interfaces, researchers currently employ *two different approaches*. The *first* approach is to obtain more information on the structural organisation and the working principles of neuronal networks and their function, as has recently been demonstrated for the mechanisms of grasping and movement intention (Carpenter 2002; Cattaneo et al. 2005; Fogassi and Luppino 2005). Another example in that line has inspired much enthusiasm in the scientific community. The experiment, conducted by researchers at the University of California in Berkeley, involved neuronal signals from 117 neurons in a relay station of the visual pathway close to the thalamus (lateral geniculate ganglion, LGL) in a cat. The LGL is connected directly to the cat's eyes via the optic nerve. Each of its cells is programmed to respond to certain features in the cat's field of view. Some cells "fire" when they record an edge in the cat's vision, others when they see lines or different patterns at certain angles. Using a technique the researchers describe as a "linear decoding" to reconstruct an image from their data, they saw natural scenes with recognisable moving objects (Stanley et al. 1999). Research at the same laboratory also demonstrated that it is possible to map non-linear neuronal responses to visual stimuli in the visual cortex (Lau et al. 2002). Knowledge on these response characteristics can be applied to identify the major input/output pathways of a specific functional pathway in the brain.

Frank Ohl of the Leibniz Institute for Neurobiology has extensively studied the functional organisation of the auditory cortex in gerbils. His research group recorded electrical brain activity in response to rising and falling "tones". When the auditory cortex itself was stimulated with a similar electrical signal, the animals were able to discriminate rising and falling tones created by direct electrical stimulation in the absence of any sound presentation (Ohl et al. 2001).

The *second* approach actually builds upon the former by attempting to model neurobiological structures that have already been extensively studied before ("morphing"). One example is the recent development of an artificial retina. "Visio1", a silicon-based microchip that includes 3600 output "cells" simulating the response characteristics to light stimulation of the four major clusters of retinal ganglion cells, was designed and built at the University of Pennsylvania in 2001. With their axonal processes, these cells account for 90% of the fibres of the optic nerve (Zaghloul and Boahen 2004a; Zaghloul and Boahen 2004b). The "neuromorphic" chip needs only 60mW electrical power – one thousandth of the power required by a regular PC. This chip may pave the way to a complete ocular prosthesis, including camera, processor, and stimulator.

In a similar way, "neural morphing" may be employed to simulate the input/output-functions of other neuronal networks, such as the auditory system, without the need to adhere strictly to the biological principles realised within a neuronal network. It has been demonstrated that the tone pitch gradients of the cochlear nucleus – an assembly of neurons in the brain stem – can be accessed through electrical stimulation with microelectrodes on the brain's surface (McCreery et al. 1998; McCreery et al. 2000). Similarly, more complex brain circuits and functions may be accessible for establishing a "dialogue" between a computer and the brain in the future (Ohl et al. 2000, Ohl et al. 2003a).

One of the most ambitious projects in this respect combines methods of computational neuroscience with computer engineering to "morph" functions of the hippocampus with computer hardware and software. Theodore Berger, a professor of biomedical engineering at the University of Southern California, and his team succeeded in simulating some basic non-linear functions of this complex structure with computer equipment (Gholmieh et al. 2001; Chauvet and Berger 2002; Gholmieh et al. 2004; Berger et al. 2005). Their ultimate goal is an "artificial hippocampus" that could restore or even enhance memory.

Unlike devices such as cochlear implants, which merely stimulate brain activity, this chip implant would have to perform the same processes as the damaged part of the brain it is replacing. It would have to receive input from the brain and to deliver its output to the brain. At present, it is hard to see how such an interface could be established. Also, human memory is not static. It is based on continuous changes in the efficacy and qualities of cellular and molecular processes, so the implant device may need to adapt to such changes. Considering the complexity of the task, it will probably be a long way from Berger's initial results to the actual re-establishment of lost memory function, not to mention enhancement of memory in perfectly healthy people.

In the meantime, clinical applications of electrical brain stimulation have gained world-wide acceptance in the treatment of movement disorders. Indications have been extended and Medtronic Inc., the major manufacturer of such implants, uses its products in clinical tests to pulse the thalamus for the treatment of epilepsy; another region of the deep brain to treat migraines, depression, and obsessive-compulsive disorder; the hypoglossal nerve in the neck to treat sleep apnea; the sacral nerve to treat bowel disorders; and the stomach to treat obesity. Parallel to the efforts of modelling and duplicating neural networks, efforts are underway to establish improved connections between electrodes and neurons.

Microtechnology now allows the electrodes to be miniaturised, and their active surface can be enlarged by laser treatment. Coating of the electrodes with growth factors appears to improve the electrical contact to the neural structures, and conductive tarnish with nanoparticles reduces the breakdown of electrodes by living tissue. Neurons cultured on nanofibres develop neurite extensions and the artificial material counteract astrocytic scar formation, at the same time (McKenzie et al. 2004; Webster 2004). Also, neural cells can be grown onto silicon chips, contact them, and promote fibre growth connecting the implant to the nervous system.

Neural implants capable of communicating with the nervous system on a chemical rather than electrical basis (electro-osmosis) are being developed at the University of Stanford. Such "microfluidic" chips can serve both as neural prosthesis (artificial retina) and focal drug delivery systems. The way they are set up is a combination of electronic implants as described earlier, with more or less mechanical actuators capable of releasing a variety of different chemicals, e.g. neurotransmitters or drugs, in a very small volume of biological tissue. Medication could be delivered topically through micropumps implanted over the cerebral cortex where it is released in response to intracortically detected changes in the electroencephalogram (EEG) that may predict an incipient seizure in epileptic patients.

To prevent a generalised seizure it may also be possible to stimulate electrically a cortical brain area upon EEG changes – in fact, a system with eight electrodes connecting to "hot spots" of epileptic activity has already been implanted at Rush University in Chicago in 2004 (NeuroPace Inc., Mountain View, California, USA) (Worrell et al. 2005). For these purposes, passive implants will be replaced by active ones that have microprocessors connected to the implanted unit or even directly adjacent to the electrodes.

Enhancement

> *Although implants resulting in enhancement are not part of today's clinical reality, they are a realistic future option for which we should be ethically prepared.*
>
> *Sven Ove Hansson*[14]

While current technology with neural implants based on electrode (or electro-osmotic) – tissue interfaces may be of help for patients to overcome a severe neurological impairment, their potential to damage normal tissue has so far prevented application in healthy persons, with a few exceptions involving human self-experimentation (Warwick 2002; Warwick et al. 2003; Warwick 2005).

However, as efficient electrical and microfluidic implants become available, the next step after therapy may be enhancement. The definition of the term "enhancement" is not unequivocal. Hall refers to neuroenhancement as "the use of drugs or other interventions to modify brain processes with the aim of enhancing memory, mood and attention in people who are not impaired by illness or disorder" (Hall 2004). This definition, however, does not cover sensory and motor enhancement with neural electronics. Moreover, neural implants (as opposed to drugs) would not necessarily have to "modify brain processes" to improve human performance. They would rather build on the normal function, and access input and output, of per se unmodified neuronal networks. In this context, a "modification" of brain function would rather appear to be a side effect of such an implant.

The Council on Bioethics to the U.S. President offers a different definition by stating that "'enhancement', by contrast (to therapy), is the directed use of biotechnological power to alter, by direct intervention, not disease processes but the 'normal' workings of the human body and psyche, to augment or improve their native capacities and performances" – only to question this definition later on and dismiss the whole concept of enhancement as being "finally inadequate to the moral analysis" (PCB 2003). Indeed, making a distinction between "therapy" and "enhancement" may be problematic as long as one does not limit the latter term to "non-therapeutic enhancement", i.e. enhancement of healthy persons. For this chapter, we will stick with this distinction for the sake of simplicity, and add some clarification on its uses and interpretation whenever necessary. We will therefore go along with the terminology laid down by Eric Juengst and Erik Parens in 1998 and apply the term *enhancement* to characterise "interventions designed to

[14] Philosophy Unit of the Royal Institute of Technology, Stockholm, Sweden.

improve human form or functioning beyond what is necessary to sustain or restore good health" (Parens 1995a; Juengst 1998). This concept will also require us to lead the ethical discussion of the concept of enhancement on at least two different levels: the individual level (including the ethics of self-improvement), and the societal level (including the goals of medicine and the goals of society).

As opposed to psychopharmacology (see Chapter 1), there is no method of enhancement by neural implants that is already in use, although technologically, as one can see from the recent developments in the field described above, it would be possible today: Artificial limbs can be controlled even with non-invasive Human Machine Interfaces "by thought alone"; non-verbal, invisible communication can be achieved with Human Computer Interfaces; and by electrical stimulation of specific areas in the brain, mood can be altered and confidence be boosted. One of the reasons why such direct brain-computer interfaces are not yet being considered in normal humans is that these technologies still require a more or less invasive approach and relatively coarse arrays of electrodes implanted inside the human central nervous system.

With the improvement of telemetric stimulation, avoiding the necessity of a direct electrode-tissue contact, sensory enhancement may be not so far-fetched an idea anymore. While some sensory enhancements do not have to involve invasive approaches at all (like ultrasound hearing or infrared vision) and will only be accepted in form of implants if they are absolutely safe, any effective cognitive or memory enhancement may be a different story both in terms of its technical establishment and of the acceptance of involved risks.

An important issue will be the reversibility of such an enhancement. Electrical stimulation can be interrupted at any given time by the implanted person him- or herself, provided that the stimulation has not led to side effects that make it impossible for the carrier of the implant to use the appropriate external switch.

Another issue that will have its part in the discussion is intention. With every new step in the development of technologies, there will be a potential for abuse. To many, enhancement by connecting electronic devices to the human body and brain will appear, at least prima facie, morally suspect. Others have argued that these technologies offer an opportunity to make life even more worth living by getting smarter, being happier, living longer – provided that society would respond democratically to the implicit social challenges (Hughes 2004).

3.5 Ethical Implications

3.5.1 Treatment

Initially people thought heart transplants were an abomination because they assumed that having the heart you were born with was an important part of who you are.

Joel Anderson[15]

Any organ that a nerve can influence – that is every organ in the body – can be affected using this technology.

Ali Rezai[16]

Although the borderline between repair and enhancement is not a strict one, the concept of "normal" is not precise, and the definition of "health" a matter of ongoing debate, we attempt to address these problematic fields in this section since there are important ethical issues involved, both on the individual and the societal level. With respect to central neural implants, once we have defined a measure as "treatment" or "prevention", the measure can usually be regarded as legitimate.

The major ethical issues involved in central neural implantation as a treatment, therefore, are not exactly new and mainly relate to the *risk-benefit-cost complex* as well as the *availability complex*. Leaving aside the impracticable WHO definition of health as a "state of complete physical, mental, and social well-being", we will rather go along with a moderate version of Norman Daniels "Normal Function Model" (Daniels 2000), according to which disease and disability are "departures from species-typical normal functional organization or functioning", always being aware that "normality" is a rather undefined concept when it comes to human beings (Parens 1998) and raises the issue of "diversity" at the same time. In this context, "health" would be referred to as the absence of disease, and the goal of health care would be to prevent, maintain, restore and compensate for loss of function. In more general (and more problematic) terms, the goal of medicine would be to provide people with "normal" function (within a range of diversity) so they have "equal" opportunities to pursue their life plans.

While there is little question that the basic neural prostheses in clinical use today, such as the cochlear implant, are beneficial to their users and that these benefits by far outweigh the risk involved, this does not exempt future implant technologies for the central nervous system from an extremely thorough risk assessment.

Beyond the surgical risks involved in the procedures (damage to healthy structures, infection, etc.), there are at least three major reasons for concern with direct interfaces to the central nervous system: *Firstly*, there may be

---

[15] Ethicist at Washington University St. Louis – http://www.newscientist.com/article.ns?id=dn3488, accessed on December 12th, 2006.

[16] Director of the Department of Functional Neurosurgery, Cleveland Clinic.

direct interference with higher nervous functions. The more central the electrodes are placed in the nervous system, the higher the amount of information processing that occurs at the specific level.

A simple example is the hearing system. The most peripheral prosthesis for the hearing system would be a hearing aid placed behind the ear to amplify the incoming sound from the environment. One would not suspect any specific peril for the bearer of such a hearing aid to have his personality transformed in one way or the other. At most, the restoration of his hearing might make him return to some of his former habits with respect to social life that have been impaired by hearing loss. When electrodes are placed at the level of the cochlea – the neural signal processor in the inner ear that transforms sound into electrical activity which is passed on to the brain – there is also little cause for concern, since the connection of the cochlea is limited to the hearing nerve, a purely conductive neural structure. If the nerve is damaged, too, and the electrodes of an implant have to be placed at the level of the brainstem to partially restore hearing for a person, the picture begins to change. The electric stimulation of such an "auditory brainstem implant" is targeted at the second neuron of the hearing pathway – the cochlear nucleus. This is a structure of a few millimetres in size, located at the periphery of the brainstem. It is surrounded by other densely packed neural systems which supply the somatosensory system (sensation of touch, temperature, vibration, pain etc.), the balance system, the so-called "reticular formation" – a neural system concerned with sleep, general arousal and states of consciousness – and others. Because of the spread of electricity occurring at all conductive layers, including the coverings of the brain (pia mater)[26], surface electrodes placed over the cochlear nucleus may stimulate other neural systems as a side effect. Consequently, users of an Auditory Brainstem Implant (ABI) have reported sensations of vibration of their whole body, tingling in the legs and vertigo when their implants were switched on for the first time (Laszig et al. 1997; Matthies et al. 2000; Otto et al. 2002).

Because of non-satisfactory results of surface implants at the brainstem, needle-shaped microelectrodes have been devised which penetrate the brainstem to reach deeper parts of the cochlear nucleus (McCreery et al. 2000; Rosahl et al. 2001). Electrodes for higher centres in the brainstem (inferior colliculus) are being developed (Rosahl et al. 2004) and a group of neuroscientists conducted a series of experiments to electrically stimulate the auditory cortex in gerbils with an 18-channel implant (Ohl et a. 2003a; Ohl et al. 2003b).

In humans these areas are related to speech perception, and they are located in close proximity to brain centres responsible for memory, social behaviour, language processing and spatial orientation. These areas also vary considerably in location, may overlap be hard to pinpoint even with functional imaging. An attempt to place any kind of electrically active implant at a cortical site concerned with speech perception is likely to produce side effects related to other cortical functions.

Secondly, electrical stimulation of neural structures does not just cause electrical signals to travel from one end of the line to the other, similar to making a phone call (see Section 3.1). Neurons along their neuritic processes receive thousands of messages from other neurons at the chemical interfaces – the synapses – and their axonal processes in turn make such contacts with yet other neurons. In this way sophisticated networks are built, in which synaptic transmission at one point can cause "synaptic spread" to areas in the brain that are not primarily intended as a target of stimulation.

The neurosciences have studied precisely the mechanisms involved in coordination of this spread and labelled them forward activation, lateral inhibition, backward masking or afferent feedback, to name only a few. The cerebral cortex is organised in modules that function on these principles to form wide-spread distributed systems. It is not hard to see that interference with one part of such an interconnected system will lead to changes – however subtle – in other parts, too.

Thirdly, just because the stimulation with neural prostheses and neuromodulatory devices commonly occurs via electrical impulses this does not mean that the effects of such stimulation also remain purely electrical in nature. Changes in the electrical activity of a neural system cause release of neurotransmitters. Neurotransmitters in turn cause ion channels in the membrane of neurons and their supporting cell system – the glia – to be opened. Release of ions in larger amounts can change the internal milieu of a larger neural network and may effect the steady state in regions farther apart from the target region of external stimulation. Hormonal systems can be activated via receptor-mediated feedback and effect gross changes in the emotional and mental status of a person, leading to behavioural changes in due turn.

Even with one of the simplest implantable neurostimulators – the vagal nerve stimulator that is connected to a cranial nerve far outside the brain to reduce the frequency of grand mal seizures – we do not fully oversee effects on processes like attention, arousal and facilitation and inhibition of higher cortical functions. Such a stimulator is actually *designed* to interfere with the neural activity in the cerebral cortex, even if it is implanted at a distance of more than twenty centimetres from the brain. The very same stimulators have recently been approved for the treatment of depression (Carpenter et al. 2003). What is more, there is a vast amount of psychophysiological data showing that subtle bodily changes via feedback through the autonomous nervous system even influence performance in mental tasks. Against this background it seems justified to assume that electrical stimulation at any level of the central nervous system has the potential to interfere with a person's mental and emotional status (Bothe and Engel 1998). However, as long as it is possible to pinpoint a specific lesion and restrict the intervention to that specific defective circuit of the brain, as is the case with sensory neural prostheses, alteration of the psyche save changes in personal identity are extremely unlikely to occur.

With devices for neural stimulation that are meant to influence psychological states (e.g. mood disorders) or higher nervous system functions like mental performance and memory, large parts and information processing systems of the brain are going to be involved and ethical as well as legal consequences will become more challenging even if the use of these implants should strictly be limited to treatment and restoration of lost function. Hansson argued that "treatments for neural dysfunction, including neuroimplants, cell transplantation in the brain, and neuropharmacological treatments, may also lead to changes in a patient's personality, other than those leading back to a previous state" (Hansson 2005).

On a societal level, distributive issues will be in the foreground of the political debate, especially in view of decreasing health care budgets and increasing costs for medical implants. The less severe the functional loss restored by an implant, the more the implantation will be compared to cosmetic surgery and other interventions that are situated at the borderline between treatment and enhancement by society, and by health insurance companies and other financial providers in turn. Authorities will almost certainly be faced with decisions in situations of conflicting interests between the principle of equal access and equal availability of health care services, on the one hand, and limitations of financial resources, on the other.

A second societal issue in neuroelectronic implants relates to the fact that these devices include the potential to influence the status and behaviour of an individual in the human community or subcultures.

Even the cochlear implant a current central neural prosthesis that is intended as a treatment rather than an enhancement, and its use in pre-lingually deaf children have been heavily criticised by members of the so-called "Deaf community" – a linguistic and cultural minority group – for undermining their individual way of living (Crouch 1997; Lane and Grodin 1997, Lane and Bahan 1998; Englert 2006). The Deaf community holds a positive view of deafness, claiming that deaf children are normal children who just happen to use a different language (Nunes 2001). This community regards itself as a minority culture with a special language and individual customs, attitudes and values. Its members claim that large scale cochlear implantation of children would withdraw their basis to exist and flourish as a minority. In fact, deaf activists refer to the ethical principle that minority cultures should be preserved and the term "genocide" has been brought up with regard to the prospect of diminishing the deaf population by making deaf children hear (Lane and Bahan 1998).

While the Deaf World argument against cochlear implants may conflict with established principles of medical ethics, such as the physicians' responsibility towards the individual patient versus the claims of a subculture that needs to recruit new members, there may be lessons to be learnt from this discussion. In particular, it shows that the ethical debate on medical implantation should take into account the social and cultural notions of disease, human diversity and the conditions under which patients will live both with and without implants (Hansson 2005; Englert 2006) in order to avoid social discrimination.

It is utterly possible that other neural implants will be rejected by different social groups. On similar grounds, neuroenhancement will not readily be embraced by all members of the human society.

3.5.2 Enhancement

There's no question there will be a tremendous number of advances in the future that will include devices, whether electrical or mechanical, which will enhance the function of our organs.
Steve Goldstein[17]

Humanity's ability to alter its own brain function might well shape history as powerfully as the development of metallurgy in the Iron Age.
Martha Farah[18]

At least in principle, technical devices can be constructed to improve functions in healthy humans beyond normal levels. However, a variety of science fiction scenarios involving cyborgs and the imminent transformation of the human race into a semi-electronic species have left the public rather perplexed and provoked over-reactions directed against any scientific progress in the field of neural prosthetics. To avoid even more confusion, ethical analysis should strive to separate realistic forecasts from the more speculative ones. Still, one should also be aware of the accelerating pace of implant technology, driven mainly by the current trends in microcomputing, neuroscience and medicine (see sections on the technological basis of central neural prosthesis above).

From a physician's point of view, it would be an obvious reaction to dismiss the possibility of enhancement with reference to the traditional task of medicine, which is to treat and prevent diseases, not to improve humanity in general. But, as mentioned before, the distinction between "disease" and "health" or "normal" and "abnormal" is not as clear as it may appear. The definition of "normality" and "diversity" largely depends on social values (see Chapter 6).

> Some conditions previously regarded as diseases are now thought of as normal states of the mind or body. Others that were previously perceived as variations of normality are now regarded as diseases. Homosexuality is an example of the former, attention deficit hyperactivity disorder of the latter. (Hansson 2005)

---

[17] Professor of Orthopedic Surgery and Bioengineering at the University of Michigan (2003).

[18] Farah 2004.

Several factors contribute to our understanding and intuitions about whether treatment should be offered for a condition. Short stature has often been cited as an example. One child can be short because of his genotype, the other owing to some identified dysfunction such as growth hormone deficiency. While both may suffer equally from short stature, insurance companies have chosen to pay for growth hormone treatment only for the child with diagnosable growth hormone deficiency – a position that appears hard to defend from an ethical point of view (Daniels 2000) as long as growth hormone is just regarded as a growth factor leaving its other functions in the body aside.

Visual impairment as a function of older age (presbyopia) is treated as a matter of course and no one questions that glasses are being paid for by health insurance. Would we assume the same view if a neural prosthesis became available for the treatment of age-related cognitive decline?

The "normality" concept does not always appear to be helpful in deciding what measures are acceptable as treatments. On the other hand, this does not mean that all kinds of enhancement should be readily accepted. If side effects are known to be severe for a specific method of enhancement, the method will probably be rejected. An implant that enhances attention, but reduces to three the number of hours the implanted person is awake during day-time, will not be regarded as desirable by everybody.

The argument that some methods of enhancements may not be acceptable, however, is no objection against neural enhancement as such. A variety of questions immediately come to mind when discussing this issue:

- What do we intend by "enhancing" human beings?
- What does "perfectibility of human beings" mean?
- Is enhancement of human capabilities by invasive measures desirable at all?
- Should the decision to enhance one's bodily or mental capabilities be left to the individual's desire?
- Does personal identity change as a "side effect" with electronic implants in the brain?
- Should "lifestyle implants" or commodity devices be allowed to enhance the well-being of healthy people?
- Will the feeling of happiness be provided by electrical stimulation in the central nervous system? Will addiction be the consequence?
- Will all enhancing implants have only reversible impact on the human body and/or in the human psyche and how can reversibility be preserved?
- Are memory-enhancing implants acceptable if they improve selected memories on cost of erasing others?
- Does a human being cease to be human if some parts of his or her brain are supplemented by electronic implants?
- How far can electronic brain interfaces give an individual, or a group, specific capabilities that could become a threat to society?

- Should future people be stronger and more intelligent than contemporary people?
- Provided an enhancement is universally and equally available to everybody, should it be prohibited or encouraged in a competitive situation?
- Will there be need for new legislation to regulate competition and societal rules in a community that is populated with temporary and/or permanently enhanced human beings.
- Is there a difference between enhancing basic (e.g. attention, arousal, decision-making, lust) and specific cognitive functions (e.g. short-term memory, mathematical or musical skills)?
- If a particular intervention for enhancement results in side effects that require treatment, should the cost of this treatment be covered by insurance? Should insurance companies offer special options at additional costs to customers to cover the risks of enhancement?

The list could be continued almost endlessly and there will hardly be a societal consensus on upcoming enhancement technologies in the near future. Moreover, a variety of normative, legal, and specific philosophical issues related to personal identity is involved in this context which will be addressed in Chapters 5 and 6.

At this point, however, it would appear possible to touch on some basic principles that should be respected with regard to enhancement by central neural interfaces. First of all, a stringent risk assessment must be available before implementing a new enhancement technique. While all new technologies potentially have side effects, manipulation of the human mind clearly raises the stakes and should not be performed without full awareness of the consequences.

In 2005, the European Group on Ethics, an advisory group to the European Commission stated that implantation should be excluded if there are less invasive and less risky ways to achieve the same goal (Hermerén et al. 2005). However, one could easily imagine circumstances when an implant might be more acceptable than an external device even if the effect of both systems were identical. There is certainly no uni-dimensional answer to the question to what extent it would be reasonable to improve human capabilities by neuroelectronic implants.

Whatever one's personal opinion on this issue, it should be clear that enhancing implants will probably not be equally available to everybody from the outset. It is also hard to see how their costs could be covered by public financial resources. While treatment of patients with neural prostheses may level social imbalances and re-establish equal chances for the patient, enhancement with similar implants could potentially lead to the formation of elites and a considerable social bias (Parens 1995b; Maguire and McGee 1999; Roskies 2002).

One may speculate on the social consequences of an enhancement of larger groups of human beings, including global issues with respect to a transformation of the whole human race by all sorts of technologies (Kurzweil 1992, Kurzweil 2000; Hughes 2004; Kurzweil 2006), but despite a tremendous potential there is no clear technological basis for such a discussion at this point of time. Still it is conceivable that persons who have received certain enhancing interventions may form subcultures. Enhancement may also change our concept of normality. "Non-enhanced" people may be regarded as "less than normal". These people may feel a pressure to become enhanced as well and follow a coercive drive while struggling not to fall behind their fellows (Hansson 2005).

Therefore, issues of distributive and procedural justice with respect to such enhancements should be part of a discussion that anticipates the future development in this field (see our chapter on recommendations).

3.6 Futuristic Scenarios

By the end of this century, I don't think there will be a clear distinction between human and machine.

...some people have expressed the wish to remain 'unenhanced' while at the same time keeping their place at the top of the intellectual food chain.

Ray Kurzweil

Looking into the future, it may be predicted that telerecording and telestimulation of the brain will be widely used.

José Delgado

Is it more important to remain 'human' or that we are 'persons'?

James Hughes (in "Citizen Cyborg")

The interaction between the brain and a computer or any electro-biomechanical system via an electrode interface does already allow for controlling machines "by thought alone". In principle, similar interfaces working in the opposite direction can be installed to evoke feelings and thoughts in human beings by electrical stimulation. They could also be established as commodity devices e.g. to instil pleasure or – in abuse – to control the mood and the emotions of the recipient.

These real possibilities have stimulated science fiction writers and movie makers all over the world. Their fantasies in turn have appealed to the military, which currently spends several fortunes in the creation of soldiers with enhanced abilities, and raised considerable debate (Maguire and McGee 1999; Altmann 2004). Transhumanists and computer visionaries paint the picture of a future in which many or all humans are enhanced, multiplying our powers by sensors, actuators, additional memory, and computational capacity. It is speculated that our minds will be scanned, uploaded to a computer and transferred onto "cyborgs". Apart from the question of the motivation behind this and apart from the fact that all this is hypothetical today, those scenarios are not irrelevant to the ethical discussion. Experience from other areas has shown that the development of neuroimplants may easily become subject to non-reflected counterreactions feeding from dangers presumably posed by technologically created cyber monsters. This may lead to the blocking of financial resources for any research in the field.

A common fear is that, if temptations like sensory enhancement and external manipulation by neuronal implants come into consideration, ethical boundaries are likely to be overrun with ease.

In 2002 Kevin Warwick, a professor of cybernetics at the University of Reading, U.K., has (probably not deliberately) fuelled those fears when he connected an advanced computer chip to a nerve and implanted it into his arm. When Warwick bended the index finger, the amplified nerve signals delivered by the chip and transmitted via the internet were sufficient to remote-control an artificial device several thousand miles away. As Warwick was experimenting on himself, permission from a formal ethics board was not required for the experiment. Scientifically, if we consider speech or Morse code, long-distance transfer of human signals per se is not a novelty. It can be done with any other human sign, even with EEG activity derived from the brain.

What is new, however, is that Warwick has established a direct interface to his nervous system connecting electrodes to nerves by an invasive procedure. This is publicly regarded as a first step to mould humans with technical parts to become what is known from science fiction as "cyborgs".

A retinal implant is not confined to detect only the visible spectrum of light. Once the technology works it may well be used to transform infrared light waves and provide its recipient with night vision. Ultraviolet light may also be "seen" by a retinal implant user as well as ultrasound be "heard" by means of an auditory implant. Blinding effects by bright light or extreme noise may be controlled by the electronics integrated in a sensory implant, and visual time resolution may be enhanced significantly, providing Mr. Superhuman with a clear advantage over his non-implanted contemporaries. In addition, he will receive an artificial hippocampus to booster his memory capacity.

He will be equipped with implants in his central nervous system that can act both ways: to remote-control technical devices (telekinesis) and to modulate his brain activity in order to bestow him with confidence as well as enhanced attention and drive.

He receives information from remote places via transcranial magnetic stimulation without the need for verbal communication or direct electrical interfaces to his brain and he controls an army of "cyborgs" by mind switches and thought translation devices. By external scanning devices he can "read" the mind of his fellows and enemies before they are even aware of their own thoughts.

It is conceivable that not everyone is thrilled at these prospects. It must be kept in mind, however, that while no reasonable mechanisms have been proposed for most of the plots involving "cyborg" technology, the human race already commands a range of simple and efficient means to control and manipulate people (Hansson 2005).

While there is certainly no point in trying to stop the development of central neural implants, an early and thoughtful discussion of their potential benefits and risks will lay the ground for a responsible application of this very promising technology.

3.7 Summary

Connecting electronic devices with the central nervous system already is routine medical practice. At the same time, the technology holds

- promise for future medical applications,
- a potential for enhancing human capabilities and
- room for a lot of pure speculation reflected in science fiction stories and movies.

To distinguish clearly between these aspects and to analyse scientifically the controversial positions in the current public debate on possible social consequences, there are two excellent advisers: history and current trends in neural electronics.

Although we have known since the days of Galvani and Volta in the late 18th century that nerves could be excited by electric current, it was not until the 1960s, before computer technology created the possibility to manufacture miniaturised electronic devices that could be implanted in their completeness into the human body, omitting the need for wired connections to large laboratory equipment. It almost seems natural that the first patients to be considered candidates for such implants were those who suffered from loss of an entire sense: the profoundly deaf. The cochlear implant, transforming the sound detected by a microphone into electrical stimulation conveyed to the hearing nerve by more than 20 electrodes, today is the most successful neural prosthesis with more than 200,000 carriers worldwide, a majority of them capable of communicating via telephone (if only to a limited extent when compared to normal-hearing people).

In fact, the implant today has been improved to such an extent that some patients have been fitted with a cochlear implant on one side and a conventional hearing aid to improve hearing remnants on the contralateral side. In these patients an artificial sensory channel "cooperates" with a severely impaired, but still functioning physiological channel on the opposite side – a true "cyborg" scenario. Technology has advanced to create similar implants that connect directly to the brainstem. Hearing quality with these devices, however, is far worse than with cochlear implants.

Complete loss of vision was another challenge, and retinal implants are now capable of delivering the whole range of light intensity visible to man. A current subretinal implant (40x40 elements on a 3x3 mm chip) can provide a spatial resolution of 0.6 degrees, a visual field of about 12 degrees and a visual acuity of 0.1. Clinical trials with similar subretinal and with epiretinal implants in blind patients are under way. Cortical visual implants have progressed to a point where discrimination of shapes and localisation of objects appears to be an achievable goal, allowing selected blind patients a rough orientation in the environment. In a wider sense, these implants connecting an electronic device to the cortex – the thin neural layer on the brain's surface – are actually human-computer interfaces (HCIs) – devices that can restore lost motor or sensory-motor function. This term, however, is now exclusively used for neuroelectronic interfaces that do not stimulate, but pick up the brain's electrical activity and utilise it to give paralysed patients control of robotic limbs or communication devices such as a computer.

The non-invasive variant of the HCI has often been referred to as brain-computer interface (BCI), but it is the invasive brain-machine interface (BMI) with its advantage of utilising localised and fast neuronal electrical activity that has recently attracted most public attention. In 2005, a 96-electrode array penetrating into the so-called "arm knob", an area in the brain's motor cortex that controls movement of the arm and the hand, was implanted in a tetraplegic patient at Duke University. Decoders allow the patient to open e-mails and operate devices such as a television set, even while conversing. He can also open and close a prosthetic hand, and perform simple actions with a multi-jointed robotic arm.

Of course these achievements, primarily intended to provide medical help when all other treatment options fail, spark imagination and even scientific projects to enhance performance of healthy human beings. With the risks of electrode implantation and device failures becoming increasingly manageable, it is at least conceivable to provide humans with additional artificial limbs which could be controlled by voluntarily generated electrical brain activity. Non-verbal, invisible communication could be accomplished with HCIs, mood could be altered, and confidence could be boosted by electrical stimulation of specific areas in the brain or to some extent – with fewer potential risks – by stimulation of the vagal nerve. One of the reasons why such direct HCIs are not considered for "normal" humans is that these technologies still require a more or less invasive approach and relatively coarse arrays of electrodes implanted into the human CNS.

With the improvement of telemetric stimulation, avoiding the necessity of direct electrode-tissue contact, sensory enhancement may be not so far-fetched an idea anymore. Even nowadays, some forms of sensory enhancements do not have to involve invasive approaches (like ultrasound hearing with sonar equipment or infrared vision with night sensing glasses). Implants to achieve the same effect will only be accepted if they are absolutely safe. An implant that could effectively and significantly enhance cognitive capacities like memory, which today is far from feasible, may be more readily accepted – even with considerable risks and side effects involved. If there were ever a way to extend human cognitive capacity by directly connecting the central nervous system to an artificial device at a very low-risk ("memory chip"), it is hard to see why people would not want to take advantage of such possibility, especially if it were based on electronic interfaces that can be turned off at any time.

With every new step in the development of electronic neural implants, there will be a potential for abuse. To many, enhancement by connecting electronic devices to the human brain will appear, at least prima facie, morally suspect. A variety of science fiction scenarios involving cyborgs and the imminent transformation of the human race into a semi-electronic species have left the public rather perplexed and provoked over-reactions directed against any scientific progress in the field of neural prosthetics. There will be others to argue that these technologies offer an opportunity to make life even more worth living – provided that society will respond to the implicit social challenges inherent to all novel methods of intervening in the brain.

4 Electrical Brain Stimulation for Psychiatric Disorders[19]

4.1 *Focal High Frequency Electrical Brain Stimulation*

During the past decades focal high frequency electrical stimulation of the human brain has been used in order to treat the symptoms of several neurological disorders, including Parkinson's disease, essential tremor, dystonia, epilepsy and Tourette's syndrome. In the human brain neuronal circuitries have been detected which are responsible for motor control, others enable reception of information from the different sense organs (vision, hearing, sensation, taste, smell), still others are responsible for emotion, sexual behaviour, intelligence, memory etc. These circuitries do not simply exist in parallel to one another. Rather, there exist important connections in between them. Transmission of information runs via action potentials within one neuron and via neurotransmitters being released at the synapses in between neurons. Action potentials are transient electrical depolarisations of the cell membrane which propagate the signal from one place to another in the cell. Technically, it is possible to intervene with the electrical activity of a neuron by simply administering in the neighbourhood of that neuron an electrical field, which changes over time at a frequency in clinical practice usually between about 50 to 180 Hz (figure 4.1). In patients, this treatment is performed by means of implanting an electrode in a certain area of the brain. The electrode can be connected to an extension cable and an external current source. The extension cable and current source may be externalised in order to test the effectiveness of the treatment. Once short term efficacy of the treatment is proven, the stimulation system may be internalised. In many centres, the external phase is bypassed because of the risk of infection and because a high number of patients proceed to internalisation anyway.

Typically, the neurostimulator is implanted subcutaneously in the chest or in the abdomen and the extension cable runs below the skin passing behind the ear, connecting electrode and neurostimulator. There are new stimulators, currently under development (but not yet on the market), which are much smaller in size and which may be implanted subcuta-

---

[19] The principal author of this chapter, B. N., would like to thank Prof. Paul Cosyns, Dr. Loes Gabriëls, Dr. Kris van Kuyck, Mr. John Das, Mrs. Marleen Welkenhuysen, Dr. Herwig Neefs, Prof. Jan Gybels, the members of the international obsessive-compulsive-disorder-deep-brain-stimulation-collaborative-group, the members of the commission for neurosurgery for psychiatric disorders, the patients, their families and their psychiatrists for their collaboration.
The Research Council of the KU Leuven (project nr OT-98-31, project OT-03-57 and project VIS-02-007), the FWO (project nr G. 0273.97.N) and the SBO (project nr 50151, 2005) provided financial support. Medtronic Inc., QUEST program (L1170) provided the stimulating devices.

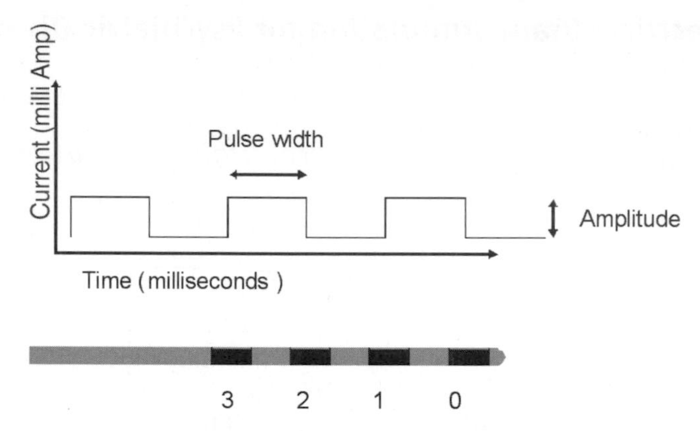

Figure 4.1: Current Applied via a DBS Electrode over Time

Above: the current changes over time. Sometimes instead of the current the potential difference (expressed in voltage) is used, but in this case the impedance should be known.

Below: illustration of a quadripolar electrode, which is implanted inside the brain.

neously on the cranium itself. Interaction with the stimulator becomes feasible through an external device which communicates with the implanted stimulator by means of a wireless connection. Thereby it is possible to vary different stimulation parameters (frequency, amplitude, pulse width etc.), to change the separate electrical contacts into anode, cathode or neutral and to obtain the history of the stimulation and the battery life. Radio-frequency systems, which obviate the need to replace the stimulator once the battery is empty, also exist, but are no longer frequently used because with this system an antenna is stuck to the skin on top of the implanted stimulator. This antenna is connected to an external stimulator via a wire. The patient can then only receive stimulation when carrying the external stimulator, wire and antenna, meaning that stimulation cannot be continued, for example, when bathing or swimming. It may also lead to skin irritation above the implanted stimulator. Rechargeable implantable systems for deep brain stimulation (DBS) are not yet available on the market, but the system is already used in spinal cord stimulation to treat chronic neuropathic pain.

Electrical brain stimulation was primarily used to treat pain and spasticity. The application of electrical brain stimulation for the symptomatic treatment of Parkinson's disease, which is best known to the public, came only later. Parkinson's disease is a disorder characterised by akinesia (the inability to start a movement), rigidity (an increased tone due to a lesion in the basal ganglia), tremor and postural instability. Many of those patients also have other symptoms such as problems with speech, writing, cognition, etc. The underlying basis is a degeneration of dopaminergic neurons in the substantia nigra. The first treatment of Parkinson's disease is antiparkinson medication. Dyskinesia and on-off fluctuations are the most common side effects of the treatment, which usually arise after three to five years of using such drugs. If tremor is the main symptom and the side effects become too severe or if the medication does not help sufficiently, then a lesion can be produced in a specific brain region and in a controlled manner by thermocoagulation in order to diminish the tremor. This is done by stereotactic insertion of an electrode in the ventral intermediate nucleus of the thalamus (Vim). The temperature of the tip of that electrode is subsequently increased (usually to 80°C) for a certain amount of time (usually one minute). The consequence of this procedure is a burn lesion in the thalamus or thalamotomy. The advantage of such lesion surgery is that, after surgery, the signs and symptoms are gone and no further continuing administration of current is necessary. However, in case of side effects (e.g. ataxia, dysarthria, paresis) one can only hope that those side effects diminish with time due to a healing process, but occasionally the side effects remain. It sometimes also happens that the effect of the lesion vanishes, which then calls for an iterative surgery.

In the 1980s researchers in Grenoble conducted extensive studies into the possibility of continuous high frequency electrical stimulation of the Vim (Benabid et al. 1991). Although the mechanism through which electrical brain stimulation acts is not entirely known, several possible mechanisms have been proposed (Benabid et al. 2005). Whilst the current is being administered to the brain tissue, the symptom tremor disappears. However, as soon as the current supply is switched off, the tremor reappears. The disadvantage of this system is the continuous need for current supply and the subsequent need for the replacement of batteries when they are depleted. By contrast, the main advantages of this system are the reversibility and adaptability of stimulation parameters in case of side effects, or in case of evolution of the disease and an aggravation of the symptoms. In these cases, the stimulation parameters, and in particular the amplitude, can be increased. If unwanted side effects arise, the stimulation parameters may be altered and, in the worst case, the whole stimulation system can be removed.

Besides the treatment of parkinsonian tremor, Vim stimulation is also beneficial for the treatment of essential tremor, tremor in the case of multiple sclerosis and posttraumatic tremor. For all these conditions, both the lesioning procedure and electrical stimulation of the Vim induce similar beneficial effects.

In addition, many symptoms of Parkinson's disease can be abolished by performing a pallidotomy (a lesion in the internal part of the globus pallidus, GPi) or electrical stimulation of the GPi. However, the beneficial effects of the electrical stimulation of the subthalamic nucleus (STN) on most of those symptoms seem to be superior to the effects induced by pallidal stimulation. STN stimulation is now the most frequently performed surgical intervention in patients suffering from Parkinson's disease. The Vim, GPi and STN are all nuclei that are connected with each other as parts of one motor circuitry, which also explains why electrical stimulation of these different structures may produce similar effects in terms of symptom relief. Very recently, another target, the pedunculo-pontine nucleus (PPN), has been addressed (Plaha and Gill 2005; Mazzone et al. 2005), which seems to improve symptoms such as freezing during the ON period and gait problems, which are not alleviated by STN stimulation. The striking aspect of this new target is that, according to the physiological data provided by animal experiments, the improvement is obtained at low frequency, therefore meaning that the nucleus has to be excited, instead of being inhibited. In clinical practice this may mean that four electrodes are implanted in a patient suffering from Parkinson's disease with freezing in the ON period: two in the STN driven at high frequency, and two in PPN stimulated at low frequency.

For the treatment of dystonia, both pallidotomy and electrical stimulation of the GPi have been performed with moderate to good results. Preliminary data have been reported on the clinical application of high frequency stimulation of the STN, and the old thalamic target used by Irving Cooper in the fifties is now being reconsidered. At present, most neurosurgeons believe that, in general, electrical stimulation is the way to proceed because of the reversibility and adaptability of the treatment. There are some observations pointing in the direction of an increased risk of suicide resulting from STN stimulation (although there is no real proof of a causal link between STN stimulation and suicide at this moment). Recent data would tend to support the hypothesis that suicidal tendencies result from a multiplicity of factors, from the strong withdrawal effects caused by the decreases in drug dosage, which are facilitated by STN stimulation, to societal changes secondary to the major, and rather sudden, improvement experienced by the patients, without ruling out a possible involvement of the limbic part of STN. In line with the role of societal factors, one might mention that suicides have been reported in the case of other highly successful surgeries, such as temporal lobectomies to treat intractable epilepsy, as well as in cardiac bypass surgery. The neurosurgical team in Leuven had one STN stimulated Parkinson's disease patient with suicidal thoughts, which decreased upon changing the stimulation parameters.

Technological innovations in brain stimulation are currently under development in various research projects, but are not, as yet, ready for clinical application. These include the miniaturisation of electrodes and stimulators, the use of nanotechnology, telemonitoring, telemedicine and telecontrol. In the case of telecontrol, the development of safety requirements is crucial to counter the risk of unwanted manipulation of stimulation parameters by unauthorised people.

4.2 Electrical Brain Stimulation for Psychiatric Disorders

Based upon the fact that both the production of a focal brain lesion and the administration of high frequency electrical current to the same target (e.g. Vim) induce similar beneficial effects in Parkinson's sufferers, and given that lesions in certain brain sites seem to benefit some psychiatric patients, collaborating groups in Belgium and Sweden have hypothesised that electrical stimulation would also lead to improvements in the symptoms of psychiatric patients resistant to all other therapies except lesioning procedures. However, several comments need to be made about this hypothesis:

1. Lesioning procedures have been made in different brain regions. The first such procedure developed was the lobotomy, for which Egaz Moniz received the Nobel prize in the last century. Several variants of this operation have since been developed. Lobotomies are now no longer performed because of the unpredictable response and the high morbidity of this procedure, as well as the profound and irreversible cognitive consequences. The procedure was not always performed on the request of a psychiatric team, nor under careful supervision of this team. Later, the film "One Flew Over the Cuckoo's Nest" gave a very unattractive portrayal of "psychosurgery". Stereotactic neurosurgeons have continued to optimise the brain target and nowadays the surgical interventions most frequently performed are the anterior capsulotomy (figure 4.2), the sub-

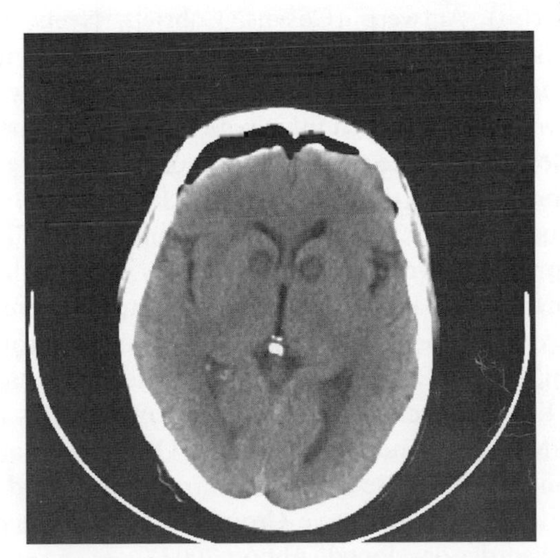

Figure 4.2: CT-scan of the Brain after Capsulotomy
Transverse computerised tomography (CT) scan of the brain, taken the day after a bilateral anterior capsulotomy was performed. The black moon-like structure in the upper part of the figure is air, which will disappear spontaneously after some days. The two "eyes" inside the brain are the two brain lesions.

caudate tractotomy, the cingulotomy and the limbic leucotomy. Those procedures, which are usually performed bilaterally, are efficient for treatment-resistant obsessive compulsive disorder (OCD) and serious treatment-resistant depression. These are also used for other disorders, but less frequently.

2. The term psychosurgery became associated with almost unacceptable surgical procedures. Consequently, the term psychosurgery is now infrequently used. In fact, the surgeon does not operate on the psyche, but on the brain, which has consequences on the behaviour of the patient. Therefore, one now describes the surgery as "neurosurgery for psychiatric disorders".
3. Thanks to the work of psychiatrist Per Mindus, the neurosurgeon Björn Meyerson, and their teams in the Karolinska hospital in Stockholm (Sweden), a lot of information was obtained about human anterior capsulotomy. Bodo Lippitz, who worked with Meyerson, has published findings on the relationship between the location of the burn lesion and the degree of beneficial effects obtained in OCD patients (Lippitz et al. 1999). The fact that the lesion was well described, provided a starting point for the Belgian/Swedish team to try to mimic the effects of a burn lesion in treatment-resistant OCD patients through the implantation of electrodes at the same spot. This work turned out to be a collaboration between groups in Leuven (van Kuyck, Van Laere, Dupont, Sunaert, Demeulemeester, Gybels, Tousseyn, Dewil, Vandenbroeck, Brak, Das, Vanlaer, Arckens, Nuttin), Antwerp (Cosyns, Gabriëls, Neefs, Vankerckhoven, Cluydts) and Karolinska (Meyerson, Mindus, Andréewitch, Linderoth, Rück). Discussions were held with A. Benabid before the first implantations in order to have as much information as possible on the experience of the development of electrical stimulation in movement disorders. A close collaboration with the industry (especially Medtronic Inc. and certain individuals – Mullett, Gielen, Rise, Stypulkowski and Langevin) was essential in order to have the correct devices, as well as to have those freely available for the first patients. Later-on, other teams were involved: Rasmussen, Greenberg and Friehs at Brown University, Providence, Rhode Island; Rezai, Malone and Montgomery at the Cleveland Clinic, Ohio; Sturm and Klosterkötter in Cologne, Germany; Curtis and Abelson at Ann Arbor, Michigan; and Goodman and Okun in Orlando, Florida. A collaboration between these different centres evolved and the deep brain stimulation (DBS) Collaborative Group for the treatment of obsessive compulsive disorder developed (Abbott 2002).
4. It seems to be the case that the administration of high frequency electrical current stimulation and the production of a focal brain lesion in Vim induce similar effects in patients suffering from Parkinson's disease. This is also correct for lesioning and stimulating the globus pallidus (GPi) for parkinsonian and dystonic patients, for STN in parkinsonian patients,

but not for stimulating or lesioning the posterior limb of the internal capsule. In the case of stimulating the internal capsule a dystonic contraction is induced and, after a stroke in the same region, a paralysis is observed. It is also not true for stimulating and lesioning the motor cortex. In the case of stimulation, patients with chronic neuropathic pain have less pain and patients with a movement disorder seem to have less abnormal movements.[20] At higher amplitudes, motor contractions can be induced and at still higher amplitudes an epileptic fit is induced. However, if the motor cortex is involved in a stroke, a flaccid paralysis is induced. Therefore, the general statement that the effects of electrical high frequency stimulation of a certain brain structure mimic the effects of a lesion in the same structure seems to apply so far only to structures that are compounds of a cluster of cells, such as the basal ganglia and the thalamus, but cannot be extended to other structures such as fibrillary structures (tracts, bundles, nerves), to structures combining large amounts of neurons and fibres, such as the cortex, or reticulated nuclei such as the lateral hypothalamus. It seems at least to depend on the brain structure involved, and also on the stimulation parameters used.

5. Electrical stimulation of the limbic system in rats is known to induce kindling, which means that the more one stimulates, the lower the threshold becomes for epileptic fits. The Leuven group has electrically stimulated the nucleus accumbens in rats, using stimulation parameters which are used for electrical stimulation of the Vim, the globus pallidus and the STN, in the case of movement disorders, and of the ventro-posteromedial and ventro-posterolateral nucleus of the thalamus in patients with chronic neuropathic pain. They found no kindling with those classical stimulation parameters. Similarly, there is no report of such kindling in the now large experience of stimulating at high frequency basal ganglia, with follow-ups as long as 19 years.

With those comments in mind, it was hypothesised that the electrical stimulation of a potentially effective heat lesion in the brain would induce symptomatic improvement in patients who suffer from very severe OCD and who are resistant to all other therapies, with the exception of a lesion procedure.

The study protocol was approved by the ethics committees of the three different hospitals involved (Universitaire Ziekenhuizen Leuven, Universiteit Antwerpen, Karolinska Hospital) and was in accordance with Helsinki Declaration of 1975 (and its 1983 revision). The selection criteria for surgical, bilateral implantation of electrodes into the anterior limbs of the internal capsules were initially the same as those for performing a capsulotomy (Cosyns et al. 1994; Meyerson 1998).

[20] Although this is still in an experimental phase, and is being investigated by the team in Nantes and Creteil led by J. P. Nguyen and Y. Keravel.

We will briefly mention the inclusion criteria used by these research groups, here. All patients suffered from *long-standing, severe, highly disabling* OCD and fulfilled the criteria for OCD (300.30) according to the Diagnostic and Statistical Manual of Mental Disorders 4th edition (DSM IV). Patients scored at least 30 out of 40 on the Yale-Brown Obsessive-Compulsive Scale (YBOCS) and 45 or less on the Global Assessment of Functioning (GAF) Scale. The level of impairment had to persist for a minimum of five years (but most patients operated on had been severely disabled for more than ten years). Reports were required on the ineffectiveness or intolerance to adequate trials of at least three selective serotonin reuptake inhibitors (SSRIs) and clomipramine augmentation strategies with antipsychotics, and cognitive behaviour therapy (CBT). Patients had to be between 18 and 60 years of age. They had to be able to understand and comply with instructions and provide their own written informed consent.

Exclusion criteria were a current or past psychotic disorder, any clinically significant disorder or medical illness affecting brain function or structure (other than motor tics or Tourette's syndrome), and current, or unstably remitted, substance abuse. If the patient did not improve after one year of capsular stimulation, the option of anterior capsulotomy would be reconsidered.

The third patient on whom the Leuven group operated will be presented as an example. She is a woman of 39 who experienced the onset of symptoms at the age of 16 and has a family history conducive to OCD. She remained single and has no children. She worked in the administrative sector until the age of 32 but lost her job due to the severity of her obsessive compulsive symptoms. She became completely non-functional and returned home to live with her parents. She had excessive toilet, washing and counting rituals, intrusive sexual thoughts and impulses and the compelling urge to touch everything. She had no tics. She was preoccupied by the thought that objects and things might not be real and might not exist. These thoughts coincided with high levels of anxiety and she developed a whole series of compulsions to ensure that objects and persons were really there. She had recurrent comorbid depressive episodes and panic attacks. She fulfilled criteria for dependent personality disorder and felt utterly dependent on significant others. Former psychopharmacological treatment included four SSRIs, clomipramine, augmentation with haloperidol, buspirone, pindolol and many benzodiazepines. She had eight years of psychoanalytic therapy and four years of cognitive behaviour therapy. During the weeks before surgery her YBOCS was 30 on 40, which would indicate severe OCD (Gabriëls 2004).

An advisory board for neurosurgery for psychiatric disorders reviewed the patients and decided upon the surgical indication for each patient. This advisory board was composed of, amongst others, psychiatrists, representatives from ethics review boards and neurosurgeons. It has an advisory

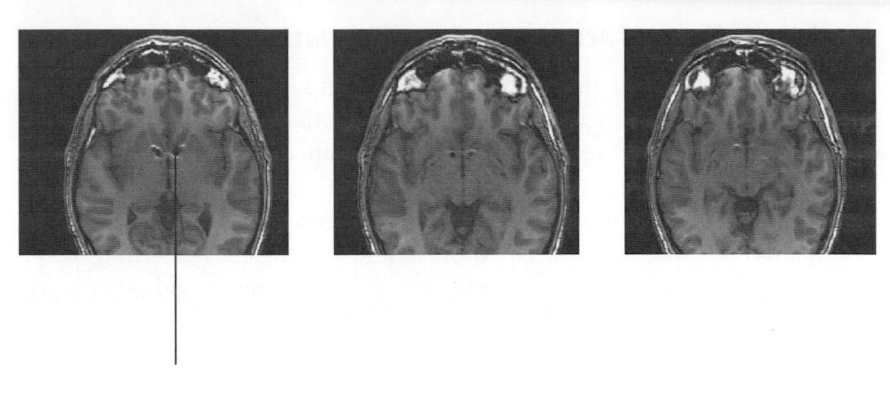

Figure 4.3: Postoperative MRI-scan of the Brain
Axial T1-weighted magnetic resonance imaging (MRI) scans in patient 8 from the Leuven-Antwerp group, showing the position of the electrodes in the brain.

role, but the decisions of this board have no legal consequences at this moment. As patients were under their treatment, psychiatrists referred patients for neurosurgical intervention. The psychiatrist was invited to present the psychiatric problem, but was not always able to attend. The patient and a close family member were repeatedly and fully informed on advantages and disadvantages of both capsulotomy and electrical brain stimulation by the psychiatrist and the surgeon independently. The patient could chose between those two interventions. The standard risks were explained.

A pisces quad compact electrode (Medtronic Inc. 3887) was bilaterally implanted in the anterior limbs of the internal capsules (figure 4.3). The distal part of the electrode entered the grey matter just below the internal capsule, because it was the experience of many neurosurgeons that this part of the brain in particular needed to be lesioned in order to obtain beneficial results when producing a burn lesion. At the time of this book's completion, the Leuven-Antwerp team had carried out implantation procedures on 14 treatment-refractory OCD patients. As far as the authors are aware, there are probably about 50 such patients world-wide.

4.3 The Clinical Effects of Stimulation

In this section, we will discuss the beneficial effects of both acute (seconds, minutes, hours or days of stimulation) and chronic (stimulation during more than two weeks) electrical stimulation. In addition, we will present some of the potential side effects and complications arising out of such procedures.

4.3.1 The Effects of Acute Electrical Stimulation

In the first two patients that were operated on in Leuven no clear beneficial effects were noticed. However, in patient three, at that time a 39 year old lady, the research team observed the following acute effects arising from bilateral electrical capsular stimulation. Without stimulation, she was sitting in front of the surgeon, motionless, with a facial expression indicative of depression and anxiety. Beside her were her mother and father. She was afraid of the surgeon and would not talk spontaneously to him. Some seconds after starting the stimulation, she stood up, approached the surgeon and started to talk to the surgeon in a less inhibited manner and in a louder voice than usual. When the stimulation was turned off, she went back to her chair and took back the same immobile posture as before. When she was stimulated again, she became talkative and started laughing and joking with the other people in the room. During this session, neither the parents, nor the patient herself, knew when and how she was being stimulated. She then received high frequency stimulation for two weeks, during which time she did not know she was being stimulated. At the end of this period, the surgeon questioned the patient, her father and her mother independently. They all responded, that more than 90% of her obsessions and compulsions had disappeared and that she had not been depressed nor anxious, but that she was sad, because she now realised that she had wasted so much time due to her compulsions over the previous 20 years. As all those observations in this one patient could still be due to coincidence or luck, a further, thorough study was made in this patient.

The stimulator was randomly on during six conditions and off during another six conditions. During four of the six stimulator-on conditions (0-1-2-3-case+, contact 0 being the most caudal of the four contacts, and case being the contact at the level of the stimulator box; pulse width 200 μsec; frequency 100 Hz; amplitude 4.7 V), the patient was unable to know whether the stimulator was on or off, according to the patient's own report. During the other two of the six stimulator-on conditions (5V), the patient felt a headache upon switching the stimulator on, but the headache disappeared after around ten seconds. During each condition, three small tests were performed (Profile of Mood States [POMS], "show that you are ..." and a Bourdon-Wiersma test). The psychiatrist and the psychologist, who were present when the surgeon changed the stimulation parameters, but who were unaware of the precise stimulation condition (the patient was of course also unaware of this) were asked independently from each other at the end of the session in which these twelve conditions had been all administered, when they thought the stimulator had been on or off. The answers of both observers were totally correct in all twelve conditions, and these questions were asked *before* they analysed the tests which the patient had taken. They could guess the condition just by watching the patient. This means that changes in the behaviour induced in the patient by means of anterior capsular stimulation can be clearly observed, just like the disappearance of tremor upon switching on a thalamic stimulator in a tremor patient.

The whole afternoon session was videotaped and each condition was shown in a random order to independent resident psychiatrists who had to rate different outcome parameters from 0 (not present) to 3 (clearly present), while they were unaware of the condition. In this patient, they rated the social contact, communication, flow of ideas, assertiveness and mobility to be significantly increased (median: off 1, on 2) and the doubt was significantly decreased during electrical stimulation (Off 2, On 1, $p<0.05$, Mann Whitney *U* test and Kendall's coefficient of concordance)[i]. The residents in psychiatry guessed on/off-position correctly in 93% of the evaluations.

Those results show beneficial effects in this patient with treatment resistant OCD. However, these results of acute testing do not describe the effects on obsession and compulsion, depression and anxiety, which are important outcome parameters in OCD treatment. Therefore, chronic evaluations were performed which will be described later.

Having observed these effects in patient 3, the research team went back to patients 1 and 2 with the knowledge of the stimulation parameters which had reduced symptoms in patient 3. In patient 1, there were only some limited beneficial effects, but these were not significant enough to be able to state that this patient clearly improved as a result of the treatment. In patient 2, however, symptom reduction could be induced. In order to illustrate the effects induced by capsular stimulation in this patient, a video was made during an exposure session to document the changes in patient behaviour between the stimulator being on and the stimulator being off. One of this patient's problems, amongst many other much more important problems, was that she was convinced that when she touched a plant, it would emit fluids that would intoxicate other people. She was convinced that plants with white stripes were particularly toxic, but she thought the most toxic plants of all were those with red leaves. During the exposure session, she was progressively presented with these plants. She was initially asked to look at a plant and then touch it. Later she was asked to do the same with the plant with white stripes etc. When the stimulator was off, she clearly had lots of difficulty touching these plants and repeatedly asked the question whether it was dangerous to touch them. Her face and voice expressed sadness and anxiety. When the stimulator was turned on, the sadness and anxiety disappeared, she spoke like a normal person and she started to touch the plants spontaneously and even cleaned them and removed the dead leaves. When she was asked to crush the leaves in her hands she had no problem doing so. She even subsequently licked the fluid from her hand, and when she found out she had a small red leaf from the red plant in her mouth she did not care and swallowed it.

This case shows that the symptoms disappeared, but that the stimulation parameters were set such that she did not even realise that the leaf she ate might actually have been poisonous. This, however, was not the case when the stimulation amplitude was slightly decreased. It shows that a person can actually receive too much electrical stimulation (meaning too high an amplitude, an incorrect pulse width or frequency, or a combination of those factors). The adverse effects of this may be a change in behaviour. This situation can be compared with drug treatment: a certain pathological condition may react to drug treatment only if a sufficient quantity of the drug is administered. However, if too much of the drug is administered, the patient may experience adverse effects. The excessively high amplitude in patient 2 actually induced an overconfidence, which was clearly a side effect. It should be clear for the reader that the examples of symptoms mentioned here were not the main reason for the operation per se. The reason for the surgery was the extremely severe treatment-resistant suffering of the patient over many years. In addition, all these patients met the inclusion and exclusion criteria as mentioned above.

Since the above experiments were conducted, the Leuven team has been able to induce at least some small beneficial effects through this type of stimulation in all electrode-implanted patients up till now. However, this does not necessarily mean that they consider them all to be good responders, as this presupposes at least a certain degree of beneficial effects. As another example of the acute effects of electrical stimulation of the anterior limbs of the internal capsule, we will present the results experienced by OCD patient 8. One of the problems of this patient was the disgust for fat. He would not eat a hamburger, would not eat butter, would not touch butter or even talk about butter etc. Once he had fully awoken from the surgical implantation of the electrodes, he was asked under several conditions how tense he felt, and to give his answer on a scale between 0 and 10 (a rating on the Subjective Units of Distress Scale [SUDS]). At first he was not stimulated. A small transparent pot filled with butter was presented to him. His SUDS-score was 8 and was lower than during the preoperative period and can be interpreted as an effect of the damage, induced by the insertion of the electrode, which can be called a capsulotomy effect. This can be compared with a thalamotomy effect after implantation of an electrode in the Vim for the treatment of tremor. In movement disorders, the beneficial effect due to the insertion of the electrode, without the administration of an electrical current, almost always disappears. When the right stimulator was switched on, without the patient's knowledge, he replied that he had the impression he had experienced a placebo effect. He said he was surprised that the pot with butter did not really disturb him anymore. His SUDS-score was 3. When he was stimulated with the left stimulator only, his SUDS-score was between 6 and 7. It turned out later-on that he has better effects induced by the right than by the left stimulator, an effect that was observed in several of the Leuven patients. When he was subsequently stimulated on the right side, his SUDS-scores immediately dropped to 2 or 3, which confirms the previous finding. These are, of course, only simple descriptions of observed effects but they are nonetheless illustrative of the type of effect one can expect. At this moment in time, it is still not clear whether the left-right differences are due to asymmetrical implantations or due to real differences in the functions of the left and right sides of the brain. It must also be remembered that a disgust for fat was only one of the many problems from which this patient suffered.

The final case study that will be detailed here is that of patient 10, in whom electrical stimulation *during* the implantation of the electrodes (under local anaesthetic) induced a contralateral smile and a feeling of well-being. The patient also experienced a transient reddening of the face, began to sweat and became more talkative (Okun et al. 2004). Initially she was only stimulated at a very low amplitude. However, on day 10 she was stimulated at 3V, 120 µsec, 130 Hz, 0-case+. This stimulation induced for a period of about two minutes a laughter which caused the other people in the room to laugh as well. She felt really good. However, after leaving her on the same stimulation parameters for around 15 minutes she felt her heart beat and she started to cry. In addition, she said she still had obsessions. Only after several weeks of stimulation were the obsessions and compulsions completely abolished and she is said to be leading a normal life since.

4.3.2 The Effects of Chronic Electrical Stimulation

In Leuven and Antwerp eight patients were subjected to randomised double-blind cross-over design tests (table 4.1, figure 4.4). The main aim was to show to the patients themselves, and to the treating physicians, the degree of effect in a

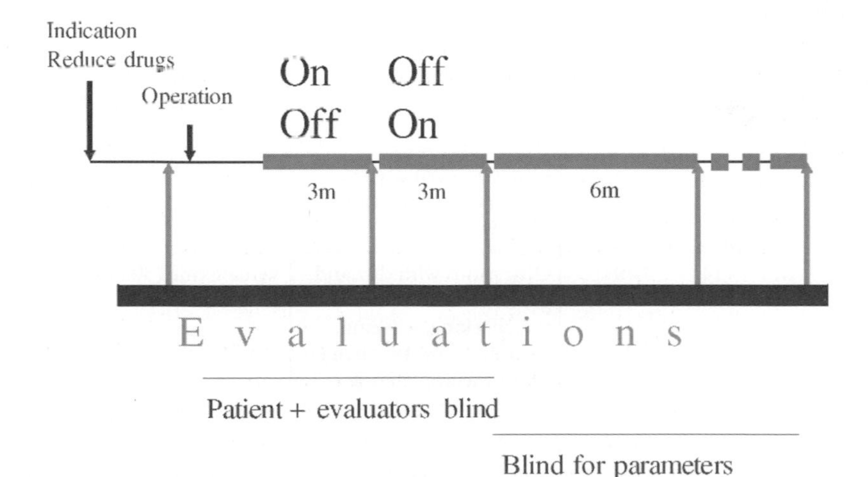

Figure 4.4: Experimental Design
Randomised double blind cross-over design used in the Leuven-Antwerp study.

Table 4.1: Patient Description. Adapted with Minor Modifications from Gabriëls (2004)
Short description of the eight OCD patients that received electrode implants and were subjected to the randomised double-blind cross-over test. M/F = male to female ratio; C1 to C8 = case 1 to case 8.

	M/F	Age of onset OCD	Age at surgery	Most severe OCD symptoms at surgery	Psychopharmacologic treatment at surgery
C1	M	12	35	Obsession with the "sound of silence", fear of hair growth	Lormetazepam (0.5mg)
C2	F	24	52	Contamination, poisonous plants, checking, asking questions	Sertraline (150mg/d) Prazepam (60mg/d) Diazepam (10mg/d) Trazodone (100mg/d)
C3	F	16	38	Obsession with whether things actually exist or not, touching things, counting, washing rituals	Fluoxetine (20mg/d) Clomipramine (50mg/d) Lorazepam (3.75mg/d)
C4	M	12	35	Extreme fear of poisoning others, obsessed with failing to assist people in need, checking, hand washing, cleaning rituals	Clomipramine (150mg/d) Risperidone (6mg/d) Alprazolam (4mg/d) Lormetazepam (2mg/d)
C5	F	14	40	Contamination (urine, faeces, sperm), washing rituals, toilet routine, repeating sentences and questions, hoarding	Fluoxetine (40mg/d) Thioridazine (50mg/d) Alprazolam (4mg/d)
C6	M	16	37	Intrusive aggressive behaviour, checking behaviour	Clomipramine (225mg/d) Olanzapine (20mg/d)
C7	F	20	39	Order and symmetry, cleaning rituals, incompleteness	Clomipramine (75mg/d)
C8	M	14	40	Obsessions with dirt and grease, order and symmetry, checking, washing, cleaning, repeating behaviours, incompleteness	Venlafaxine (300mg)

controlled manner. Once the advisory board for neurosurgery and psychiatric disorders had approved the surgery, drug intake was reduced to a level which was bearable for the patient. Having optimised the stimulation parameters, the patients entered a cross-over design experiment, in which they were stimulated for three months, followed by a period of three months without stimulation. In other patients, the sequence was the other way around: three months of stimulation followed after three months without stimulation. The patients were randomly assigned to these groups through the toss of a coin. The evaluators (psychiatrists and psychologists), as well as the patients, were kept unaware of the stimulation condition, and they could decide to shorten the period of 3 months if the patient was in great distress. Extensive psychiatric and neuropsychological testing was performed before surgery and at the end of each three month segment of the trial. A description of all measured parameters during both the period of stimulation and the period of non-stimulation can be found in several references (Gabriëls et al. 2003; Nuttin et al. 2003b). The primary means of measuring the outcomes was the Yale-Brown Obsessive-Compulsive Scale (YBOCS), a scale of 40 which measures obsession and compulsion. A score of less than 30/40 was used as the cut off point at which patients were excluded from surgery. Before surgery, the mean of all eight YBOCS-scores was 33, at the end of the no stimulation condition the score remained 33. However, at the end of the period of stimulation, the mean YBOCS-score decreased to 17. Six of the eight patients were considered to have responded well to their treatment, because their YBOCS-score dropped by at least 35% during stimulation. In this group of patients the level of their depression, as measured by the Hamilton Depression Scale, decreased with 50%. The patients who were operated in 1998 and experienced a good effect due to the stimulation are still benefiting from the results of stimulation treatment today (2006).

4.3.3 Side Effects and Complications

When introducing a new therapy, as much attention must be paid to the possible side effects as well as the beneficial effects. As far as we know, there are no publications available on the possible side effects and complications of this type of therapy apart from those published by Leuven-Antwerp. Therefore, only those issues uncovered by the Leuven-Antwerp group will be discussed here (Nuttin et al. 2003a; Nuttin and van Kuyck 2002; Nuttin et al. 2000; Cosyns et al. 2003).

1. Technical problems due to the limited life of batteries. The most important problem the Leuven-Antwerp team was confronted with initially was the battery power source of the stimulation devices. It needed to be replaced surgically every four to twelve months. This kind of surgery can be undertaken as outpatient treatment and under local anaesthetic, but puts the patient at risk of infections and can damage the extension cables. In patients 7, 9 and 10 the amplitudes employed approached the level of amplitudes used for the electrical brain stimulation in movement disorders and chronic pain. However, it is too early to state that the battery problem has been solved. On the other hand, Medtronic Inc. has built a stimulator with a rechargeable battery, which is being tested in patients with chronic neuropathic pain, and which could be recharged by wearing a belt now and then for a period of

patients but no clear beneficial effects have been observed. The reason for this is unclear but may be because of a slightly different electrode position. The other centres of the DBS-OCD-collaborative group have found similar effects arising from acute and chronic electrical stimulation in 26 patients as those described above. Some of these results have already been published (Sturm et al. 2003; Abelson et al. 2005) and others will be published soon. Several papers describing the effects of electrical brain stimulation in one or two cases have been published recently in the international literature on a variety of psychiatric disorders (Anderson and Ahmed 2003; Canterbury 2003; Aouizerate et al. 2004; Cosgrove 2004). For instance, a group from Paris has implanted electrodes in the STN in two parkinsonian patients who also suffered from OCD. The symptoms of both Parkinson's disease and OCD improved as a result of electrical STN stimulation (Mallet et al. 2002). These findings have been confirmed in another centre (Fontaine et al. 2004) and are currently the subject of a multicentre trial in France. Moreover, stimulating another target, the inferior thalamic peduncle, seems to decrease the symptoms of OCD.[21] All those targets are part of the limbic circuitry which is affected in OCD.

Based on the findings of the Leuven-Antwerp group that both depression and anxiety were influenced to a large extent by electrical brain stimulation in OCD patients, the logical step was to study the effects of electrical brain stimulation in patients with severe anxiety and/or depression. In Cologne, Sturm et al. found clear beneficial effects in patients suffering from anxiety. In addition, a group based in Toronto has published some promising initial results on the treatment of major depression (Mayberg et al. 2005). This group determined their target based on positron emission tomographic data. The members of the DBS-OCD collaborative group have also started to study the treatment of major depression and twelve patients have been operated on so far within this collaborative group.

In France, neurosurgery for psychiatric disorders has not been performed in the last decades. In 2002 the "Comité Consultatif National d'Ethique pour les Sciences de la Vie et de la Santé" has decided, in response to a question posed by A. Benabid (Grenoble), that lesioning procedures still may not be performed in France. However, the committee has allowed research into the use of DBS for the treatment of OCD to proceed, because of the reversibility and adaptability of the treatment (Comité Consultatif National d'Ethique pour les sciences de la vie et de la santé 2002; Goodman 2002; Gybels et al. 2002).

Looking back to the development of DBS in movement and psychiatric disorders, the research community did not know much about the basic mechanisms involved in treating these conditions, but was confronted with the severe suffering of certain patients and was looking for a reversible treatment. These two reasons were the major drives for the development of the

[21] Personal communication with Francisco Velasco, meeting of the European Society for Stereotactic and Functional Neurosurgery in Vienna, June 2004.

treatments. For the development of DBS for Parkinson's disease there was also the fact that intra-operative electrical brain stimulation had already been used for a long time to determine the site of the lesion to be made while performing a thalamotomy. A partial insight into the basic mechanisms involved in the use of DBS treatment in movement disorders followed later. For DBS in psychiatric disorders, lots of the mechanisms are still unknown. In many fields, medicine proceeds in precisely this way. One needs to have an idea of the possible risks and benefits for a patient to be treated with a new kind of therapy. However, in the initial stages at least, it is probably not essential that one understands completely how the therapy works.

Neurosurgeons are stimulating abnormally functioning networks for different conditions: for OCD one stimulates the anterior limbs of the internal capsules, the nucleus accumbens, the bed nucleus of the stria terminalis, or the limbic part of GPi (figure 4.5). All those structures are, in one way or another, connected with each other and are part of the so-called limbic system. Electrical stimulation in one of those nuclei has already been shown to

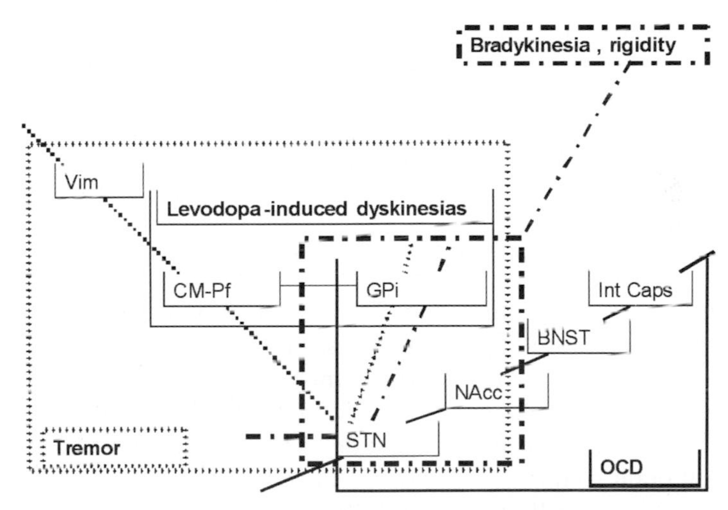

Figure 4.5: Networks
An example of different abnormally functioning networks: for OCD the anterior limbs of the internal capsules (Int Caps), the nucleus accumbens (NAcc), the bed nucleus of the stria terminalis (BNST), or the limbic part of globus pallidus (GPi) have been stimulated electrically with beneficial effects in at least one patient. All those structures are in one way or another interconnected: for bradykinesia and rigidity GPi and subthalamic nucleus (STN), for levodopa-induced dyskinesia GPi and centrum medianum-parafascicular nucleus (CM) and for tremor ventral intermediate nucleus (Vim), CM, STN and GPi.

(Figure taken with permission and adapted from Benabid, personal communication in the Europäische Akademie, March 3, 2006)

have at least some effect on the OCD-symptoms in at least one patient. Depending on which of the nuclei is stimulated, one symptom may be influenced more than another one. However, other networks exist, like the motor circuitry and this motor circuitry differs depending on which motor activity one looks at, for instance levodopa-induced dyskinesia's, tremor, bradykinesia and rigidity. As those networks do not always lie next to each other, but are interconnected, one can understand that psychiatric symptoms may arise when one is stimulating a motor network. The subthalamic nucleus is a good example. It is composed of a motor part, a limbic part and at least one other part, which is not relevant in this discussion. When treating a patient with Parkinson's disease with electrical subthalamic high frequency stimulation, the motor symptoms may improve, but this may lead to the creation of new symptoms (like confusion or euphoria) induced by the electrical stimulation of a perhaps previously normally functioning limbic network. On the other hand, electrical stimulation of the GPi or STN may be performed to treat either a motor disorder or a psychiatric disorder (e.g. OCD).

The indication for DBS in Parkinson's disease has widened over the years, as it became gradually clearer that the disadvantages of the surgery did not outweigh its possible advantages in less severe cases of Parkinson's disease. At this moment, the indication for DBS in psychiatric patients has not yet widened, but it is not impossible that a similar evolution will occur, depending on the risks and benefits of this treatment, observed in well controlled clinical trials.

4.5 Transcranial Magnetic Stimulation

In transcranial magnetic stimulation (TMS) magnetic pulses are applied to a certain region of the head by a handheld stimulating coil. This coil is connected to a stimulator, which generates those pulses. The magnetic field, which changes in time, induces an electrical current in the skin, the deeper tissue and, most interestingly of all, in different brain structures. As opposed to electrical brain stimulation described above, this technique is non-invasive. It is possible to deliver single, paired or repetitive magnetic pulses. In the latter case, one uses the term repetitive transcranial magnetic stimulation (rTMS). As an example of an effect induced by TMS, we can state that muscle contractions can be obtained above the motor cortex. Most studies have looked at effects of TMS on superficially lying brain structures.

Both electrical brain stimulation and TMS were developed in the clinic itself and only later on were basic neurobiological data obtained in order to understand some of the underlying mechanisms. TMS seems to be a safe technique. Safety guidelines have been developed and, taking into account those guidelines, TMS rarely provokes seizures and the auditory threshold does not change. The application of TMS may cause local pain resulting from the direct stimulation of those muscles directly underlying the coil and from the stimulation of facial and scalp nerves. Between 5 and 20% of patients experience headaches after rTMS sessions. Some transient cognitive changes have been observed. However, there is no indication that TMS causes brain damage. rTMS on the dorsolateral prefrontal cortex has been used in healthy subjects to elucidate the basic neurophysiology of mood modulation. In depressed patients, antidepressant effects of rTMS are transitory and, therefore, a maintenance strategy needs to be developed in order to make rTMS useful in a clinical setting. As a research tool, though, rTMS definitely seems to be a promising technique.

Therapeutic seizure induction has a strong and reliable effect on depression. Electroconvulsive therapy (ECT) is now routinely being used in several psychiatric clinics. At this moment, it is not at all clear that rTMS is better than ECT. rTMS at convulsive levels is now being developed as a more targeted form of convulsive therapy (Schlaepfer et al. 2006).

4.6 Comments on the Published Guidelines on Electrical Brain Stimulation for Psychiatric Disorders

What follows is the summary of an interview, dating from June 2005, by Mrs. Allison Abbott (Nature) with 2 of the OCD patients operated on in Leuven, who received DBS (Abbott 2005). The patients did not hear each other's answers, but the answers were in essence the same. Question 1: How severe was your disease before the operation? Answer: I would surely have committed suicide if the surgery hadn't taken place. Question 2: Do you think the surgery has changed anything? Answer: After surgery there was a major change in my life. I can enjoy life again, which was impossible before. My compulsions and obsessions are greatly reduced. They do not bother me so much anymore and I can now live with them. I am neither depressed nor anxious anymore. Question 3: Would you advise anyone else, who has the same degree of illness as you, to have the surgery? Answer (immediately, without any hesitation): Yes, without any doubt. Question 4: Don't you find it an ethical problem that an artificial stimulating device rules your life and makes you feel better? Answer (immediately): I don't see the ethical problem. It makes me feel better and I like to be better. If this is an ethical problem, then any medical treatment to improve the condition of a patient is an ethical problem.

The authors of the guidelines are the OCD-DBS collaborative group (Nuttin et al. 2002; Nuttin et al. 2003c). When they started with DBS for the treatment of OCD, they were afraid that something similar could happen as has occurred with the lobotomies for psychiatric disorders in the past. There were only general rules and the group decided to develop self-regulating guidelines that would serve as a basis for possible future of neurosurgery in the case of psychiatric disorders. The main drive for the development of DBS for OCD was the existence of very seriously ill OCD patients that need treatment. The main difference with the lesions being produced in this case is the reversibility and adaptability of the treatment. However, doctors still influence patients' behaviour and this could be conceived of as brain manipulation. This thought alone may lead the public to demand an end to the implantation of electrodes in the brain to treat psychiatric disorders. However, doctors also influence the patients' behaviour when performing much more mundane tasks such as prescribing antidepressants to those suffering from depression. Similarly, doctors may also alter the behaviour of patients simply by telling them to make lifestyle changes such as giving up smoking. Therefore, it is not necessarily bad to change the behaviour of a patient. In the case of refractory obsessive compulsive disorder, the patient suffers so much that in many cases suicide is the only alternative. If death is the outcome of the disease, then most people will not bother with a surgical intervention that aims to diminish suffering, even if the behaviour of the patient is changed. In fact, a change of behaviour is a wanted response, because obsessions and compulsions are unwanted behaviours, and if one wants to remove those, one has to change the behaviour of the patient anyway. There are many examples where behaviour is irreversibly changed due to surgical interventions. A very clear example of this is surgery for epilepsy, where a large part of the temporal lobe is removed in order to stop epileptic fits, but which often results in (irreversible) behavioural changes.

In *severe* cases of major depression, it is well known that the patient may suffer so much that suicide seems to be their only alternative. The first trials with DBS for major depression now indicate that, when the amplitude of stimulation is increased relatively quickly, hypomania may arise as an unwanted side effect. This does not occur in all patients and can be controlled. However, further clinical research is necessary to develop strategies to diminish the chance of developing hypomania. If it turns out to be impossible to avoid hypomania altogether, then it may be the case that DBS is not the best alternative for the treatment of major depression.

In order to try to prevent DBS from being used as a routine treatment at this moment without the necessary further research, the DBS-OCD collaborative group has decided to publish guidelines on "Electrical brain stimulation for psychiatric disorders". At this moment these are the only published guidelines and these will be explained in the following paragraphs. If somebody were to disagree with those guidelines, the logical step would be for that person to publish a new set of guidelines, so that these could be compared with the existing ones. It is also clear that guidelines may change over time with progress and experience.

One of the statements is: "Treatment of psychiatric patients with DBS remains investigational, however, and is *not* considered standard therapy" (Nuttin et al. 2002, 2003c). The aim of the collaborative group is to optimise the therapy before it is routinely used. The DBS-OCD collaborative group recommended that the following minimum requirements be met by those considering the application of DBS in the case of psychiatric conditions:

1. An ethics committee (e.g., the Institutional Review Board in the United States) that will have ongoing oversight of the project should approve the investigational protocol.
2. A patient assessment committee should evaluate each patient as a possible candidate for inclusion in the protocol. The role of this committee is to ensure that potential candidates meet certain medical and psychiatric criteria and are appropriate for inclusion in the study and to monitor the adequacy of the consent process. Patient assessment committees should be constituted broadly to achieve an ethically valid consensus, and they should have the opportunity to obtain independent capacity assessments when indicated. (ibid.)

In the case of the Leuven Antwerp group, this assessment committee was a self appointed advisory board and not an official committee, installed by a higher authority with legal standing.

3. Candidates for DBS surgery should meet defined criteria for severity, chronicity, disability and treatment-refractoriness. (ibid.)

   These criteria should be described in the research protocol.

4. The use of DBS should be limited solely to those patients with decision making capacity who are able to provide their own informed consent. Patient consent should be maintained and monitored throughout the process, and patients should be free to halt their participation voluntarily. (ibid.)

One of the ways this patient freedom can be dealt with is to provide the patient with a handheld programmer, which will allow the patient to switch the stimulator on or off whenever he/she wishes. It would also be possible for the patient to change stimulation amplitude, pulse width and/or frequency if the doctor agrees to this. The doctor can set the stimulation thresholds to ensure that the current remains high enough to achieve the desired beneficial effects but low enough to avoid any side effects. It is possible for the doctor not to let the patient change any stimulation parameters, but at this moment it is not possible to prevent the patient from switching the stimulator on or off, as long as the patient has a well functioning handheld programmer. Currently, the programmer is not given to the patient during the blinded periods of stimulation, because the programmer would provide a tool that could reveal to the patient whether or not he is being stimulated. However, in all protocols until now, these blinded periods are limited in time and are followed by a period of open stimulation, where the patients know the stimulator is switched on. One possible way to solve this issue could be to provide the patient the right to ask for a programmer and at least to be able to switch the stimulator on or off. This gives the patient the same freedom as when medication is prescribed: the patient can decide to take medication or not to take it. In fact, it gives them even more freedom: when a patient is admitted to the hospital, a doctor prescribes drugs which are often not explained to the patient. With the stimulation the patient will need to have given informed consent and will always be able to stop the stimulation after the blinded trial period. During the blinded period, when the patient has no handheld programmer, the patient still has the ability to withdraw from the study at any time.

On the other hand, this concept of allowing patients to change the parameters of their stimulation in order to fulfil his freedom is a double edged sword, as the patient lacks the training for programming and may end up with an inappropriately programmed system, which may open him/her up to the risk of unwanted, inefficient stimulation, which can be unpredictable and possibly harmful. The patient may even inadvertently switch the stimulator off without wanting to do so. Therefore, we do not want to impose that it is necessary to give patients such a handheld programmer.

5. Patient selection, surgical treatment, device programming, and comprehensive, regular psychiatric follow-up should be conducted at or supervised by a clinical research centre.
6. The investigative team should include specialists from the following disciplines, and they should work in close collaboration:
   a. A functional neurosurgical team with established experience in DBS.
   b. A team of psychiatrists with extensive experience in the psychiatric condition under investigation.
   c. Preferably, both of the preceding groups should have some experience in neurosurgical treatment for psychiatric disorders. If not, close consultation with experienced centres is indicated.
7. Investigators must disclose potential conflicts of interest to regulatory bodies such as ethics committees or institutional review boards and to potential enrollees during the informed consent process.
8. The surgery should be performed only to restore normal function and relieve patients' distress and suffering. (Nuttin et al. 2002, 2003c)

This last statement was included to avoid the possibility that people would try to develop DBS procedures for the purpose of improving certain mental capacities (e.g. memory) in normal, healthy individuals. As far as we know, no such surgery exists today. The reason why the DBS-OCD collaborative group imposed an opposition to such developments on themselves is that in the normal person, the advantages of the surgery are not proportional to the possible risks involved in the surgery. Moreover, being a healthy person, and having had a successful DBS procedure to change one's memory, one would have an unfair advantage over other people who did not have this surgery for this superior memory. This could lead to other people wishing to have this surgery, putting them too at an unnecessary risk. It may become an unwanted rush for the best operation and the value of a normal person without DBS might be endangered.

Continuous critical analysis of medical and ethical issues in the field of neurosurgery for psychiatric disorders should be conducted by those research centres performing such interventions in order to avoid the type of development seen in the time of Walter Freeman (Kopell and Rezai 2003).

9. The procedure should be performed to improve patients' lives and never for political, law enforcement, or social purposes." (ibid.)

This statement is in line with the previous paragraph and tries to avoid the history of "psychosurgery" repeating itself. In the case of abnormal auto- or heteroaggression, in particular, one should always distinguish the advantages of surgery for the patient and for their surroundings. This is especially so in the case of children. For further elaboration on this topic we refer to Chapter 6.

> In our experience, embarking on this type of research requires a major commitment of time, energy, and resources across disciplines before and after device implantation. DBS has the potential to offer hope for severely ill patients, but investigations in this area should proceed cautiously to maintain the public trust necessary for scientific progress. (ibid.)

With regard to TMS, rTMS and rTMS at convulsive levels, we think that, as there are very few side effects, the advantages of their use may, in several cases, seem greater than the disadvantages. However, well designed clinical studies are still needed in this field. The use of TMS or rTMS for enhancement purposes should not necessarily be disregarded on the grounds of safety. However, many complex issues arise out of this potential use of these techniques. For an in depth discussion of these issues, we refer the reader to Chapter 6, which specifically talks about the question of enhancement procedures. At this stage it suffices to note that at this time neither TMS nor rTMS are routinely used for enhancement purposes.

4.7 Summary

In electrical brain stimulation, electrodes are inserted into the brain and a high-frequency electrical current is applied directly to the brain tissue, thus reducing the symptoms of patients suffering from motor disorders (such as Parkinson's disease) or severe psychiatric diseases refractory to pharmacological treatment. While in former times surgical techniques were often used to locally destroy deep brain nervous tissue, most neurosurgeons currently prefer electrical stimulation because of the reversibility and the adaptability of the treatment.

Obsessive-compulsive disorder (OCD) and major depression are the two psychiatric indications for which electrical brain stimulation has now been shown to be successful. However, even for these two indications the technique is still in an experimental stage. The main drive for the development of electrical brain stimulation for OCD and major depression was the existence of very seriously ill patients in desperate need of treatment.

In transcranial magnetic stimulation (TMS), magnetic pulses are applied to a certain region of the head by a handheld stimulating coil. This coil is connected to a stimulator, which generates those pulses. The magnetic field, which changes over time, induces an electrical current in different brain structures. As opposed to electrical brain stimulation, this technique is non-invasive. Both electrical brain stimulation and TMS were developed in clinic practise. Only later were basic neurobiological data obtained helping to understand at least some of the underlying mechanisms responsible for their effectiveness.

Patients with deep brain electrodes can be equipped with a handheld programmer in order to enable them to decide when to receive stimulation or not. This on-/off-switch provides a practical way to counter concerns that stimulation techniques might be used to manipulate patients. However, the idea of safeguarding the patient's autonomy by allowing him or her to change stimulation parameters is a double edged sword, as the patient lacks training in programming the stimulation device. Patients themselves do not seem to consider it an ethical problem that an artificial stimulating device influences their mind as long as it makes them feel better. They compare the device with other implantable devices, such as pacemakers, which are used for the treatment of other diseases like heart disease.

Electrical stimulation devices are being inserted into the brain by means of surgical interventions. The term "psychosurgery" is nowadays being replaced by "neurosurgery for psychiatric disorders". In France, this kind of surgery has not been performed in the last decades. In 2002 the "Comité Consultatif National d'Ethique pour les Sciences de la Vie et de la Santé" decided to maintain the ban on lesioning procedures for psychiatric disorders. However, the Comité has agreed to allow electrical brain stimulation for OCD in research centres as part of a research protocol because of the reversibility and adaptability of the treatment. A collaborative group trying to optimise electrical brain stimulation for OCD has decided to develop self-regulating guidelines that can serve as an example as to how the application of neurosurgery in psychiatric disorders may be regulated in a responsible way. Furthermore, it is already common practice to have an advisory board for neurosurgery in psychiatric disorders review the patients and decide upon the suitability of surgery for each patient.

Technological innovations for brain stimulation are on the horizon in laboratory conditions and in research projects, but not yet in the clinic. These include the miniaturisation of electrodes and stimulators, the use of nanotechnology, telemonitoring, telemedicine and telecontrol. The future possibility of telecontrol, in particular, necessitates the development of safety requirements.

Part II
Societal, Ethical, and Legal Challenges

5 Person, Personal Identity, and Personality

5.1 *Preliminaries*

It was mentioned in the introduction that one of the major types of concerns related to new methods of intervening in the brain is expressed in the question whether the identity of those persons they are applied to is put at risk. Worries of this kind have already been voiced in the past with respect to traditional intervention techniques used in neurosurgery, psychopharmacology, and even (non-invasive) psychotherapy. However, the availability of new techniques like neural grafting, neuroprosthetics and electrical brain stimulation endows those old concerns with new socio-political vigour.[22] In this preliminary section we will attempt to disambiguate the fears of those who would regard certain techniques for intervening in the brain as a potential threat to personal identity. In doing so, it will turn out that, while some particular worries falling within this category need not be dealt with at great length, others require a clarification of the concepts of identity in general, of personal identity in particular, and of related concepts like personhood and personality before a comprehensible assessment of possible hazards can be given for different techniques.

As an example of the type of concern that can be dismissed relatively easily, we bring to mind a rather peculiar worry pertaining specifically to the technique of neural grafting: Some people seem to worry that certain of a donor's personality traits, which might be encoded in a neural graft, could get transferred to the graft recipient. The reason why this particular concern can be put aside without much ado is that it is based on an all too naïve picture of the brain's functioning, on the one hand, and of the technique of neural grafting, on the other. Even though, in a sense, there is truth to the claim that certain delimited parts of the human brain are specifically involved in the implementation of certain psychic functions, the brain doesn't work like a construction kit with neatly separable modules for each of a person's functional traits. In any case, such brain parts could certainly not confer "alien" personality traits when dissected from *immature* brains and inserted in a topologically analogous *mature*, but malfunctioning site in the skull of a person (Boer 1999:470). But *this* (not a transplantation of brain parts of other persons) is exactly what is done through the technique of neural grafting. Considering, for instance, the actual experimental treatment of

---

[22] While this concern pertains *mutatis mutandis* to all new techniques for intervening in the psyche, in recent years it has been widely discussed especially with regard to brain tissue transplantation. See Boer 1994, 1996, 1999; Franz 1996; Hildt 1996, 1999a, 1999b; Jelden 1996; Linke 1993; Metzinger 1996; Northoff 1995, 1996a, 1996b, 2001; Quante 1996.

Parkinson's disease by means of neural grafts, the danger of alien thoughts, memories, preferences, etc. intruding a recipient's mind and undermining his identity becomes utterly elusive since the sole source for acquiring neuronal grafts at present are electively aborted human foetuses or pig foetuses.

However, even if there is no reason to expect a donor's psychic traits encroaching upon the personality of the respective recipient, the inserted material might still act as a disintegrating force on a recipient's personal identity – in the sense of leading either to a breakdown of personhood itself or to an alteration of his personality so radical that, in the end, he would be "no longer the same". Let's take a closer look at both of these possible perils[23] in turn. The expression "breakdown of personhood" is meant to describe a situation in which following an intervention a patient can no longer be said to be a person. Whether one takes this to be an actual possibility will depend on one's general understanding of personhood. For there is an old tradition according to which the use of the concept of a person doesn't allow for human beings to be deprived of personhood. This tradition, which is deeply rooted in medieval theological thinking, acknowledges the possibility of nonhumans being persons (e.g. angels), but on the other hand holds that there can be no human being which for any reason or at any time in its life is not to be considered as a person.[24] According to a second – distinctively modern and secular – strand of tradition, though, human beings do not qualify in and of themselves as persons, but rather by virtue of certain capacities. We will see later on that there is some disagreement among the proponents of this view as to *which* capacities are those that are essential for personhood. However, usually these capacities are taken to be such that no human being already possesses them at the time of birth (s. e.g. Quante 2002:20) and that for any person there is some likelihood to lose these capacities again (either permanently or for some period during their lives).

To illustrate the dissent between the two traditions, let us consider, for a moment, the case of human beings living in a *persistent vegetative state* (PVS). Being in such a wakeful yet unconscious state, they more or less lack all the characteristics (like e.g. awareness and self-consciousness) deemed to be constitutive for being a person by followers of the second tradition. Still, adherents of the first tradition would take offence at the claim that humans trapped in PVS are not to be considered as persons. The reason for their uneasiness is that they conceive of personhood as the distinctive status of beings deserving moral concern. Given this assumption, conceding that human beings lose personhood by entering into PVS implies that they forfeit

---

[23] Please note that "possible" here does just mean that the occurrence of such effects cannot be ruled out by a priori arguments. It does *not* mean that they are empirically established "possible side effects" of the technique.

[24] Accordingly, most contemporary philosophers who subscribe to this view have a strong affinity to theology, see for instance Ford (2002) and Spaemann (1996).

their right to respectful treatment.[25] The idea of (living) human beings devoid of any rights and discriminated against in medical care is as unacceptable to us as it is to the objectors of non-personal human beings. Still, in this chapter we will develop an account of personhood along the lines of the second tradition, that is, we acknowledge the possibility of human beings which are not persons. The reason for this is that for a *serious* consideration of concerns regarding the identity of persons that undergo a new kind of medical intervention this approach is without alternative. After all, if one presupposes along the lines of the first tradition mentioned above that "person" is just another word for "human being", then it becomes a trivial truth that nothing that you can do with a person's psyche will change her identity. For no matter how thoroughly you change the personality of a human being, it will still remain the same individual of the species *homo sapiens sapiens*. However, to forestall misconceptions we would like to emphasise from the outset that we do *not* require holders of moral or legal rights to be persons. Instead, we will argue that personhood is a prerequisite just for the ascription of *duties*, but not for the recognition of *rights*.

Coming back to where we started, the expression "breakdown of personhood" can be used to refer to the situation of patients that – due to some medical intervention or for other reasons – end up being no longer a person. Of course, if there was a higher than negligible risk for patients undergoing a particular kind of intervention to be bereft of necessary capabilities for being regarded as persons, then the procedure in question would not be employed. In this respect, science and medical practice has obviously learned from the history of psychosurgical interventions in the brain. For instance, in the early 1950s lobotomies were still performed at a rate of 5.000 per year in the United States notwithstanding their side effects, which include inertia, apathy, decreased attention, social inappropriateness, and seizures (Missa 1998:737). How drastic a change in personality can result from brain surgery has been famously depicted by Jack Nicholson in Milos Forman's movie "One Flew Over the Cuckoo's Nest" (1975). Nicholson played McMurphy, a rebellious patient in a psychiatric ward, who in the end is subdued by lobotomy, thereby turned into an apathetic wreck.

With Nicholson's performance in mind one might wonder if a person's identity can get "extinguished" without it being replaced by a new one, but also without the person ceasing to exist altogether as is the case with PVS. Let us suppose that after the lobotomy McMurphy still knows who and where he is though he doesn't care much about it, furthermore, that he is still able to

[25] This would then, of course, include medical care. On this background, especially considering the crimes committed by physicians under the Third Reich, the concern of medical practitioners is fully understandable: Normatively loaded terms like "person" could potentially be misused to discriminate against certain patients, and should therefore, in practice, be either avoided or applied indiscriminately to all human beings (as potential patients).

other spatial objects). Therefore, the relation of numerical identity is such that each object has it to itself and to nothing else. Accordingly, "*t*" and "*s*" in the formula $t=s$ do not indicate different objects, but just are different linguistic means referring to one and the same object.[30] In ordinary language, sentences stating identity can be more than mere tautologies though, since it is not at all obvious in every case that two names or descriptions refer to the same thing, as in Gottlob Frege's famous example of an informative statement of identity "The morning star is the evening star".

5.2.2 Identity Through Change: Perdurantism

Having expounded the relation of logical identity like we did above, one might raise doubts whether it ever makes sense to claim numerical identity when talking about temporal objects, so called *continuants*[31]. For all such objects – not to mention persons, who from childhood to old age can be expected to be in a more or less constant flux with respect to their "personality" – there is always the possibility of a change in attributes over time. Now it seems that, according to the principle of indiscernibility of identicals, things before and after having undergone any kind of change could no longer count as identical. It is important to see that – for a number of reasons – we can't just bite this bullet, simply give in and, consequently, restrict the notion of identity to "timeless, unchanging objects" like, e.g., numbers. Such a conception would be at odds with the most fundamental presuppositions upon which the very frame of our languages (natural and formal alike) is based: By using names we subscribe to the conviction that things can be re-identified in various situations at different times as the *same*. If there was no object permanence, the use of a name more than once could never be correct. Furthermore, if there was no chance to recognise objects as one and the same, all natural laws/equations which functionally describe a change in

[30] As objects are counted by identity, it is often remarked (and rightly so) that certain natural-language formulations of the principles governing identity are unfortunate insofar as they seem to presuppose that the "objects" the identity of which is stated are in fact "two". The most obvious slip would be "If two objects *t* and *s* are identical, then …", which in the antecedent clause assumes a manifest contradiction. And in one of the formulations of the principle of substitution we cited above, we wrote: "For *t* and *s* to be identical, *they* must be indiscernible." However, inconveniences like this can easily be avoided in a more canonical mode of speech, in which we may avoid using anaphoric cross-references or other constructions grammatically demanding plural form. Fir instance, "if *t* is identical to *s*, then *t* is indiscernible from *s*" would be perfectly fine.

[31] This term has been coined by W. E. Johnson (1924) because it is unburdened by the problematic connotations of the term "substance". He introduced it against the backdrop of the classical metaphysical dichotomy of "event" and "substance", indicating that continuants are objects which persist through change, whereas events do not change, but rather consist of changes.

state of given objects over time – like the law of free fall – would be false.[32] "Strictly speaking", objects would never change, but rather continuously pop into and out of existence. For any practical purpose it would, obviously, be impossible to handle the infinite explosion of the number of objects which abandoning the idea of object permanence would entail.

The way out of this predicament has been shown by David Lewis (and others – but see especially Lewis 1983: "Survival and Identity"). The basic assumption is that, as soon as one is talking about a continuant, any predicate *Q* expressing a property liable to change is implicitly relating the object to a point in time, such that the *same* object can be *Q* at one time *t* and *not Q* at another time *t'* without violating the principle of substitution. As a matter of coherence, *spatial* objects have therefore to be regarded as extended not only in space, but also in time: they are "4-dimensional". Or, in more general terms, all continuants (e.g. events) are *at least* extended in time, and spatial continuants are extended in *both* space and time. That entails that continuants have temporal parts, so called *stages.*[33]

---

[32] This raises the question whether object permanence is a condition of the possibility of scientific experience or even of experience in general. That this is indeed the case is argued for by Immanuel Kant in his "Kritik der reinen Vernunft" (1904/11 [AA III]: B 178). We will have to put the presentation of the argument on hold, however, until Section 5.3, where it will be part of our analysis of what is entailed by the assumption that some being is a person.

[33] Antagonistic to the position we adopt here is the view that continuants are at all times "wholly present" (see e.g. Zimmerman 1998). Often, the two competing positions are terminologically highlighted by saying that according to the "4-dimensionalists" continuants *perdure,* whereas according to the "wholly-presentists" they *endure.* Sometimes, the very term "continuant" is reserved for the endurantists – which then, of course, implies that the perdurantists *deny* the existence of continuants. This, however, is unfortunate as many perdurantists – like e.g. Lewis – explicitly use the term "continuant" for the 4-dimensional objects they conceive of. Anyway, we fail to see how the endurantist can solve the problem of continuants as changing and at the same time "enduring" without committing a violation of Leibniz's principles, which we saw are logical truths and therefore not open to revision. Maybe the best way to approach the endurantist's position is to lay open the intuition motivating his rejection of "4-dimensionalism" and then show how this intuition, however sound, is employed incorrectly. The sound intuition is that, in the world we live in, we are able to perceive continuants. However (so it is argued), if a continuant was a perduring object, we could never perceive or otherwise have contact with it – all we could perceive or have contact with would be temporal stages of it. Hence, to perceive a continuant, it must be "fully present" at all times. What is wrong with this argument is that, according to the same logic, we would also never perceive an *enduring* spatial object, as, for instance, we always only see some very small spatial part of it, namely the surface-part which is presented to us. And from this, we could then (again by the same line of reasoning) infer that, as we really *do* see spatial objects, they must be "wholly subsistent" in all their visible parts. But of course this is all but a conceptual confusion. To dispel it, we have to distinguish between two ways of using the expression "to see": one use according to which we always see$_1$ just certain parts of an object, but never the whole object, and a second use according to which we always see$_2$ objects simpliciter. And the relation between these two usages is very simple: whenever one does see$_1$ an arbitrary surface-part of an object, one does see$_2$ that object. And along the very same lines, one does of course see$_2$ it, if one does see$_1$ a surface-part of one of its stages.

However, this concept of continuants is still not sufficiently elaborate. For unless one puts further restrictions on the identity of objects over time, continuants would have to be thought of as *eternal* inasmuch as no change (short of "complete vanishing") would ever end their existence. The first step in resolving this further puzzle is to distinguish between two ways of talking about "existence". One kind of sentences stating the existence of something can be analysed using the existential quantifier of predicate logic. Only because of their superficial grammatical form, sentences in natural languages like "Lipid-soluble toxic substances exist" seem to attribute a property ("existence") to objects. But their logical form is revealed by reading them "For at least one *x* holds that ...". In a second sense, however, the verb "to exist" is indeed used as a predicate proper. In sentences of the respective kind, it can be exchanged by predicates such as "alive", "enduring", "present", etc. So, if someone (implausibly) stated "Adolf Hitler still *exists*" he would thereby claim that Hitler was still *alive*.

Sometimes both ways of talking about existence are used together. Take, for example, the sentence, "There is a painting of Titian that was destroyed in a fire and so no longer exists today." In analysing the formal structure of this sentence one needs to use the existential quantifier. If this would imply attributing a property, then the first and the last part of the sentence would contradict each other. Actually, the existential quantifier could not at all be employed to formalise statements about things long gone if it stood in for a predicate. But its function is rather to indicate the *reference* of a statement. We can understand what someone uttering the above sentence is talking about, no matter whether any painting of Titian ever was destroyed in a fire. On the one hand everything we can at all talk about *exists* "timelessly" in the sense that the semantic relation of reference is itself timeless. On the other hand we can talk – in the second sense specified above – about the existence of continuants over certain timespans. In order to avoid confusion we shall use the verb "to persist" when we will be talking in the "non-timeless" or attributive sense of existence. For instance, from the statement, "Napoleon is to be considered the greatest military strategist of all times" it follows that there is someone who is to be considered the greatest strategist *now*, but not that this someone does also *persist* now.

As said above, criteria of identity of objects over time are needed to allow the possibility that continuants can actually cease to persist. Furthermore, such criteria are also required to decide, in the first place, whether any given two "stages" at different times are stages of the same continuant or not. And here we are again homing in, in a most general form, on the main topic of this chapter, the question whether "snapshots" of a human being, taken before and after an intervention, might not belong to the same person. A few quite fundamental philosophical remarks might help the reader to get a better understanding of that question.

First of all, objects do not exist "in themselves". They are constituted by our distinguishing them through means of general concepts. In an important sense, language actually constitutes our world. Certainly, not all the linguistic means I might use to describe an object are of equal importance with respect to its constitution. I might describe the thing standing in front of me as "relatively big", "stained", "ugly", as "a present from my mother in law" and as "made of porcelain", but still you would not know really what I am talking about. It would have been of great help to you if I had told you in the first place that I am talking about "the cup" standing in front of me. In a way, all the other properties I attributed to that cup by applying those various descriptive expressions to it happen to be merely "accidental". The cup could be rather small, clean and pretty, and it would still remain a cup. Its being-a-cup, on the other hand, one might call its "essential property". This dichotomy has been established by Aristotle, who also referred to an object's essential property as to its "form". But we would like to avoid these expressions as we do not want to endorse *ontological essentialism.* Without going into details, the distinctive difference between our way of thinking compared to Aristotle's essentialism is that we consider the "essentiality" of a property as *being relative to a description,* which in turn will, generally, be justified only in relation to its "fit" with respect to the goals pursued within the discourse in question. To emphasise the context- and language-dependence of our approach we will talk about *constitutive predicates,* rather than about essential properties.

Having said this, we hope it is still comprehensible for us to maintain that, for any given object distinguished by us as such, there will be a constitutive predicate. Since every object is constituted by the application of a constitutive predicate, a necessary condition for any object to persist (rather than to perish or to be transformed into another object) is that this predicate "keeps on applying". If we stick to the example given above, and consider the predicate "cup" as constitutive for a certain thing, then it may be painted differently or lose its handle and still remain "the" cup. However, if it breaks, what remains is not a cup anymore and so that particular continuant has ceased to persist.

5.2.3 Material Identity and Material Continuity

Introducing the concept of constitutive predicates into logic brings another noteworthy consequence: Unless we adopt it, there is for any *P* which is also *Q* always an *identical Q* which is also *P*. This is no longer the case if we bring constitutive predicates into play to avoid having all objects existing (persisting) eternally. Certainly, if we are faced with a constituted *P* that happens to be *Q*, we can still say that there's also a constituted *Q* which is, accidentally, *P*. However, on logical grounds of the substitution principle alone, "the *P*" need not be identical to "the *Q*", namely, if there is a time where the *P* does still/already persist while the *Q* has ceased/not yet begun to do so (and *vice versa).* Imagine, for instance, a little boy who moulded a toy dog from plasticine. As long as he is playing with the dog he will typically treat it as a dog, being totally oblivious to the fact that it is made of plasticine. Let's say, after having done with it, the boy tosses the toy dog into some box. Then, after some time, he might feel again like playing with plasticine. When eventually he finds the discarded plasticine dog he may treat it as nothing but a blob of plasticine, quickly squeezing it beyond recognition. – This innocent example illustrates how what is taken to be constitutive of an object as against to what is deemed to be accidental can change with the attitude that is taken towards that object. Furthermore, it becomes clear that the continuant we referred to as the "toy dog" is not identical to the plasticine it consists of, since the latter is there before the former comes into persistence and after it ceased to persist.

This last insight can be generalised: *No* material object will be identical to the matter it consists of. First of all, this obviously holds true for all those things of which one can remove or replace some material part, or which can lose or exchange some amount of the matter they consist of, without thereby changing their identity. Actually, there are not many things whose identity is constituted rigorously by the exact amount of matter they consist of, to the extent that they would not count as the same when some tiny fraction was removed. A notable exception could be the prototype for introducing the international mass unit kilogram – a cylinder made of platinum-iridium-alloy stored in the "Bureau International des Poids et Mesures" in Sèvres near Paris. In this case one could argue that the prototype's identity is actually changed if you scrape off just the tiniest part of it. But even then, the continuant we refer to by the definite description "the prototype for the kilogram" is *not* identical to the noble metal it consists of, since – once again – the latter clearly was there before the former was introduced in a meticulously controlled production process.

By arguing that "the *P*", in general, is not identical to "the *Q*" it consists of, we refute the view that for spatiotemporal continuants identity as such is constituted by *material identity*. To further illustrate this point, we will now consider the persistence conditions for human bodies, for this will prepare the subsequent discussion of personal identity. Regarding the identity of a human body, two of the hard questions one can ask are: When exactly does it come into being? And when exactly does it perish? Fortunately enough, these are questions we need not answer here, but at least we would plead for a pragmatic way of approaching them. In our opinion, there is not just one *true* answer to each of them. It rather depends on practical purposes what answer can be taken to be *appropriate* in a certain context. Long before the arrival of modern imaging techniques, which today provide us with various insights into a mother's womb, it was a known fact that human bodies do come into persistence *before* they are born. Even today, though, the difficulty is to tell *at what time* in between conception and birth they come into being. On the one hand, thinking of the continuity of this development, it seems quite arbitrary to pick out any particular stage of embryonic development as a "starting point" for the body. On the other hand, however, it seems rather odd to choose the fertilised egg as a starting point, since it bears absolutely no similarity to the human body that later on we identify by its traits as one and the same in spite of all its changes. We find ourselves in a similar kind of quandary when it comes to the exact stage of decomposition from which onwards it is no longer appropriate to call the mortal remains of a human a human body. The important point is that, apart from particular practical contexts for which the answer to this kind of questions would actually make a difference, we do not have any criteria to judge the "absolute" appropriateness of different possible answers.

So, considering the human body as a continuant, it is not easy to specify a starting and an end point for this 4-dimensional entity. However, no matter how this problem is settled, one will find support for the assumption that the relationship between any particular human body and the matter it consists of is not one of identity. Much to the contrary, regarding its material substrate the human body offers a striking example for identity through change. Assuming the (living) body's material substrate means its chemical composition, it is well known that the body is in permanent metabolic exchange with its environment via assimilation of nutrients, excretion, etc. Consequently, there probably is not a single molecule – or cell for that matter – that is part of a particular body from its elusive start till its elusive end. However, the example of the human body also indicates that it would be premature to move to the opposite extreme by claiming that the identity of material objects wasn't constrained in any way by conditions regarding their material substrates. For, regardless of the human body being in a permanent reconstruction process, we seem to require some sort of material *continuity* between two body stages if we are to accept that both of them belong to one and the same body. To grasp this point, just imagine teletransportation was actually possible in the following way[34]: In one place all the information about a human body is encoded and then transmitted to another location

[34] Readers who are not familiar with what is called "thought experiments" in philosophy may be somewhat alienated by what seems to be a lengthy discussion, not of empirically relevant facts or possibilities, but of far-fetched science-fiction scenarios. However, it is important for the reader to understand that the reason for the regular occurrence of such examples within philosophy is *not* that philosophers take a special, escapist liking to science fiction or weird things in general, which would have no relation to, or bearing on the urgent problems we face in real life. Rather, such discussions of counterfactual situations are part of the philosopher's genuine task of analysing and clarifying the meaning of concepts. Thought experiments invoking radically counterfactual (but logically consistent) situations are a valuable tool for elucidating the meaning of a concept (including its links to other concepts) because they allow testing of its *limits*. With respect to any proposal that the meaning of a concept should be taken to consist in "such-and-so", thought experiments will test whether that proposal is "robust" with regard to the entire range of possible experience with which future developments may or may not confront us, or whether it implicitly draws on the stability of contingent facts.

where it is used to create an exact copy of the original body, which itself is destroyed in the process. Despite its exact similarity we cannot admit that the copy-stage belongs to the original body. For imagine the last step of destroying the original body was omitted: Then we were faced with two exactly similar human bodies, the stages of only one would be counted as belonging to the body prior to the process of teletransportation – the one which bears the relation of material continuity with the body prior to teletransportation. Thus, in "teletransportation" the copy is nothing but a copy, regardless of whether the original body is destroyed or not.[35]

One may still think there is something puzzling about material continuity as a necessary[36] criterion of identity for human bodies: Take on the one hand two stages of one and the same human body separated by a long stretch of time and compare the relationship they bear to each other with the relationship between one stage of a human body immediately prior to teletransportation and one stage of this body's copy immediately subsequent to that process. According to what we stated above, in both cases you might not find a single molecule or cell that establishes a direct material connection between the two respective body stages. What is more, in the first case the two stages look very dissimilar, while in the latter case they look strikingly similar. But still it seems plausible to maintain that only in the first case the two stages belong to the same human body. In order to come to terms with this "paradox" it is helpful to compare the relation between two stages of a human body, one at the beginning and one at the end of its life, with two parts of a rope at opposite ends: Even though not a single fibre runs through all the rope, so that there is no immediate connection in this sense between two parts at opposite ends, they still are obviously connected. In much the same way there is a material continuity between stages of a human body at young and old age, respectively, that is lacking between the body and its "teletransported" copy.

Quite obviously, the criterion of material continuity – allowing for persistence despite loss/exchange of matter – can be generalised to cover not

---

[35] Teletransportation violates the criterion of material continuity insofar as the "rebuilt" material parts of a "transported" object cannot, not even in principle, be considered as numerically identical to the destroyed parts. The reason is that material continuity presupposes *spatiotemporal* continuity. It follows that for "teletransportation" to be taken serious, its "theory" would have to be quite different from the one involving the trias "scanning"/"destroying"/"rebuilding". It would have to assume that (under specified circumstances) objects could pass through a fourth *genuinely spatial* dimension that directly connects regions which are only indirectly connected in three-dimensional space (for illustration, think of a paper that is folded up onto itself).

[36] Material continuity is at the same time obviously not a *sufficient* condition for the identity of the human body. For this, the constitutive predicate "human body" must remain applicable, too. (If it decomposed or transformed into another type of body, it would have ceased to persist, regardless of maintained material continuity.)

only human bodies, but at least all living bodies, i.e. organisms. Can it be generalised to cover *all* bodies? Many philosophers (mostly following Locke and Nidditch 1975:II, 27, § 3) think there is a difference between organisms and inorganic bodies in that the criterion of material continuity only applies with respect to organic bodies, while an analogous (necessary) criterion of identity over time for inorganic bodies would be material identity.[37] Though it is obvious that the latter criterion would eventually have to be relaxed (otherwise the removal or exchange of the tiniest part would again change the identity of inorganic bodies), the overall proposal has indeed a certain plausibility to it: Assume, for instance, my wife had once bought me a tripartite lamp consisting of a frame, a shade and a bulb. Over the years, I exchanged the bulb, then the shade, and eventually the frame. It would ring rather peculiar if I nevertheless would insist that what I've got there hanging in my room is still the lamp my wife once bought me – even if in exchanging parts I had kept to the same brand and model. For if I had given the original parts to a friend who eventually put them together again, *his* would be considered to be the lamp my wife had once bought me.

To put to test the hypothesis regarding the range of application of the criteria of material continuity and material identity, let's see how they fare with respect to the famous puzzle of the "ship of Theseus". This puzzle, which traces back to Plutarch, runs as follows: Over time, worn planks of the ship of Theseus are replaced, bit by bit, by new ones, so that eventually none of the original planks remain in it. Meanwhile, however, the worn planks are used to build a "new" ship by assembling them in just the way they were arranged in the original ship. After completion of this reconstruction process, there are two ships looking pretty much alike except that one is made of new planks (ship 2) while the other is made of worn planks (ship 3). And now the question is *which* of them is identical to Theseus' original ship (ship 1).[38] This being a good puzzle, no answer is completely satisfying. On the one hand, only ship 3 satisfies the requirement of *material identity* as it is made of the very same parts that constituted Theseus' original ship – thereby making a good case for claiming that this is indeed the same ship. On the other hand, replacing a worn plank is obviously not enough to end the persistence of a ship and create a new one instead. But if that is so, then persistence must be preserved through *each single such step* and, hence, ship 2 must eventually inherit identity with ship 1. Now, if we ask what it is that connects ship 2 (but *not* ship 3!) to ship 1, we find that it is in fact the relation of *mate-*

---

[37] It is clear that, insofar as "material identity" means "consisting of the same material", one will eventually have to face the task to define the criteria of identity for *that*.

[38] More precisely, the question is which of these stages (2 or 3) is a stage of the ship which stage 1 belonged to (as the different stages cannot be identical anyway). However, for the sake of convenience, in the following we will use this precise formulation only if otherwise there would ensue pseudo-problems.

rial continuity – which seems to make a strong case here even if Theseus' ship is an inanimate object.

While searching for the one true answer to this puzzle will give the metaphysician a serious headache, we once again opt for context-specific solutions. For example, a practical need for a straight answer to the question as to whether ship 2 or ship 3 is identical to ship 1 could be constituted by a legal interest to settle the question of ownership. If, for instance, Theseus sold the replaced pieces of his ship to a scavenger who then came up with the idea of reconstructing her, then it is blatantly clear that Theseus is the owner of ship 2, but not of ship 3 – and thus ship 2, but not ship 3, would be regarded as identical to ship 1 in this context. To see the problem from another context, consider the following clever modification of the Theseus puzzle, borrowed from S. Marc Cohen[39]: This time Theseus' ship is not replaced during its journeys, but, having been put out of service, displayed in a museum. Suppose now some thieves are trying to steal the ship by removing its pieces one at a time. In the museum, the stolen pieces are replaced with look-alikes while they are secretly reassembled elsewhere in the original way. In this modified case it seems quite clear that only the ship in the thieves' hideout may be considered to be identical to the original ship whereas the ship finally left in the museum is a fake. Even though our legal intuitions point into opposite directions in the two cases discussed here, the respective judgments seem fairly obvious. The lesson is that questions regarding identity that are bewildering as long as they are posed "out of context" frequently may be settled quite agreeably in the light of concrete practical purposes. We will have to keep this lesson in mind when it comes to the real, serious concerns pertaining to personal identity associated with the medical procedures that are the principal topic of this study.

To avoid narrowing the scope for finding practical solutions for identity issues, we deliberately refrain from setting very strict criteria for persistence through change. For instance, the way we determined the concepts of identity and persistence of continuants in general still *leaves open* the logical possibility that at least some kinds of things can cease to persist and then later begin to persist again. Consider once again the example of the plasticine dog. Say, while your child is playing with that dog you inadvertently step on it, squashing it completely and leaving him crying his heart out. To console him you take up the task of moulding "the same" dog until at least your boy is convinced that "here it is again". It is not that important whether *you* would actually accept this as a genuine case of "resurrection" or rather think by yourself, "well, it is a different dog looking more or less similar and made of the same material". In every individual context we may have good reasons to

[39] "Identity, Persistence, and the Ship of Theseus", http://faculty.washington.edu/smcohen/320/theseus.html, accessed on December 8th, 2006.

treat such cases one way or the other[40]. So it turns out as an advantage rather than a shortcoming of our account that resurrection is not a priori ruled out for *conceptual* reasons. If required, constraints of "unbroken continuity" could easily be introduced to further regulate the identity of certain types of objects – like we suggested in the case of organisms.

Another theoretical advantage of our account is that it does not enforce an affirmative answer to the question whether differences in *modal properties* rule out identity. Modal predicates such as "is *necessarily* mistaken" or "is *possibly* harmful" are sometimes considered to ascribe to objects a special kind of properties called "modal properties". If one subscribes to this *(de re)* conception of modal expressions it seems natural to maintain that – according to Leibniz's laws – objects differing in nothing but their modal properties must nevertheless be different. In our view, however, modal statements are *not* statements about objects, but statements about statements *(de dicto)*. The reason is that the *de-re* view together with the principle of substitution must inevitably lead to absurdities. For example, if the statement, "It is necessary that 9>5" is taken as ascribing a "modal property" to 9, then from its combination with the true sentence, "The number of planets of our solar system=9" one could infer via the substitution principle: "It is necessary that the number of planets of our solar system >5". While we still may talk in a derivative sense about the modal properties of *objects*, we always have to keep in mind that an object does not have its "modal properties" *independent of the expressions used to refer to it*. Accordingly, differences in modal properties do not *per se* exclude identity.

The motif behind the inclusion of modal properties by some philosophers is the fear that, otherwise, different objects might not be discerned, for example a cup might falsely be considered identical to the porcelain it consists of, in cases where both would come into existence and vanish simultaneously. However, to us it appears that, apart from a possibly different timespan of persistence, there are always other *actual* differences to be found: The Rosenthal-cup, for example, is worth 20 Euro, but the "mere material worth" of the porcelain is much less (think of the longstanding debate regarding customs duty on CDs or diskettes).

5.2.4 Perdurantism Refined and Defended

Let's now return to the main question of how the riddles surrounding the concept of identity through change can be resolved. Our first step was to introduce the concept of a continuant with stages as temporal parts. This led

---

[40] Maybe the best example for a field where talking of "resurrection" is the common mode of speech is the context of historical buildings. During its history, a bridge, a castle or a city hall may have been not only enlarged, restored or relocated, but even destroyed and later rebuilt. It is also quite obvious that it would be futile to search for definitive ontological criteria with respect to the question of whether buildings "really" persist through such-and-such changes or not.

to a reconciliation of identity (in the strict logical sense) with change. The second step was the introduction of constitutive predicates, which allowed for continuants to cease to persist. Above we said that, for a continuant to persist, at the very least the constitutive predicate has to "keep on applying". It is now time to reveal that this, if taken *a la lettre,* is either circular or not quite penetrating to the fundamentals. This can be easily seen if we ask *to what* the constitutive predicate is supposed to "keep on applying". Obviously, if we speak in those terms, we presuppose *having already constituted* some "subsisting" continuant. For example, if we would agree upon material continuity (implying spatiotemporal continuity) as a necessary and sufficient criterion for *bodies,* we could then say that "this cup" persists as long as the constitutive predicate "cup" applies to "this body". But even though it is indeed true that bodies are, in a certain way, the primary continuants[41], neither can all continuants be thought of as constituted through bodies in this way (e.g. events cannot), nor do the persistence conditions for all sorts of continuants presuppose that some other, subsisting continuant must persist at least as long (e.g. for a traffic congestion to persist there does not have to be one individual car involved in it *all* the time). Fortunately, there is a non-circular, even if somewhat roundabout way to formulate our criterion of the "continuously applying constitutive predicate": With respect to any given continuant-stage that exemplifies some continuant through a constitutive predicate (e.g. "this cup"), only such later continuant-stages to which at least the constitutive predicate (i.e. "cup") applies can be considered as possible continuations of *that same* continuant. From this formulation it immediately becomes clear that there must be stronger criteria for really fixing the identity of continuants over time. For many (though, as we will learn from the example of persons, not for all) embodied continuants, these criteria often conceptually involve the identity of the subsisting bodies over time, and thus their spatiotemporal continuity (which is implied both by the criterion of material continuity and by the criterion of material identity).

However, even in conjunction with continuous application of the constitutive predicate these criteria often do not suffice. Imagine, for example, I start out with an 80386 IBM computer which I gradually change over the years, replacing the motherboard, the case, the monitor, the mouse etc., eventually ending up with a Pentium IV with flat screen. In this situation, the constitutive predicate "computer" obviously still applies to the object I am working with. But is it really still the "same computer", just very fancily changed? Maybe we wouldn't want to say so and accordingly would need to agree on stronger criteria for "persistence of computer identity". Maybe, insofar as the central processing unit (CPU) can be considered to be a computer's "brain", one would

[41] They constitute space and thus our universal frame of reference, in relation to which all other continuants get located directly (like lightning) or indirectly (like a smile or an itch).

want to argue that after replacing the CPU with one of a different type a computer is no longer the same (in our example, a 80386 is turned into a Pentium IV), while changes at the periphery (mouse, monitor etc.) do not interfere with a computer's identity. Once again, this prosaic example seems fit to bolster our general point of view that questions regarding identity should be handled as pragmatic rather than as "metaphysical" issues. But what's even more important is that the example also shows that, in general, what is needed in addition to a continuously applying constitutive predicate *P* are criteria stating which *further* predicates *Q* must hold for any specific *P* to stay the "same *P*".

In the next section we will turn to the task of setting out what it means if the constitutive predicate "person" applies to a continuant. Thereafter we will propose criteria that further specify what mustn't change for a person to stay the "same" person. But before doing so, we would like to discuss a few more theoretical issues concerning identity of continuants in general that might appear somewhat idle to non-philosophers, but play an important role in the technical literature. One such issue, which some presume to offer an objection to four-dimensionalism, is typically addressed by the keyword "overpopulation". It is usually exposed by talking about persons, but we prefer to address it by talking about "cups" so as to emphasise its relevance for the notion of identity of continuants in general.

The main strand of arguments referring to overpopulation relates to the problem of individuating continuants. If you were a philosopher sitting in front of a cup you might wonder how many cups you are actually facing. Is it just one cup? Or maybe two cups, one with a handle and then the same cup again, but this time counted without the handle? Or are there even more of them? Concerns of that kind can be resolved by stipulating that continuants are "maximal" in space. So, for situations in which *n Ps* are to be counted, if a certain *P* (say *a*) is counted once, no "further" *P* is to be counted which is constituted of just part of the matter that makes up *a*.[42] Similarly, but less trivially, continuants are maximal with respect to time as well. That is, no temporal stage of a cup is *another* cup.

Thought experiments involving amoeba-like "splitting" also give rise to concerns regarding the concept of a continuant. Actually, the case of amoebas itself can be used to discuss the issue (the advantage being that this is *not* a mere thought experiment): Suppose, an amoeba is dividing, with an end result of two alike but numerically different amoebas. This is what in the literature is called a case of "fission"[43], in which we are confronted with three

[42] As always, we must not forget that criteria like this must be understood as pragmatic, not as metaphysical truths. There are contexts where we might want to use criteria of counting that disregard maximality. For example, we might prefer to stick with the habit of saying that *two* animals are shown in the famous ambiguous duck/hare-picture.

[43] Usually exemplified by thought experiments using "duplicators" or "teletransportation going wrong".

things: one previous to the fission point (amoeba 1), and two of them in different places subsequent to it (amoebas 2 & 2'), indiscernible from each other except for their spatial properties. Certainly, this indistinguishability may be limited to the time frame immediately before and after the fission point – for instance, one of the two resultant amoebas might get injured shortly after the fission. But still, other than in the case of the ship of Theseus there is (at least *ex hypothesi*) no difference whatsoever regarding the material properties of amoeba 2 and amoeba 2'. Therefore, the question as to which of them is "identical to" past amoeba 1 seems even more intractable. One might argue as follows here: "In the case of fission, amoeba 2 and amoeba 2' can't be both identical with amoeba 1, because then they would (per transitivity of identity) also be identical to one another.[44] That would mean neither amoeba 2 nor amoeba 2' should be regarded as identical with amoeba 1. Amoeba 2 and amoeba 2' are "new" whereas amoeba 1 simply ceased to persist. But that, in turn, must eventually lead us to the generalised conclusion that *never* should *any* object be taken to be identical to some earlier object, as persistence clearly shouldn't depend on the totally *accidental* ("external") issue of whether (in the meantime) a fission has *de facto* occurred or not." – There must be something wrong with this train of thought since it implies that no object can survive the shortest stretch of time, a notion already found untenable above.

To solve the problem, the so-called "best candidate theory" was proposed (see e.g. Nozick 1981). According to this view, in the case of fission one has to pick the object which is the "best candidate" with respect to the claim of being identical with the object that was there before the fission occurred. For example, if teletransportation fails in the sense that, while a copy of the object actually appears elsewhere, the object is not destroyed at the original location, the object at the original location would be the "best candidate" because it alone bears the relations of material and spatio-temporal continuity with the object before the fission point. Only if no "best candidate" can be found, the object prior to the fission point has ceased to persist (as it has been replaced by at least two "new" objects). It has to be conceded that the "best candidate" theory contains some grain of truth, but only insofar as there indeed have to be independent criteria for deciding whether two stages belong to one-and-the-same continuant or not. If some object stage S_t does not pass the test with respect to another object stage $Z_{t-\Delta t}$, while another

[44] This argument can be couched in terms of fusion, too. To avoid the realm of thought experiments, one has to draw on examples of symbiotic or parasitic fusion (e.g. the case of sperm/ovum, the hypothetical development of mitochondria etc.). Sperm and ovum cannot both be counted as identical with the "fused" zygote, for then they would have to be identical to one another, too – which is not the case. However, the argument from fusion does not yield any surprising or unsettling results as, according to common intuition, things are usually not expected to "survive" fusion anyway.

"candidate" S'_t does, then S'_t, but not S_t is to be regarded as a continuation of $Z_{t-\Delta t}$. Still, the "best candidate" theory fails insofar as it entails more than that, namely that in fission there *either* is one "best" candidate, which then will count as the continuation of the original object, *or* there are at least two equally good candidates, in which case the original object ceased to persist. A "fission type" thought experiment, originally devised by Wiggins (1967) and since then often recycled and modified by others (e.g. Parfit 1984:ch. 12, sec. 89), can be used to show that this leads to (conceptually) absurd consequences: Imagine brain transplantation would be possible and a (most probably mad) neurosurgeon was about to transplant the two hemispheres of your brain into different new bodies. Let's assume, for the sake of argument, that the new bodies are exact copies of your old body (Parfit invites us to assume they are in fact the bodies of your two brain-dead triplet brothers), and also that both hemispheres are (maybe deficient, but) equally good candidates for being continuations of your brain as it was before.[45] Now, as in such a case the "best candidate" theory *ex hypothesi* decrees that the original person ("you") will cease to persist, it would be very rational for you to bribe a nurse to destroy one of your brain-hemispheres so that only the other gets transplanted (in this vein e.g. Noonan ²2003:ch. 12.5). For in *this* case, there would remain a "best candidate" and you would survive! It is very obvious from this that the verdicts of "best candidate" theory are too arbitrary to be of help in solving fission-related problems regarding the concept of "continuants". Some better solution has to be found.[46]

Luckily, we do not have to look very far. Our diagnosis is that fission engenders problems only if it is addressed by the wrong question: As objects *themselves* are extended in time, the seemingly innocent question, "Is object

---

[45] This is allegedly true for at least some individuals where none of the usual functional asymmetries between hemispheres is to be found. Functional asymmetries tend to be strongest in right-handed males and much less in females and left-handed people.

[46] Holding on to the "best candidate" approach, Derek Parfit (1984) takes these considerations to show that *"identity is not what matters in survival"*. Of course, this view is extremely counterintuitive, and not *just* because, taken literally, it is incoherent: If it's not *me* at a later stage, then I didn't *survive*. What Parfit means, however, is that "division" thought experiments can be used to show that what we care for is not that *we* will still be there later, but rather that there are future persons (at least one) which are, in a sense, *continuers* of us. For – as, *in truth*, we would find the idea of bribing the neurosurgeon into destroying one of our brain hemispheres extremely inappropriate – what we are interested in *cannot* be our literal survival. It is easy to see from this that the whole argument *presupposes* best candidate theory to be correct (this has been shown in all desirable clarity by Harold W. Noonan [²2003:ch. 9]). So, in the face of the undisputable fact that the assumption of a lack of interest on our part in *our* survival is extremely counter-intuitive, this very consequence of "division" thought experiments rather seems to show the absurdity of the "best candidate" approach once more. In any case, if there are rival theories regarding the persistence of continuants which do *not* imply that we lack interest in our survival, they clearly should be preferred.

O1 at t_1 identical with object *O2* at t_2?", does not properly confer the meaning that is commonly intended. To consider an object at a certain time means to consider a *stage* of that object. However, stages *at different times* are never identical anyway, so the question in question would, strictly speaking, *always* have to be answered to the negative! However, it makes perfect sense to ask "Is *O1* identical to *O2*?", or "Are *O1* at t_1 and *O2* at t_2 both stages of the *same* object?" Here, the negative answer is not obligatory. It only is if objects *O1* and *O2* are discernible at (at least) *some* point in time *t* – and this is how it should be. Such a distinction between objects *O1* and *O2* would have to be registered, for instance, if there is any point in time for which their spatial location differs.[47]

The decisive point, however, which still has to be made, is this: Regarding the correct questions, there is the (logical) possibility that amoeba 1 and amoeba 2 are stages of the same object and *also* that amoeba 1 and amoeba 2' are stages of the same object. This does *not* imply that amoeba 2 and amoeba 2', too, are stages of the same object![48] (In fact – due to their different spatial locations after the fission point – we *know* that they are not). Generally put: Two different objects (that is, objects which aren't identical) may nevertheless *share stages before or after a certain point in time.* And, of course, these points will be fission or fusion points.

But, while this clearly "defuses" the threat that fission presents to the concept of continuants and their persistence in time (thereby also doing away with the need to resort to "best candidate" theory[49]), we now seem to be faced with the problem of "overpopulation" again, in the sense that where a fission occurs there apparently have been *two* objects before the fission point even though we thought there was only one. But, of course, before the fission point in question is actually reached, it makes no sense to distinguish two things (as, before that point in time, they are literally indistinguishable). So, in our example, before

---

[47] Of course, any spatial object is such that spatial parts of it do occupy different regions in space. So, if one feels inclined to ask why a spatiotemporal object cannot occupy two *distinct* spaces at the same time, the question needs to relate to the object as a *whole.* Under this reading, the assumption that an object occupies two distinct spaces at the same time would bring about logical and categorical mishaps: Suppose, for example, there were two spatially distinct "occurrences" of "one-and-the-same" marble, then the resultant discontinuous object taken as a whole could no longer be called a marble at all.

[48] This is in sharp contrast to the results yielded by the wrongly put question in which stages were confused with the objects they belong to. By mistakenly asking which "later" objects are *identical* to some "earlier" one, one is unavoidably led to the problem of transitivity of identity.

[49] In this way we also avoid the nasty consequence of that theory, namely that our literal survival does ("in truth") not matter to us. For, in cases of real fission, *no one* ceases to persist – and *this* is the reason why, under the (idealised) circumstances of Wiggins' thought experiment, the idea of bribing the mad neurosurgeon into destroying one of our brain hemispheres before the transplantation doesn't appeal to us (and *not* some alleged indifference with respect to our literal survival).

the amoeba has divided there *are no* two amoebas. To better understand how this is still in step with our view that different objects could share stages before a fission or after a fusion point, it is helpful here to distinguish between two kinds of situations in which to use the expression "before". It is one thing to talk about events happening before a time t^* while t^* has not yet arrived, and quite another to talk about what was before t^* when t^* has passed. After the fission we might think differently about amoeba 1, with which we were acquainted before. Alluding to Arthur C. Danto (1985: especially ch. VIII), one might say that, in a way, the future can change the past.[50] However, it may come as a relief to those who feel uneasy with the last statements that even after t^* we are not necessarily obliged to say that "two" things (amoeba 2 and amoeba 2') existed before t^*. In order to come to terms with cases of fission and fusion, David Lewis (1983: "Survival and Identity") introduced the notion of *tensed identity*. According to his proposal, things are to be counted by *identity-at-t* instead by identity simpliciter[51]: a and b are identical at t if they are indistinguishable at that time. So, even if we have two amoebas which share stages before the fission point t^*, there still is at any point before the fission point t^* just *one* amoeba, which "becomes" *two* amoebas only afterwards.

5.3 Persons

In the last section we discussed quite arcane issues, which sometimes may even seem to be "off topic". However, we had to face these issues and puzzles as they regularly confuse the discussions about persons and personal identity in the (philosophical) literature. Our aim was to disentangle questions that may be dealt with by clarifying the notion of identity in general from questions that are specifically related to the notion of person and personal identity. We can breath more freely now, after having shown how many issues can be resolved by adopting the view of perduring objects as 4-dimensional continuants.

The present section is devoted to the question as to what conditions a continuant needs to fulfil to be recognised as a person. We require an account of these conditions in order to judge whether certain forms of intervention, by affecting particular capabilities, could deprive persons of personhood.[52] As mentioned in the introductory section, the case that a person is

[50] After a fission point, our very language changes, as we have *two* names at our disposal then where there used to be only one. It is this "new" language that enables us to give a different account of the past.

[51] Note that this is extremely plausible. For, else, to correctly count objects, we would have to know the future!

[52] It seems obvious that the reasons *why* we have to be able to judge effects of interventions on personhood ultimately have to do with the very foundations of ethics itself. Roughly, the connection to ethics is this: a) persons usually hold the very conditions securing their own persistence *as* persons in high esteem and b) it is *persons* who discuss, decide on and are addressed by moral and legal norms.

annihilated because constitutive conditions for personhood no longer obtain needs to be distinguished from the case that a person is annihilated because of a change of personal identity. In both cases the existence of a person comes to an end, but only in the second case a new person (however deficient) comes into existence. By acknowledging the possibility of a genuine change in personal identity it is clear that the *criteria of persistence for persons* (specifying the conditions under which a person can be said to remain the "same") will differ from the *criteria of personhood* (the conditions for applying the constitutive predicate "person"). For only given these differences we can imagine that, after having undergone an intervention, someone still may be considered to be a person even though his or her former identity has been wiped out. So, we will tackle the question of the criteria of personhood in this section, while in the next we will frame the criteria of persistence for persons.

5.3.1 "To Consider Oneself as Oneself" – A Transcendental Analysis of the Concept of a Person

We won't live up to the conceptual challenge at hand by just enumerating certain conditions we feel someone has to fulfil to count as a person. This approach would be too *ad hoc*. Rather, we should first answer the question what the concept of a person is actually needed for, what it is supposed to *distinguish*. Having answered this we may then *derive* the different aspects which, otherwise, we would only enumerate.[53] The starting point for our analysis will be the one that has been constitutive for the philosophical debate on the concept of a person in modern times. The core ideas of the modern history of deliberation about persons and their identity have been laid down by John Locke in his "Essay Concerning Human Understanding" (1975 [1689]). First of all, Locke clearly distinguishes *human beings* ("man") from *persons*, the identity of the former being founded in their living bodies (1975:II, 27, §6), while the identity of the latter is constituted by "consciousness" (ibid.:§9). Locke's second important insight is that "person" is a "forensic term" or, as we shall prefer to say, a *moral category*, "appropriating actions and their merit" (ibid.:§26).[54] Basically, a person is a being that can be held *responsible* for its actions. Therefore, it is not surprising that the concept of a person will always be encountered in contexts of rights, duties and law.

[53] Also, a mere enumeration would always leave open the question of its completeness. On the other hand, while every list of conceptually derived aspects too may be open to further enlargement, that would not be a defect: for there would be clear criteria for whether an aspect has to be included in the list or not.

[54] Locke was not the first to frame this idea, but he is still a particularly important historical warrantor, since much of the contemporary thinking on persons traces back to the enormous influence of his work. For historical surveys on the person concept see e. g. Noonan (^{2}2003) and Sturma (1997).

It follows from Locke's distinction that there can be persons that are not humans and humans that are not persons. As we already pointed out in the introduction to this chapter, the latter does, of course, not at all mean that such humans – like babies – don't have *rights*. On the contrary: as "person" is tied to "responsibility", babies will just have no *duties*. In this context it should be of interest to note that "human", too, is in fact not a purely descriptive category (like "homo sapiens sapiens"). However, it rather conveys *rights* than duties and so we e.g. speak of "human rights" and not of "person rights". Think of the concept of a "legal person" applied to abstract entities like companies: the main reason for applying the concept "person" to them is that thereby they can be held responsible e.g. by being *sued*. Babies, on the other hand, can neither be sued nor prosecuted or convicted.

From the *form* of the concept of responsibility alone, we can already derive some interesting aspects of what being a person implies: On the one hand, *one* is responsible *for* one's actions, but, on the other, all this would not make any sense if this being responsible was not a responsibility one has *to* someone. So the relation of responsibility is three-place: x is responsible for H to y.[55] The question, of course, is what goes into the place of y. There may be cultures in which certain people owe responsibility only to particular groups or even just to themselves ("god-kings"), but in our modern societies, which have their roots in the universal ideas of the Enlightenment, a person is held *legally* responsible for her deeds by the whole of the community of persons falling under the laws and jurisdiction in question (usually institutionalised as a state), and held *morally* responsible for her deeds by the (ideal) community of *all other* persons. However, the question as to what degree responsibility is universalisable has no bearing on the simple fact that for someone to be held responsible for their deeds they at least must fulfil the cognitive *prerequisites* for acquiring the concept of responsibility (if we do not want to postulate that persons must necessarily *have* that concept already). These prerequisites are that one must be able to *regard oneself as oneself* and so to *attribute one's actions to oneself*. That is, a person will not only have *consciousness* (certain mental states and capabilities which are presupposed by the sheer ability to act and which we will consider in more detail later), but *self*-consciousness (having a concept of oneself as the one *having* these mental states and *doing* those actions). That is what Immanuel Kant meant with his notion of the "transcendental unity of apperception", the "I think", which "must be able to accompany all my representations" ("Kritik der reinen Vernunft", 1904/11 [AA III]:B 131).

---

[55] Even those who would be inclined to think that persons are responsible for their actions *simpliciter*, usually *do* have some surrogate for the third argument place in the relation of responsibility: "responsibility simplicter" is responsibility to "God" or to "Nature" etc.

So, to make use of language and to confer meaning is not a private affair; it rather presupposes being part of a *community*. Consequently, being a person ultimately presupposes the acknowledgement of other persons besides oneself. This has an immediate consequence which will again deserve our attention later on in Section 5.4: for it entails that persons must be able to recognise (identify) each other. Hence, as subjects of experiences, persons do not only experience the "objective world" from their different "subjective perspectives", but – even more important – they are the *objects* of the experience of *other* persons with whom, by communication, they intersubjectively constitute a common objective world.[61] That is, persons mutually constitute each other as inhabitants of a common objective world, and as such they must be locatable within the objective space-time framework too, running their course as long as they persist.

Starting with the rather parsimonious supposition that a person must be able to at least *acquire* the concept of responsibility, we came a long way in deriving a number of further conditions a being has to fulfil for being recognised as a person: Above all, it must have a concept of *itself*, which in turn demands cognitive capacities to such an extent that it can be said to be a subject of experiential knowledge, a participant in a community of language users, and as such locatable within the common objective world the community intersubjectively constitutes. It may come as a surprise to find that, in the end, this result comes very close to Locke's straightforward definition of a person as "a thinking intelligent Being, that has reason and reflection, and can consider it self as it self, the same thinking thing in different times and places" (Locke 1975:II, 27, §9).

[61] It becomes obvious now that the concept of objectivity featured throughout this text does not entail realism, but rather is neutral regarding this issue. While some authors (most prominently, the "early" Husserl of the "Logische Untersuchungen" [1900/1901]) indeed endorse a realistic understanding of objects of experience, they can be just as well understood as being constituted in their "objective being" as an outcome of discourse among subjects of differing experiences, i.e. persons. Objectivity in this sense is properly understood as *intersubjectivity*. And, though in the opinion of Kant and Husserl the feat is to be accomplished via general *conditions* regarding the subjects of experience rather than by discourse among them, intersubjectivity is also the sense in which both (Husserl since the "Ideas" [1913]) conceived of the "objectivity" of intentional objects of experience. While this, at first glance, may seem to be at odds with Kant's famous distinction between "things in themselves" and "things as they appear", it is important to realise that in writing on objectivity as secured by the categories of the understanding (in the "Transzendentale Analytik"), Kant wasn't concerned at all with arguing for the existence of inexperiencable "things in themselves" outside of the realm of the "Anschauung", but for the fact of objectivity *within* that empirical realm itself. (It is remarkable that the only – fairly weak – argument regarding the additional existence of "things in themselves" *outside* the realm of experience is given in the preface to the 2nd edition of the "Critique of Pure Reason". It bluntly states that we have to assume the existence of things in themselves to avoid the "contradiction" of there being "appearances" without anything that is appearing.)

5.3.2 "Being Capable of Having One's Actions Imputed to Oneself" – Further Cognitive, Motivational and Emotive Requirements of Personhood

In the following, we will try to dig a bit deeper still. That is, we will mainly talk *in more detail* about the cognitive capacities which we established above as conditions of personhood, and we will broaden the scope by considering motivational and emotive capacities as well. To this end, we once more begin with Kant, who confirms the forensic account of personhood by stating: "Person ist dasjenige Subjekt, dessen Handlungen einer Zurechnung fähig sind."[62] Kant stipulates *freedom of the will* or *autonomy* as a decisive prerequisite for the kind of imputability that he is considering to be constitutive for personhood. Autonomy stands for the freedom of rational agents to subject only to laws they adopt themselves by exercising reason. And reason, in turn, is viewed by him as located *outside* the causally determined realm of experience, even if it is – indirectly – operating on it. At this point it may seem as if we could not avoid entering the gargantuan field of debate about free will and its relation to the rival positions of (causal) determinism and anti-determinism. But fortunately we can. Most extant determinists are so-called *compatibilists*. Still, compatibilist determinists and incompatibilist libertarians *agree* that there is free will and responsibility and that the former is a necessary condition of the latter.[63] This opens up the possibility of formulating a position which is *neutral* with respect to the metaphysical issue of whether determinism is true or not.[64] In the following, we shall examine in neutral

---

[62] "Metaphysik der Sitten" (Kant 1907/14 [AA VI]:223) – "A person is a subject who is capable of having his actions imputed to him" (translation by W. Hastie). – Taken at face value, this quote might seem to imply that persons are subjects of a certain kind, i.e. constituting a subclass of subjects. However, this interpretation does not fit into the general frame of Kant's philosophy. The way he uses the two terms rather lends itself to the interpretation that all subjects (at least insofar as being a subject is meant to entail being capable of arriving at experiential knowledge) are persons. According to our own analysis, it furthermore seems that "person" and "subject" are not only coextensional predicates, but semantically necessarily so, that is, they in fact express the same concept. Their usage differs only insofar that the expression "subject" emphasises epistemological (theoretical) aspects, while "person" indicates that attention is to be focussed on moral (practical) aspects.

[63] That is because compatibilism holds that free will and responsibility are *compatible* with determinism. Only a minute fraction of philosophers contend that determinism is true and *hence* there is no free will and *hence* no one bears responsibility for his or her actions. Sometimes, these philosophers then advocate radical changes in our legal and juridical system to the effect that people should not be sentenced and punished according to "obsolete" categories like guilt, retribution or penance, but rather with respect to the chances of their resocialisation (i.e. the probability of them abstaining from committing crimes in the future). Of course, one cannot but wonder what performative sense such appeals to reform do make against the background that, if determinism is true, what is bound to happen will happen anyway.

[64] In Hartmann (2000/2005) it is argued that determinism is in fact false.

to respond) discriminatively to a presently given difference, then we may say that it *perceives* that difference. And if we can *account* for a being's responses towards a presently given difference only by assuming that it has been exposed to it before, then we may draw the conclusion that the being *recognises* that difference.[68]

In fact, most if not all perceptions involve recognition, and recognition is in turn the most basic function of the faculty of memory, be it in the form of recognition of *types* of situation ("*F* again") or of objects ("*a* again")[69]. If a being does not have recognitional capacities, it is not a person, not so much because there is a direct connection between recognitional capacities and executive virtues (though there is), but rather because a being that does not perceive/recognise much of what is going on around it will not be able to exercise very subtle forms of behaviour, let alone action. Still, obviously perception and recognition do not exhaust what is required for personhood. Taking responsibility for one's deeds presupposes another form of memory, the ability to remember *what one did*. For example, a decision one made is an event in one's life. If one cannot remember such events, how is one *ever* to act out one's decisions? Occasionally, we blame persons specifically for their forgetfulness, for instance when someone forgets having given a promise. But this is because we assume that the person would have remembered if she had only exercised some care. On the other hand, beings which cannot ever remember what they have done in the past will not be treated as responsible for their responses at all. Not only will they not be able to commit themselves to anything by promise or assent (because they will forget at once that they did); they will obviously be unable to lead any form of autonomous life. So, persons need to be able to recall their actions and, more generally, past experiences, that is they need to have *episodic memories*:

IIb) Persons need to be endowed with episodic memory.

Closely related to memory is another requisite for personhood:

IIc) Persons need to be endowed with learning abilities.

Quite often it is only a matter of point of view whether we refer to a being's memory abilities or its learning abilities in order to explain its responses. If we want to emphasise the process of *acquisition* of a behav-

---

[68] See Hartmann (1998:II.2.1) and Galert (2005:Ch. 2) for a more elaborate account. One important advantage of that account is that it provides a fairly clear understanding of how to ascribe these psychic functions to a being even in situations where (because of a lack of communicative abilities on the part of the respective being) it is not possible to simply ask it what or whether it is perceiving or recognising.

[69] It is important to see that (despite the examples in brackets) these basic functions of recognition do not yet presuppose the use of language. That is, "recognition" in this usage does convey the same meaning as the German "wiedererkennen", but not the same as "erkennen" in the sense which results in "Erkenntnis" ("knowledge"). The latter has to be of propositional structure and is therefore bound to language.

ioural modification (in the widest sense), we talk about learning. If, on the other hand, we want to emphasise the *retention* and *retrieval* of a behavioural modification, we talk about memory. A recourse to basic forms of learning is already involved at least in the *scientific* ascription of discriminative abilities as expounded above under IIa – for it is primarily in the context of learning (conditioning) experiments that we can acquire data that semantically warrant the ascription of specific abilities of perception and recognition.[70]

Neither discriminative abilities, nor simple forms of learning and memory require possession of language on the part of the discriminating/learning/remembering being. Even episodic memories need not necessarily assume a linguistic form. On the contrary, we would find it rather strange if we could "tell" what we did, but would lack any accompanying *re*-presentations in the visual, tactual, auditory or olfactory modes of imagination. However, there are nevertheless independent reasons for stating that:

IId) Persons need to be endowed with language abilities.

To hold a being responsible for what it does we need to assume some understanding of what it means to be responsible for one's deeds on the part of that being. One important aspect of being "capable of having one's actions imputed on oneself" is to be able to get engaged in the kind of interaction that is constitutive of *interpersonal relationships*. These relationships comprise, *inter alia*, the assertion and justification of claims against each other, the making of commitments, the granting of rights, the exchange of reasons for one's actions, the justification or questioning of actions with respect to rules, or the justification and questioning of those rules themselves. All these features of interpersonal exchange require the medium of a shared language,[71] however keeping in mind that the possession of language abilities is not to be equated with the ability to speak. The different systems of sign language for deaf mutes, for instance, basically fit the same purposes as do spoken and written forms of language.

Finally, language abilities are indispensable for persons as they are the decisive prerequisite for a final cognitive ability that we consider to be a necessary condition for personhood:

IIe) Persons need to be endowed with deliberative abilities.

---

[70] For a more general account of different forms of learning see Hartmann (1998:II.1.1.2). The relationship between the psychology of learning and the psychology of memory is dealt with ibid.:II.2.5.

[71] For the purposes at hand we do not need a clear-cut distinction between mere *communicative* abilities and *language* abilities in the strict sense. For a tentative account of some distinctive features of language see Hartmann (1998:167–168). However, it is clear from the examples given in the text that the communicative abilities of (at the very least) most animals lack the complexity required for typical interpersonal interaction.

No doubt, there are theoreticians who stand up for the possibility of thought without language (see e. g. Weiskrantz 1988). Once again, we cannot delve here into the reasons why we consider this position to be ill-founded, but we set them forth elsewhere (see Hartmann 1998:172–176). The need for deliberative abilities is already implied by what we just said concerning interpersonal relationships. So, we only would like to add that it is mostly *by deliberation* that persons arrive at decisions to act in spite of internal or external hindrances, or at decisions to refrain from acting in spite of certain immediate satisfactions or benefits that an action might bring about.

Considering the cognitive requirements for personhood we deduced above, it is obvious that animals will hardly qualify as persons and that infants are not *yet* persons. Animals as well as infants may be considered to have "personalities" in the weak sense that they can have individual character traits, that is certain relatively stable bundles of dispositions for behaviour of a certain kind (especially traits that are traditionally regarded as constituting the "temper", like aggressiveness, irritability, anxiousness, curiosity etc. – see Section 5.4.3 for more on this). But we will limit our use of the term "personality" to the character of persons. Our account of the cognitive criteria for personhood also explains why, in the introductory section of this chapter, we came to the conclusion that human beings in persistent vegetative state can no longer be regarded as persons. For these people as well as severely mentally challenged people do not fulfil most of the conditions we found to be constitutive for personhood. However, there is no doubt that, according to our criteria, most people who are considered to suffer from some mental disability will have to be regarded as persons as long as they are able to get engaged in social interactions to such an extent that they can grasp the meaning of responsibilities and mutual obligations. After all, a requirement like the demand of language abilities is not to be understood in such a way that a person would need to be able to comply with the highest standards of linguistic perfection. Finally, we also would like to reinforce the point we made above that by denying a human being the status of a person he or she is deprived of all *duties* and *responsibilities*, but not of his or her moral and juridical *rights.*[72] A common way of stating this is to say that the range of *moral objects* is broader than the range of *moral subjects*. Furthermore, it should be noted that by distinguishing between the moral category "person" and the biological category "human" the possibility is left open for there to be persons that are not humans as well. It is only a contingent fact that so far we never came across any nonhuman beings that would fulfil the cognitive criteria for personhood.

With our account of the cognitive prerequisites for personhood completed, we will ask what else might be required of persons besides these cog-

[72] Except, of course, such rights whose execution entails one's taking over certain duties – for example the right to negotiate and submit to a contract.

nitive abilities. We already stated that being a person is by no means a private affair, and now we would like to add that it is no ghostly affair either:

III) Persons need to be embodied.

This provision in fact follows from what we established already in this chapter, namely that persons must be locatable within the frame of objective space-time through which they run their course as long as they persist. The embodiment condition might seem trivial to some, but facing the long standing debate on persons as immaterial souls it certainly is not. However, given that persons are moral agents in the sense that they are capable of having their actions imputed on them, embodiment is obviously indispensable for being a person: Even if we grant, for the moment, that immaterial beings could effectuate changes in the material world, this would at once confront us with insurmountable problems in the context of actually *ascribing* such changes to mere spirits. If you think of a typical ghost story featuring some invisible poltergeist tossing down books from the shelves and so on, how are we to hold a *particular* poltergeist responsible for these nasty deeds? After all, it could be a dozen of them! By adding some recognisable ghostly voice coming out of nowhere and commenting on the deeds, the scenario certainly gets more "personish" (and scary), but it nevertheless won't be a candidate for serious consideration, because we would still lack the means for establishing a reliable connection between the invisible source of the voice and the intangible originator of the "actions".

The requirement of a body does, however, *not* presuppose even a remote resemblance to the human body. The body of a person may be of any matter, structure, shape and size as long as it is endowed with sense organs (not necessarily ours) and executive organs that allow actions in general and linguistic interactions *with us* (i.e. the community of human persons) in particular. We need not even assume the existence of a brain, although – at present – we don't know of any structure other than a brain that could warrant implementation of the functional requirements we postulated before.[73] We emphasised the indeterminacy of condition (III) in order to counterbalance any impression of "species chauvinism" that our account of the cognitive prerequisites for personhood might have created. On the other hand, since this study deals with interventions in human beings, the question of which degrees of freedom there are with respect to the way persons can be embodied is not of great relevance for the purposes at hand.

We will now inquire if there are – beyond the cognitive prerequisites and the embodiment condition – motivational and emotional prerequisites as well. Let's first consider whether a person necessarily needs to have certain

[73] But maybe we can at least *conceive* of possible designs for intelligent "no-brainers". Think, for instance, of a being with a web of ganglia (or just ganglia-*like* structures) evenly pervading its body.

This account is attractive to many because of its straightforward simplicity, but the bodily criterion for personal identity still fails.[87] This is shown by the following thought experiment: Let's assume science had developed to a stage where neurosurgeons would do successful brain transplantations. Let's assume further that, after an accident leaving the brain of a person *P* intact, but damaging the rest of its body *B* beyond any hope of recovery, *P*'s brain is transplanted into a living "donor body" *B'* (say the body of a former person *P'* which suffered brain death). While our strong intuition would be that, under these circumstances, *P* would still persist embodied by *B'*, *P* would have ceased to persist according to the persistence criterion of bodily identity.

Thought experiments like that have led most philosophers who favour a physical criterion for personal identity to drop the criterion of identity of the *body* and adopt a criterion of identity of the *brain* instead: Person stage x at time t is a stage of the same person P as person stage y at time $t+\Delta t$ if and only if the corresponding brain stages $b(x)$ at time t and $b(y)$ at time $t+\Delta t$ belong to the same brain B.

Unfortunately (perhaps), the criterion of brain identity fails as well. This can be shown by a thought experiment originally devised by Bernard Williams (1973)[88]: Assume we could scan the brain of a person with respect to all the relevant information regarding states and traits of her psyche, like episodic memories, cognitive capabilities and character traits.[89] Let's further assume that, for purposes of treatment or prevention of certain degenerative processes, we actually could replace (at first only relatively minor) parts of the brain by bio- and/or electronic implants and that we could overcome the problem of preserving the information residing in the parts to be replaced by suitably modifying our implants according to the information derived from a pre-surgery brain-scan.[90] This would certainly be a most welcome scientific breakthrough. If such interventions involving the replacement of minor parts of the brain proved successful in the sense that all original psychic functions were actually preserved, we would not dream of saying that after the surgery we do not deal

[87] Psychiatrists may want to raise the objection that the bodily criterion cannot account adequately for the concept of dissociative identity disorder (DID), formerly known as "multiple personality disorder". We can leave this issue undiscussed as the bodily criterion of personal identity also fails for other reasons.

[88] Actually, we are embellishing the original thought experiment of Williams quite considerably in order to make more obvious and striking its connection and relevance to the topic of new methods of intervening in the psyche.

[89] It is worth noting that *especially* those who would want to identify the self with the brain should conceive of this as possible at least *in principle* as they would hold that the self is the brain *precisely* because all psychic functions are encoded in the brain.

[90] This must not be read as meaning that information pertinent to the psyche is stored away in various parts of the brain like dishes in various drawers of a cupboard. Instead, information may "reside in" a part of the brain in the sense that via its mode of connection to other parts the part in question modulates or contributes to the overall information processing in a *specific way*.

with the *same* persons as before the surgery. But if this is so, then there is absolutely no reason for judging differently if such interventions eventually were extended to a point where brain-identity was not preserved anymore.[91] Think, for example, of the successive replacement of considerable parts of the brain by bio- or electronic implants, or by a mix of such implants, while – *ex hypothesi* – preserving all psychic functions. A most radical, empirically improbable, but still conceptually possible case would be the transplantation of a wholly new brain, thoroughly modified to match the results of the brain scan of the original brain. It follows from these considerations that identity of the brain as the criterion for personal identity over time has to be discarded.

5.4.2 Psychological Criteria of Personal Identity I: Memory

The reason why the brain was considered as pertinent to personal identity in the first place is that we (correctly, in all probability) assume that it embodies the psychic functions we are looking for: cognitive abilities and character traits. Accordingly, our investigation so far shows that it is rather these abilities and traits themselves we have to consider, not their contingent physical implementation.

We therefore continue by addressing ourselves to psychological criteria of personal identity. Again, Locke was the first to embrace this approach by suggesting "sameness of consciousness" as the criterion for personal identity over time (see e.g. Locke, 1975:II, 27, §23). Although consciousness encompasses much more, episodic memory is certainly the key to understanding this criterion insofar as consciousness according to Locke involves knowledge of one's thoughts and actions. "Sameness of consciousness" is constituted by the knowledge of thoughts and actions shared by earlier and later stages of a person via episodic memory. Therefore, even though Locke does not explicitly use the term in presenting his position, he is correctly regarded as trying to give a criterion for personal identity over time in terms of episodic memory. The difficulty is, however, to state the criterion in such a way that certain more or less tricky problems can be avoided. In order to gain insight into the problems to be avoided by an adequate memory-based criterion of personal identity, it is helpful to mention and discuss briefly the main strands of critique with which Locke's approach was historically confronted.

First, there is the so-called "circularity objection". It goes back to bishop Joseph Butler and can be stated like this[92]: A person *P1*'s memory of a past experience cannot be used as a criterion for *P1* being the person *P2* who originally had the experience in question because to establish that *P1* really *remembers* having had the experience, it would already have to be verified independently that *P1*=*P2*. The point is that, according to common usage,

[91] Or at least not according to any non-trivialising criterion for "identity of the brain".

[92] In the original writings of Butler, the objection itself is not presented in a very clear way. A contemporary reconstruction can be found in Shoemaker (1970).

"to remember" is a "success-verb", whose application is correct only if the remembered event really took place. This in turn engenders that, if what is remembered is an *experience*, (i.e. an episode from the first-person perspective), that experience must have been had by *oneself*.

It is quite obvious that the problem encountered here is a mere technicality. To avoid it we need a concept which in all save one aspect behaves like the concept of (episodic) memory: For its correct application it must not presuppose that the episode to be remembered actually happened to the person remembering it. Sidney Shoemaker (1970) coined the term "quasi-memory" for this concept. So, if we could "transplant" episodic memories (or if, in Lamarckian fashion, some episodic memories of parents could be inherited by their offspring), then the persons receiving the memories would quasi-memorise these episodes.[93]

A second problem with memory-based criteria for personal identity was pointed out by Thomas Reid (1983 [1785]). It draws on a strict reading of Locke's "sameness of consciousness" criterion, where "sameness" as constituted through knowledge *shared* by earlier and later stages is taken to imply that for various person-stages to belong to the same person the later stages have to faithfully retain the experiential contents of the earlier ones. If succeeding person stages *x*, *y*, *z* are such that *x* and *y* share some experiential content *E*, but *z* and *x* do *not* share that content as well, then – according to Locke's criterion in its strict interpretation – they do not constitute the same consciousness.

With his now famous "paradox of the 'brave officer'" Reid illustrates that this has quite unwelcome consequences[94]: Imagine a brave officer, who had been flogged for some mischief when he was still a boy, has taken a standard from the enemy during his first campaign as a young officer, and was eventually, at advanced age, promoted to rank of general. Further assume that he still could remember the flogging by the time he took the standard, and that he could remember taking the standard when he was made general, but by then had lost all memory of the flogging. According to Reid, it follows from Locke's account of personal identity that the boy and the young officer are the same person, as are the young officer and the general, whereas the boy and the general are not – and this would obviously be at odds with the transitivity of the relation of identity.

Reid's argument has to be disentangled a bit as his presentation is marred by the fact that he confuses continuants with stages. Only because of this the conflict with the transitivity of identity arises. We saw in Section 5.2.4 that different stages cannot be identical anyway, so that questions regarding the identity of continuants encountered at different times have to be put this

---

93 In fact, if wholesale Lamarckian inheritance of parental episodic memory would be the standard, our understanding of the life of persons would probably be very different (for the result would be a very complex network of psychological fusions and fissions pervading different organisms).

94 See Reid (1983):Ch. 6 of "Of Memory".

way: "Are $O1$ at t_1 and $O2$ at t_2 both stages of the *same* continuant?" Hence, what Reid *should* have argued is that according to Locke's theory (in its strict interpretation) the boy and the young officer are both stages of some person P, and the young officer and the general are both stages of a person P'. But as – again according to Locke's criterion for sameness of consciousness – P and P' do not *share* all their stages (the boy-stage belongs to person P, but not to P'), it follows that $P \neq P'$. And even though this is *not* logically inconsistent, Reid has indeed a point in claiming that this result shows Locke's criterion of personal identity to be inadequate. For, of course, all three stages – boy, young officer and general – should belong to *one* person.

What this means is that an adequate (quasi-)memory based criterion for personal identity over time has to take into account that persons may *forget*. This is achieved by defining a transitive relation of *(quasi-)memory continuity*.[95] As this relation is logically complex, the definition has to be broken down into several steps[96]:

(R*-Def.) Let R^*xy stand in for the following relation: y can *quasi-memorise* at least one episode of experience of x from the x-perspective (i.e. the first person perspective).

The range of x and y are person-stages.[97] As mentioned above, as is the case for memory proper, quasi-memory has to be veridical in the sense that the episodes recalled by person-stage y really happened to person-stage x, but unlike memory proper, it does not presuppose that x and y are stages of the same person. It is an indispensable proviso that the episodes are recallable from the first person-perspective of x. Else, if I can recall episodes I saw happening to my father, and my father at that time was able to recall episodes he saw happening to *his* father, the intended definition of "memory continuity" building on R^* would yield continuity between the respective stages of my grandfather, my father and me. And as "memory continuity" is supposed to provide a criterion for personal identity, this would eventually lead to the absurd result that there is a person P of which these three stages are temporal parts. Note that for the relation R^* to hold between x and y, y does not *actually* have to recall an episode happening to x, but just has to be able to do

[95] Using Locke's terminology, we could say that "sameness of consciousness" is constituted by *continuity* of knowledge about one's past experiences rather than by actually *shared* knowledge.

[96] Usually this is done by employing the apparatus of formal logic to make fully transparent the pertinent structural and inferential properties of the concepts to be defined. However, for the benefit of readers who don't have a background in formal logic, we just introduce a few symbols standing in for the concepts we are talking about (for the purpose of convenient cross-referencing) and otherwise give the account in plain English.

[97] As such they have to be embodied. However, having abandoned physical persistence criteria, we do *not* postulate here and in the following that these stages must share the same body or brain.

so.[98] Note also that, for convenience's sake, we did not attach time-indices to the stages x and y in the above definition. But it is implicit in the definition of R^* that x and y can only stand in the relation R^*xy if it is true for times $t(x)$ and $t(y)$ that $t(x)<t(y)$.[99] For if $t(x)>t(y)$, then we would not speak of "memory", but rather of something like "precognition". The case $t(x)=t(y)$ is ruled out by the following considerations: Either $x_t=y_t$ or $x_t \neq y_t$. If $x_t \neq y_t$, then these person-stages count as embodiments of different persons anyway (and y's capacity to "recall" something experienced by x would be considered as some kind of "clairvoyance"). If $x_t=y_t$, then the person-stage in question cannot, strictly speaking, experience something and *at the same time* recall it already.

R^* is irreflexive and asymmetrical.[100] Above all, it is not transitive. We now (recursively) define a transitive relation R using R^* as follows:

---

[98] This too must not be read in too strict a sense. For example, while someone is asleep at night he may be considered to be "able" to memorise episodes of the day in the sense that *if* we wake him up and ask him, he will tell us about it. (Generally, this dispositional reading should go for all capacities deemed constitutive for personhood – cf. Quante 2002:20.)

[99] It is important to note that the times t have to be taken to be (conveniently small) time spans, *not* points in time. The reason for this is that stages have to be spatiotemporal *parts* of continuants. If one successively divides a spatial object into ever smaller parts, the parts will still remain extended. The same has to hold for the division of a continuant into temporal parts. For convenience's sake in what follows we just consider a division of time into "small" stretches of like duration leading to what could be called "standard stages" as smallest units. But of course any temporal part of a person may count as a "stage". This does not at all affect the validity of the arguments in the main text, as long as we disregard stage overlaps or stage inclusions – where the terminology of "later"/ "earlier"/"simultaneous" becomes muddled. The ensuing problems could be solved by providing a mereological theory, but more easily they can be avoided by observing the convention that in theoretical contexts the breakdown of continuants into stages should always be carried out such that the resultant stages do not overlap (that is, instead of two overlapping stages we would consider three continuous stages, etc.).

[100] For readers not familiar with the terminology regarding structural properties of relations, we explain at least those types of relations used by us in the text: A two-place relation Rxy is *reflexive* if on the range of objects that can stand in the relation R *every* object must bear the relation R to itself. For example, every object that at all has a length has the same length as itself. R is *non-reflexive* if there could possibly be objects that do not bear R to itself. E.g. perhaps not everyone loves himself. R is *irreflexive* if no object can stand in the relation R to itself. For example no object can be longer than itself. R is *symmetric* in case that if x stands in the relation R to y, then so will y to x. For example if Fritz is of equal height as Hans, then Hans got to be of equal height as Fritz. R is *non-symmetric* if there can be pairs of objects x,y with Rxy, but not Ryx. For example, Fritz may like Hans, and yet Hans may not like Fritz. R is *asymmetric* in case that if Rxy, then it can never hold the other way round, too. For example, if x is taller than y, then y can't be taller than x. Finally, R is *transitive* just in case that if Rxy and Ryz, then we must also have Rxz. For example if Bill is taller than Jacques, and Jacques is taller than Fritz, then Bill got to be taller than Fritz. R is *non-transitive* if that doesn't have to be the case. For example, if Anna is befriended to Lisa, and Lisa befriended to Wendy, then Anna may or may not be befriended to Wendy. R is *intransitive* if this *can't* be the case. For example, if x is father of y and y is father of z, then x can't be father of z. The way we explained these structural properties, they have to be understood as determined by the *meaning* of the very concepts R in question.

(R-Def.) Let Rxy stand in for the following relation: The person-stage y is *indirectly linked* via (quasi-)memory to the person-stage x. R is to hold between x and y if and only if there is a finite chain of person stages beginning with x and ending with y where each link is connected to the next through the relation of quasi-memorisability R^*.

We can now define the relation of *(quasi-)memory continuity* C:

(C-Def.) Let Cxy stand in for the following relation: Two person-stages x and y stand in the relation of *(quasi-)memory continuity.* C is to hold between x and y if and only if y is indirectly linked through (quasi-)memory to x (i.e. Rxy), or x is indirectly linked through (quasi-)memory to y (i.e. Ryx), or x and y are the same stage (i.e. $x=y$).

C is a so-called "similarity relation", characterised by being reflexive and symmetric, yet not transitive. Using the relation C of (quasi-)memory continuity, we can now finally proceed to define what it means (within the framework of theories drawing on psychological continuity criteria) for a conglomerate of person-stages to constitute a person:

(P-Def.) Let Px stand in for the predicate "x is a *person*". P is to hold with respect to a conglomerate p of person-stages if and only if
1) all person-stages belonging to p as temporal parts are continuous (C) to one another and
2) p is *maximal* in the sense that if some person-stage is continuous to all stages belonging to p as temporal parts, then it is itself a temporal part of p.

From this it follows as a *necessary* criterion of personal identity over time that if two person-stages encountered at different times both belong to some (the same) person, then they must be continuous; and more generally:

(MemCrit1) *If the members of a set of person-stages M all belong as temporal parts to some (the same) person p, then they must all be continuous to one another.*

Regarding the relation between personal identity and persistence, based on the definition (P-Def.) given above, the question of whether a certain person p persists at a certain time t is rendered trivial: it boils down to the question of whether there is a person stage at t belonging to p.[101]

---

[101] In line with what we said in Section 2, this definition does not rule out the possibility of "reincarnation", i.e. that a person persists during a certain time span, then ceases to persist, then persists again later. To exclude this possibility, one would have to incorporate into the definition that for any two stages x and y belonging to p with $t(x)<t(y)$, $t(y)$ is either the direct successor of $t(x)$ (with respect to our division of time into standard durations) or there is a stage z also belonging to p and $t(x)<t(z)<t(y)$.

process persons can persist in spite of *considerable* loss of episodic memory. In this, it is an important stabilising factor that their character-traits remain suitably stable for their social contacts to "recognise" and anticipate their "typical" actions and behaviour. However, this "robustness" of personal identity does not extend as far as to cover also the final stages of the disease where episodic memory is eventually too attenuated and disintegrated to still provide for suitable interaction – think of the stages when the patients don't recognise their relatives and friends anymore.

5.4.3 Psychological Criteria of Personal Identity II: Personality/Character

Now the crucial question is: Is (episodic) memory continuity not only necessary, but also sufficient for personal identity over time?[106] Instances of radical personality change, as most strikingly exemplified by the fictional character(s) "Dr. Jekyll and Mr. Hyde", render this doubtful: In Stevenson's novel, episodic memory seems to remain unaffected through the back and forth transformations between Jekyll and Hyde. After all, Dr. Jekyll at least initially takes delight in living out his "dark side", which could hardly be explained had he forgotten everything he did as Mr. Hyde. Still, it seems natural enough to suggest that we are faced in the story with altogether different *persons* rather than with one person repeatedly undergoing *personality changes.* Admittedly, it is by no means crystal clear how this case and related – less dramatic, but non-fictional – cases are to be judged.[107] But, tellingly, our intuitions are not as unambiguous as in the thought-experiments destined to explore whether memory continuity is *necessary* for personal identity. We do not say: "Well, *of course* they must be one and the same person, for they stand in the relation of memory continuity!"

---

[106] In some way it is *certainly* not a sufficient criterion because it is stated much to liberally. The antecedent of MemCrit2 could already be fulfilled if there is just one single isolated quasi-memory connecting me to someone else. However, this is not a decisive argument against memory continuity *as such.* It merely shows that, to be sufficient, the relation R would still have to be strengthened. Doing this by adding constraints on the *amount* of quasi-memories or their causal *origin* (as promoted by some philosophers) is not very promising. Rather, it is their *content* that needs to be further specified. Instead of being isolated entities, memories usually are connected to other memories, so that each of them has a distinctive "place" within the network of one's memories as a whole. If the quasi-memories of a person-stage y connecting it with the experiences of a person-stage x do not "fit in" with the whole of y's network of memories, they may not offer sufficient evidence for establishing that there is a person the stages x and y both belong to. However, we will not attempt to specify the criterion of content-connectedness of memories any further here. The reason is twofold: firstly, we will see that a criterion of memory-continuity cannot be sufficient for personal identity anyway, and secondly, the sort of connectedness we just referred to is much better explained within the "narrative account" of personal identity, which we will expound later.

[107] As a convenient litmus test for our intuitions we may ask ourselves whether we would tend to hold Dr. Jekyll responsible for Mr. Hyde's deeds. If they are the same person, we certainly should do so.

So, when it comes to the question what is *sufficient* for personal identity, then, in addition to memory-continuity, personality-traits seem to be relevant, too. As additional evidence for this observation one may cite the common way of talking about the "identity" of persons, in which the term is more or less synonymous with, or at least closely related to what is called "personality".[108] This would be not at all mere coincidence if (aspects of) personality should turn out to contribute in a pertinent way to questions regarding the persistence of persons. However, in order to see how exactly we may refer to it in framing criteria for personal identity, we need to analyse the notion of personality in somewhat more detail.

What ever personality is, it surely is not to be understood as a simple property. Therefore, we first try to analyse the complex bundle of interacting traits (p-traits, for short) personality seems to consist of. To get a grip on the question as to what p-traits are and what distinguishes them from other traits persons may have, we set out by defining the comparatively unsophisticated concept of "habit": Habits are dispositions to behave or act in a certain way in certain types of situations. Dispositions themselves may be established and disestablished again, and there is no constraint on how long a disposition can or must hold to count as one. But habits not only are "relatively stable" – that is the underlying associations between types of situation and types of action or behaviour have to hold over a suitable length of time –, but they also have to manifest themselves suitably often.[109] Habits are not themselves p-traits, however: e.g. the habit to brush one's teeth, drink coffee in the morning or raise one's hat to greet people one encounters would not count as p-traits (or character-traits). A single p-trait is not just a stable disposition to act/behave, but rather comprises a wide range of dispositions of a certain more general kind. Instead of trying to define this more precisely, we settle for giving examples: For instance, the p-trait of "friendliness" will comprise habits like greeting people, giving polite answers to questions, readily offering help when needed etc. Or the p-trait of "being conservative" will comprise various dispositions favouring established or well-tried situations, procedures and institutions over new alternatives. It is far from easy to categorise such traits. According to the well-

---

[108] We already alluded to this usage that is sometimes picked up by psychology too when discussing the case of McMurphy in the introductory section where we found that, in this way of talking about "identity", more emphasis is given to those personality traits which make the person in question differ from other persons, i.e. those which – in their combination – make him "unique".

[109] What length of time and what frequency of occurrence are to be regarded "suitable" depends on the context at hand. A mayfly during its short life might be said to have had the habit to fly in the direction of light-sources. On the other hand, I probably can't be said to have had the "habit" of coming home late last week, or throughout my life to have had the habit of visiting my parents on turns of centuries. It seems to be futile here to try being much more precise than that.

known classification[110] by Joy Paul Guilford, we would have the following categories: temper, attitude, interests, needs, abilities (talents), morphological traits and physiological traits. Out of these we would dismiss morphological traits (e.g. skin-colour) and physiological traits (e.g. being prone to sweat) right away as it seems not to be adequate to regard them as p-traits in a strict sense (even though they may under certain circumstances very well causally condition, interact with or "favour" certain p-traits in the more strict sense).

Temper is the oldest known category of p-traits. Temper comprises long-term emotional dispositions.[111] Hippocrates – the "father of medicine" – sorted these into typical bundles, constituting the sanguineous, choleric, phlegmatic and melancholic personality types. Based on similar considerations by Wilhelm Wundt (1903), Hans J. Eysenck (1965) postulated two dimensions – introverted/extroverted and stable/unstable – in which all traits belonging to temper are supposed to be locatable.[112] If the dimensions are graphically represented as orthogonal lines defining a plane, the four sections comprise temper-traits belonging to the classical four tempers distinguished by Hippocrates: introverted-stable=phlegmatic, introverted-unstable=melancholic, extroverted-stable=sanguineous, extroverted-unstable= choleric. Accordingly, "depressed" (German: "bedrückt") – the typical attribute of the melancholic type – is about equally accounted for by "introversion" and "instability". On the other hand, "anxious" and "unsociable" also belong to the melancholic personality, but "anxious" loads higher on instability than on introversion, while for "unsociable" it's the other way around.

---

[110] There are other classifications, of course. We especially mention Guilford's because it is not only one of the most prominent classifications, and probably the most exhaustive, it is also the easiest to start from, with the goal of conceptual clarification in mind.

[111] One may be in an aggressive *mood* without having an aggressive *temper*. One could say that the temper of an individual is characterised by those moods – relatively short term dispositions to feel (and thus act) in a certain way – which are "chronic" in that individual, that is, occur so often and/or last so long as to pervade the life of the individual, shaping the whole of its behaviour and agency.

[112] For the reader to grasp Eysenck's model, we have to explain briefly the basic features of so called "factor analysis". Factor analysis is a mathematical method (developed by the psychologist Charles Spearman at the beginning of the twentieth century) for grouping variables according to their mutual correlations. But instead of just putting the variables into *categories*, new variables – "factors" – are abstracted ("extracted") from the correlation-data, and then used to describe the original variables and their relations: For every variable and factor, there is the measure of how much the variable is "loaded" with the factor. The higher the loading, the higher the contribution of the factor to the value of the variable. The goals are to find factors which are "orthogonal", i.e. uncorrelated to one another, to have as few factors as possible that still allow for a most exhaustive description of the relations among the original variables, and – last but not least – to keep the factors easily interpretable. Eysenck's dimensions "introverted/extroverted" and "stable/unstable" are just such orthogonal factors.

By his category, “needs”, Guilford does not address “universal needs” like the need of food or fluid intake for survival, as such needs do not differ in any interesting way between persons.[113] Rather, the traits he has in mind would belong to a broader category comprising *basic long-term motifs* (interests, goals, values) which persons may or may not have, or may have in varying degrees. Guilford’s “interests” category (to be understood in the common way of “taking an interest in specific activities” – such as “thinking”, “chatting”, “doing needlework”, “climbing mountains”, etc.) would also fall under that broad category as long as they are long-term and basic in the sense that they are executed for their own sake (not just as means to *other* goals).

“Attitudes” towards all kinds of issues (things, facts, proposals, norms etc.), while quite correctly being associated with personality, at first may not seem to constitute an independent group insofar as they are analytically bound to motifs via mediation of one’s (long-term) beliefs: If my goals include getting good education for my offspring, and my beliefs include that college *C* is substandard, then – all other things being equal[114] – my attitude regarding the idea to have my daughter attend college *C* is already fixed. However, beliefs are *themselves* (propositional) attitudes. And while certain beliefs may be “favoured” by one’s motifs, and certain motifs by one’s beliefs, no group can be reduced to the other. Hence, *basic* (=non-derivative) *long-term propositional attitudes* indeed form a category of their own that in conjunction with the category of motifs determines a person’s attitudes in the wider sense.

Finally, what about *talents?* A talent for *X* is an innate[115] and, compared to the average, increased capacity[116] to learn whatever is required to successfully perform the kinds of actions related to *X*. Are talents p-traits? Or do they just interact with the personality?[117] Considering the common use of “personal-

[113] When inquiring about someone’s *personality*, we would find it rather strange to be informed that the person in question has got to eat, drink and sleep on a regular basis.

[114] Meaning that in the complex net of purposes and beliefs no other purpose-belief connections serve to outweigh or override this connection.

[115] Although one can indeed acquire talents – by maturing –, and though one may be fostered in this process of maturing, it would be wrong to claim that talents themselves can be “learned”. By which actions could someone learn not merely how to play the violin well, but rather the *talent*, i.e. the increased capacity to learn to play the violin well?

[116] “Increased capacity” does first and foremost mean that the achievable *level of success* is higher than in non-talented competitors. Though this does most often include the ability to achieve levels *faster*, this ability is usually not to be identified with the talent itself. To be sure, someone *may* be said to have the “talent” to get into the very basics of certain things extremely fast (and then be forever stuck there). In that case, however, the description of the respective talent would have to mention that, explicitly.

[117] There are certain usages of the word “character” by which talents would not be regarded as part of the character, namely when “character” is restricted to such traits – like “reliability” or “greed” – that are subject to moral judgements. This usage comes to the fore in phrases like “she has character”, “he’s got a bad charac-

ity" it seems that talents do not just interact with, but rather are to be considered an integral part of the personality of a person. For example, could one adequately describe the personality of Einstein without mentioning his knack for physics? But then again, what about latent and unused talents? Could it be that only fully developed talents form a part of one's personality? We think this should be answered to the negative, at least if one does not want to exclude a person's *potentials* from the p-traits of that person. A person may never have gone into politics, but he or she nevertheless may have had all the prerequisites of becoming a great social reformer (and if this does not count as information about personality, then what does?).[118]

In a nutshell, our analysis of personality in terms of the character-traits it seems to consist of yields the result that personality is the system of interacting *temper*-traits, (long-term) *motifs*, (long-term) *propositional attitudes* and *talents*. Regarding the quest for a not only necessary, but also sufficient condition for personal identity over time, one could now try to augment the requirement of memory continuity by postulating that, additionally, a certain yet to be specified relation pertaining to personality (character) has to hold between two person stages for them to belong to one (the same) person.

It is quite easy to see that a mere relation of "character continuity" (defined in formal analogy to memory continuity[119]) will not do the job: Just compare the logically possible case where – for whatever reason – a character-change occurs continuously, but radically, in a matter of days (or maybe hours), with the case that – somewhere within the same time period – an equivalent result is brought about "abruptly" (non-continuously). Whatever we would decide regarding the question of personal identity in such cases,

---

ter" etc. But if we consider that traits of temper *definitely* belong to character, this already goes to show that a purely moral usage of "character" is too narrow, as certainly many temper-traits are neutral in that regard – e.g. to be anxious is *per se* neither a virtue nor a vice.

[118] However, it is worth noting that from the inclusion of talents into the range of p-traits it does not follow that the concrete abilities (psychic or physical) one acquires in using a talent are themselves p-traits. This would indeed stretch the use of "personality" or "character" beyond what is adequate. A person may have the talent to do maths, but only that talent, not the particular ability to solve quadratic equations is part of her personality.

[119] One would start out with a basic relation of "(sufficient) character overlap", where two stages have (a certain minimum amount of) p-traits in common. One then would go on defining that two person stages stand in the relation of "character continuity" if they are indirectly linked via a chain of stages where each two succeeding stages stand in the relation of "(sufficient) character overlap". Eventually, one would arrive at a definition stating that a conglomerate of person-stages constitutes a person if and only if the stages all stand in the relations of (quasi-)memory continuity *and* character continuity to one another, and the conglomerate is maximal. According to such a definition, each relation would provide a necessary criterion for personal identity, while together they would (purport to) yield a sufficient criterion.

we would most probably not treat the two cases *differently;* and even *if* we did so, then definitely not *because* the change was "continuous" in the first case and "non-continuous" in the second.

A lesson which, one may think, has to be learned from this is that a character-based criterion has to draw on a demand for a certain "stability" of a person's character over time rather than on continuity. On the other hand, it is clear from the outset that at least the most straightforward form of such a demand – namely that a person's character should *not at all* change – would be blatantly false (pace Schopenhauer). Hence, even while stability of character and (quasi-)memory continuity combined would maybe *suffice* for personal identity over time, this is achieved only on pain of that combined condition not being *necessary* anymore because one ingredient (character-stability) is not necessary for a person's persistence. Nothing is more obvious than the observation that not every change in personality already amounts to identity change.[120] For good or bad, the personality of persons is bound to develop throughout their lives. Hence, an adequate criterion for personal identity over time must leave room for personality changes. More than that: it is also futile to single out any specific *subset* of p-traits from the categories *temper, motifs, attitudes* and *talents* which is such that at least *its* members have to remain stable for a person to "survive" as the person she is. For there is no such set: All else being equal, any given p-trait may at some point during a person's life be subject to change without the person ceasing to persist.[121]

So what are we to do with this? As a last try one could seek to reconcile the conflicting demands for continuity and stability by proposing a criterion of

[120] While this statement hardly seems to require justification, let us give one reason (just in case): If a person's character could – for conceptual reasons – never change, then any observed change in personality would imply that a person (the one who used to be there prior to change) has actually ceased to persist, giving way to another, the "post-change" person (both being successively embodied by the same organism). This in turn would imply that one could, for example, not be convicted for a crime after a personality change, for the crime would have been committed by someone else entirely (namely the pre-change person) – which of course is absurd.

[121] What if one suggested that, while every single p-trait may indeed change, the character "as a whole" must not change beyond a certain degree (say 50% of the p-traits) for still being able to talk about "the same" person? This is, of course, totally out of the question as it is open to "Reid"-type objections: Imagine our brave officer changing about 25% of his character-traits from boyhood to young adulthood, and then again such that in the end somewhat more than 50% of the p-traits have changed along the way from boyhood to old age. Again we would have the undesirable case that boy and young officer constitute one person, and young officer and general *another* – with the young officer belonging to *both.* But this is not where it ends: Definitions in this vein could split up one person into a whole bunch of "overlapping" persons, depending on *where* one cuts out phases just satisfying the criterion (looking continuously back in time from the old age undoes certain changes, which in turn gives room for taking in more of the boyhood personality – and *vice versa).*

character continuity with "relatively slow" overall character change – calling this "relative character stability". – But this would be intolerably vague, if not really desperate. How leisurely paced would we like character change to proceed so as not to endanger personal identity? We confess that we cannot see any non-arbitrary answer to this. Even *if* we would resort to just setting certain constraints by decision (of the sort that there must not be more than n p-trait changes for two person stages that are less than a certain stretch of time Δt apart), this would not help at all. The reason is that every such notion of "relative character stability" would still have a continuity relation built into it. With reference to that "ingredient", it can always be challenged by imagining some Methuselah who fulfils the relevant criteria for being a person all through his age-long life, but – while all stages satisfy the combined criteria of (quasi-)memory continuity *and* relative character stability (whichever way the latter may be spelled out) – the late stages bear *no* direct relation, neither memory- nor character-wise, to the early stages. Wouldn't we be inclined to say that in such a case the early stages and the late stages constitute different persons? In fact we do not have to decide this question to see the inadequacy of "relative character stability". It suffices to note that the Methuselah case is setting the stage for the very same objection we've already discussed above with respect to the relation of "mere" character continuity: If we compare two "Methuselahs", where in both cases the late stages are radically different from the early ones, we would not dream of treating them differently with respect to questions pertaining to personal identity (like whether we could hold the old men responsible for crimes they committed during their youth) just because we were told that in one case the intermediary stages all satisfy the requirements of "relative character stability", while in the other case there had occurred a more "rapid" character-change somewhere along the way.

The message to be taken from this discussion is that psychological continuity relations – whether drawing on memory, p-traits or a combination of both – will *never* provide sufficient criteria for personal identity, but at best necessary ones (like quasimemory continuity).[122] On the other hand, any strengthening of (quasi-)memory continuity by way of combining it with some strict psychological equivalence relation[123] (like "sameness of charac-

---

[122] Indeed, in its original context, the "Methuselah" example (as discussed by Lewis 1983: "Survival and Identity", IV) does not deal with character, and rather should be viewed as arguing for the inadequacy of any mere continuity relation for providing a sufficient criterion of personal identity. We therefore could have used the "Methuselah" example already above to support the argument that (quasi-)memory continuity is by itself not a sufficient criterion for personal identity. The reason that we didn't do so, but rather drew attention to the possible overriding force of radical character change, is that the full strength of the "Methuselah" example is only exploited if it is used to show that even (quasi-)memory continuity and character continuity combined do not yield a sufficient criterion.

[123] Equivalence relations are reflexive, symmetric and transitive.

ter") will *at best* provide a sufficient criterion, however on pain of not being a necessary one anymore.

5.4.4 A Narrative Approach to Personality

Alas, it is time to admit defeat on this particular battlefield and look out for a whole new tack on the issue. What we tried to do until now was to specify necessary and/or sufficient conditions that persons needs to fulfil in order to remain who they are over a course of time. The failure of all these attempts could be taken to indicate that, as a matter of principle, this type of criteriological approach will not yield a satisfying account of personal identity. This is because its feasibility critically hinges on the assumption that problems of personal persistence may be settled by referring to changes in psychic traits that can be qualified without further reference to the specific *situation* in which these changes occur. In this way, we feel entitled to say, for example, that *whenever* a being suffers a total loss of its language abilities it cannot be considered a person afterwards. However, there is a conspicuous difference between situations in which a being's person-status is in question and situations in which we come to decide cases of identity change. While in the former situations the affected being will hardly "raise its voice" on its own behalf[124], in the latter cases we are considering persons that have a stake in their being recognised as still or no longer the same and as such will themselves *participate* in the process of deciding about the pertinence of the kind of change they underwent. Maybe it is due to its participatory nature that the social process that mediates our mutual recognition as one-and-the-same in different situations cannot be adequately analysed in terms of context-invariant criteria. To further investigate the plausibility of this reasoning, our next step will be to develop a theoretical account of the process of challenging and defending claims for or against personal persistence that promises to do better justice to its inherent context-sensitivity.

In order to attain a reasonable distinction between gradual personality changes, on the one hand, and outright changes of personal identity, on the other, we first need to establish a more adequate understanding of personality. Up to now we treated personality more or less as a mere aggregate of p-traits. This account would be adequate with regard to the character of animals or pre-personal toddlers. In the previous section we stated that many character traits can be ascribed to non-personal beings, provided they display suitably complex behaviour with stable long-term dispositions. Their *character* is nothing over and above the sum total of these ascriptions of character traits. Still, the difference with regard to *personality* is not just that next to these character traits persons also possess some further (or, for that

[124] If it does, this will of course suffice to falsify the hypothesis that it is not a person we are dealing with. Please also keep in mind what we said in the previous section about personhood, namely that having "language abilities" does not presuppose the ability to *speak* (i.e. using the larynx).

matter, even *many)* p-traits that cannot be ascribed to beings that aren't persons because of them lacking certain abilities. In this vein it would be right to say that a person, but not an animal can be virtuous or courteous as these traits require a conceptual grasp of certain values or norms that is beyond reach for any known animal mind. However, compared to character as it may be attributed to beings which are not persons, personality is not merely a construct with some extra dimensions. Rather, there is a qualitative difference due to the fact that persons are self-referential beings, who not only *have* character traits, but, moreover, hold a set of beliefs *about* these traits as well.[125]

What persons believe about their own p-traits is part of a more complex system of self-related beliefs (and, as we will see, motifs) that constitutes their *self-concept.* When, in the third section, we found that persons as moral agents need to have a concept of them*selves* being members of a community of "others like them", we brought to bear the concept of a self in a most general form. Actually, all individual persons at any given time of their persistence entertain a much more colourful self-concept, which they may – under inviting circumstances – disclose by numerous statements involving the personal pronoun "I". However, by no means all self-related statements constitute part and parcel of a person's self-concept. For instance, I do not reveal anything about how I understand myself by stating "I had a bad night's sleep." Just like personality, the self-concept does not represent how a person is at the present moment or how she thinks about herself today, but rather it offers a more general or long-term account. Tentatively, we can single out the relevant statements by postulating that they may be uttered in response to the question "Who are you?" Of course, when confronted with this somewhat dubious question, we usually make do with saying our name. But suppose our opponent is not satisfied with our reply, and provided we take a sincere interest in presenting a comprehensible picture of who we are, then we may start telling a more detailed story including distinguishing features of various kinds: As said before, we may express opinions on our p-traits. Given the way we introduced these traits, this includes statements about our values, preferences, and what we appreciate in life ("I hate injustice", "I am a soccer maniac" etc.). However, a person's self-concept is not exhausted by beliefs on his or her p-traits. For instance, while we excluded morphological and physiological traits in our review of Guilford's account of personality, *beliefs* about traits of these kinds may very well form part of personal self-concepts ("I am a particularly handsome and good looking guy", "The root cause of all my problems with others is that I am not attractive", etc.). Even though we took pains to conceptually discern persons from their bodies, it cannot be neglected that in talking about themselves persons frequently refer

[125] This is (or anyway should be taken as) already implicit in that part of Locke's definition of "person" according to which a person can *consider itself as itself.* If a person can do this, she will necessarily have what we will call a "self-concept" and expound in the paragraphs to follow.

to their bodies. Furthermore, in the stories they tell about who they are, persons like to include pieces of information that relate to their social position by specifying e.g. their occupation or certain of their achievements ("I am a member of parliament", "I am a father of six children" etc.). Finally and most peculiarly, who a person is in part determined by who he or she *wants* to be.[126] That is, a person's self-concept includes her projects of "self-creation".[127] In summary, we don't want to be very restrictive regarding the question as to what kinds of self-related beliefs persons may incorporate in their self-concepts. Everything persons consider to be "typical" or significant for their individual "way of being" can be a proper part of their self-concept.

Statements by which persons seem to express their self-concepts can be untrue in two different ways: Firstly, as a matter of fact, persons at times deliberately deceive others about their personality. For various reasons (too obvious to mention), people sometimes want others to believe that they have certain p traits which they actually lack. Usually, when persons deliberately give false information about their personality, they will (at those occasions) also try to act accordingly, so that those they are trying to cheat will more readily believe that they really are the kind of person they claim to be. Of course, it would be wrong to say that persons express their self-concept by statements that are uttered to deceive others. A person's self-concept is constituted only by those beliefs that he or she honestly considers to be true. By deceitful self-related statements and by those actions that should render them credible persons actively create *images* of themselves.[128] It seems quite safe to claim that, next to their self-concept, most persons entertain one or more images fitting different purposes and contexts. Now, to unmask images, it is not enough to find out that the information persons convey about their personality is not correct – after all they may honestly believe

---

[126] This is what in psychology is called the "ideal self-(image)". My ideal self does not consist in how I see myself, but rather how I *want* to be or *become*. It could be said that one's ideal self is the *normative dimension* of one's self-concept.

[127] This particular aspect of personhood has been analysed with great care by Jonathan Glover (1988).

[128] Since the dichotomy of self-concept versus image is of paramount importance for psychotherapy, numerous terms in different languages (that frequently are not readily translatable) have been introduced to address it. In English, the term "persona(e)" is sometimes used to refer to the social role(s) a person may play. However, we decided for the more neutral term "image" in order to avoid the baggage "persona" carries due to its origin in archetypal psychology. To avoid possible misreading of our discussion about "images" in the main text above, it is in order, however, to point out some more things pertaining to ideal self-images: Just as the ideal self-image does not describe how I actually see myself, it also must not be confused with how I want others to see me – in those mere "images" I may create of myself. Persons also try to act according to their ideal self-image, just like in the case of a mere "image". However, in doing this, they do normally *not* want to deceive others about their p-traits, but just to attain these traits as habits. In fact, people are often perfectly *honest* about these things ("I always try to be friendly, but once I'm under stress, I tend to lose my temper").

that they really are as they are claiming to be. So how can one know what is genuine self-concept and what is image in these cases? Well, as the saying goes, you can fool some people all the time, and you can fool all people some of the time, but you can't fool all people all the time. In contrast to acting in accord with one's p-traits, pretending needs some amount of effort. It is not quite that easy to live up to other's various expectations by compromising one's genuine self-concept without anyone ever noticing. If a person tries to convey the information that he or she has a particular p-trait in a certain type of situation and to certain other people only, such that at other occasions she does not care to act as if she herself believed she got the trait in question – then that is the sure sign of an image.[129]

The second way in which self-related statements can go wrong is that persons may simply err with regard to who they are. Someone may think he is quite self-composed, yet, his short-tempered way of reacting may reveal his choleric temper. Numerous psychological studies have shown that we are by no means completely transparent to ourselves. Much to the contrary, we can be mistaken with respect to almost each and every aspect of ourselves. So, even though only honest convictions should be considered part of a person's self-concept, it can (and usually will) contain false beliefs as well as true ones.

Self-related beliefs are false if they do not appropriately represent the way the person is who holds them. In other words: false components of a person's self-concept do not match with her *personality*. Whenever someone offers an account of another person's personality, they basically try to answer the same question we found to be constitutive for personal self-concepts, namely *who that particular person is* compared to other persons. Self-concepts represent subjective points of view on personalities. Their subjectivity, however, lies not in their being independent from other persons' points of view on the same object. Much to the contrary, the way persons come to think about their personality is deeply influenced by what others think about who they are.[130] Rather, a self-concept is subjective in the sense that it comprises *the person's* thinking about what marks him or her off from other persons, no matter whether it truly represents the person's personality or not. Consider, for instance, an anorexic young woman who is utterly convinced to be too fat even though she is in fact close to starving. It is a genuine part of her self-concept that she considers herself to be too fat. However, in giving a faithful account of her personality one cannot refer to her being (too) fat, for the simple reason that she is not. All we can say with respect to an anorexic woman's personality is that it is a salient feature of her that she holds

[129] Of course, sometimes, especially when confronted with inconsistencies between self-related statements and their behaviour, persons may even openly admit that their words or deeds are founded in a consciously designed image.

[130] Actually, an important way of learning words for p-traits is to understand how others (most prominently parents) respond to ones own behaviour by the ascription of p-traits (e.g. "You are a naughty boy"). In this way, others already exert an influence on a person's self-concept before she acquires the means to make up her own mind about who she is.

wrong beliefs with regard to her outward appearance, or that she has got a disturbed perception of her own body.

Another way to misunderstand the notion of subjectivity in relation to personal self-concepts would be to think that nobody but each individual person is in a position to know what makes up the contents of her self-concept. Most intuitions indicating a particular *epistemic authority* of persons regarding their self-concepts are based on the conviction that it is a *private affair* how a person thinks about herself[131]. In order to see that this is not quite right, just imagine a human resources manager who publicly purports to have a decent egalitarian attitude with respect to racial differences. Suppose he is so cautious not to reveal his prejudice against black people that he will never communicate it to anyone. However, in the privacy of his office he visits racist websites and enjoys laughing at jokes mocking black people. Now *if* this behaviour got revealed beyond doubt (for instance by a hidden camera in his office), this would be sufficient evidence to conclude that having racial prejudices is not only one of his p-traits, but indeed also a part of his own self-concept. This diagnosis could even prove robust against any later efforts of his to hold up his egalitarian image by trying to "explain away" the evidence in question once he got confronted with it ("I was just trying to get information in order to better be able to fight racism" etc.). What the example shows is that there can be good reason to attribute beliefs to a person's self-concept even if that person consistently denies holding them. Of course, if the example is found to be convincing, then this is because a person simply cannot *avoid* being/becoming aware of his holding of racial prejudices if he really spends a good deal of time in active search for racist jokes which he then finds himself smirking, giggling or outright laughing about. To be sure, it has been established in a number of studies, employing *inter alia* "Implicit Association Tests", that white personnel managers may be unconsciously biased against black applicants.[132] However, unconscious bias needs to be distinguished from covert (but nevertheless conscious) prejudice, and only the *latter* can be part of personal self-concepts the way we want to conceive of them here.[133] Of course, aspects of the self-

[131] Private in the sense that, as a matter of principle, only I myself have access to and, hence, can really *know* about it – while others always have to rely on my information.

[132] The classical experiment has been conducted by Word et al. (1974). For a host of further references see the "Project Implicit" website at http://projectimplicit.net, accessed on December 8th, 2006.

[133] Which is: as the actual "self-*understandings*" of persons, as the ways persons actually do "consider themselves as themselves", and *not* as some part of their psyche that – however important – is unavailable or intransparent to them. What e.g. a psychoanalyst does is (in a first step) to help people in *becoming aware* of repressed beliefs, goals, conflicts etc. and thus to help them in descriptively *adjusting* (not discovering!) their self-concept. Only on the basis of such "insights" on the part of the clients, further progress can be made towards resolving psychic conflicts and any symptoms possibly connected to them. This will most often involve a change of the ideal self-image of the client, too.

concept a person entertains may very well remain private in the harmless sense that they will *de facto* never be known by anyone else (maybe the covert racism of the manager really goes unnoticed). What doesn't make sense, though, are privacy assumptions along the line that – "as a matter of principle" – no one but the person in question can *ever* know about aspects of her self-concept.

What we just dealt with (and refuted) was the claim that a self-concept is a private entity, one which only the person who actually has it has access to, and that therefore persons have epistemic authority with respect to what *is* contained in their self-concept and what *not*. This has to be sharply distinguished from the even more radical claim that knowledge about the truth of the self-related beliefs that actually *are* contained in a person's self-concept is *itself* a private affair – bestowing the person having the self-concept in question with epistemic authority regarding not just her self-concept, but her personality as a whole. One could summarise this in statements like, "No one can know myself better than me" or, "In the end, only I *know* what I am really like." In order to avoid such exaggerated ideas with respect to an alleged privacy of self-concepts, one must not forget that a self-concept is a linguistic entity. The expressions persons use to characterise themselves (like "anxious", "daring", "musically skilled", "striving to become a surgeon", "being convinced that everyone can make it if he only tries hard enough") are part of the language they share with their speech community. Consequently there are "public" (i.e. intersubjective) criteria for their correct usage (cf. our condensed account of Wittgenstein's argument against the possibility of "private" languages in Section 3.1). Of course, constituents of personal self-concepts rarely ever are so blatantly false as in the examples of an anorexic person claiming to be fat or of a person of our times claiming to be Napoleon. But for any (even the must subtle) utterance, be it self-related or not, to be meaningful, there need to be intersubjectively testable conditions under which it can be refuted. The only reason to, nevertheless, grant persons a somewhat privileged position in deciding the truth of parts of their own self-concept lies in the fact that they – in a way – have the most complete survey of the pertinent evidence for these beliefs. Since, usually, the relevant statements are unrestricted with respect to the period of time for which they claim to hold true, their empirical basis is nothing less than the sum total of what the respective person says and does. Sure enough, for each person she herself will be the only one who can claim to be *always* present when she does or says something. Therefore, it makes good sense to grant persons benefit of the doubt regarding matters of their personality as expressed in their own self-concepts. However, once there is reason to question the trustworthiness of persons, the reliability of their memory, their capacity of unbiased judgment etc., their self related statements will be scrutinised more closely. Given the many reasons for persons to lie with respect to who they really are and the various ways in which episodic memory may delude them, the most complete familiarity with the empirical data does – just by itself – not warrant the most reliable knowledge[134].

This we have tried to make quite clear: If you want to know about a person's personality, it is not enough to just ask her about it. Still less, however, can you *do without* asking, because each and every statement persons issue about their own personality is of significance for an account of it in some way: If there is reason to assume deceptive intent, statements may indicate an image the person deliberately creates of herself. In such cases, for an adequate understanding of her personality, one has to investigate what kind of image the person sustains by the insincere statement, and in which situations and for what reasons she does so. If a statement faithfully represents a person's self-concept, it needs to be included in a comprehensive account of her personality in any case, be it right or wrong. The reason for this is not just that the ways in which a person is mistaken with respect to herself may again permit conclusions on her *actual* personality, but rather that a person's self-concept itself constitutes an important *part* of her personality, and therefore must not be omitted in an adequate account of it. Thus, any change in a person's honest beliefs on who she essentially is deserves to be regarded as a change in her personality, no matter whether the propositional contents of her new self-related beliefs are in fact true or not.

For the sake of illustration, imagine Tom who is smug about his extraordinary intelligence. At least it is part of his self-concept that he considers himself to be much smarter than most people around. Actually, the people who know Tom well would not describe him as being of above average intelligence – but who cares and who knows for sure? One day, however, Tom decides to participate in a clinical trial for a new enhancement technique that is supposed to boost general intelligence by means of a single irreversible intervention. In order to measure the effect of the enhancement participants are subjected to a number of the most carefully validated IQ tests prior and at regular intervals subsequent to the intervention. On request, the participants are told about their initial scores, but for the duration of the long-term follow-up investigation they are blinded with regard to their test results after the intervention. It is revealed to Tom that his IQ at the begin-

[134] There is some truth in saying that it is easier to assess the personality of others than one's own: If one's actions are very much out of sync with one's "ideal self", then admitting the facts about oneself can be very painful. In such situations, the subconscious temptation to rather reduce the cognitive dissonance by "rationalising" one's actions may be hard to resist. As one usually does not have to deal with *such* obstacles in assessing the personality of others, this may very well result in more objective judgement here. Everyone knows the case of people who, while totally blind with respect to their own problems and shortcomings, nevertheless have a sharp and analytical eye when it comes to assessing the personality, problems and faults of others.

ning of the study (with respect to different tests) is slightly *below* average – and it doesn't change due to the intervention, for he is a member of the placebo control group. In the end, the only lasting result of the trial is a change of Tom's self-concept, because after the disappointing disclosure of his initial test scores he no longer prides himself on his intelligence. In the light of what we said about the relationship between personal self-concepts and personality, Tom's case should be described as follows: Given Tom's IQ scores prior to the alleged enhancement, he had entertained a false belief regarding his intelligence – he thought it was above average while in fact it was not. As his scores did not change, it would have been wrong all along to describe Tom's personality by stating that he stood out against others with respect to his intelligence. However, it would have been perfectly *right*, before the clinical trial, to refer to his wrong belief on his outstanding intelligence in describing his personality by stating that this belief constitutes a part of his *self-concept*. Since participating in the study adjusted Tom's self-concept, his personality changed (in an advantageous way) even though his intelligence did not.

Nobody can claim to be the last authority with respect to the question who a person is compared to others – not even (as we saw) the person whose personality is actually under scrutiny. Nevertheless, given conflicting views on particular aspects of a person's character, it is not that difficult in many cases to decide which view is true in an unambiguous sense. Questions regarding personality traits can often be settled with reference to (more or less) generally acknowledged standards like IQ tests. However, tools of that kind just offer particularly sophisticated ways to generate and analyse evidence about questions concerning personality. Ultimately, the truth of both, first *and* third person statements purporting to describe a person's personality, must be decided in the light of how the person acts (including speech acts) and behaves. Given the complexity of this evidence, however, there is a point in saying that it will not be possible for each pair of inconsistent statements on a person's character to single out one as definitely true (or definitely false). Nevertheless, one of these conflicting statements may still be more convincing than the other. For example, there may be reason to accept one of the statements by virtue of this resulting in a more coherent overall picture of a person's personality.

To further flesh out this new aspect of "coherence" that shall prepare our final word on the issue of personal identity, it will be helpful to envision the way how persons express their self-concepts. Usually, a person's account of who she considers herself to be does not assume the form of a warrant of apprehension in that she would simply enumerate traits of herself that she considers to be salient. Rather, persons convey their self-concepts in a *narrative* form by telling coherent stories of how they came to be who they are. Again, rather than merely *conveying* something they already got in their pocket, so to speak, they actually *create* their self-concepts by telling stories about who they are.[135] Since we recognised that a person's self-concept is an integral part of her personality, *in a limited sense* persons can be said to thereby create their personalities as well. This careful wording is required as talking about a "narrative approach" may evoke associations of the seemingly limitless freedom of authors of works of fiction. To counter this impression we would like to point out again that in many ways we find ourselves *endowed* with a particular personality. This holds true for most of the p-traits we introduced above. For instance, we explicitly mentioned that talents are innate in that there is nothing a person can do to acquire one set of talents rather than another. All we are left with is to decide whether or not to make the best of our given talents. In much the same way, choleric persons do not *choose* to be overly irritable. However, they may be free to adopt different attitudes towards their tetchy nature. In general, persons can exert a reinforcing, inhibiting or shaping influence on the p-traits they find themselves endowed with by the particular way they integrate p-traits into their self-concept (especially with respect to their ideal self).

The most conspicuous difference between the narrative situation of persons developing their self-concepts on the one hand, and authors of fiction on the other is, of course, that the former are supposed to be true to the facts of their life in their storytelling. They share this particular claim of giving a faithful account of a life's course with the authors of biographies. However, as opposed to biographers, persons who give a narrative account of themselves will be expected to be true to their word in the way they lead their life after having finished telling their story – finished *for the time being*, one should add, because the stories themselves by which personal self-concepts are constituted will never come to an end for as long as a person continues to persist. In a nutshell, at each given point in time a person's former way of life,

[135] Far from new, this narrative approach to personality and "personal identity" (here in the sense of individuality) has been pioneered in different directions by a number of theoreticians, among them Taylor 1989, MacIntyre ²1985, Dennett 1992, and Glover 1988. However, as Quante (2002:22) points out correctly, personal identity over time is not the same concept as personality. Consequently, if "personal identity" is used by prominent proponents of narrativity, this is not to be understood as meaning (diachronic) numerical identity. So the way in which we address the question of personal identity over time, and thus the question of the criteria for the *persistence* of persons, by adopting a narrative approach is novel. The reason why it was not explored before presumably lies in the tacit (and premature) conclusion that the different usage of "personal identity" in prominent narrative approaches means that such a kind of approach *can not* be used to address the problem of personal identity over time. It is this tacit conclusion too which leads Quante – despite his clear understanding of the importance of biographical self-concepts (ibid.:Ch. 5) – astray: Having already predecided (ibid.:26) that problems of "personal identity" in the sense of persistence and of personality have to be strictly kept apart and solved separately, he later inevitably finds that the question of personal identity is without an adequate answer – and thus has to be substituted with a related (but different) question, namely about the persistence of human beings as organisms (ibid.:54).

as specified by her verbal and nonverbal actions as well as her behaviour, does determine the framework for credible stories on who that person is. Likewise, a person's present self-concept, and especially those parts of it declaring her projects of self-creation, determine her future actions, provided the person wants to remain credible.

Whether a person meets all the claims she (more or less consciously) raises by expressing her self-concept will be observed by the different recipients or addressees of self-constituting narratives. That these narratives do have addressees is, again, one of the noteworthy similarities to more common situations of composing narratives. However, what's special is the active part that addressees of stories through which persons express their self-concepts tend to play. Far from merely listening to what a person has to say, these addressees sometimes even qualify for co-authorship. This will mainly (though not only) be the case when persons get in a sense "lost" in their own stories about who they are. For instance, a person may be at a loss to account for some deeds of herself that do not fit at all with her self-concept. In such cases sympathetic listeners can provide support to "retrieve the storyline" by pointing out coherences the "main author" may have missed or by hinting at former actions that are in good accord with the recent disturbing ones, thereby recommending a revision of the person's self-concept in some particular aspect. In some cases, others will even take on most or all of the storytelling in place of a person whose way of being is at issue, and this is not just the case if the person in question is dead or missing: There are persons who, for a variety of reasons, will not indulge in ambitious storytelling or at least not spend many words on themselves. However, not to express your self-concept is by itself a particularly *telling* way to show character. And, what's most important: even the most reticent person, who remains imperturbably close-mouthed whenever others approach her with their unbidden characterisations, cannot avoid to confirm or refute the stories they tell about her through her deeds.[136]

Because in our earlier discussion about the relationship between self-concepts and personalities we rather stressed the *critical* function the commu-

[136] It is worth mentioning this particular type of person, for in this way we demonstrate that Galen Strawson's recently raised objections "Against Narrativity" (2004) do not hit our account. Neither do we adopt the "Narrativity thesis" in its descriptive "psychological" form, claiming that all persons do look at their lives as some sort of narrative or have the habit of telling stories about themselves. Nor do we adhere to the "ethical Narrativity thesis", which would propagate self-constituting storytelling as the most auspicious way for leading a good, satisfying life. All we contend is that persons essentially have a self-concept and that this will require them *to be able* to make narrative sense of the events of their lives and to comment on stories that others may tell about them. By the way, Strawson does more than enough to prove that he himself is entertaining a self-concept in the required sense by avowing himself an "Episodic" (i.e. one of those persons "who are likely to have no particular tendency to see their life in Narrative terms" [2004:430]).

nity of persons exhibits with respect to its individual members' understanding of themselves, it was high time to finally mention also the *supportive* part other persons (friends, relatives, colleagues etc.) may play with respect to a person's efforts to come to grips with who she is. For sure, both functions, the supportive and the critical, are complementary aspects of the same process, namely the social process of interpersonal exchange in which self-concepts as well as accounts of personalities are constituted[137]: By taking stock of what they did and what they experienced, persons develop a sense of individuality or even uniqueness over the course of their persistence. Most persons do occasionally or even habitually share their self-concepts with others by telling stories about what they consider to be special about themselves given their past lives and their plans for the future. In the light of what the addressees of these stories know about the storyteller's past and present way of life, they may come to their own conclusions about who that person is compared to other persons. More or less frankly and more or less sympathetically they may share their doubts or objections with the person whose self-concept is at issue. In turn, the person may either defend her self-concept so that everyone involved is eventually convinced by it[138], or she may acknowledge the observed inconsistencies and modify her self-concept accordingly. However, it is not always possible to settle dissension in a manner which is agreeable to all. If the result of interpersonal exchange on a particular person's self-concept is that it got things wrong in some particular respect, then the "official" account of that person's personality will diverge from that of her self-concept. There can be many different stories around which all purport to represent a person's personality, including the one that is told by that person herself expressing her *self-concept.* However, her *personality* is what is represented in the most *intersubjectively convincing* story of who that particular person actually is when compared to others.

5.4.5 A Narrative Approach to Personal Identity

What we have so far is a narrative approach to *personality.* So, what is it good for with respect to the problems of *personal identity?* First of all, it offers a new line of reasoning to explain the significance of episodic memory for the persistence of persons. The point is that the raw material for those stories we tell about ourselves is provided by the faculty of episodic memory. More pre-

[137] It is a distinguishing feature of narrative accounts to put emphasis on the social constitution of the self; see e.g. Taylor (1989:I.2.2.) and Quante (2002:170).

[138] We would just like to mention a few ways how a person may defend her self-concept once it is challenged in some particular aspect. Let's assume someone is pointing out an episode of my life that is at odds with how I claim to be like. First of all, I may deny the truth of his account of what I did. If I have to admit its truth, I may give some reason why I did not act in line with my general disposition in that particular situation. Or, I simply may try to outvote him by citing a number of counter-examples that support my claim.

cisely, the availability of episodic memories is a condition of the possibility of the kind of storytelling by which persons generate their self-concepts. Hence, if episodic memory is wiped out completely, as in severe cases of retrograde amnesia, then a sufficient condition for a change of personal identity to occur is fulfilled. This, of course, is perfectly in line with our earlier result that some sort of episodic memory continuity (as specified in MemCrit1) between person-stages is indeed a necessary condition for them to belong to the same person.

The episodic memories of persons provide the raw material for the communicative process whose narrative outcome is an intersubjectively approved account of their personalities – including a critical appraisal of their self-concepts. We consider it indispensable for an adequate understanding of persons' characters to make allowance for their narratively constituted self-concept. Only in this way one can make sure not to miss anything that is pertinent for deciding questions regarding the persistence of a particular person. By just following a highly schematised check-list in describing personalities one cannot do justice to individual variations of the contents of personal self-concepts. These variations are due to the fact that persons refer to vastly differing properties in composing their self-concepts. But even this does not account for all the variety: something quite pertinent is left out if one does not pay attention to a person's particular *narrative style* in expressing her self-concept. Some persons seem to follow the aesthetic ideal of a classic coming-of-age novel in that they see every event worth mentioning in the light of how it contributed to the eventual achievement of one overarching *telos*. Quite to the contrary, others may cultivate a thoroughly "episodic" stance towards life, avoiding the assumption of any overarching *telos*, seeing their lives as a conglomeration of independent phases which would have to be characterised by nothing so much as the contingent circumstances and tasks they were confronted with at the respective times.

It will be illuminating at this point to take a closer look at possible cases of change in a person's narrative style: Can a person who is there after a transition to an episodic outlook on herself still be considered as the same person who formerly used to think of her life as proceeding towards some *telos?* Well, why not? For instance, after some deep disappointment a person loses all her faith in a deeper meaning of life. As a consequence, she may begin to live her life from one day to the next, from year to year, thereby just changing her behaviour along with the circumstances, opportunities and roles presenting themselves to her. But it still would be *her* life. After all, she has got reasons for why her self-concept changed so radically. Others may question the consequences she has drawn from her experience of disappointment, but they will need to admit that she has got a story to tell that is worthy of consideration. As long as she cares a bit – maybe not for herself, but for others –, as long as she is ready to take responsibility for what she does and for what she did prior to her "identity crisis", there is no reason to doubt that she is still the same person, even though profoundly changed in her personality in general and in her self-concept in particular.

We now consider a more radical change in "narrative style", from *telos*-style narration to one which maybe could be labelled "radical deconstructivist": When questioned about his self-concept, the radical deconstructivist will say "I don't have a self-concept, there is nothing but ever-fleeting images of myself." He considers "personal persistence" to be an illusion, too: Every morning he will wake up thinking "Let's see *who there is* today". Consequently, he will refuse taking responsibility for "his" actions. He may say, "I know someone did something yesterday, but that has nothing to do with…", and after a pause he may continue by saying "who cares!" Well, the others will certainly care! If this "deconstructivist stance" turns out to be nothing but a superficial "attitude", as some sort of transitory digestive trouble possibly caused by reading philosophical or spiritual literature of a certain kind, it has to count as nothing but a very weird and rather phoney sort of image in the end. The person in question will therefore be held responsible for everything he does (or did, earlier) – whether he likes it or not. If, on the other hand, his opinions are considered genuine (this presupposes that his behaviour is properly erratic), he most likely will be considered to suffer from a severe depersonalisation disorder and will be treated accordingly. This means that rather than describing the transition of the "coming-of-age person" into the "radical deconstructivist" as a change of personal identity, one would describe it as a person going so insane as to lose personhood. But why? The reason seems to be not so much that the deconstructivist story is not convincing (though in fact it is not, as it does not even *try* to account for anything, least of all the transition from the "*telos*-style" to the "deconstructivist" one). Rather, it does not count as a story in the first place (and thus the "deconstructivist style" in truth is not just one "narrative style" among others).

Quite obviously not every sequence of utterances can count as a story, but what the criteria for "story-ness" are is a harder question. There are some *minimal requirements* with respect to coherence that any narrative *with a claim to truth* (and so *a fortiori* any narrative defence or modification of a self-concept) needs to fulfil. These requirements are such that violating them in particular instances means that – with respect to the goal of intersubjective agreement – there is something not quite correct yet about the story, which has to be amended to get it "right". Violating them more often, however, does rather result in the breakdown of "story-ness" itself.

The first requirement we want to draw attention to is that inconsistencies with respect to the time-order in which a person places the events of her story cannot be tolerated. This does of course not mean that the order in which events are to be reported has to be the order in which they actually occurred. This would be a just demand on chronicles, but not on all sorts of stories with a claim to truth. Quite to the contrary, depending on context and purpose, such stories may present us with a whole lot of very helpful flashbacks or anticipations of things yet to come. What *can* be justly demanded, however, is that the order of events in a story with a claim to truth can be consistently deduced from it. In other words: If, according to the story, some event is both to happen and not to happen at a certain relative place in the time-line, then this is definitely something calling for amendment. It should be clear that if you have an increasing amount of inconsistencies in the time-line of a story, it will, at some point, eventually break down as a whole. Just as a bunch of "timeless" statements (like e.g. Euclid's axioms) doesn't make a story, a bunch of statements about events that cannot be ordered even partially is no story, either (even if terms like "post-modern", "deconstructivist" or whatever are invoked).[139]

The second requirement we would mention has to do with the observation that a mere concatenation of event-stating sentences does not make up a story either – even if the time-line is correct and the sentences are all true.[140] The coherence of a story thus must consist in more than just a consistent time-line: There has to be some sort of "connectedness" of its statements beyond that. To be sure, a story must feature certain recurrent objects and "themes", but in general it would be quite futile to try getting a grip on the pertinent kind of connectedness in question by looking for purely syntactical or even semantical criteria. To get closer to the heart of the matter, it is crucial to realise in a first step that a story's claim to truth (if it has such claim) is never just "to report something that happened", nor "to tell it all" or "to tell it most exactly". Rather, for every story, there is an explicit or implicit background of goals against which objects, events and levels of descriptive detail and completeness are judged pertinent or irrelevant.[141] So, ideally, what is told in a story is relevant with respect to "what it is about". This very general observation can be elaborated a bit further by taking into account that, even with respect to the specific goals which determine what the story is about (and what not), a story's claim to truth (again, if it makes such claim) is never just to *report what happened*, but also in a way to *make sense of it*. This in turn can be understood in a variety of ways, the most prominent being the intentional explanation of actions and the causal explanation of other events ("Why did Stalin offer the reunification of Germany in 1953?",

[139] Here and in the following we would ask the reader to keep in mind that we are talking about stories that claim to be true. We do not want to say that e.g. deconstructivist movies are worthless as pieces of art.

[140] See Danto (1985:117). His counter-example: "Naram-Sin built the Sun Temple at Sippar; then Philipp III exiled the Moriscos; then Urguiza defeated the forces of Buenos Aires at Cepada; then Arthur Danto awoke on the stroke of seven, 20 October 1961."

[141] Again Danto (1985:131) has a nice example to illustrate the point: "Suppose I'd wish to know what happened at a court trial. [...] I should be dismayed if [...] he were to tell me how many flies there were in the courtroom, and show me a complicated map of the precise orbits in which they flew, a vast tangle of epicycles."

"Why did the dinosaurs become extinct?").[142] For example, a self-conceptualising story should provide us with something which a simple listing of p-traits ("social, serious, open-minded …") cannot provide: an answer to the question "Who are you?" in the sense entailing questions like: "How did you *become* who you are?", "Why did you *change* in this way?" Bearing this in mind, the relevance of parts of a story can be assessed through questions like "Does this set the stage for, or contribute to the understanding of something else which the story is essentially about?", "Is this something we can take for granted or rather something that should be explained?", etc. Again, "ideally", every part of a story would be relevant in the sense that it serves a function with respect to the descriptive and explanative goals associated with the story. The function of the respective part would be its *significance*, which is why we are speaking of the "requirement of significance".[143] As with the requirement of consistency of the time-line, single violations of the requirement of significance, while sticking out like sore thumbs calling for band-aid ("Why did you tell us about that watch of your father, the one which you accidentally broke?"), will not threaten "story-ness" – but an increasing amount eventually *will* do.[144]

The third and last requirement to be mentioned here is, actually, a generalised version of the first one: Keeping a consistent time-line means an instance of following the more general requirement of keeping truth-claiming stories free from contradictions. Therefore, the addressees of self-conceptualising stories actually have the right to object to *any* inconsistency they notice. And again we can state that, whereas truth-claiming stories are

---

[142] To be sure, a satisfying story does not have to (and usually in fact does not) give all these answers by way of mentioning explicitly all the pertinent maxims or causal laws. However, for the story to be satisfying, they must be, in principle, distillable from it – at least to the extent of providing an explanation *schema*.

[143] To forestall any misunderstandings, it is extremely important to point out that the requirement of significance does not mean that, in their self-conceptualising enterprise, persons should try to give "meaning" to every miniscule episode or even to a major part of the episodes of their lifes (this could be called a "theodicy-style" narrative). Rather, the requirement just says that significance is to be given to every episode which *is* actually making the cut, showing up in the story constituting a person's self-concept. Note also that this does not demand or even favour *telos*-style narration (i.e. that the significance of any part of a story lies in its contribution to the same final goal).

[144] Though we maintain that the goal of "making sense" and the requirement of significance also hold with respect to stories that do *not* have a claim to truth (especially novels), we of course acknowledge that this may interact with other goals here. For instance, it may be extremely boring and shallow if the significance of every scene is too obvious. It even may be especially praiseworthy if the significance of many events is left unclear until the last moment, or proves to be quite different than it seemed at first ("twist"), or if the story as a whole is open to more than one "interpretation". Again, not even a "deconstructivist story" is ruled out as a possibly subtle and worthy work of art – it is just ruled out as a *story*.

"robust" with respect to singular, isolatable contradictions, they can take only so much of these before eventually breaking down wholesale.[145]

Of course, the internal consistency of a story is not enough to make it a true story. To this end, a story also has to be "consistent with the facts". Regarding self-conceptualising stories, there can be more or less obvious conflict between what a person *says* and what she *does*. We already saw how to deal with "external" inconsistencies of this kind. If they can't be "explained away" (i.e. if it can't be shown that they just *seemed* to contradict the facts), they can be explained with reference to an image that a person may consciously create in order to fool others about her true self-concept, or with reference to a discrepancy between how a person thinks about herself and how she actually is. As a special variant of the latter case those numberless situations are worth mentioning in which persons fail to act in accordance with their "ideal self-image". The important thing here is, though, that no amount of external inconsistencies will ever lead to a breakdown of "storyness". As long as it is internally consistent, a story may be as blatantly and impudently wrong as you dare to imagine – it will still be a story. So, contrary to what we found with respect to *internal* inconsistencies, the coherence of self-constituting stories, and hence the stability of self-concepts, is never threatened by *external* inconsistencies. Thus, the maniac who thinks he can take on the world all on his own *has* a self-concept, however "off-target", while the "radical deconstructivist" has none at all.

Having dealt with structural criteria which stories (with a claim to truth) must fulfil as such (and good stories in particular), we revert attention back to our example of a person going from *telos*-style to episodic style self-conceptualisation. What are the general lessons such examples may teach us about the distinction between personality changes and changes of personal identity? Well, we came to the conclusion that persons may persist through very profound changes of their personalities *including* their self-conceptualisations. This seems only to confirm our earlier result that it is not possible to establish adequate character-based criteria for personal persistence: If all we have got with respect to two person stages at different times are two most comprehensive descriptions of personalities, including the respective self-concepts in every detail, then it will not be possible to tell whether the two person-stages they describe belong to the same person. However, by putting things this way something quite essential is missed: As we have seen by now, a person's self-conceptualisation is not exhausted by opinions stating whether she has or has not certain p-traits. Rather, it is also constituted by narratively structured opinions[146]

---

[145] In this we of course accept that standard logics are wrong in assuming that from a contradiction *every* proposition follows – in that case a single contradiction would suffice to make a story worthless.

[146] This may be a good place to state that it does not matter so much whether the "stories" a person has to tell about herself are explicit in the sense that she actually

regarding how the person acquired these traits and, consequently, by likewise structured opinions about how her self-concept *itself* has developed and about how it came to change, maybe profoundly, throughout her life. That is, a later stage of a person is connected to the earlier ones by way of narrative integration of the personalities of the earlier stages. Though this is only possible by recourse to episodic memory, it is nevertheless a much stronger link than mere memory continuity provides: In narratives, memories are arranged within a wider time-frame, and they are interlinked with respect to their content by recurrent objects and themes. By including episodic memories in a story-line or by leaving them out as "irrelevant", storytellers valuate their contents, and they give a certain "meaning" (in the sense of "significance") to them by putting them at certain, specific places within the story.

In this way a story can do several things a mere episodic memory, or even a string of such memories, cannot: Firstly, it can in a way incorporate stages which are not directly accessible by episodic memory anymore. For example, I may have no recollection at all of what I did on the 13th of February, 1984, but if I know where to place that date within the larger frame of "my story", I will nevertheless have a pretty good idea about what kind of guy I was back then: what my temper, goals, opinions and talents were – even what I used to think of myself. The second important thing a story (as against a string of memories) can do is to tell what happened and at the same time *give an account of it, make sense of it, explain it.* This is so strong a tool that it even can deal reflectively with, and account for changes occurring over time in the story *itself.* What we have in mind here goes way beyond those trivial changes due to the mere addition of ever new parts with the advance of time: For example, a story could change in that it picks up events which were left out as irrelevant in earlier versions, or leaves out or qualifies elements which were formerly considered of special import. Maybe some seemingly inconsequential action of mine proved to be one of earth-shattering consequence much later; or what I thought was the root of all my problems was in fact important only in that it diverted my attention from my real, however repressed conflicts. In both cases, the later story would in a way explain (or try to explain) what was wrong with the earlier version, and thus would incorporate the "story of the old story" into the new story-line ("I used to tell myself that my moodiness was due to too much stress at work until I eventually realised, when my uncle died, that it had much more to do with ..."). As we have seen in the example about the person turning from *telos*-style to episodic narration, a story could even

---

told them to someone, or e.g. wrote them down in a diary, or rather implicit in the sense that they could be elicited by prodding her in the right way, asking the right questions etc. What counts is that she actually has a set of opinions about herself, about her life and development as a person, which together exhibit a narrative structure.

change its overall narrative style – and such a change, too, could be accounted for in the new story.[147]

We are now in a position to state more clearly what is required for a decision as to whether two person stages (at different times) that exhibit more or less different personalities do nevertheless belong to the *same* person at different times of her life: Two person stages x and y belong as temporal parts to some (the same) person p if and only if they are continuous and the narratively structured self-concept of the later stage y does plausibly integrate stage x. Before we pause to talk about a host of issues regarding this criterion (like the meaning of "plausibly integrate"), we first propose a generalised version[148]:

(PI-Crit) The members of a set of person-stages M all belong as temporal parts to some (the same) person p if and only if they are all continuous to one another and for every stage whose narratively structured self-concept does not plausibly integrate all earlier stages there is a later stage which does so.

The criterion has now the form of a biconditional ("if and only if"). That is, if we manage to hold on to it, we finally got the necessary and sufficient condition for personal identity we have been after for so long. So let's begin to discuss it.

Firstly, it may be questioned why the criterion is focussing on the self-concept of the individual. After all, didn't we make quite a fuss about the *intersubjectivity* of the stories about personality, speaking about "co-authorship" and such, denying the individual person epistemic authority? But our focussing on the individual's self-concept has nothing to do with epistemic authority. Rather, if the question of personal identity is put, one has to focus on certain capacities of the person (stages) under consideration, namely their capacities of memory and narratively structured self-conceptualisation. Thus, the criterion does not involve in any way that a person stage is, by definition, itself the ultimate authoritative judge about the question of what earlier stages belong to it or not, even though the objective (i.e. intersubjectively validated) answer to this question directly depends on its subjective capability of relating itself to those other stages.

[147] According to Danto (1981), works of art are like symbols in that they have meaning, but – unlike other symbolic representations – manage to say something about their subject matter through their mode of representation itself. In this vein, the narrative style of a story *itself* "tells" something about how the storyteller conceives of the subject matter of his story. In other words: the narrative style of a story constituting a self-concept is itself *expressing* something about how the storyteller sees himself. The content expressed in this way is therefore itself part of his self-concept (provided the storyteller could, in principle, make corresponding explicit statements – otherwise we would have to treat his narrative style as a *symptom* for a p-trait which he is not himself aware of).

[148] This is necessary for two reasons: Firstly, the case of two stages does not imply anything regarding the case of n stages. Secondly, only the generalised version will allow us to incorporate an important *liberalisation*.

Secondly, one may ask why the criterion does not include the liberalizing provision that later stages only have to integrate such earlier stages with regard to which they can *directly* quasi-memorise any episodes of experience from the first-person perspective. The answer to this was implicitly given above: Though episodic memory is a prerequisite for narrative self-conceptualisation, the latter transcends the former. I may not remember anything I experienced on a certain day, but as I can locate that day within the wider frame of my life, I nevertheless should have a concept of "who I was" at that time – what my temper, goals, beliefs and talents were like, what I thought of myself, and even which opportunities and hardships I was confronted with that I think were bound to have an impact on my further "story". This is a relation I should by some measure have to *all* earlier stages of mine, even to those with regard to which I am not able to directly recall any specific experiential episodes.

Thirdly, one may wonder whether, on the other hand, the criterion is too liberal. Why don't we require every stage to integrate *all* earlier ones? Why did we add the provision that, in case of failure, things are "saved" by a later stage doing the integrating? Now, let's assume we have consecutive person stages *a*, *b*, *c* belonging to the same human body *B*, and things be such that the person at *b* suffers a "crisis" in that she is not able to integrate the earlier stage *a*, but then overcomes the crisis at *c* so that she can integrate again both *a* and *b*. Now, had we formulated our criterion more strictly, we would face the following situation: *b* and *c* would belong to one person, as would *a* and *c*, but *not a* and *b*. Therefore, we would have not one person, but *two* which just share stage *c* (and all following ones) – a case of "psychological fusion". This would certainly be an artefact of the criterion being too strict, and it is proof of the adequacy of PI-Crit as given above that we can describe this example as the case of a *single* person recovering from a crisis.

For further illumination, let's compare the issue to the case where we have to deal with a phase of retrograde amnesia at *b* which is eventually overcome at *c*. Here, we may count the stage *b* as belonging to the same person as *a* and *c without* having to tamper with the definition of memory continuity, because the modal formulation "can (quasi-)memorise" provides us with the leeway we need: We already mentioned that while someone is asleep at night, he may be considered to be "able to memorise" episodes of the day before in the sense that *if* we wake him up and ask him, he will tell us something about it. In a very similar sense we may (and actually in practice do) treat a transient phase of retrograde amnesia: *If* the specific contingent obstacles that were eventually removed for *c* would have been already removed for *b*, then this stage would have remembered something. The point is that this strategy is only licit if we restrict ourselves to true conditionals which are not analytic trivialities (in the vein of "if we would have made him remember, he would have remembered") and, furthermore, if we have an "if"-clause which is not just logically, but also empirically possible (by this provision we exclude conditionals such as "if we had a *perpetuum mobile*, then we could save big on resources"). In the case of the overcome amnesia, the mere *fact that it was overcome* already provides the required backing for the assumption that it was empirically *possible* to overcome the amnesia after all.[149] It is important to note that this elegant way out is not transferable to the case where someone's narratively structured self-concept is not able to integrate his earlier self, for this would amount to translate "does plausibly integrate" into "would do so if it were different".

Now we address ourselves to the most critical question: What is "plausibly integrate" supposed to mean. First of all, the expression is to convey that it is *not* required for pieces of narrative self-conceptualisation to represent the "true story" in the sense that they would need to explain all the changes in personality in the most intersubjectively convincing way. Positively, and in the most general way, "plausibly integrate" means:

a) there is a story (i.e. a structure which satisfies at least the basic criteria for "story-ness") relating the earlier stages and the pertinent changes to the actually "present" stage and
b) this story is sufficiently grounded in episodic memory to be counted as genuine.

Apart from this, the threshold for "plausible integration" will, however, not be the same *tout court*, but differ widely with context. The strongest demands will be put on the coherence of a story when there is reason to doubt that all pertinent person stages are represented by the same body. Even though *conceptually* we consider it to be possible that a person may wake up one morning in a different body, there certainly is no empirically accredited case of one person showing up in different bodies at different times. However, sometimes it so happens that a person claims to be someone who had disappeared for a long time. Especially in the past (before the advent of DNA-testing), it quite often was impossible to settle allegations of that kind by checking physical continuity between the person who had disappeared and the person claiming to be him. If the present person lays claim on the property of the person who had disappeared and if others who knew that person are affected by these claims, then we have a type of conflict on which various novels and movies are based. In situations of that kind, the claimant

---

[149] That is why cases of ongoing amnesia have to be treated with some agnostic care. For example, it is reasonable that a court does, at the one hand, *not* subject a person suffering from total retrograde amnesia to punishment for a crime committed during her "former life". For maybe the amnesia is total, the episodic memory "wiped out" once and for all, the band of psychological continuity severed, never to be mended again. Such a person would in fact be "someone else". However, it is also reasonable that the court will not let the amnesiac simply go free either: he will still be submitted to punishment, should the amnesia be overcome, and as long as there *is* a chance for this, the accused also has to be treated like a person with a disorder rather than a "new" person.

needs to tell a particularly convincing story about how and why he disappeared and about where he has been and what he did in the meantime. On the other hand, those who take an interest in unmasking an impostor will give close scrutiny to the requirement of sufficient grounding in episodic memory – typically by asking tricky questions the correct answers to which an impostor would be highly unlikely to know ("Your great-aunt told our investigators that you had a nickname for that sleigh you were so fond of as a child – how did you call it?").[150]

If, on the other hand, physical continuity between two person stages is unquestionable, there is strong *prima facie* reason to suppose that both stages belong to the same person. Therefore, the demands on the plausibility of stories by which person stages are integrated are much lower here. Actually, the onus of proof is on those who want to argue that two person stages that are represented by the same body are *not* stages of the same person. This becomes obvious when one considers court cases where a person is accused of some felony. Here we have got a profound public interest that the person who is sentenced is actually the person who committed the crime. If a defendant's physical continuity with the criminal offender is established, then we may get one of the extremely rare instances where someone takes an interest in arguing that he emanated from a change of personal identity, so that "he is no longer the person" who committed the felony.[151] Sometimes defendants try to argue in this vein if the crime has been committed long ago and if – in the meantime before their apprehension – their personality has changed very favourably, so that they wouldn't be likely to commit such a felony now.

---

[150] Just for the record: Such scenarios of investigation would in principle also apply if it was (or became) empirically possible for persons to survive their bodies, be it by continuous transmogrification into different bodies or by more discontinuous means of replacement (including "reincarnation"). In the end, it all comes down to the question under what circumstances we would *accept* someone *as* someone. These circumstances are, we argue, related to someone's capability of memory-grounded storytelling. Assuming this *is* true, then if certain phenomena became rather common (instead of just being explored in novels and movies), society would eventually begin to *treat* them as cases of reincarnation or body switching. To make this more palpable, imagine someone would show up claiming he were in fact the reincarnation of your long dead brother. Of course, you would react most sceptically, to say the least. But now imagine he would not only show the characteristic personality traits of your brother, but would also be able to recount and relate to all the things you experienced together, and could do the same, consistently, for all other members of your family. Wouldn't you and your family eventually begin to accept him? At the very least – we dare to predict – you would do so if that sort of phenomenon, rather than being unheard of, would actually be a more common thing for which society had already developed certain traditions of coping.

[151] The inverted commas express reservation against this wording, for if "he" is to denote the person that appears in court and if actually an identity change occurred in the meantime, then *he* never was the person who committed the felony.

However, as we saw in our discussions about "character stability" and "character continuity", character change alone – however drastic – is by no means a sufficient condition for a change of personal identity. Even a most radical and abrupt change in character may leave a person's capability of narratively integrating that change untouched.[152] Consequently, on the basis of our narrative account of personal identity, the defendant's best chance would be that his lawyers provide convincing evidence that he suffers from complete retrograde amnesia. In this case he will not be able to accomplish narrative integration of the person stages before onset of amnesia, thus not satisfying PI-Crit with respect to those stages. And while he will[153] not really be acknowledged as a "new person" because of this, but rather as a person with a certain form of dissociative disorder (dissociative amnesia), he would (or at least should) not be submitted to punishment until he does recover (if he ever does).[154] Now if the defendant does *not* suffer from dissociative amnesia, but actually *does* remember the deed, he will have a comparably harder time proving that he is not the one who is to be held responsible for it. However, even this is not impossible in principle: What the defendant would probably claim in such a case is that he remembers that "someone else" with his body committed the felony, and his lawyers would try to rack up sufficient evidence that he is suffering from DID (dissociative identity disorder, previously also called multiple personality disorder). In this case, the set of person stages associated with one and the same body can in principle be regarded as divided into several mutually exclusive subsets which are characterised by the fact that every stage x is only able to integrate those prior stages which belong to the set x itself belongs to. The subsets correspond to the different (usually *very* different) "personalities" that take turns in "surfacing" for certain periods of time. It is even more clear here than in the case of dissociative amnesia that this situation will not in fact result in an official acknowledge-

[152] This also has implications for cases where, in countries with capital punishment, people sometimes change their character in a favourable way while spending years on "death row". It is *not* a good idea to argue, for someone of that kind, that he shouldn't be punished because he "is no longer the one who committed the crime". For when people change from "criminal" to "good citizen", they usually got that character change firmly integrated into their self-concept, and even make a special *point* of telling the story of that change. Thus, rather than taking recourse to an alleged "identity change", arguments for the reprieve of these people would have to draw on the inhumanity of delivering capital punishment after years of incarceration. (Here is a last comment on the inadequacy of trying to argue for identity change through character change: If drastic character change would *indeed* all by itself count as a change in personal identity, then this would have to be acknowledged also if such a change in character had taken an *unfavourable* direction!).

[153] By most courts, in all countries, as far as we know, and according to extant law.

[154] It is known that retrograde amnesia can be caused by traumatizing events, and the felony *itself* could be just such an event. However, in such cases there is also a good chance for the memory eventually to return.

ment of "several persons" – DID is a disorder after all. Instead it will (or should) result in suspension of punishment.[155]

The two examples given above (potentially different bodies with a claim to personal identity vs. one and the same body with a claim to a change in personal identity) were supposed to make clear that, and which way, the criteria for "plausible integration" of person stages in identity-preserving stories can systematically vary with the general type of situation and claim we are confronted with. Both examples were set in the context of a "court trial", though, because we wanted to show that our narrative account of personal identity is not in danger to relegate questions of personal identity into the realm of subjective opinion (like matters of taste), but, on the contrary, can be applied to and makes a difference in situations where we want to settle such questions according to objective (i.e. intersubjective) standards of truth. On the other hand, questions of personal identity obviously do not only occur and play a role in situations where public interest is at stake. For example, a marriage may come to an end because one of the partners insists (even in these words) that the other is "not the person anymore she fell in love with" – and maybe the partner even agrees to that. Or, to give another example, some listeners may find it fully acceptable when a person accentuates a profound change of his personality by changing his name from Saulus to Paulus, and explains the change with reference to the "epiphany" of another person that passed away some time earlier. These examples show that the narrative account is also at work if there is no public interest at stake – just that what is considered "plausible integration" is then defined to a large part by more "particularistic" standards agreed by storytellers and recipients in particular narrative situations.

This should suffice for now to establish the general framework of the narrative account of personality that in our view is most apt to resolve questions concerning personal identity. We don't need to summarise it at this stage, as this will be done in the next section. Also, its consequences for the normative issues at hand will receive more attention there.

---

[155] In fact, things can be really complicated with DID. For instance, sometimes the different "persons" associated with the body of a patient with DID do not know of each other and, consequently, can't recall events that are experienced by those "other persons" – in which case we have to deal with forms of amnesia too. Sometimes they only partially or asymmetrically recall each other. If they do, they may have opinions about and emotions towards each other, and sometimes they seem to be able to "communicate". Furthermore, with the progress of time, some "persons" may dissolve and others "arise". If the courts would take it on themselves to treat DID-phenomena as anything *other* than a disorder, they would have a hard time to disentangle things. And even if they could, there would result a host of practically unsolvable problems. For example, if the person who committed the felony is still among the set of alternating persons, how could one punish *this* person without at the same time unduly punishing the others?

5.5 Summary and Consequences

In this last section of the chapter we will deal with the import the results of our analysis of the concepts of person, personality and personal identity have for a normative evaluation of the techniques of intervening in the brain presented and discussed in this book. Finally unburdened by the need for argumentative backing and discussion of rival theories, we will briefly summarise the main results of the foregoing sections and point out, for each result, *why* it is important.[156] On this background, we will eventually arrive at some specific recommendations to be included in the last chapter of this book.

5.5.1 Summing Up

But first things first: Let us turn to the promised summary of the main results achieved so far and the exposition of their import for the normative aims of this project. Our investigation started with looking into the concept of identity in general. Identity is a purely logical relation (i.e. definable within logic itself): objects *a* and *b* are identical if and only if all properties of *a* are also properties of *b* and *vice versa*. This raises a first non-trivial conceptual problem once *continuants* are taken into account, i.e. temporal objects that can change through time. For if an object *O* undergoes a change at time t, then *O* at $t''>t$ will not share all properties of *O* at $t'<t$. How can we, on the background of the definition of identity, then still coherently talk about encountering the same object *O* at *t′* and *t″*? Given that a presuppositional analysis of the conditions of the possibility of experience shows the very concept of object permanence to be indispensable, the only solution to this problem is to adopt the position that in talking about continuants any predicate is implicitly relating the continuant to a point in time, such that the *same* object can be *Q* at one time *t* and *not Q* at another time *t’* without violating the definition of identity. This in turn entails that continuants are to be conceived of as extended in time and, consequentially, spatial continuants (i.e. "material objects") *both* in space and in time. In other words: material objects have not only spatial, but also temporal parts, so called *stages.* To avoid certain logical confusions (especially, but not only, pertaining to cases of "fission" or "fusion" of continuants), the question whether an object O_1 encountered at *t* is actually the same object as an object O_2 encountered at *t′*

[156] This procedure will especially benefit those readers who are – for whatever reasons – not interested in the arguments themselves, but would just like to learn about our general train of thought, the claims we come to maintain and their connection to our eventual recommendations. However, even the mere *results* of the philosophical discussion cannot be just "listed", but have to be arranged in an order that reflects their place within the systematic structure of questions, arguments and results. Therefore we must warn *urgently* against any temptations to mistake the raw sketches and outlines of argumentative structures to be found in this section for the arguments *themselves* establishing the presented results.

has to be conceived of as the question of whether the *stages* encountered at t and t' both belong to one (the same) object as temporal parts. To answer this question, one needs criteria: the criteria of identity over time for the sort of continuants in question (where the criteria can be different for different sorts of continuants).

The concept of a continuant as an object related to points in time logically allows for continuants to survive change, but as we do not want them to have to persist "eternally" (i.e. never ceasing to persist, but just ever changing) either, the criteria of identity over time have to be such as to also allow for an answer to the question of whether a continuant O at a certain time t has ceased to persist rather than just changed. In a first step this is achieved by means of *constitutive predicates*, those predicates by which objects are identified and re-identified. For instance, "this cup" may undergo various changes, but if a change results in undermining the conditions of ascribing the (here constitutive) predicate "cup", then "this cup" has ceased to persist rather than changed. It follows that the persistence criteria for continuants will vary with the predicates serving as constitutive, and hence the continuant "this cup" will not be identical to "this amount of porcelain" – even if "this cup" at a certain time consists of that amount of porcelain. An intuitive way to phrase the persistence condition for a continuant that is based on its constitutive predicate is to say that, for the continuant to persist, its constitutive predicate has to "keep on applying". However, to avoid a certain sort of circularity built into this phrasing, the exact formulation of the criterion has to be more technical: With respect to any given continuant-stage that exemplifies some continuant through a constitutive predicate (e.g. "this cup"), only such later continuant-stages to which at least the constitutive predicate (i.e. "cup") applies can be considered as possible continuations of *that same* continuant. From this formulation it immediately becomes clear that there must be stronger criteria for really *fixing* the identity of continuants over time. For many (though not for all) sorts of embodied continuants, these criteria will conceptually involve the identity of the subsisting bodies over time, and thus their spatiotemporal continuity. However, even this will in many contexts only provide a *necessary* criterion for the object in question to still persist as "the same", and so – depending on the sort of continuants in question – there may be various reasons to formulate even stronger criteria. For example, continuously upgrading a computer by exchanging all its parts one by one (thus ensuring spatiotemporal continuity between stages) may result in us wanting to maintain, eventually, that it is *not* literally "the same" computer we originally started out with, even though, at all intermediary points in time, the constitutive predicate "computer" actually applied to the system.

The reason why these results regarding the identity of continuants in general are of utmost importance with respect to our project is the fact that *persons are continuants*: they can (and indeed are expected to) change through time while still surviving as the persons they are. It immediately follows that the specific criteria of *personal* identity over time have to be clarified in order to be able to assess possible risks for personal survival involved in certain techniques of intervening in the brain. This is even more urgent on the background that – as the persistence criteria for continuants vary with the constitutive predicates employed to identify them – the criteria for the identity of "this person" may very well *not* be the same as those for "this human body". In other words: the mere fact that an intervention does not touch upon the identity of a *human body* is not in itself sufficient insurance that, after the intervention, it is still the same *person* we are dealing with. What's more, even the continuous applicability of the constitutive predicate "person" will not by itself ensure this, for the criteria for personal *identity* have to be stronger than those for personhood.

Still, before the issue of the criteria of personal identity can be resolved, the criteria for the predicate "person", i.e. the criteria of personhood, have to be made explicit. Rather than to just enumerate ad hoc certain capacities that are commonly associated with personhood, a more systematic and integrated approach of delimiting the range of pertinent capacities is in order. The starting point for this is that, since the times of Locke, the role of the concept "person" is that of a moral rather than just a descriptive category. Basically, in the philosophical debate since Locke "person" is used to classify those living beings which can be held responsible for their actions (which is why the concept is pre-eminently encountered in contexts of rights, duties and law).

This is, of course, *very* important since it entails that the concept of a person is *not* coextensive with the concept of a human: There can be persons that are not humans and humans that are not persons. As was stressed earlier in this chapter, the latter does of course not mean that such humans – say babies – have no rights. On the contrary: as "person" is tied to "responsibility", babies, for instance, will just have no duties. In this context it is helpful to realise that the concept "human", too, is not a purely descriptive category (as "homo sapiens sapiens" is). However, the concept "human" rather conveys rights than duties. Hence we speak of "human rights", not of "person rights". Compare this to the concept of a "legal person". The main reason for widening the concept "person" so as to include abstract entities, e.g. companies, is *exactly* that this implies that they can be held responsible and, for instance, be sued. Babies, on the other hand, cannot be sued, prosecuted or convicted. Apart from these issues, it is of utmost importance to realise that for a serious consideration of concerns regarding the identity of persons which undergo a new kind of medical intervention it is *indispensable* to not just regard "person" as another word for "human being". For on such a basis, it would be true by mere linguistic convention that *nothing* that is done to a person's psyche could negatively affect her identity, as no matter how thoroughly one changes the personality or character of a human being it will still remain the same individual of the species *homo sapiens sapiens*.

Now, for someone to be a person, i.e. to be held responsible for their actions, they must fulfil at least the cognitive prerequisites for acquiring an understanding of the concept of responsibility: the ability to *regard oneself as oneself* and so to *attribute one's actions to oneself.* That is, a person does not only have *consciousness* (certain mental states and capabilities which are presupposed by the sheer ability to act), but *self*-consciousness (having a concept of oneself as the one *having* these mental states and *doing* those actions). That a being which is a person must have a concept of *itself* in turn presupposes cognitive capacities on its part to the extent that it is a subject of experiential knowledge and a participant in a community of language users. From this follows the non-cognitive (but nevertheless important) requirement that a person must be locatable within the common objective world. In the end, all these results may be regarded as summed up quite nicely in Locke's famous definition of a person as "a thinking intelligent Being, that has reason and reflection, and can consider it self as it self, the same thinking thing in different times and places".

Given these quite general results, and shifting focus to the observation that persons, to be responsible for their actions, require *free will* in the sense that they are able to *refrain from actions* as well as able to *act out decisions to act,* further and more specific cognitive, emotive and motivational prerequisites for personhood can be established through presuppositional analysis. In particular, persons need to be endowed with *discriminative abilities* (perception and recognition), *episodic memory, learning abilities,* abilities of *language* and *deliberation,* with *purposes,* a disposition to satisfy their *natural needs,* and with *sensations* of *like* and *dislike.* Apart from these "mental" requirements, it can be established that persons need to have a *body.*

In a way, the reason why these results are of importance regarding the evaluation of techniques of intervening in the brain is quite trivial: It should be made sure that their application does not – by way of side effect – eradicate any of those capacities constitutive for personhood. However, a more subtle point is that the techniques should also, at least ideally, have no negative effects on these capacities *below* the threshold of utter eradication, because such effects would have to count as "undermining" personhood. So, if with respect to an intervention technique there are certain possible side effects of that kind, this deserves special consideration in risk/benefit-weighing.

Just like the debate on the concept of a person, the modern debate on the question of personal identity can be traced back to John Locke. Since his times, the question of personal identity is the question about the criteria of persistence of particular continuants, namely persons. Even though the origin is often forgotten, talk of "personal identity" within psychology and everyday life descends from philosophical debate. In the contexts of morals and jurisdiction it is more or less obvious that the question of personal identity is important, as we attribute actions to persons and so we have to make sure that the persons we praise or condemn or convict are the same persons that carried out the actions we praise, condemn or convict them for. However, the issue of personal identity is also of special interest with regard to the project pursued in this book, because *we* – i.e. the community of persons – *ourselves* are the objects under investigation. Thus any issues pertaining to the question of whether techniques of intervening in the brain could bear a potential risk of undermining the conditions laid down by the criteria of personal identity and persistence will be relevant insofar as persons are interested in (and have a right to) their own continued survival.

The first step towards establishing such criteria is the insight, following from the discussion of the role of constitutive predicates for the identity of continuants in general, that the continuing applicability of the constitutive predicate "person" is a necessary condition for a person's persistence. However, it is also obvious that fulfilment of this condition alone is not sufficient to establish that it is really the *same* person we're dealing with at different times. Candidates for the required additional criteria determining personal identity are usually categorised into two groups, "physical" and "psychological" criteria. In the discussion of the previous section it turned out that the physical criteria (namely personal identity as bodily identity or brain identity) are too strong and therefore not adequate. Although, at first blush, it may seem so, it would be a mistake to think that this result has no direct bearing on the normative dimension of the debate about present techniques of intervening in the brain.[157] On the contrary: As nowadays most people (quite correctly) assume that their psychic states and functions are not independent of states of their body, especially their CNS, there is an intuitive fear among the general public that interventions involving neurografting or neuroprosthetics should be *per se* regarded as bound to destroy or at least gravely endanger the personal identity of those who would be subjected to such techniques (think of the "Borg" of the popular Star-Trek universe, which can be seen as a fictional manifestation of such fears). The reason why the brain is indeed germane to personal identity is that it embodies the pertinent psychic functions (cognitive abilities and personality traits). But it is of utmost importance to recognise that it is therefore rather these abilities and traits *themselves* which have to be considered with respect to the question of personal identity, *not* their contingent physical "implementation". If the crucial psychic functions are preserved, persons would survive, as the persons they are, even massive interventions involving neurolesioning, neurografting or

[157] The reason why one may be inclined to think so is probably this: "Techniques" discussed in the pertinent thought experiments, like scanning and reimplementation of psychic functions, are neither available, nor does it seem likely (as of now) that they ever will. Hence, the failure of physical criteria of identity *at best* seems to show that, though empirically improbable or even impossible, a host of novels or movies employing scenarios in which personal identity is retained through, let's say a complete transformation of body (like in Kafka's "Die Verwandlung" ["The Metamorphosis"]), are nevertheless conceptually coherent (in contrast e.g. to stories involving time travel).

neuroprosthetics, resulting in a brain that is quite literally not the same anymore. It is hence *not* true that intervention techniques of that kind are "by their very nature" (i.e. *as* techniques that do alter structures of or connections in the brain) bound to destroy personal identity.

Of course, this still leaves open the question of which psychic functions are the ones crucial to personal identity, i.e. the question of what are the "psychological" criteria of personal identity. Unfortunately, the most prominent candidates – criteria of psychological *continuity* – also encounter insurmountable difficulties. At most it can be shown that continuity of *episodic memory* is indeed another *necessary* criterion for personal identity. While this is undoubtedly a major result insofar as it clearly implies that intervention techniques have to be checked against possible amnestic side effects, it can be shown that continuity of episodic memory does, on the other hand, not provide a *sufficient* criterion for personal identity. Even worse, further analysis shows that the "natural" idea to upgrade the criterion to a necessary *and* sufficient one by including further reference to continuity or stability of *personality traits* (of the categories temper, motifs, propositional attitudes and talents) leads nowhere. On the contrary, it turns out that continuity criteria must always fail as sufficient criteria for personal identity (while "stability criteria" always fail as necessary criteria).

Therefore another approach to personal identity has to be found. To this, the key lies in the insight that the personality of a person is not merely the aggregate of all her p-traits as they may be described from a third person's perspective. This aggregate view of character is valid only for non-personal beings that are incapable of holding and communicating opinions of their own with regard to the way others describe what's special about them by ascribing character traits to them. Persons, on the other hand, are self-referential beings, who not only *have* character traits, but, moreover, hold a set of beliefs *about* these traits as well. What persons believe about their own p-traits is part of a more complex system of self-related beliefs and motifs that constitutes their *self-concept.* As self-referential beings, persons try to make sense, on their own behalf, of their actions and behaviour in a way that sheds light on who they are as against other persons. At any given time of their persistence persons may look back from their first person perspective on how they acted and reacted in various situations in order to identify those features in which they are unlike others. In a process of constant exchange with others like them persons weigh these bits and pieces of self-observation and self-interpretation and include the more significant ones in their self-concepts. Since any change of a person's self-concept clearly manifests a change of her personality, the self-concept actually constitutes a part of the personality. Therefore, rather than merely *having* a personality that at most would need to be *discovered* by a person during the course of her life, persons – at least to some extent – actively *create* their personalities by composing their self-concepts.

The process through which personal self-concepts take shape bears significant similarities to the process of composing a narrative. To begin with, this comparison is helpful in expounding the structural properties that a set of self-related beliefs needs to possess for it to be recognised as constituting a self-concept. Since self-concepts are expressed in narratives that claim to be *true* (to the facts of a person's life and, especially, personality traits) they need to fulfil certain minimal requirements governing all stories that are associated with a claim to truth. These requirements are such that violating them in particular instances just means that – with respect to the goal of truth – there is something not quite correct yet about the story, which has to be amended to get it "right". Violating them more often, however, does eventually result in the breakdown of "story-ness" itself. The first requirement is that, ideally, truth-claiming narratives should be free from contradictions in general; and, in particular, it should be possible to arrange all the events mentioned in a story of this kind in a consistent temporal sequence. Another structural requirement can be derived from the general fact that stories are told with certain goals in mind. For every story, there is an explicit or implicit background of goals against which objects, events and levels of descriptive detail and completeness are judged pertinent or irrelevant. So what is told in a story should be relevant with regard to "what it is about". This can be elaborated further by taking into account that, even with respect to the specific goals that determine what the story is about, a story's claim to truth is never just to *report what happened*, but also, in a way, to *make sense of it*. To varying degrees of explicitness and detail (ranging from "elaborate" to "sketchy" and "implicit"), this will include the *intentional* explanation of actions as well as the *causal* explanation of other pertinent events. Ideally, every part of a story would be *significant* in the sense that it serves a function as regards the descriptive and explanative goals that are associated with the story. Consequently, the relevance of parts of a story can be assessed through questions like: "Does this part of the story set the stage for or contribute to the understanding of something else which the story essentially is about?", "Is this something we can take for granted or rather something that should be explained?", etc. Self-constituting narratives are told with a particular goal in mind, namely to convey how the storytellers became the persons they conceive themselves to be now. If someone is unable to distinguish the significance of their self-related beliefs with respect to this goal, they obviously lack a clear-cut concept of who they are.

Whether someone's self-related statements satisfy these requirements so that they constitute a coherent self-concept can be decided without knowing the actual truth of any of these statements. Of course, the internal coherence and consistency of a story is not *enough* to make it true. To this end, a story also has to be "consistent with the facts". Once we know more about a person than what she tells us about herself, we will therefore start scrutinising the whole of her self-related statements in a different way: By drawing on immediate acquaintance with her actions or on independent reports about what she did in different situations we have a chance to question the truth of parts of a person's self-constituting narratives. A person's way of describing her past development may be distorted by inaccuracies of memory or by deliberate efforts to gloss over the past. In much the same way, inconsistencies between a person's account of who she is and her actual behaviour can be explained either by her misapprehension of what marks her off from others or with reference to some image that the person intentionally created to conform to others' expectations. Finally, a person's statements about her future projects of self-creation can be proven wrong by failure to put them into action. The final result of the social process in which inconsistencies between the stories a person tells about herself and her actual way of being are first identified and then explained along these various lines is an *intersubjectively recognised account* of who that person is: A person's personality is represented by the most coherent story that persons could agree upon with respect to who she is, given the available knowledge about her past and present life, including her plans for future personal development.

According to this narrative account of personality, not only changes in a person's actions and behaviour affecting *temper*, basic long-term *motifs*, basic long-term propositional *attitudes* and *talents* need to be regarded as changes of her personality, but also changes in her narratively structured self concept. However, none of these different types of personality changes necessarily amounts to a change of personal identity. Rather, a person is persisting as the person she is if and only if she is (not always immediately, but eventually) able to plausibly integrate personality changes (including changes of her self-concept itself) into her ever developing self-concept. "Plausibly integrate" does *not* mean that the narratively structured self-concept of a person has to be a true representation of her personality, but (to put it in the most general way) that there *is* a "story" relating earlier person stages and the pertinent changes to the actually "present" person stage and that this story is sufficiently grounded in episodic memory to be counted as at least genuine.

Apart from this, the threshold for "plausible integration" will, however, differ widely with context. To address the most problematic case first: the strongest demands would be put on the coherence of a story when there is serious reason to doubt that the person stages in question are represented by the same body. In our present day societies, reasoning about personal identity is strongly guided by the intuition that physical continuity is necessary for personal persistence, and even though in Section 5.4.1 this could not be established as a *conceptual* truth, it may well be true *empirically*. Anyway, if two person stages are *known* to not belong to the same body, then only the most coherent and detailed story – one that would pass closest scrutiny regarding the requirement of sufficient grounding in episodic memory (typically tested through tricky questions that an impostor would be highly unlikely to answer correctly) – would have a chance to eventually lead us to accept the identity claim despite of this knowledge. (Probably, that claim would not even be considered as a residual possibility, if the "case" at hand was to remain a singularity.) If, on the other hand, physical continuity between two person stages is unquestionable, there is strong *prima facie* reason to suppose that they indeed belong to the same person. Therefore, in such cases the demands on the plausibility of stories by which the earlier stage is integrated by the later one are so much lower that, actually, the onus of proof is on those who would argue that the two person stages do *not* belong to the same person. According to our narrative account of personal identity, only complete retrograde amnesia and DID would make strong cases here. However, because there is usually at least a *chance* of recovery, these are (reasonably) treated, in practice, as cases of *one* person having a *disorder*, and *not* acknowledged as two or more persons in succession "occupying" one body. (Things would probably be handled differently if such cases were more frequent, stable and irreversible.)

There are several points with respect to which the narrative account of personal identity is of import for the evaluation of techniques of intervening in the brain: First of all, the narrative approach offers no grounds to state *in advance* what changes of his or her personality a person may successfully integrate into a coherent identity-preserving narrative. Not even on the basis of the most comprehensive knowledge of a person's personality at some given point in time is it possible to come to any *prognoses* that a certain change of personality *must* result in a change of personal identity. Secondly, the narrative account implies that any changes in personal identity an intervention may cause would *never* go unnoticed, but would become openly manifest as severe dissociative disorders. This consequence deserves particular emphasis because it should assuage public fears that intervention techniques possibly could cause identity changes that may not be detectable. Such fears are usually based on dualistic intuitions paired with the view that scientists can only access "the Objective" (behaviour and other publicly observable data), but not "the Subjective" (the mind, the person itself).[158]

[158] Fears regarding the possibility of unnoticeable identity changes even receive (probably inadvertent) theoretical backing by an influential philosophical position: the "simple view of personal identity", according to which persons are immaterial thinking substances. As a consequence of their dualism, proponents of the simple view claim that empirical data may at best provide "evidence" for matters of personal identity, but *never* criteria in the strict sense. The simple view therefore allows for the logico-semantical possibility that a person (the immaterial substance associated with a human body) may be replaced by someone else (another immaterial thinking substance), and even for the possibility that the person vanishes, leaving the body behind as an organism still living, but no longer associated with a person (immaterial substance). For a refutation of the simple view, see Section 5.4.2.

5.5.2 Consequences

On the basis of our exposition of the normative import the results of this chapter bear on the discussion of intervening in the brain, we are finally able to formulate and justify certain ethico-political recommendations regarding research on, and application of the techniques involved. For this set of recommendations we will not claim completeness – not even with regard to issues pertaining to personality or personal identity. The recommendations will be *specific*, though, in the sense that they pre-eminently deal with such issues, and they will be *general*, at the same time, in the sense that they do not deal with any intervention technique specifically.

By the very nature of recommendations directed to a field of research on, or application of certain techniques, these recommendations will for the most part involve the specification of situations where a certain *caution* is in order. Let us make it clear from the outset: Our general stance regarding the techniques presented and discussed in this book is positive, and this should not come as much of a surprise. After all, if there were not such promise in this field, without the prospect of finding new and more effective kinds of *treatment* for old diseases and disabilities, this whole study would most likely not have been undertaken.

We are in favour of the continuation and even extension of the funding of the *research* done in the field under consideration. In our opinion, the therapeutic benefits alone suffice to warrant this statement, regardless of how one may think about the issue of enhancement. The argument for this is rather trivial and well known: As *everything* can be misused, the mere fact that something *could* be misused towards unjustified goals cannot count as an argument against it (or we would have to object to even the most banal artefacts, such as hammers). With the question of funding in mind, one may think there are certain fields of research on techniques of intervening in the brain which are more treatment-oriented, while others are more enhancement-oriented. But, in fact, this is not the case. Rather, it seems that the same techniques *mutatis mutandis* can be used in situations of treatment as well as enhancement.

The aforementioned general positive stance on the new techniques does not mean, though, that our approval is without reflection, or uncritical. This will become evident from the recommendations to follow, which deal with the detection and prevention of certain *side effects.*

A side effect is any unintended effect of an intervention (that was carried out correctly). The purpose of the proviso "carried out correctly" is to terminologically distinguish side effects related to a technique as such from the effects of *accidents* that may occur in an attempt of its application. If, for instance, a surgeon performing a prostate operation accidentally cuts the patient's ureter, this would not be classified correctly as a "possible side effect" of the respective operating technique. While – for any given surgical technique – certain accidents may occur contingently (e.g. when the scalpel of the surgeon slips because of a sudden cramp in his hand), there may also be a considerable *probability* for a certain *type* of accident to occur when applying the technique in question. With regard to risk/benefit weighing, such accidents are, for all intents and purposes, treated just like possible side effects in the strict sense of the term. Consequently, for the sake of clarity, we are going to address these types of possible accidents under the general heading of "side effects", too (to avoid cumbersome differentiation as "possible side effects *and* possible accidents significantly correlated with the application of a certain intervention technique").

Because a side effect is an unintended effect, the decision about what is or is not counted a side effect will depend on the goals *and* there may be positive (welcome) side effects of an intervention as well as negative (adverse) ones. In the following, we will not discuss positive side effects any further, and we will also just consider such side effects which are considered negative with respect to the whole range of morally and legally licit goals of intervention. These side effects can be broken down into sub-classes in a variety of ways. For the following we propose:

- biological death
- somatic diseases (e.g. ulcer, cancer)
- motor or sensory disabilities (e.g. paralysis, deafness)
- psychic (i.e. cognitive, emotive and motivational) diseases and disabilities (e.g. depression, schizophrenia, aphasia, amnesia, sociopathy)
- personality changes (i.e. changes in temper, motifs, propositional attitudes, talents and self-concept)
- psychological death (i.e. loss of personhood or identity change)

Obviously, not all of these classes are mutually exclusive. For instance, certain somatic diseases can underlie psychic dysfunctions; a sensory disability is – via the cognitive aspect of perception – also a psychic disability; psychological death will be accompanied either by grave psychic disabilities or personality changes, etc. However, as rough as it may be, this classification should still be of some use.

Furthermore, our classes of side effects do not specifically address interventions in the psyche, but can also be applied (regarding the intended effects) to somatic interventions. There is a wide range of well established surgical procedures or medicinal drugs coming with a non-negligible – but, with respect to risk/benefit weighing, acceptable – lethality rate (death), infection risk (organic disease), or risk of other complications, which, like e.g. apoplexy, can be correlated with possible further effects like aphasia (psychic disability), loss of certain talents (personality change) or even irreversible coma (psychological death). That the subclasses of side effects given above also apply to somatic interventions should not be an objection to them, but rather a vindication: after all, the difference between somatic interventions and interventions in the psyche is *not* that the latter deal with a different kind of substance than the former. On the contrary, interventions in the psyche (at least those we discuss in this book) are carried out as somatic interventions too. The only difference is that interventions in the psyche are such somatic interventions (usually in the CNS) that are conducted with the explicit *goal* to thereby influence certain psychic functions, whereas "ordinary" somatic interventions are conducted with more or less *exclusively* somatic goals in mind. In any case, the class of possible side effects is essentially the same for both kinds of intervention.

However, it is to be expected that because the somatic targets of interventions in the psyche are structures which implement psychic capacities or at least directly interact with such structures, certain kinds of side effects should be more prominent here than in the case of "mere" somatic interventions. Indeed, the risk of having a psyche-related side effect in, say, podiatric surgery is quite obviously much lower than in neurosurgery.

Finally, one may wonder whether side effects regarding personality changes actually belong here in the sense that they are always considered negative. One has to be very cautious here: We cannot, for instance, just suppose that a personality change is per se warranted if its direction is socially accepted or even valued. Even less does the mere fact that personality changes anyway all through life gives license to ignore or tolerate side effects on personality associated with an intervention, even if they should turn out to be on the socially acceptable side. Rather, an unintended personality change can only count as a "positive" side effect if the person undergoing the intervention would have welcomed that change *beforehand*.[159] But if that is indeed the case, then we were just very lucky, and that is why personality changes qua side effects have to appear on this list.

Before we go a step further towards recommendations, there is another, quite different, but nevertheless important way of dividing the class of possible side effects that has to be mentioned: the division of side effects into *conspicuous* and *subtle* ones.[160] Conspicuous side effects are those that will rarely go unnoticed even if no or little effort is made to check for their presence. Subtle side effects on the other hand are those that may go unnoticed (at least for a while) if not specifically checked upon. It is important to note that the distinction between conspicuous and subtle side effects is by no means co-extensive with that between major and minor ones, which already

[159] This can be tricky to test after the fact. The p-trait change itself can have an effect on a person's attitude towards that particular p-trait. Let's say a person was rather introverted before an intervention and is much more outgoing and social afterwards. It is quite possible (or even trivial) that the newly extroverted person approves of this trait, but what would be the value of such approval?

[160] While this distinction as such is not new, there seems to be no terminological convention governing it – calling the classes "conspicuous" and "subtle" is our own proposal.

Not all of these procedures are equally available at present, be it for technical, practical, or legal reasons. However, some of them, in particular various means of pharmaceutical intervention, are, at least to some extent, already part of our modern way of life. Other such procedures will become so in the foreseeable future. Nevertheless, the impression is hard to avoid that some descriptions of the present state, and future potential, of these procedures is a loose, and perhaps overly optimistic, mixture of science and fiction. This refers, in particular, to some of the expected or alleged developments in neuroprosthetic procedures and in brain-computer interfaces. Some accounts of the future possibilities for altering certain mental features through genetic interventions also bear a greater resemblance to fantasy than to scientific indications of a new approach in clinical practice. However, apart from the fact that there are also remarkable exceptions[164], the somewhat speculative nature of some of those perspectives does not dispense us from the task of clarifying as soon as possible the normative issues, which arise out of these actual or potential developments.

Each of these (potential) means of interventions into the mental life of human beings were originally developed due to their expected clinical application. However, many of them were quickly identified as holding potential, not only for the purposes of psychotherapy, but also for the enhancement of the mental state of by and large healthy people. Four forms of such a mental enhancement can be distinguished:

- Enhancement of cognition, i.e. of cognitive abilities in the widest sense,
- enhancement of emotional states, such as mood,
- enhancement of motivational and/or conative states, and
- enhancement of "autonomic states", i.e. mental states emerging from autonomic functions of the CNS and, like these functions themselves, not subject to volitional control, such as dreaming, proprioceptive awareness, or sexual arousal.

These distinctions must be kept in mind. They seem to be of importance for the specific purpose of our investigation, namely the clarification of the underlying and accompanying normative problems that arise out of this type of procedure. These three kinds of enhancement pose, as one might expect, ethical and legal problems of diverging significance and difficulty. We will explore these issues in due course.

[164] For a review on recent advances of brain-machine interfaces and neural prostheses cf. Agar (2004); Berger et al. (2005); see also Stieglitz (2006); as to genetic interventions cf. Donoghue (2002); Kennedy Institute of Ethics Journal (15(1), 2005) for several lengthy essays on the prospects of "genetic enhancement"; for the genetics of psychiatric disorders see van Belzen and Heutink (2006); for a review of research on genomics of learning and memory see Paratore et al. (2006); for a case of genetic enhancement of learning and memory in mice cf. Tang et al. (1999).

Presently, however, it is the pharmacological methods of mental enhancement that are (and will increasingly be) the subject of large scale social demand. Expanding markets have already been established for such products. Prozac® (fluoxetine), which belongs to the pharmacological class of selective serotonin reuptake inhibitors (SSRIs), serves as a telling example. Originally developed as an anti-depressant, it has, at least in the United States of America, assumed the role of a lifestyle drug for mood enhancement (Kramer 1993; Barondes 2003; Elliott and Chambers 2004). In Germany, it is marketed under the proprietary name of "Fluctin", and is currently meeting the demands of a quickly expanding circle of consumers. The figures of the sale of the drug, both in Germany and the USA, demonstrate *ad oculos* that it is being used by more and more people for less and less serious mental indispositions or disorders. The market for so-called nootropic substances is also growing rapidly in Europe as well as in the United States (although the latter is considerably further ahead in this development). These are stimulants aimed at the enhancement of cognitive abilities (in a wide and functionally fundamental sense), such as memory, attention, vigilance, and other learning preconditions (cf. Ingvar et al. 1997; Caldwell et al. 2000; Wesensten et al. 2001; Yesavage et al. 2002; Turner et al. 2003; Jones et al. 2005). Most notably of all, Methylphenidate (Ritalin®), prescribed for some time in the treatment of attention deficit hyperactivity disorder (ADHD) in children, has ceased to be a purely therapeutic device and is increasingly being used as a so-called *smart drug* whose aim is the cognitive enhancement (of an apparently growing number of people) via an induced expansion of their attentive potential (Diller 1998; Cooper 2005:249).

The change in the social function of these medications from therapies to enhancement tools has been accelerated by the fact that their use seems to be largely free of danger and lacking even in immediate or unpleasant physiological side effects. However, the following *caveats* must be added to the above, the former relating to the potential effects on the psychological well being of the individual and the latter to the potential effect of the use of these substances on society as a whole. First, the long term risks and the potentially lasting impact of the use of such substances on the structure of the brain are not fully understood. Indeed, far from excluding the possibility of such side effects, the physiological impact of those substances on the neuronal microstructure of the brain has been well documented in existing research (Hyman 2002; cf. also Gazzaniga 2005:78). Second, the potential effect of widespread, long term use of psychotropic substances for non-clinical purposes on the "state of mind" of the entire society is barely understood. These concerns do not relate primarily to the immediate consequences that mass enhancements of psychic capacities might have. Rather, what is at issue here is the indirect effect of these procedures on other parts of society, grounded in, and ordered by, complex textures of legal, ethical, aesthetical, and prudential norms, and thus the possible impacts on these

We will follow this line of analysis and investigate the problems of these two spheres separately and, in due course, we will draw some more distinctions within their respective conceptual and normative scope.

In a somewhat different but related way, one could also differentiate between, on the one hand, the view of the individual whose possible enhancement is being debated, and, on the other hand, of society as a whole. These two perspectives are themselves loosely affiliated to a normative distinction between the ethics of individual action and the area of public policy. We will keep this way of differentiating within reach and will turn to it on occasion.

It is fairly obvious that both parts of our basic distinction go along with a *prima facie* suggestion of strong normative implications. We will turn to these later. At this point, however, it is important to note that those implications, whatever their content, are not founded upon exactly the same normative principles. Roughly speaking, if a specific act of enhancement is "in itself" judged to be morally reprehensible according to ethical criteria of individual acting, it should certainly not be part of professional medicine. Nor should it be part of the basic package of care that the social system of medicine is supposed to offer to every member of society. What is individually forbidden cannot be a legitimate part of the public service of medicine. In this respect, the normative ground for both spheres is identical. However, this does not hold the other way around. For not every possible and potentially useful medical intervention that lies beyond the proper limits of medicine must, simply for this reason, transgress the limits of what an individual person may do to and with herself on grounds of morally good or acceptable reasons. Medicine as a social system obviously needs to observe principles of distributive justice over and beyond the maxims of individual ethics. The provision of medicine is a scarce and expensive public good that should be subject to fair distribution. Therefore, many cut-off points must be drawn that do not follow from moral criteria of individual action but only from those of distributive justice. This is, of course, especially true for enhancements. The fact that they – for reasons of justice and scarcity – may not be a legitimate part of the basic package of care offered by the social system of medicine does not mean that they are not morally acceptable for the individual person who is willing and able to pay for them.

Furthermore, it should be clear that most of what belongs to a normatively well-founded package of basic care in medicine is not just permissable, but is obligatory for a well ordered society, while most of what is morally allowed as individual behaviour with respect to one's own body or mind is, of course, discretionary for the respective individual. There is, to be sure, the Kantian notion of (moral) "duties to oneself", and, in Kant's view, practices by which one improves one's physical or mental capacities certainly belong to the realm of those duties (cf. Kant 1907/14 [AA VI]:417-447; id. 1903/11 [AA IV]:428). We will return to the question of such duties to oneself later.

These considerations lead to a related issue. There is a second body of normative principles, beyond those governing individual behaviour, that any sensible attempt to delineate the limits of proper medicine has to take into account: principles that regulate social behaviour and, therefore, contribute to the stabilisation (or the erosion) of collectively shared values, ideas, and other symbolic forms of life of a society. To be morally acceptable, individual behaviour must not always rely on those collectively oriented principles. But certainly the social practice of medicine must.

Obviously these two spheres of partly diverging normative entitlements and obligations (whatever their exact content) may conflict with each other. An individual may have good reasons to enhance him- or herself by a psychopharmacologic intervention, or may at least have reasons that are unobjectionable from a moral or legal point of view. Consequently, the enhancing measure would be essentially a matter of his or her personal liberty. On the other hand, decisions like the one in question may, if taken on a large scale by large numbers of individuals, possibly affect society as a whole in an undesired way. In that case, we would encounter difficult problems of normative trade-offs between the different spheres of rights and interests at stake. What are the exact criteria by which to judge whether an individual act that does not in itself harm anybody might, nevertheless, be morally inappropriate and even legally forbidden for the simple fact that it might contribute to the risk of an undesired societal development? What complicates this question even further is the fact that it remains uncertain whether any such negative side effects will be brought about. Furthermore, this unwelcome development will result, if at all, not from the individual whose psychic state will be enhanced but, instead, from the behaviour of people other than the individual enhancer himself. Important parts of this problem also run as deep as the fundamental issues of social justice. They, therefore, share the notorious difficulties and intricacies of the philosophical debates in this area. We will return to these questions and try to assess some of their difficulties.

6.3 Problems of Delineating the "Proper Limits of Medicine" by Employing the Concept of Enhancement

6.3.1 Preliminary Conceptual Clarifications

As far as the demarcation of the proper limits of medicine as a social system[166] is concerned, "enhancement," in its common usage, functions as a negative boundary concept, comparable to the often cited concept of a "futile treatment". Consequently, it bears *prima facie* normative weight. Since conceptually it fulfills a negative function, it is meant to circumscribe what should not be the case. That is:

---

[166] Henceforth, for the purpose of abbreviation, we will refer simply to the "proper limits of medicine" or the "limits of proper medicine".

- what should not be part of the professional services of medical practitioners (of a basic package of care), as far as these services are publicly financed by either a social-security system or through general taxation,
- and, consequently, what should not be covered by health insurance systems based on public financing,
- and, finally, what should not be an objective of any publicly funded biomedical research,[167]

A preliminary remark is required at this juncture on the conceptual relationship of "enhancement" and "improvement". An enhancement of particular human features and properties certainly does imply an "improvement" of the respective feature. There is no enhancement which does not at the same time improve at least something for someone.[168] But the improvement implied by an enhancement is relative in at least two senses. First, what counts as an enhancement, viz improvement, depends on the standpoint from which the desired enhanced state is defined as advantageous, relative to certain values. These values do not necessarily have to be shared by other people. In extreme cases, they could even be rejected by everybody else. An enhancement in that particular, value-relative context may, therefore, not appear to be an enhancement for anybody else, or could even amount to a worsening or a disadvantage from the point of view of other people. Second, enhancements can be, and often are, relative to particular contexts and/or particular times in the life of a person. What is an enhancement/improvement at one time and in one context, may not be so at other times and in other situations in that same person's life. Take the example of memory enhancement. Advantageous as it might be for person X in most contexts of her life, it may not be so after a severe traumatic experience that X urgently wishes to forget or suppress in her memory. An inability to forget such an incident may cause her considerable suffering, and may even give rise to a serious form of psychological illness (cf. Fields 2005; Glannon 2006a; President's Council on Bioethics 2003:218).

In using "enhancement" as a negative concept, one obviously needs to draw a line between what counts as enhancement and what does not. This is commonly done by contrasting it with the concept of treatment. Once again, we regard "enhancement" as being negatively defined by its conceptual

[167] This refers only to research directed at the development and application of enhancements, not to research aiming at the elucidation of chemical, physiological or mental processes, induced or influenced by enhancing means, for other purposes. Both research areas may, of course, in part overlap. (Similar research on dangerous and prohibited drugs does not aim at furthering drug distribution, even though it may partly overlap with research serving just that purpose.)

[168] Not all improvements, of course, are enhancements. Successful treatments of diseases lead to improvements in the condition of the patient without being an enhancement in the sense in which the term is employed here, i.e. that of moving beyond a merely healthy state.

opposition to treatment. Enhancement will be considered to be any physically or psychologically efficient, or possibly efficient, effort to improve the human condition that cannot be considered medical treatment. As such, enhancement is not part of proper medicine. When used as a boundary concept like this, "enhancement" has both descriptive and normative features and functions. By employing it, we can identify and label efforts as either treatment or enhancement. Furthermore, we can characterise such efforts as either a legitimate part of proper medicine or not. This of course raises familiar problems.

6.3.2 A Third Category: Prevention

We do as yet not have a clear understanding of what can plausibly count as treatment and what cannot. That poses problems of a primarily conceptual nature and highlights several other semantic fields whose boundaries are also not very clearly defined, such as those of "health" and "disease". But even before approaching these questions, one encounters another problem with a clear-cut distinction in the dualistic scheme of treatment and enhancement: It does not seem to do justice to strategies of prevention. Vaccination provides us with a particularly clear example of preventive medicine, but practices of prescribing and taking statins to reduce the likelihood of stroke and myocardial infarction, and other such preventive strategies could be cited as well. Nobody doubts that vaccination, and similar preventive measures of the said kind, are a sensible and legitimate part of medicine and medical research. On the other hand, they cannot properly be labeled "treatments", not even "anticipated treatments". Rather, they are something directed against treatment, viz. designed specifically to avoid its future necessity. Considered just in themselves, they amount to a strengthening of the human organism and therefore a certain type of enhancement.

One could certainly settle this conceptual difficulty by simply introducing prevention as a third category besides those of treatment and enhancement, and then just include it into the legitimate sphere of medical practice by relying on a self-evident intuition. Disease-related prevention is an integral element not only of the practical reality of modern medicine, but also of its moral image.[169] As part of proper medicine in this sense, prevention is connected to treatment insofar as it functions as a

[169] We use the term "disease-related prevention" to hint at the fact that there are other forms of prevention of unwanted states of affairs which could also possibly employ new techniques of intervening in the psyche. What we mean here are forms of prevention that could be called "sociopathy-related", destined, for instance, to prevent someone from developing a disposition to criminal behaviour. From a normative point of view, these latter forms are, in general, a lot more problematic than the former. Presently, we use "prevention" only in its disease-related sense. However, we will deal with problems of sociopathy-related preventions when we tackle the questions of treating or enhancing mental states of prison detainees.

way of anticipating and circumventing the otherwise impending necessity of the latter. In a normative perspective, i.e. considering questions of legitimacy, this is perfectly plausible. Both concepts, treatment as well as prevention, are related to, or oriented towards, "fighting off" or controlling diseases, i.e. states of physical or mental well-being below a certain standard judged as "healthy" by the relevant criteria within a given society (regardless of what these relevant criteria are and how they are being derived.)[170] The term "fighting" is metaphorically indicative of the common normative ground of both concepts: The task of both treatment and prevention is to *confront* disease by preventing, removing, reducing, or at least confining and controlling it.[171]

The crucial point is that, from a normative perspective, "prevention" bears a close affinity to, or in some sense may even be coterminous with, the concept of treatment. On the other hand, from a descriptive or phenomenological perspective, some forms of prevention, such as vaccination or taking statins, are a specific form of enhancement, aiming at enhanced immunity from disease. To be sure, not all preventive medicine is enhancement. Perhaps only a small part of it is.[172] But even this small part is sufficient to blur the lines between what is "proper medicine" and what is not, which had offered itself as a normative corollary of the distinction between treatment and enhancement. For even if vaccination against major diseases results in a super-normal strength of human immune systems, it remains a perfectly sensible medical measure and should therefore be considered a legitimate part of proper medicine (Juengst 1998). This casts a first doubt on the widespread contention that this distinction, holds decisive normative force and is, therefore, able to inform us about what forms of intervention are ethically permissible, or even obligatory, (treatment) and those which are not (enhancement). This is quite obviously a crude simplification, with respect to both the purely descriptive demarcation and the normative guidance it is supposedly able to provide.

To complicate the picture, one might even add a fourth category: physical or psychic interventions that cannot be considered treatment, prevention or enhancement, but which do, nevertheless, have a close connection to the sphere of medicine. Their relation to medicine is threefold. First, they can be adequately performed only by trained physicians. Second, there is a strong societal demand for them as services to be provided for by

[170] For our present purposes, "disease" is meant to encompass any pathological state, including disability. There are, of course, differences between disease and disability and some of them certainly bear normative weight, though not for the distinctions we are trying to establish here. For disability, no less than disease, is subject to legitimate treatment within the sphere of proper medicine.

[171] This, of course, points to familiar problems in the long-standing debate about the concept of disease. We will touch these problems in the following section (*sub* 6.3.3).

[172] For instance, preventive screenings for late-onset diseases are certainly not.

physicians. Third, their individual refusal may lead to a considerable amount of suffering, or conversely, their provision to relief from considerable burdens. Abortion would be an example of such a procedure. Normatively speaking, it is probably closer to enhancement (even though lexically it hardly belongs to the scope of meaning of this concept). Far from being a disease in need of treatment, pregnancy is, in fact, proof that a woman is in good physical condition. Still one may doubt this by saying that – at least from the subjective point of view of the pregnant woman – an unwanted pregnancy puts her in a potentially "harmful" physical state, even though some might consider this a rather strange aberration from the common meaning of "harm".[173] Abortion aside, it is not easy to think of any other example of a procedure that would fit this final category, except perhaps the related, but largely harmless, medical practice of prescribing female contraceptives.[174] So it seems that we can, without a major risk of missing important insights, neglect this final category in the context of our analysis.

6.3.3 Basic Models of Health and Disease

But apart from its *prima facie* plausibility, our trichotomy of treatment – prevention – enhancement is unable to solve all the conceptual problems that arise here, let alone the normative questions that follow in their wake. The next issue to address is how we ought to develop and clarify the difference between interventions that count as treatments (and perhaps preventions) and others that must be considered *only* enhancements (without being of a disease-preventive character). What basic account of health, disease and treatment should inform our definitions of treatment and enhancement? What is treatment from one perspective may not count as treatment from another. The same holds true for enhancements as well. Take for example a form of psychotherapy aimed at liberating a person from her natural shyness from which she might suffer considerably. In a system where shyness has been sufficiently "medicalised", perhaps simply for the fact that it can be treated like other disorders that certainly count as diseases, shyness can be considered an illness. In a different system where the range of medicalisation does not extend to cover "habit variations" of various sorts, shyness might be considered simply a form of behaviour or a

[173] Still, consider the following, admittedly somewhat wild, imaginary case. During a regular appendectomy on a woman, the doctor maliciously, and without the patient's consent, implants the in-vitro-fertilised embryo of another woman completely unknown to the patient, thus causing her to become pregnant. It certainly does not seem too far-fetched to call this the intentional infliction of a physical harm.

[174] We ignore the fundamentally different practice of lethal injections by medical doctors in some countries that retain capital punishment. Apart from questions about the legitimacy of capital punishment itself, this practice seems, by all ethical criteria, to amount to a patent misuse of professional medical expertise.

disposition within the normal spectrum of human character traits. In yet a third system where the notion of "illness" is defined by criteria of subjective suffering and potential treatability, we might again consider unusual forms of shyness a disease in need of medical treatment. If we couple this problem with the question of the bounds of legitimate medical practice, we can employ our distinguishing criterion to demarcate the limits of medical necessity as well.

All of this invokes the well-known and long-standing problem of the concept of disease. The labyrinthine subtleties of the recent debate, spanning a period of more than three decades, cannot, and need not, be explored in detail here.[175] It is obvious that a concept of disease must fulfill different functions in different contexts of both theory and practice. Consequently, it may also assume different meanings according to the respective context in which it appears.[176] For our current purposes, we need, on a very abstract level, a concept of disease which allows us to elucidate the criteria by which we can define the proper limits of medicine as a system of public health (or, on the macro-level, a system of organised medical services). This can only be done by connecting the concept of disease to certain fundamental elements of social justice, which has been the subject of a much longer and much more extensive debate spanning almost the entire history of western philosophy since the time of Aristotle. Despite the longevity of such debates, nothing like a basic consensus has emerged among moral, legal, and political philosophers on the most fundamental questions of social justice. Certainly, it is beyond the scope of the current paper to add to this already extensive literature by arguing for our own principled conception of social justice. Our intention is, instead, to sketch briefly some basic considerations and abstract criteria for what we believe any reasonable attempt to draw macro-level limits to the health care system must take into account. This will yield a fairly well delineated model of health, disease, and treatment that we consider preferable to others as a basic orientation for a system of public health.

[175] There is a vast literature on this topic. For a "naturalist" ("realist", "descriptivist") account see the seminal papers of Boorse (1975; 1977; 1997); for a "normativist" ("value laden") account Khushf (1997); Stempsey (2000); Fulford (2001); finally for a differentiating and mediatory account Hofmann (2001); illuminating collections of essays are Caplan et al. (1981) and Humber and Almeder (1997).

[176] For instance, a doctor confronted with a patient suffering from some unclear – perhaps organic, perhaps "only" psychogenic or even hypochondriac – cause will probably try to help and, thus, consider the patient's state "diseased", no matter what turns out to be its real cause. For the psychogenic or hypochondriac case, this might be viewed differently by, say, a legislator trying to delineate what is to be part of proper medicine and, therefore, to be covered by social security. Similarly, it might be seen differently again from a judicial court deciding on that question. Nevertheless, all three are dealing with the concept of disease. (And probably none of them would claim that what the other two have to say about this concept was simply mistaken.)

6.3.4 Deriving a Normative Standard for the Distribution of Healthcare Services

Health is not an ordinary good among others. Instead, it is, philosophically speaking, a "transcendental" good[177]: It has, in a very fundamental sense, an enabling function. This means, it is a precondition for practically any individual life plan based on whatever personal preferences someone may have. It is a universalisable human interest.[178] This enabling, quasi-transcendental function – together with the plain empirical fact that nobody can reasonably expect to be spared every disease throughout his or her entire lifetime – makes medical services one of the "primary" (or "basic") goods of a society, and a genuine object of distributive justice.[179] To be sure, health is a "primary good" in an even more encompassing sense. It is an enabling condition not only for social life, but also for almost any imaginable "natural" life too. Thus, it must be considered a "natural primary good" as well. As a social primary good, however, it remains a pivotal object of justice. Hence, a society unable or unwilling to organise a (largely) egalitarian provision of basic medical care – according to whatever standards – lacks a fundamental feature of a well-ordered community.

Understanding publicly organised medical services as a primary social good in that sense subordinates them to limiting criteria that must, in the first instance, be *objective* in kind. Genuine matters of distributive social justice cannot plausibly be conceived of as matters of subjective personal preferences. The general public, being not only the recipient but also the financier of costly medical services, has a right to the development and application of criteria which organise the distribution of those services according to objective and general standards of human need, not along the lines of individual preferences and desires. For the latter are in principle not suited to establish criteria of social justice (Kersting 2002:149). With regard to the philosophical debate over the adequate concept of disease, one may formu-

[177] We do not want to imply any aspects of the meaning that are being ascribed to the technical term "transcendental" in metaphysics. We just use the term, somewhat loosely, to point out that health (or significant aspects of it) is one of the most important empirical – not, of course, metaphysical – "preconditions of the possibility" (to employ the Kantian use of "transcendental") of a good life.

[178] Cf. Kersting 2002:144; see also Buchanan et al. 2000:122. This "transcendental character" is nicely illustrated by the old proverb "Health isn't everything, but without health everything is nothing."

[179] To be more precise, it is actually the legally founded and, if necessary, enforceable *claims* to basic medical care (rather than the practical services provided by doctors) that are the primary goods to be distributed justly. The concept of a primary social good is, of course, one of the well-known fundamental concepts in John Rawls' "A Theory of Justice" (cf. Rawls 1971:§§ 11, 15, 67; see also Rawls 1993:II. 5. §§ 3, 4), even though Rawls himself does not include public health services in his list of primary goods. This omission can be (and has been) criticized for various reasons, even from a Rawlsian standpoint: see for instance Daniels' "extension" to Rawls' theory (Daniels 1996:191); for an (only partly convincing) explanation of Rawls' omission see Pogge (1994:68).

late the following as its first premise: Only a concept of disease that is modeled on objective standards (of whatever kind) can plausibly serve as the primary criterion for a distribution of health services based on principles of justice. This function cannot be fulfilled by subjective definitions of well-being and of disease, nor by immediate demands on public health services not tied to disease at all, but grounded only in subjective needs and personal desires for certain medical benefits.

6.3.4.1 Three Basic Accounts of the Scope of Health Care, and the One to be Preferred

The question, of course, is how and from what basis to derive these objective standards that dictate the tasks and the limits of a social health care system. Precisely what is it that should be distributed fairly by a health care system? Roughly following a conception developed by *Norman Daniels*, we distinguish three basic models one could refer to in trying to answer these questions:[180]

- *disease-based accounts*, where "disease" is understood in terms of human *normal functioning* – or rather, in terms of aberrations from it – which are assessed in purely medical or biological terms.
- *capability based accounts*, that is, accounts based on constraints of personal capabilities not chosen by the respective individual;
- *welfare based accounts*, that is, accounts based on (unchosen) constraints of the personal potential for happiness, or of subjective capabilities for pursuing individual life plans. These constraints could be delineated in two ways: first, in terms of impediments of personal choices; second, in terms of a failure to meet some normative criteria, based on a social consensus about the necessities of individual welfare. According to this latter kind of reasoning, the concept of personal welfare and of disease-like deviations from it is not a matter to be decided by any naturalistic or subjective-individualistic criteria, but by social conventions or, as some would have it, by social construction alone.

The second and the third demarcation strategies listed above obviously widen the semantic scope of "treatment/prevention"[181] – as opposed to "enhancement" – beyond a strict disease-based limit. Therefore, they also possibly extend the normative scope of this distinction, i.e. the realm of what is *prima facie* morally obligatory for a society to provide at the macro-level of public health. Perhaps it is not only necessary to "fight disease" in the strict sense, but also to "fight" other unchosen constraints beyond the realm

---

[180] Daniels (1996:232) with J. E. Sabin. This does not mean that we endorse Daniels' contention that the objective concept of disease can also be developed in purely naturalistic (i.e. non-normative) terms.

[181] For the purpose of clarifying our conceptual distinctions, we will henceforth, employ only the term "treatment". Just keep in mind that in the normative perspective "prevention" is closely affiliated with it.

of health that keep physical and mental capabilities below a certain level. It could also be extended to include even unchosen constraints on physical or mental potential for happiness. This widening of the scope of "treatment" relies on tacit normative assumptions. Whatever reasons could be given for such a widening, they could hardly be of a purely descriptive, but must obviously be of an essentially normative character. We *should*, the message seems to be, include practices aimed at fighting any unchosen physical or mental restraint on the pursuit of a satisfying individual life.

However, this is far from convincing. In the light of the above considerations on health care services as a primary social good and a pivotal subject of distributive justice it is clear that welfare-based accounts of disease, at the very least, cannot plausibly be based on principles of justice as this would mean health care services cease to be considered matters of distributive justice, but begin, instead, to be treated as a welfare issue. And this is not what health care services in a liberal society should become. If they did, the distinction between treatment and enhancement would lose its descriptive as well as its *prima facie* normative significance and the lines between them would be blurred. There are no good ethical reasons to widen the scope of social justice beyond the boundaries of universalisable, "transcendental" human interests into the sphere of personal, subjective preferences. On the contrary, the maximisation of health care claims by equating them in principle with personal preferences would, given the potential boundlessness of those preferences and the steady development of new medical processes, absorb a growing amount of resources that are presently devoted to other social purposes. Such a tendency of monopolising resources in the health care system is neither ethical nor just, and, in liberal societies, hardly acceptable (cf. Engelhardt 1996:376–402; Beauchamp and Childress 2001:239–250). This is true even if one considers the compensation of undeserved individual disadvantages resulting from the "natural lottery" of physical and psychic traits in principle a matter of justice. For this holds only to the extent that those disadvantages impair the most basic "enabling" conditions of human existence. Above and beyond those fundamentals, the compensation of natural inequalities should not be subjected to the principles and institutions of distributive justice, even though they may produce gravely differing chances of fulfillment in life. With regard to these "normal," natural inequalities, a society has no moral obligation to take responsibility for compensation.[182]

[182] This is, as one might expect, a strongly contested thesis. However, it clearly seems to be prevalent in the international debate on social justice and health care. For a rather different position, based on "individual well-being as the fundamental value", cf. Segev (2005:231–260) (containing numerous further references); also critical of the "normal-functioning approach", from a different point of view, Stark (2006:31–84). We cannot evaluate even the major arguments that figure prominently in this principled debate about justice. We content ourselves with the stating of our own – and the internationally prevalent – position.

Most of the above also holds true for our second type accounts: those based on personal capabilities where "capability" is not understood in the sketched ("transcendental") sense of universalisability, but in terms of means for subjectively defined ends. If, on the other hand, one understands "capabilities" in the sense of basic physical and psychic functions that belong to the enabling preconditions of any conceivable human life-plan, then it is plausible to regard any deviation from such basic functions as a disease, thus subsuming the remaining "capability-based accounts" under the heading of "disease-based accounts".

What this leaves us with is only the disease-based accounts as a well-founded, basic model for a just distribution of health care services.[183] It undertakes to distinguish measures of treatment from strategies of enhancement with regard to the problems to which they respond. These problems are defined as deviations in pure medical and/or biological terms, considering simply the factual state of one's body and one's mind. This corresponds roughly to one of the primary tasks of the liberal state with regard to the protection of constitutional rights. In Germany the respective basic right is Art. 2, § 2, 1 of the Constitution ("Grundgesetz"), which states: "Everybody has the right to life and physical integrity." There is a practically undisputed consensus among constitutional lawyers that this right not only contains a negative (defensive) dimension, granting protection against killing or physical harm perpetrated or sponsored by the state itself.[184] Rather, it also grants the citizen a positive claim on the state to take protective measures to ensure "life and limb" against attacks by fellow citizens and, within specific limits, against "attacks" (i.e. dangers or potential harms) of natural origin. "Life and physical integrity" – nothing beyond that![185] This strongly suggests that only the protection of those "transcendental" enabling physical conditions which are of universal interest to every human being, and consequently only the respective health care services, are covered by the protective force of constitutional law (cf. Gethmann et al. 2005:146–158). To be sure, this conception

[183] Of course, the entire scope of problems of health care allocation encompasses a lot more than we have touched upon here. Following Norman Daniels, one might distinguish between five basic questions that, to a varying degree, concern or involve health care allocation decisions: (1) >What kind of health care services will exist in a society? (2) >Who will receive them and on what basis? (3) >Who will deliver them? (4) >How will the burden of financing them be distributed? (5) >How will the power and control of these services be distributed? (cf. Daniels 1985:2). We have only elaborated on matters of topic (2) and on a few aspects of topic (4). The discussion of the other topics is of no particular importance to our purposes here.

[184] However, there is the obvious exception of law-enforcement rights and of principled emergency rights (such as self-defense or necessity).

[185] In our present context we are, of course, only concerned with the protection of body-related claims, i.e. only with the possible objectives of the services of medicine and not with the numerous other constitutional rights which citizens in liberal democracies usually have.

includes the possibility of a few additional minor constraints on citizens' rights to medical services: not all negative deviations from the regular standard of normal health may give rise to claims to treatment. Sometimes the burden of a physical malfunction may fall below a threshold of significance where it no longer creates a plausible normative demand on the financial solidarity of others.

What this conception definitely excludes from the realm of constitutional obligations of a state towards its citizens is the protection of any particular precondition for a purely subjective life-plan or a demand for personal fulfillment. This does not, of course, rule out the legitimacy of ordinary legal provisions widening the scope of individual claims to medical treatments beyond the line just sketched, if this stays in accordance with the financial and economic capabilities of a society. Still, there is no such thing as a duty of a state to legally provide for it, even if that state could financially afford the said expansion of health care. In other liberal democracies, the constitutional situation is certainly not profoundly different from that of Germany.

Note that all of this does not provide us with a mechanism to answer any concrete question as to what specific services must or should be included in a disease-based account of macro-level health care services. That, of course, depends on a whole range of historical, political, legal, cultural, and economical (and possibly other) preconditions that may vary considerably from state to state and from society to society. What our basic model does provide is the conceptual framework within which such concrete questions should be located, and in which answers to these questions should be sought. Stated briefly, it's only "disease" that entitles one to medical services. However, what counts as "disease" is left open by this observation.

Norman Daniels suggests that disease ought to be defined by the (allegedly) naturalistic criterion of "normality", i.e. the "species-typical functioning" of physical and/or mental human systems, features, and qualities (Daniels 1996:185; 242). That is in principle a plausible conception. However, contrary to what Daniels seems to claim, this criterion does not entail purely descriptive or naturalistic (biological) features. It contains an unavoidably normative element. More precisely, the clarification of its meaning relies on normative criteria in at least two respects. First, what is to count as "species-typical normality" is not merely a biological matter. In the last instance, it depends to a considerable extent on *decisions* that each society must take for itself. Such collective decisions are taken by the relevant institutions of a society, mainly social policy networks, legislatures, and the judiciary, but also other competent bodies that influence the complex process of decision-making.[186] Decisions are, of

[186] In the German legislature, for instance, "illness" or "disease" is the one and only legal prerequisite for an entitlement to the coverage of medical services by the health-insurance system of social security (§ 27 SGB ["Sozialgesetzbuch", i.e. Social Security Act] V). There is a huge and illustrative body of judicial decisions developing, elucidating and limiting the extension of this concept.

course, always interspersed with normative elements. Second, it is quite obvious that not all aberrations from a measure of species-typical functioning can be subsumed under the concept of "disease". To be considered such they must be, in some sense, aberrations "for the worse". After all, people like Shakespeare, Mozart, Kant, and other unusually outstanding geniuses certainly exemplify quite significant deviations from the species-typical functioning in the respective areas of their intellectual or artistic achievements.[187] However, what is to be considered a deviation "for the worse" is not always immediately obvious. In some cases it presupposes a decision and such decisions are governed by the normative criteria of what counts as a positive ("good") development of human functions, and what does not.

So, in this sense, we adhere to a normative, not a purely – or even primarily – descriptive (naturalistic) concept of a disease insofar as we take into account, and integrate into that concept, the unavoidable elements of collective decisions.[188] However, the term "normative" does not mean, nor even entails, a notion of "subjective". On the contrary, it excludes pure subjectivity as a defining force, since valid norms are just as objective as physical facts.

After this primary conceptual clarification we retain the plausible, descriptive and *prima facie* normative force of our initial distinction between treatment and enhancement. On the macro-level of medicine as a social system it identifies the distinguishing characteristics of a decent and just health care system, thus allowing us to differentiate between those services that this system is obliged to provide for its citizens, and those which it is not.

6.3.4.2 Limits of the Abstract Standard: "Hard Cases" and the Question of Individual Justice

However, this does not settle all of the problems with the treatment/enhancement distinction even on the macro-level of public health. The first difficulty may arise when it comes to what could be called "coupled phenomena", i.e. certain physical or mental features which by no means resemble a disease but may cause effects that certainly do. Then, in trying to treat or prevent the latter one must try to alter the former trait. To take some vivid examples: If having a specific physical feature – such as black skin, or a short stature, or a hooked nose, or a disposition to obesity, or to shyness, or something similar – is coupled (at least statistically) with significant disadvantages in a society, then having one of these features might predispose its possessor to psychological problems, such as depression, that we do in fact con-

[187] These positive deviations appear to be primarily (or even exclusively) mental in kind. But considering the speed of development of today's neurosciences, it is not too far fetched to ask how long it might take until we learn to what extent these deviations in talent were also deviations in brain functioning from the species-typical standard.

[188] For the ongoing debate between "naturalists" and "normativists" in the struggle over an adequate concept of disease cf. n. 175 above.

sider psychic disorders or even diseases. In this case, preventing or treating the psychological disease would mean altering a healthy physical trait, thus crossing our boundary between treatments and enhancements detailed above.

This may not be a difficult problem, as long as we have the informed consent of the person involved. What is important, one might say, is not the immediate target of the medical intervention, but, rather, its final goal. If that is a disease, then nothing stands in the way of intervening with some physical or mental feature which, in itself, does not exhibit the symptoms of the disease, but which causes them.

However, it is not at all clear whether we should consider all of the above mentioned potential interventions to be enhancements, let alone cures. In fact, such interventions can potentially be either, viz. in terms of the relationship to certain societal norms which may denigrate certain features such as those mentioned above, thus making the bearer of such a feature in some way socially disadvantaged. However, we would label such societal norms as prejudices, and we would not want to endorse them by establishing medical services which, in a certain sense, comply with those norms. That raises the problem of medicine's complicity with undesirable social norms. For complying with those is exactly the symbolic meaning such a medical intervention would exhibit. Take, for illustrative purposes, the example of genetically modifying one's skin colour, or rather the future skin colour of an embryo *in vitro*. Such a measure might well become possible in the foreseeable future. If one did that for the sole reason that in one's society one's natural skin colour is bound to convey significant disadvantages, then one is tacitly endorsing a set of unpalatable, racist social norms. Such consequences should not, of course, be part of proper medical practice.

On the other hand, given the social norms as they are, the impending threat of harmful psychological consequences, like depression, might be very real and thus presenting a solid case for medical prevention or treatment. As far as justice is concerned, it is quite unclear whether (or to what extent) we can legitimately burden an individual with the cost of fighting social prejudices by not acknowledging her very real, individual problem as one that should be treated. Of course, the same ambiguity holds the other way around. To what extent (if at all) are we entitled to help individuals whilst at the same time reinforcing an undesirable social situation which is the very cause of them demanding that help and may lead to many others facing similar individual difficulties in the future.

Still, one may deny that this is a real problem. Interventions that raise the question of complicity with dubious social norms, one can argue, are still a rather long way from becoming reality due to the current rate of progress in scientific discovery.[189] That aside, altering healthy physical or mental features

[189] Even though we are in fact not convinced at all that this is so.

in order to fight a disease caused by one of them and surfacing elsewhere in the respective human organism is simply and only a matter of the personal freedom of the (informed and consenting) individual.

But things are not always as clear cut as in the case of reshaping one's nose. Take the newly debated phenomenon of "amputees by choice": the so-called "body integrity identity disorder" (BIID), a rather unusual but nevertheless by no means extremely rare mental (and neurological) disposition urging those who have it to demand amputations of healthy limbs, or interventions like the severing of the spinal cord because they desire to be paraplegic (cf. Bayne and Levy 2005). Quite a few of these people face serious problems of depression, sometimes grave risks of suicide, if their request is constantly denied. Should this type of an amputation be considered treatment (or prevention) of a mental disease?[190] That would certainly strain our normal conception of treatment. Should it be called an enhancement (of mental features and qualities)? This, too, would somewhat strain the respective concept. The answer is not at all clear. Nor is it clear whether, in cases of serious risk of suicide, such an amputation should be included into the realm of proper medicine or not: as an intervention into the *psyche* through a surgical intervening into the body.

In the not so distant future, highly efficient strategies to correct severe deficits of psycho-social capabilities by intervening into the neural texture of the brain will probably be available. If such deficits, for instance an uncontrollable and reckless aggressiveness, are, by acknowledged diagnostic criteria, identifiable as manifest sociopathies, they might be integrated into the sphere of diseases, thus becoming legitimate objects for treatment. With respect to our "normal functioning" model of disease, that raises the question of whether or not there are criteria of a species-typical normality of such character traits as aggressiveness, in terms of positively compensating opposite traits (such as moral sensitivity, empathy and the like). This seems doubtful. It is difficult to see how the concept of a species-typical normality could be applied to human traits that are, in principle, of a limitless range. Take "moral sensitivity" as one example. Intellectual capacity (which might be significantly enhanceable in the foreseeable future) is another. Or take artistic talent or the ability to exhibit a socially graceful attitude in communicating with other people. It is hard to see what a theoretical account of species-typical functioning with respect to these "psycho-social" or intellectual capacities would look like.

But even if we managed to come to an agreement about where to draw the lower and upper limits of normality in such capacities, the species-typical-functions account would still face problems of justice: the exclusion of

[190] Bayne and Levy (2005) report two such amputations in 1997 by a Scottish surgeon named Robert Smith. The amputees' personal (psychic) lives are reported to have significantly improved after the operations.

some individuals from beneficial medical services on grounds that may become dubious in certain individual cases. Manifestations of undesired traits in a person can be the results of some species-typical malfunctioning (medically speaking), but such behaviour can also have other causes not plausibly characterised as functional deficits. Norman Fost and David Allen, more than ten years ago, came up with the following widely discussed example:

> Johnny is a short eleven-year old boy with a documented growth hormone deficiency resulting from a brain tumor. His parents are of average height. His predicted adult height without growth hormone treatment is approximately 160 cm (5 feet 3 inches). Billy is a short eleven-year-old boy with normal growth hormone-secretion [...]. However, his parents are extremely short, and (without additional growth hormone treatment) he has a predicted adult height of 160 cm. (Allen and Fost 1990:16)

Obviously it would not be easy to justify, why the undesired outcome in adult height for Johnny should be medically treated because it is the result of a deficiency in species-typical organic function, while treatment for Billy should not be granted because his condition cannot properly be labeled as malfunctioning of a species-typical physical capacity. On the contrary, seen from the individual's perspective, these criteria of line-drawing seem arbitrary and, therefore, unjust. Why should we, one might ask, be more concerned with the physiological cause of a particular condition than with the individual suffering originating from that condition?

It is not difficult to come up with examples in the field of psychic capacities. If, for instance, a boy is unable to concentrate in school for some disorder affecting the metabolism in his brain, then, on the species-typical account, we would have to acknowledge this as a malfunction deserving of medical treatment. But we would probably have to deny such acknowledgement if the same kind of inability to concentrate had its origin in certain omissions of early childhood education which the parents of the boy may be guilty of.

Two obviously real cases of that type are cited by Buchanan et al.:

> (1) An adult patient with a history of bipolar disorder had been stabilized on lithium for some years. He remained shy, however, and was referred to an out-of-plan group therapy situation, from which he clearly benefited over a period of several years. In its original benefit structure, this long-term treatment could not have been covered by HCHP (Harvard Community Health Plan, a health maintenance organization serving over 550,000 people in New England). HCHP revised its benefit structure, allowing an 'extended benefit' that would cover protracted therapy of this sort, without extensive copayments, provided the treatment was for a serious condition. But does treatment for shyness count as treatment of a serious disorder? The psychiatrist managing the Shy Bipolar's case believed that the shyness was the result of the onset of the bipolar disorder; had the disorder not interfered with the adolescent development of this man, who was normally outgoing before its onset, he would probably have been more outgoing. Consequently, the therapist reasoned, the 'extended benefit' should be given. Had the shyness not been 'diagnosed' as the result of the bipolar disorder, then even if it were comparably serious, there would have been no eligibility for an extended benefit.

(2) An intelligent, professionally successful, married father of two children sought treatment because of severe unhappiness associated with marital distress. His wife suffered from a serious mental illness that made her very difficult to live with. The 'Unhappy Husband' was committed to maintaining the marriage. A V code diagnosis ['Conditions not attributable to a mental disorder that are a focus of treatment' (DSM IIIR:359)] (marital problem) was made. In 26 sessions of psychotherapy the man was able to clarify some of the pertinent dynamic issues in his marriage, and developed a number of adaptive strategies for lessening his distress. The 26 sessions were highly productive. Unhappy Husband wished that his treatment would be covered by insurance, but he agreed that he was not suffering from an illness and that it was fair to expect him to pay. (Buchanan et al. 2000:111; cf. the further cases in Daniels 1996:237–241).

Whether or not it was really fair to expect that of the Unhappy Husband is not clear. True, the psychotherapeutic sessions he had should not, at first glance, be termed "treatment", at least not if the label is to be reserved, as we suggested it should be, for attempts to cure illnesses or disorders defined as deviations from species-typical functioning. Rather, what the man showed was a very normal (species-typical) mental reaction to stressful circumstances in his life, which he was unable to escape. So what was done with him looks more like an enhancement of his mental strength that enabled him to cope with those circumstances, and thus improved his well-being. However, seen from another possible perspective – the view that the common goal of medicine is the alleviation of suffering which results from certain physical or mental states – the exclusion of the "Unhappy Husband" from the basic, macro-level package of medical care seems arbitrary.

"Hard cases" like these certainly raise questions of justice. What they demonstrate is that even for the problem of demarcating the sphere of proper medicine the treatment/enhancement distinction is, to some extent, imprecise, and, therefore, of only limited worth. But that does not mean that it is of no worth at all. For beyond the appearance of arbitrariness in some individual cases, there are the general demands of distributive social justice that our distinction is supposed to meet and is apt to fulfill. The treatment/enhancement distinction is, primarily, an essential conceptual scheme under whose main categories we subsume the answers to the questions of what belongs to the realm of proper medicine and what does not. In addition, on the factual or material level it is a useful tool to begin the deliberations about what concrete services should be part of the basic package of care within that realm. However, we must be aware of its limited *normative* capacity: i.e. its capacity to draw a line between what is morally obligatory and what is not.

The distinction is a value laden tool, as is the concept of disease upon which it rests. We should not, therefore, misinterpret it as a criterion that could be established exclusively on empirical grounds and then deliver solutions to all problems of individual justice that might occur by simply applying scientific (bio- or physiological) means. Materially it cannot be used as an automatic and by itself decisive criterion for those problems of justice in specific individual cases. Rather, it opens an entrance to further debate in hard cases such as those detailed above. To a large extent, however, it is left to the individual decision making process within a given society to decide on which criteria these cases are to be identified in the first place, and according to which principles they should subsequently be resolved.

The important point about this process is that the democratic institutions, which have the competence to resolve these questions, have great deal of autonomy and a wide range of options open to them in developing their respective solutions. On the abstract level of legal norms, this refers primarily to the public policy process and to legislature and, on the concrete level of clarifying specific individual cases, to the judicature. Of course, the actual process of finding or drawing a line between normality and pathology in concrete cases and for concrete diseases is often significantly more complicated than is expounded by this description. This has to do with the fact that the treatment/enhancement dichotomy we have used so far is somewhat of an idealised abstraction. Both these concepts denote broad classes of activities, which might, in concrete cases, fall under the category of either treatment or enhancement to varying degrees. Thus, there will be certain cases which involve both treatment and enhancement of the individual in question. So rather than being a clear-cut distinction, the above dichotomy marks the conceptual endpoints of a wide continuum. Of course, there are plenty of clear-cut examples of treatment as well as of enhancements that we could cite. However, in between there is an unlimited range of activities that only partially fulfill the criteria of treatment or enhancement or may occupy a grey area in between. This general ambiguity could not possibly be handled by legislators and lawyers alone. So besides the legislature and the judiciary, there are other institutions involved as well that have a specific say in the process of defining these types of intervention and in drawing lines of demarcation between them. In particular, medical associations and physicians' organisations often develop guidelines for diagnostic criteria for particularly difficult or ambiguous cases. Similarly, the scientific medical community in general constantly contributes to the process of developing and sharpening such criteria. Finally, individual clinical practitioners are directly involved in deciding whether to treat a particular condition or not. And in so doing, the individual physician remains under the potential control of legal courts in reviewing his or her decision. All of these institutions and persons exert their own discretionary power within certain limits that are established and shaped by legal norms, in a complex process of defining treatment or prevention, on the one hand, from enhancement on the other.

Whatever the solutions adopted in individual cases might be, they will inevitably and legitimately be influenced by cultural, historical and, above all, economic factors. Of course, now and then this is bound to lead to individual decisions that will appear hopelessly arbitrary. (The growth-deficiency case of Johnny and Billy described above is an example.) But this is an unavoidable consequence of the discretionary power which is in an essential element of democratic structures. What may seem arbitrary in the individual case is nevertheless jusitifiable under the abstract limits to individual claims on health-services that are legitimately set up by the respective democratic processes and authorities. Whether, and to what extent, society or legislation should entrust the individual physician with certain discretionary powers to deviate, in exceptional cases, from the regular treatment/enhancement scheme and consider a medical service "treatment," even though it would not be accepted as such on the macro-level of public health, is another matter. It might be handled differently by different societies. In general, the scrutiny and perhaps revision of such individual deviations will remain the task of competent legal courts.[191]

6.4 Problems of the Treatment/Enhancement Distinction for an Ethic of Self-disposition (viz. Self-improvement)

Instead of "self-disposition" or "self-improvement", the object of our following inquiry might even, and more poignantly, be labeled "self-creation." The latter term was introduced by Jonathan Glover almost twenty years ago for similar purposes as characterise the present context and to illustrate the core conception of a particular way of dealing with one's own embodied self. Its meaning Glover defined as "consciously shaping our own characteristics" (Glover 1988:131[192]). If we relate that more specifically to mental capacities, the term graphically captures an important idea behind, and a primary feature of, such a way of self-enhancement. The idea that somebody might deliberately assume responsibility for a development of her own character going far beyond what "nature and nurture" have endowed her with. So we will keep the term, as it were, within conceptual and normative reach.

---

[191] A recent decision by the German Constitutional Court (Dec. 6th 2006) may illustrate this point. It ruled that a patient dying from an incurable illness, with no more recognised treatment options available, had a claim to a treatment of last resort that he strongly believed in and thus profited from mentally, even though it was deemed futile and useless by established medical standards. Social security, the court says, must provide financial funds even for treatments of that type of last resort with only psychological, but no physiological, effects, if there was no alternative offered by conventional medicine. The decision was criticised and rejected by the majority of commentators on grounds that its guiding principle could not be generalised, for it would be impossible to finance such a generous extension of the scope of proper medicine as a social system (cf. Francke and Hart 2006).

[192] The general notion of a person "creating" or "choosing" his or her own character is, of course, much older in the philosophical literature; cf. Aristotle, Nicomachean Ethics, Book III, Para. 7.

First of all, however, we need to draw another basic and fairly obvious distinction with regard to possible normative problems of an individual self-enhancement. This distinction is between:

- problems of enhancing *one's own physical or psychic traits,* and the
- problems of *enhancing such traits in others.*

The second point relates mainly, but not exclusively, to persons or human beings who are not in a position to give informed consent to medical procedures. This distinction obviously bears considerable normative weight. We will try to identify and deal with the major moral and legal problems in both areas.

A further clarification and specification appears to be useful. Conceptually, as well as normatively, it does not seem quite accurate to discuss the problems of enhancing somebody else's psychic features under the heading of "self-improvement" (or "self-creation"). Certainly, such interventions raise questions of enhancing a human "self". However, it is not the enhancer's *own* self. This fact causes difficult problems of its own. Consequently, we will deal with the issues arising from this constellation separately (see Section 6.4.2, infra).

6.4.1 Enhancing One's Own Traits: Preliminary Remarks and Basic Distinctions

1. The questions surfacing here appear right from the outset to be more difficult than those of the treatment-enhancement distinction discussed in the preceding sections. For, in this instance, the competence of the legislature and other democratic institutions to distinguish "robustly" along broad criteria, insensitive to particularities of individual cases, is not in place. Here, we are dealing not with a just allocation of scarce resources in a society, but with the moral, and perhaps legal, limits of self-disposition in individual cases. The normative questions, therefore, need to be clarified from top to bottom. They cannot be decided under criteria of distributive justice as the problems they raise do not belong to that domain.

To begin with, however, we want to continue to adhere to the treatment-enhancement distinction as a useful analytical tool that can again offer us a *prima facie* normative orientation. It should be noted, though, that beyond this *prima facie* perspective, we do not want to argue that the distinction maps exactly onto the boundary between what is individually permissible and what is not. Nor does it, as we have pointed out, provide the legislature, or other decision-makers in that field, with an exact tool by which to decide which measures (perhaps even certain enhancements) to include in the proper limits of health care, and which measures (perhaps even certain treatments) to exclude from it.

Recalling this premise and its limits, one gets the immediate impression that, for our present analytic purpose, the potential function of our distinction differs from the role it played in our macro-level analysis of medicine as a social system. Above all, this is for the reason that any person of sound mind may, in principle, do to and with herself what she wishes, as long as she does not harm others in so doing, and as long as she knows what she does or what she consents to. Thus, whether such an intervention is to be called treatment or enhancement does not seem to matter very much to the normative question of whether it is permissible. Rather, this question seems, on first inspection, to simply belong to the realm of personal liberty rather than being a matter of particular ethical concern.

2. However, a closer look reveals at least three important restrictions to that (somewhat rash) assumption:

(1) The first restriction is probably best envisaged by employing the Kantian notion of (moral) "duties to oneself" that every rational being is supposed to have (cf. Kant 1907/14 [AA VII]:417–447). Such duties might, if justifiable, ethically exclude the possibility of enhancing one's (healthy) physical or mental traits by massive neurophysiological interventions.[193]

(2) The second restriction concerns the fact that most legal systems put certain constraints on the justification of physical intrusions into, or injuries of, other peoples' bodies, even if those others have given their informed consent. In German law, for instance, § >228 of the Criminal Code, prohibits (and threatens with punishment any person found guilty of) the infliction of physical harm on another person if the injury inflicted amounts to a "grave affront to common ethical convictions and rules," regardless of whether the act was performed with (informed) consent of the other person .[194] Consequently, if a deep neural intervention into another person's brain to enhance his or her mental capabilities (be it by pharmaceutical, surgical, or electro-magnetical means) is to be considered a grave affront against common ethical convictions, it may well be legally forbidden and may even be considered a crime.

(3) The third *caveat*, which must be added, points to the possibility that an intervention, aiming at a substantial alteration of one's own features, which would usually be considered a matter of personal freedom, could very well have undesired social consequences when established as a common social practice and applied on a large scale by millions of people. If that were the case, practices of self-enhancement would possibly transgress the boundaries of the sphere of personal matters and individual freedom. They would raise problems of harm to others or to society as a whole.

Now, for all those three types of factual and/or normative circumstances that impose limits on the personal liberty of self-enhancement, the treatment/enhancement distinction might again prove useful, even indispensable,

[193] One obviously does not have to be a Kantian, or adhere to Kant's philosophy, to acknowledge the possibility of moral duties to oneself. However, to investigate Kant's conception certainly is a useful way to begin the analysis of the problems.

[194] A norm of similar content probably exists in most modern criminal codes.

as an instrument of our normative inquiry. However, now it assumes a role that appears different from the one it played in our macro-level analysis. Still, "enhancement" might again be used as a negative boundary concept. Since the term "enhancement" lacks clarity in many respects, for the purpose of elucidation we ought to look again at its conceptual counterpart, treatment. For whatever is to be labeled "treatment", does not seem to raise any specific normative problems (though it certainly raises conceptual ones). Mass applications of treatment measures of any kind are, of course, part of our everyday normality. Their individual permissibility is, in principle, not in doubt, regardless of whether or not they are counted to the realm of proper medicine and, therefore, covered by health insurance systems or not. New and specific problems, it seems, can only arise out of practices of self-disposition over one's own body or mind, which cannot be considered treatment.

6.4.1.1 Distinguishing Law and Ethics

Our three *caveats* above suggest some further basic distinctions for the following deliberations. Most important of all is the distinction between law and ethics.[195] Both these spheres have numerous important features in common, while at the same time exhibiting just as many, equally important, differences. The field of these questions and the respective scholarly debates are highly complex, and they encompass far more problems than need concern us here. Hence, we will set most of these aside. What is important for our purposes, though, is one very basic functional difference between law and ethics which distinguishes the tasks and goals of legal norms from those of ethical norms. Doctrines of ethics deal primarily with the problem of clarifying and justifying the conditions of "the good deed". In contrast, law in general is destined to regulate and secure the widest scope of individual freedom of action that is compatible with the same freedom of every other person. Briefly and rather crudely put, ethics clarifies the morally good, whereas law protects liberty.[196] It is one of the consequences of this basic functional difference that law and ethics have a lot more norms in common that *prohibit* a certain behaviour (stating so-called negative duties) than they have

[195] We take "ethics", in accordance with the universally prevalent use of the term (but differing from the meaning Jürgen Habermas gives it in his book "The Future of Human Nature" [2001]), to be the doctrine, or rather the various doctrines, of morals. "Morals", on the other hand, is the corpus of rules and principles themselves that govern the right and/or good human acting.

[196] Of course, there is a lot more to be said about the relations and interconnections between law and ethics. This is particularly true with regard to the normative content of the respective principles in both fields. Many, or even most, of those principles are to a large extent alike, equivalent or overlap with each other. That is why some legal philosophers consider the entire realm of law just a special instance of the so-called "general practical (i.e. normative) discourse" (cf. Alexy 1983:261). Whether this is plausible or not is of no relevance to our argument above. For here we are only concerned with the most prominent *functional difference* between law and ethics, not with their *normative overlaps* or *similarities*.

common norms that *require* a certain behaviour (stating positive duties) since intervening into the protected freedom of another person without an accepted justification (i.e. to violate a negative duty) is usually not only legally forbidden, but also morally reprehensible. On the other hand, it is very often morally, but in principle not legally required, to positively assist others.[197] To negligently fail to fulfill such a positive duty may be morally objectionable but normally it does not violate the protected freedom of the person needing that assistance. Thus, it usually does not constitute a violation of his or her legal rights.

These few remarks may suffice to point out the necessity of a clear distinction between law and ethics for the following analysis. Somebody pursuing nothing else but an enhancement of his or her mental capacities usually does not (directly) encroach upon other people's protected liberty. Therefore, the rules of law, *prima facie,* do not seem to apply to such behaviour. Of course, the boundaries of the sphere of possible legal prohibitions may be transgressed if something like a mass phenomenon of individual enhancements begins to produce unwanted consequences for society as a whole (cf. our third *caveat* above). However, a contradiction to certain *moral* principles may even be found in an individual case of such behaviour (cf. our first *caveat* above). A clearer distinction between legal and ethical considerations seems to be in place here than was the case for our previous reflections on the proper limits of medicine as a social system. This should enable us to better understand these normative interrelations and differences.

6.4.1.2 "One-party" and "Two-party" Cases

A further principled distinction is connected with our second *caveat* above. The distinction is between

- an enhancement carried out directly and personally by and on oneself,
- and an enhancement carried out with the help of, or even exclusively by, another person, usually a physician. This might be labeled "mediated enhancement".

[197] This general principle is subject to important exceptions. They are based primarily on three legal (sub)principles: First, on duties of solidarity that are necessary to keep up fundamental social institutions (for instance, duties of parents to assist and positively protect their children); Second, on a legal duty of (minimal) solidarity between all citizens in cases of acute emergency, justified only by their common status as members of one and the same legal community, amounting to a kind of mutual social insurance policy to the advantage of everyone; Third, on a kind of extension of the prohibition of harm into the sphere of positive obligations to rescue or to assist. This holds only for specific cases: If one harms another person without justification, he or she is legally obliged to prevent further harm that could possibly develop from the former. This obligation encompasses any assistance that appears necessary to save the harmed other (provided it is not beyond a (very wide) scope of reasonable proportionality).

For the sake of convenience and brevity, we will henceforth distinguish these two types as the "one-party case" and the "two-party case".[198] This distinction is of particular importance for the law for the following reason. A person may, in principle, avail herself of the help of others for almost any form of dealing with her own goods, including their destruction. As far as that competence refers to material goods (property) alone, there is no legal problem involved and no legitimate cause for the law to intervene. However, when non-material goods, like life and physical integrity, become involved, we are posed with a different and more difficult set of questions. At least as far as one's life is concerned, the above principle does not apply at all. Most legal systems contain a prohibition of what is usually called "killing on demand".[199] As far as bodily integrity is concerned, the aforementioned principle applies only with specific limitations. Therefore, the legal liberty of a person to do as she wishes with her own life and body (one-party case) reaches considerably further than her ability to seek the assistance of others in similar such activities. From the perspective of those others participants, their legal permission to assist her on request (two-party cases) is limited to the same extent. To inflict bodily harm on oneself may in some (perhaps even most) cases be morally objectionable. For the law, however, it is, in principle, of no interest. In particular the criminal law of a liberal constitutional order is not a legitimate tool with which to interfere in such matters.[200] However, as soon as one involves another person in one's self-harming, one assigns the role of a proxy harmer to the other in such an undertaking. This converts the whole process into a *social interaction*. And in that type of event the law, even the criminal law, takes a legitimate interest. Applying this to acts of self-destruction of one's life, may serve to clarify this distinction. Committing, or attempting to commit, suicide is not subject to legal prohibition in most countries with a liberal constitutional order. However, in almost all of those it is illegal to seek the assistance of others for the purpose of having one's life ended "on demand".[201] The normative reason for the prohibition is twofold. On the one hand, the law attempts to protect persons seeking to end their own life against themselves. In so doing, the law presumes a better understanding

198 Following Feinberg (1986:100).

199 This prohibition, like practically any other legal prohibition, is, of course, subject to specific exceptions in exceptionally justifying circumstances, like, for instance, necessity (the circumstances of the better-known exception of self-defence hardly being imaginable in cases of killing on demand).

200 Apart from the limited primary, freedom-protecting function of the criminal law, one of the further reasons for this is the following. Persons that inflict harm on themselves, impose at the same time a kind of natural punishment *(poena naturalis)* on themselves. An additional legal punishment would, therefore, exceed the limits of proportionality, and be unjust.

201 To be sure, that legal threat is not usually aimed at the death-seeking person but at the proxy-killer.

of the individual's own "true" and long-term interests (an attitude usually referred to as "soft paternalism"; cf. Dworkin 1971:120). On the other hand, it is the aim of the law to protect a fundamental social norm: the in-principle prohibition of (at least *actively)* killing others.[202] The latter reason accounts for the fact that in most legal systems the prohibition of killing on demand remains in force even if there are no legitimate grounds for presuming the death-seeking person to be in need of a (soft-paternalistic) protection against herself, viz in cases where her death-wish is based on well-considered and understandable reasons.[203]

Even in cases of a free decision to harm only one's *body,* most legal systems differentiate between one-party cases and two-party cases. For fairly obvious reasons, this distinction cannot be as stringent as that between suicide and killing on demand. Inflicting physical injury on another person with that person's free and informed consent certainly cannot be completely outlawed if the notion of personal autonomy is to be assigned any value at all. In most states, the criminal law prohibits a consent-based injuring of others only if the physical harm involved reaches a certain degree of seriousness and irrevocability that amounts to the level of a "grave affront to common ethical convictions" as signified by the above quoted formula of the German criminal law. In addition, some legal systems extend the threat of punishment to the infliction of physical injuries destined to serve a further illegal purpose, for instance defrauding an insurance company, or cheating in competitive sports through the use of performance enhancing drugs.

For the discussion at hand, this has an obvious significance. If certain types of mental enhancements are considered sufficiently grave and harmful intrusions into the body (i.e. the brain) or are undertaken for the purpose of entering into fraudulent activity, they might still be tolerated by the law if a person performs them herself and. without the assistance of others.[204] However, similar activities may well be legally prohibited if a physician performs them on one of his patients (or customers), even with that person's informed consent.[205]

---

[202] The "in principle", of course, points to the fact that even this fundamental norm is subject to certain exceptions in specific justifying circumstances (like, for example, self-defence).

[203] The possibility of an exceptional justification for euthanasia in cases like these poses a different question, which is notoriously answered differently in different legal systems.

[204] The said fraudulent purposes themselves, of course, remain illegal and punishable on other normative grounds than those protecting *physical* integrity.

[205] It is difficult to formulate a sufficiently selective criterion to distinguish all cases of immediate self-harming from all cases of consent-based harming of others. Still, the typical cases of these two types can be distinguished fairly well and the difficulty of drawing decisive conceptual demarcation lines in difficult individual cases, is, so to speak, the law's daily business. For our present purposes we may ignore this particular difficulty.

This distinction between self-harming and consent-based harming of others has some significance for ethical deliberations too. In this case, however, its role is less pronounced than in law. First, self-performed enhancements that do not concern the law may still be objectionable from a moral point of view. In this instance, the distinction between one-party cases and two-party cases lacks decisive ethical significance. Second, exactly for this reason, any cooperation of another party with the self-harmer (regardless of whether it has grave consequences or not) may well be considered immoral as well. It would be ethically wrong irrespective of law's tolerance in the particular case.

6.4.1.3 Issues of Concern

This should suffice to set the basic conceptual stage for the following investigations. Let us begin with a list of the most important issues at hand. We will engage with the more or less obvious concerns that accompany the prospect of a widespread use of freely available methods of intervention into the CNS for enhancement purposes. We will attempt to clarify the normative foundations, implications, and the limits of those concerns, keeping in mind our preliminary remarks and the several distinctions we have developed above. Those principle concerns referred to above are the following:

- *Safety:* in particular the risk of unforeseeable side effects or harmful long-term consequences. Closely affiliated with this issue is the problem of *informed consent* in circumstances where the possible consequences of an intervention remain uncertain.
- Linked with the informed-consent issue are matters concerning the *autonomy and authenticity* of self-related decisions. Do measures of mental self-enhancements contain a particular risk of impairing or even destroying one's autonomy and one's authentic self by having it altered substantially? Or, presuming the scenario of a widespread use of enhancement techniques, would they go along with a risk of *self-estrangement* of large numbers of people?
- Enhancement as an artificial corruption of and, therefore, a threat to the *true nature of human beings.*
- Enhancement as *corruption of the goals,* i.e. the mental improvements, themselves that are supposed to be achieved by employing enhancement measures, if such measures become a common social practice.
- *Large-scale medicalisation* of heretofore normal variants of human behaviour.
- Problems of *social justice.* If supposedly expensive enhancement-techniques become available only to wealthy people, the effect could be a significant distortion in the rules and premises of fair competition in our societies, leading to far greater differences in the distribution of wealth, social status, and fulfillment in life.

Of course, not all of these matters are of equal normative weight. Furthermore, many of them are intertwined with one another or overlap in various respects. We will keep an "analytic eye" on these interrelations too.

6.4.2 Safety Concerns

6.4.2.1 Side Effects

Effective medical drugs have side effects. At least, such side effects can never be excluded with complete certainty. They may range from mere inconveniences to grave disabilities or even death. This seems to be an almost universally confirmed empirical fact of pharmacology. This is equally true of psychiatric drugs (Stahl 2000; Davis et al. 2002; Barondes 2003:72). These may even produce peculiar risks that drugs designed for the treatment of physical disorders do not feature[206], as any effective intervention into a persons brain, by such a drug, may not only change that person's mental state, but also his or her future behaviour. This may in some, if very rare, cases have grave, unwanted consequences. The phenomenon may occur if and when the drug-metabolising functions of the consumer deviate significantly from those of the average human being (Barondes 2003:132–134). Several years ago, this sort of risk was illustrated by a landmark legal case in the United States. A federal court in Cheyenne (Wyoming) ordered the pharmaceutical company GlaxoSmithKline to pay $ 6.4 million damages to compensate the relatives of a sixty year old man named Donald Schell. After having taken paroxetine (Paxil®), a selective serotonin reuptake inhibitor (SSRI) marketed by the company, Schell had reacted in an unexpected and shocking way. He had been prescribed the drug by his doctor for depression. However, after taking just two of the pills, Schell killed his wife, his daughter, his granddaughter, and finally himself. During the court case in 2001, psychiatric experts confirmed the sufficiently high probability of a causal link between the intake of the drug and those killings. Other SSRIs, not only paroxetine, may lead to similar reactions.[207]

However, extreme and tragic cases like this provide no good reason for complete prohibition of strong psychotropic drugs like paroxetine as a failure to treat severe forms of depression, which in many cases can be effectively alleviated with SSRIs, would create grave risks to the personal and the professional life of a patient. In addition to the risks of self-harm, criminal behaviour towards other persons is a potential side effect of failing to treat depression adequately. Such risks result from the depression itself. Thus, the failure to

[206] It must be emphasised here that the eminent progress of the neurosciences in the last decades has significantly blurred the dividing line between physical and mental disorders. As the latest edition of the American "Diagnostic and Statistical Manual of Mental Disorders" (DSM IV) aptly points out: "A compelling literature documents that there is much 'physical' in 'mental' disorders. [...] The concept of mental disorders, like many other concepts in medicine, lacks a consistent operational definition that covers all situations." (quoted in Barondes 2003:90–91).

[207] The case and the outcome of the litigation in Barondes 2003:135–136.

treat this depression with appropriate psychiatric drugs can substantiate liability for any such behavioural side effects. A general ban on such drugs, therefore, is simply not an acceptable solution for the problem of their side effects.

Many of the new psychiatric drugs produce (on average) significantly fewer undesired side effects than most of the traditional drugs with similar therapeutic functions (Barondes 2003:17–59). This is true for antipsychotics as well as for antidepressants. Unfortunately, this positive development is subject to two important limitations. First, most cases are still characterised by a profound uncertainty about undesired *long-term* consequences. Second, in exceptional cases, like the Schell case in Wyoming, some of the side effects that have been observed are extremely severe for the very reason that efficient psychotropic drugs may always profoundly change behavioural dispositions too. Sometimes such a dispositional change leads to self-destructive behaviour. Recent studies have shown that the antidepressant fluoxetine (Prozac®), also an SSRI, when given to children or adolescents under 18, causes a serious increase in suicidal tendencies in around 2% of the cases. "Taking antidepressants may increase suicidal thoughts and actions in about 1 in 50 people aged 18 years or younger."[208] Adults may also face a greater risk of suicide when treated with the drug.

> Several recent scientific publications report the possibility of an increased risk for suicidal behavior in adults who are being treated with antidepressant medications. > [...] FDA is highlighting that adults being treated with antidepressant medication, particularly those being treated for depression, should be watched closely for worsening of depression and for increased suicidal thinking or behavior.[209]

It is not only *pharmacologic* interventions into the brain that cause risks of unwanted and grave side effects. The newly developed method of deep brain stimulation (DBS), with electrodes being implanted into the thalamus in order to control movement disorders (for instance Parkinson's disease), obsessive compulsive disorders and epilepsy, may produce similar risks (cf. Theodore and Fisher 2004). Finally, it is not only immediate physical or psychic harm that may result from psychotropic interventions. Some of them, if used over extended periods of time, may be connected with a considerable risk of addiction.[210]

The problem of how to deal appropriately with side effects of drugs or other therapeutic means is, of course, a general one in medicine.[211] To cope with such issues, a rich body of medical-ethical rules has been developed.

---

[208] U.S. Food and Drug Administration (FDA) Alert 7/2005. "FDA has approved fluoxetine for treating children who have depression or obsessive-compulsive disorder." (http://www.fda.gov/cder/drug/infopage/paroxetine/default.htm, accessed on 10th January, 2007).

[209] Ibid.

[210] Cf. Foster (2003).

[211] Apart from the said behaviour-specific changes of dispositions that might specifically originate from "mental interventions".

The most important of them are designed to protect research-subjects in the developmental phase and patients in the subsequent application of the respective measures. In most technically advanced states, these rules are also enforced as legal statutes. If they are cautiously observed during the process of development and marketing of a new drug, they produce an important justifying effect for the individual physician who subsequently uses or prescribes them. If he gives such a drug to an informed and consenting patient, he acts within a legitimising framework that jurists aptly label "permissible risk". This means roughly the following. If a new drug passes the manifold procedures of preclinical testing and clinical trials, and is then approved for marketing and use, according to the relevant legal provisions, responsibility for the risks of its possible side effects is taken over by society. An individual physician, therefore, does not neglect her duty of care towards the safety of her patients, even if, in exceptional cases, her prescription of the drug leads to such catastrophic consequences as in the above mentioned case in Wyoming. Those consequences now belong to the accepted, though potentially dangerous, normality of social life (or rather of its medical part). If in rare individual cases, one of these tolerated dangers materialises into an unwanted, serious harm, responsibility is not assigned to the physician. Instead, this harm is treated as a misfortune. Neither under criminal law, nor under civil law, is the physician liable to legal measures for the results of his behaviour.[212] He may have been clearly aware of the risks of such rare side effects, and therefore also the possibility of causing grave harm. However, that did not affect his legal permission to act as he did, provided, of course, that the patient was sufficiently informed about that risk in advance.[213]

---

[212] That does not, of course, mean that the physician had a *permission* to bring about those catastrophic consequences. It means only that she had permission to take certain risks. This leads, as it were, to her being legally "distanced" from the unwanted (and in themselves still prohibited) results of her acting. (Compare the case of a car driver who carefully observes all traffic rules, but still unavoidably kills a child that unforeseeably runs in front of his car. Normatively, no responsibility for the killing is assigned to the driver. However, he certainly had no permission to kill the child. One may, therefore, correctly say that he acted permissibly, and thereby killed someone. One may not say, though, that he had permission to kill someone.)

[213] To complete this statement with a look at the subjective side of such acts under "permissible risk", let us employ a somewhat remote scenario. The permission of the physician to act as described would not be altered if she, at the same time, clandestinely (and perversely) hoped for such a catastrophic outcome, i.e. if she acted with the wicked intention to take the (however minimal) chance to gravely harm someone. Such an intention would certainly prove the physician's character to be despicable. It might also suffice to turn the act itself into a *morally* reprehensible one (this being doubtful and much disputed in ethics). However, it would certainly not in the least effect the legal permissibility of the act. This is for the simple fact that the legality of this act is based on purely objective grounds and, hence, is not alterable by any accompanying subjective attitude or intent of the perpetrator. In short: if the physician is legally allowed to act as she does, she may act with whatever intent she may happen to have.

All of this holds, in principle, for any of the legally approved and licensed medical drugs and products. Thus, the fact that the problem of unwanted side effects surfaces also in the special areas of psychopharmacology or of other interventions into the CNS does not confront us with questions of any specific novelty. Therefore, we do not need to deal in great detail with the normative rules governing the handling of those problems. In addition to the general legal norms already in force, we see no plausible argument for a proposal of new and specific laws in order to control the risks of side effects of psychotropic substances for therapeutic purposes.

6.4.2.2 Informed Consent in Cases of Enhancement

If such psychotropic drugs and measures are not used for treatment, but for enhancement purposes, some important peculiarities arise. In principle, society, and in particular the law, accepts the (statistically calculable) risks of harmful side effects of drugs only in cases where a regulated process of weighing those risks with the demonstrable benefits of the respective drug has yielded the rational conviction that its use is an ethically responsible and, therefore, reasonable practice. To clarify and verify this risk-benefit ratio is what the legally regulated procedures of testing and licensing drugs are designed for. Normally, the benefit side of this calculation derives its particular force exclusively from the value of the respective drug for the treatment of diseases. Only that value accounts for the justified acceptance of even serious risks as generally "permitted".

By far less clear is the question whether the same sort of permission of the risk of side effects tied to certain drugs also applies to their use for the purpose of enhancement. Society as a whole certainly does not take over any risk of side effects that results from behaviour serving only the end of individual pleasures or idiosyncracy. Individuals acting for these purposes must take responsibility for the associated risks exclusively themselves. In such cases, three related forms of individual responsibility may be distinguished. The significant risks resulting from such idiosyncratic acts are:

- either straightforwardly prohibited if they are imposed on non-consenting others;
- or exclusively a matter of the individual actor where he imposes them only on himself (one-party cases);
- or, finally, tolerated within the previously outlined limits of the justifying power of informed consent if they are imposed on somebody else with his or her informed consent and if they will not foreseeably cause severe physical harm to, or a risk of death for, the consenting person as this

would make the respective action a "grave affront to common ethical convictions" (two-party cases).[214]

Mere enhancement uses of drugs obviously belong to the category of personal idiosyncrasies, rather than to the range of generally accepted physical or psychological necessities like treatment of diseases.[215] They have their grounds in specific preferences of the individual. Their utility in a rational risk-benefit calculation has no more weight than any other personal desire. In this respect, it is comparable to non-essential cosmetic surgery.[216] The risk-utility ratio that accounted for the official approval of the drug as a potential means of treatment does not, therefore, encompass its use as an enhancement. Responsibility for the risks of side effects of such an off-label use are not taken over by society. If, in rare cases, they lead to catastrophic consequences, these are not considered a misfortune, but something which the participating individual(s) must in some way take or share responsibility for.

This does not mean that such purely enhancing applications of psychotropic substances are legally prohibited. Neither does it mean that in the risk-benefit ratio there is no considerable counterpart to the risks anymore. For, in this type of case, the benefit at stake is the autonomy of the individual actors, their rights and liberties to self-disposition of their bodies and their behaviour. This certainly bears considerable weight. But the responsibility for harmful consequences must now be taken over by the participating individuals themselves.

How this risk is to be assigned among them, according to the circumstances of the individual case, is shown in our threefold scheme above. In one-party cases it falls exclusively on the self-enhancer.[217] In two-party cases,

[214] In various respects, a special case would be dangerous sports like boxing or motor racing. Even when performed according to the respective rules, they not only endanger the individual performing them but usually others too. Their being permitted, nevertheless, is not only due to the fact that, in societies like ours, they are enjoyed by a great number of people (i.e. they have considerable social utility) but also with the fact that they have usually developed over long periods of time rather than being enacted by any single political decision. They have simply always "been there" as part of our way of life. One must not underestimate the justifying power of such historical developments of social normality.

[215] Recall our remarks on the vague and sometimes blurred line between treatment and enhancement, particularly in the field of psychotherapy. We will return to that problem later.

[216] Hence the label "cosmetic neurology," now widely in use to describe the present and future practice of neuroenhancements (cf. Chatterjee 2004:968).

[217] Without the possibility of having recourse against anybody else. The information about possible risks on the package or insert of a drug does not normally relate to the risks of side effects in enhancement contexts. Usually, those will not be substantially different from potential side effects of treatments. If in rare cases specific side effects of enhancement uses should occur, the drug company is not liable for the related harm – except, of course, when the enhancing use was also suggested on the insert.

it regularly also falls on the enhanced, i.e. the person consenting to the enhancement. However, if the (foreseeable) resulting harm amounts to something like a "grave affront to common ethical convictions", the responsibility switches over to the physician.[218] Acts bearing the foreseeable risk of such consequences are then, of course, prohibited and even punishable. The informed consent only mitigates, but does not abolish punishment. According to present legal standards, this switch of responsibility only occurs if the foreseeable consequences consist in grave (usually irreversible) physical harm. The German Federal Court in criminal law presently demands that it be a concrete threat to the consenting person's life.[219] Dangers below this threshold remain solely a personal matter of the informed and consenting consumer of the drug.

To illustrate this point: If an officially approved drug sometimes produces the side effect of serious suicidal inclinations, and if, in a particular case, this danger materialises in the suicide of a patient, that consequence belongs to the realm of permissible risk. It is not attributed to the physician. Beside the informed consent of the patient, there is a second justification for the physician's acting: a medical indication. The latter is nothing other than the risk-benefit ratio that originally lead to the approval of the drug for therapeutic purposes, applied to a specific individual case.[220] Thus, the indication, together with the consent, lead to the take-over (acceptance) of the suicidal risk by society. However, if the suicide occurred as a side effect of an *enhancement* with exactly the same psychotropic drug, taken in exactly the dose recommended for treatment purposes, the legal consequences change remarkably. If the risk of occasional suicides was known in advance, maybe even listed among the side effects the package insert warned of, the physician may be guilty of negligent, even reckless homicide.[221]

---

[218] This is, as we have pointed out, the limit drawn in German criminal law. However, other legal orders contain comparable limiting criteria for the justifying power of informed consent. We should perhaps add that in German law this switch of responsibility only occurs if the physician *knowingly* brings about the said grave consequences. This exclusion of negligent acts on the physician's side has no good material grounds, but simply results from the wording of § 228 of the Criminal Code.

[219] In specific areas of medicine, the law provides other, usually narrower, limiting criteria for consent-based medical procedures, for instance in so-called "living donations" in transplantation medicine, The reasons for lowering the prohibition threshold of living donations significantly below life-threatening risks are manifold, reaching beyond "soft paternalistic" motives into the sphere of protected public interests. Cf. Merkel (2005).

[220] More precisely, the medical indication as the result of the official risk-benefit ratio of the drug encompasses the weighing principles that in law (and also in most ethical theories) regulate so-called states of necessity and the permitted rescuing behaviour in such a state.

[221] Not so, for materially insufficient reasons, in German law (cf. note 208 above). However, this is the case in other legal orders.

These fundamental principles not only bring forth consequences for a physician's possible liability (civil and criminal), they also aggravate his duties of information to the patient (or, rather, the consumer of a drug). For now the risk is not being taken over by society any longer, but must be shared among the individual participants along the lines we have sketched. If the doctor prescribes a drug solely for enhancement purposes he must inform the patient (consumer) to a considerably larger extent than in treatment contexts about any risk of unwanted side effects if he wants the responsibility for the potential risks involved in taking the drug to remain exclusively with the consumer.[222] Usually, the notion of informed consent is thought of as containing three basic elements and some detailing specifications (cf. Beauchamp and Childress 2001:80):

- *Preconditions* on the side of the consenting party. This has two elements: (1) competence to understand and decide, and (2) freedom of decision.
- *Information elements,* mainly on the side of the medical doctor to (1) disclose material information, (2) to recommend a therapeutic plan, and (3) to ensure the understanding of (1) and (2) by the patient.
- *consent elements,* namely: (1) decisions in favour of a plan, and (2) authorisation of the chosen plan by the consumer of the drug.[223]

In the German civil judicature it has been expressly acknowledged that for *physical* enhancements, namely for merely cosmetic surgery, the physician has considerably extended informational duties, as opposed to cases of treatment. In 1985, the Higher Regional Court ("Oberlandesgericht") in Düsseldorf ruled that a physician, having been urged by a patient to undertake a medically not indicated surgical intervention on the patient's genitals, was liable for damages, even though he had informed the patient of all risks immediately associated with the intervention as would have been sufficient had it been a medically necessary procedure. The patient's desire to have the operation was, as the doctor had realised, grounded in an idiosyncratic motive which during the litigation was classified by psychiatric experts as an "abnormal sexual attitude". The court stated that in cases like this, in which any type of medical necessity is completely lacking, the doctor is not only obligated to inform the patient of the risks directly associated with the surgery, but also to obtain the expertise of a psychologist or a psychiatrist on the risk of *future psychic harms* that might result from the intervention and to inform the patient of that risk as well.[224]

---

[222] Again, only within limits set by the "grave affronts to common ethical convictions" standard. Beyond those limits, even the most extended information and the subsequent free consent do not save him from (perhaps even criminal) liability.

[223] Legal requirements of valid informed consent usually concentrate mainly on the second basic ("information") element in our list, sometimes differentiating along other specifications (cf. for the German Law Lenckner 1989:142), thereby presupposing the "preconditions" of the first element.

[224] Oberlandesgericht Düsseldorf, Neue Juristische Wochenschrift 1985:684.

Similar considerations may play a role in cases of a medically assisted doping in sports.[225] As far as matters of informed consent are concerned, purely enhancing applications of psychotropic drugs also belong to this category. They also meet with considerably enlarged duties of information on the side of the physician.

In the framework sketched above, the treatment-enhancement distinction again plays a decisive normative role. However, in this case, the problem it raises is quite distinct from the one that engaged us in our attempt to delineate the limits of proper medicine on the macro-level.[226] In that case, its function was to render a criterion for defining and limiting the obligation of a society to provide for health care services under the primary aspect of distributive justice. This entails, as we have pointed out, a "robust" discretionary power of the state. Singular cases that may appear to be treated arbitrarily, and thus unfairly, under that criterion do not effect the justification of such generalising demarcation strategies on the macro-level.

Here, though, we are dealing with a quite different matter. First, it concerns the just distribution not of a social good (health care services), but of responsibilities for the risks of grave side effects in individual cases. Second, it involves the attempt to delineate a zone of absolute prohibition of enhancement strategies on grounds of the sheer severity of their impending side effects, the presence of an informed consent by the consumer notwithstanding. For these questions, we cannot formulate our criterion for the distinction of treatment and enhancement in that "robust" generalising manner. In this instance, it serves the function of doing justice to individual cases. Therefore, in each individual case it must be clarified under the respective particular circumstances, whether or not the medical intervention is (still) to be considered treatment or (merely) enhancement. No less in need of clarification is the magnitude of the particular risk of side effects in each individual case. Finally, the question arises whether the impending side effects amount to a "grave affront to common ethical convictions", thus strictly prohibiting "two-party cases" such as the participation of a physician or any other assisting person.

---

[225] German criminal courts tend to judge *all* (two-party) doping cases in sport to be cases of unjustified bodily harm (despite the informed consent) – and, therefore, "grave affronts to common ethical convictions" – on the side of the cooperating medical (or coaching) personnel, because of the fraudulent aims of doping. This court opinion is rejected by some legal scholars on grounds of preferable systematic arguments: There are no good reasons to include punishment for fraudulent motives into the purview, i.e. the protective function, of a norm that prohibits injuring another person's *body*.

[226] Recall that, for normative reasons, all medically reasonable measures of prevention are included into the sphere of treatment. Their concrete reasonableness must be based on a majority consensus in the scientific community. For the arguments for this inclusion, see Section 6.3.2 above.

Another important difference to the treatment-enhancement distinction on the macro-level consists in the fact that, whilst on the macro level a clear-cut line of demarcation needs to, and can, be drawn, in this instance the dividing line between treatment and enhancement is less easily definable. There exists, instead, a sliding scale or continuum of responsibility on which each individual case will be located. This is particularly true for interventions into "the psyche", designed to alter mental states. For here, a clear distinction between treatment and enhancement is even more difficult than for exclusively physical disorders.[227] Take, for instance, the difference between depression (already considered illness) and melancholic states (still considered an aspect of normal human emotions). There are no "hard scientific criteria" for distinguishing the one from the other.

Just as the question "treatment or enhancement" may be a matter of degree, so is the related question of the responsibility for side effects assigned to the actor(s) in either one of these two categories. Similarly, the extent of the physician's duty to inform a patient about potential risks may also vary from case to case, analogous to the aforesaid gradation of his responsibility. The closer an "enhancement" intervention comes to being a form of "treatment", the fewer additional duties a doctor has to inform that patient (or consumer) of even remote potential side effects and risks. Similarly, the converse equally applies: the further away this intervention is from being considered a form of treatment, the greater the doctor's informational duties.

None of these considerations provides us with anything like a formal apparatus or a strict criterion for an exact calculation of the relevant data of each individual case. This is quite obviously impossible for our problems. What our analysis has rendered, instead, is a conceptual framework that specifies important normative distinctions between certain types of intervention. The relevant circumstances of any individual case must be assessed according to that framework, viz subsumed under its concepts. This facilitates the clarification of the necessary distinctions in that individual case. The efficiency of the above framework notwithstanding, any decision of a complex case requires a considerable amount of judgment (in the Kantian sense of the term) on the side of all participating persons. The physician must exercise judgment in prescribing a psychotropic drug. Equally, the consumer must do likewise in taking it and, finally, a court, when ruling on problems of liability and punishment for serious and undesired consequences of the drug in question, must also exercise judgement.

What our analysis of safety concerns has provided us with is a differentiated set of criteria allowing us to determine the boundaries of permissible

[227] The "exclusively" points to the fact that we know today that most (possibly all) psychic diseases have physiological correlates in the brain.

risks, and for the clarification and distribution of responsibility in cases where such a risk materialises. However, it is far from providing any compelling, or even plausible, argument for a general prohibition of neuroenhancements. Such a general prohibition simply would not be justifiable for reasons of safety of the participating individuals alone. The fundamental principle of respect for the autonomy of persons is normatively decisive in this instance. Paternalistic norms that allow this autonomy to be overridden completely, through outright prohibition of a certain type of behaviour, only on grounds of the intent to safeguard the potential actor from the risks of its consequences, have no foundation, even in ethics. In law, they are patently illegitimate. As Joel Feinberg comments:

> Those who have experienced, or can experience hypothetically in their imagination, irksome constraints justified wholly on paternalistic grounds, will testify that their resentment is not mere frustration or antipathy. Rather it has the full flavor of moral indignation and outrage. Their grievance is not simply that they have been unnecessarily inconvenienced or 'irked', but rather that in some way they have been violated, invaded, belittled. (Feinberg 1986:27)

Such an intrusion into one of the most important domains of somebody's legally protected privacy is simply not acceptable. Neither is it justifiable according to moral principles grounded in mutual respect and recognition of the other as an equal. Certainly, though, the protection of individual autonomy in cases of mere enhancement has a price: the increased responsibility for unwanted consequences falling solely on the participants. But the danger of such consequences is, in itself, no sufficient reason to completely ignore or override autonomy concerns.[228]

This leaves us with two open questions. First, what preconditions must a person satisfy to be considered autonomous in cases of enhancement? Second, could seriously harmful side effects possibly impend on others outside the personal sphere of the individuals involved, perhaps on society as a whole? Both of these questions are on our list of basic concerns above. We now turn to the first of them.

6.4.3 Concerns of Autonomy and Authenticity

"Personal autonomy" is a notoriously difficult and complex concept.[229] A first, rough distinction could be drawn between autonomy as sovereignty, i.e. self-government, and autonomy as authenticity, i.e. being true to one's own nature. In addition to that (and following Feinberg 1986:27–51), we propose

[228] A different matter, though, is the question whether the costs for treating pathological side effects resulting from intervention merely for enhancement purposes should be covered by health insurance systems that are publicly financed and thus are based on a legally mandated solidarity. There is no normatively cogent answer to this question, we will return to it later under the heading of "Justice".

[229] We ignore conceptions of autonomy of larger communities, above all of states (i.e. questions of "sovereignty"). Problems of these conceptions do not, for obvious reasons, concern us here.

to distinguish between four levels of its meaning that refer respectively to four different functions of the concept:[230]

- autonomy as a basic capacity;
- autonomy as a set of factual preconditions of self-government;
- autonomy as an ideal;
- autonomy as a right.

Of these categories, "autonomy as an ideal" closely connects with "authenticity", whereas the other three categories are subdivisions of "autonomy as sovereignty". We will begin with the last point: problems concerning autonomy as a legal right with regard to our general theme, the enhancement of psychic capacities. In this context, questions of autonomy, in the juridical sense, are comparatively easy to deal with. Furthermore, in some respects they are closely connected with our reflections on safety concerns given above.

6.4.3.1 Legal Considerations

"Autonomy" as a legal concept exhibits two fundamental characteristics that are of importance for our analysis. First, and diverging from "autonomy" as a psychological concept, it is typically an "all or nothing" concept. This means that, in any specific context, autonomy of a person is, under legal criteria, either completely present or not present at all. However, this does not mean that it could not be restricted to, or reserved for, only specific contexts of life and action. Obviously this is possible, and is, in fact, quite common. One might, for instance, be legally autonomous regarding decisions over one's religious confession, but not autonomous to vote in parliamentary elections. In this case, autonomy must also be assumed either to be completely present or completely absent within that specific context. There is no such thing as a person being "partly or semi-autonomous in the specific context X" (e.g. in matters concerning her religious confession) in the legal sense.

There seems to be at least one exception to the first one of these principles, though. Many or most criminal law codes know the concept of "diminished culpability".[231] If one plausibly considers criminal culpability to be the logical reverse side of a specific form of autonomy, one must acknowledge that there is at least one possibility of a "graded autonomy" in law: that

[230] We are, of course, aware that there are quite a few other ways of conceptualising and disentangling the complex bulk of problems that questions of "autonomy" give rise to. Most of these ways, as suggested in the huge literature on the subject, have their own merits in varying theoretical perspectives and their own shortcomings in others (for a comprehensive overview and bibliograhy see Buss (2002); cf. also the illuminating collection of essays in Christman (1989). For our purposes here, Feinberg's distinctions seem to be a perfect fit.

[231] In German Law it is regulated in § 21 of the Criminal Law Code.

which makes a person responsible for his or her criminal deeds. But still, this is an exception and perhaps the only one in law.[232]

However, as we have already mentioned, this "yes-or-no" principle of legal autonomy does not mean that a person, who is legally autonomous in particular respects, must, necessarily, be autonomous in all other respects too. The question of criminal responsibility, for example, is based on other considerations than the question of whether or not that same person can already engage in valid contracts, consent to medical treatment, or has the right (i.e. the autonomy) to vote. These examples show that the law grants autonomy to persons according to various empirical circumstances and for varying purposes. Criminal culpability is usually linked with a rigid criterion of age.[233] On the other hand, in most liberal legal orders, the autonomy to give informed consent to invasive medical procedures usually depends on the factual (empirical) capability of a person to understand what is involved and which of her personal interests are at stake in the treatment in question.

Therefore, the question of whether or not a person is legally capable to give informed consent to medical measures, i.e. whether she is autonomous in that respect, may find different answers in different treatment situations, depending on the severity of the respective medical intervention and on the ability of the person to sufficiently understand what is at stake. Hence, for example, a fourteen year old girl may well be in the position to give informed consent to an appendectomy or perhaps, within the respective national statutes, to an abortion[234]. She may even be able to give informed consent, were she dying of leukemia, to the withdrawal of life-prolonging measures, even against the wish of her parents.[235] However, presuming she is physically and mentally healthy, she could certainly not validly consent to a surgical intervention destined to sterilise her.

---

[232] It has to do with the following: The "all or nothing" autonomy in civil law mainly serves the purpose of delineating the legal spheres of individual competence, personal liberty and privacy. Therefore, it must be formulated in a robust and clear-cut manner. (In criminal law, the concept of diminished culpability and, similarly, "diminished autonomy", serves the purpose of retributive justice. Therefore, it must be fine-tuned to the real psychic state of an individual perpetrator when committing his or her concrete criminal act.

[233] Most legal orders know at least two forms of *full* (cf. the previous note!) criminal responsibility: that of an adolescent and that of an adult.

[234] The opposite, i.e. legally a valid refusal to undergo an abortion, is, of course, equally possible for a 14 year old. On the bulk of rather complicated questions involved here cf. Merkel (2006:§ >218a, marginal nos. 28–31).

[235] Actually, it is more correct to say that she may be in the position to *refuse* consent to any further life-saving treatment, since it is the invasive treatment that stands in need of an informed consent in the first place, not, primarily, the withdrawal of that treatment. Another difference is that the treatment *may be given* with informed consent (but need not be under all circumstances). The latter, however, *must be omitted or stopped* (under all circumstances) after a valid refusal of consent.

For the question of consent to mental enhancements this is of great significance since, from a medical point of view, such an enhancement is not necessary. The respective intervention into the CNS, whether it is undertaken by pharmacologic or other means, appears to be comparable with the above-mentioned example of the sterilisation on demand. In both cases, there is no medical indication for the procedure to be undertaken. As we have already seen, this does not make the interventions impermissible. It only means that the immediate invasive as well as the subsequent, longer term, side effects fall exclusively on the part of the participating parties. However, in such cases the law can, and usually does, raise the demands on the physician's informational duties and, reflecting those greater demands, the preconditions for the validity of a given consent. For instance, German law requires a range of strict criteria which must be met before a castration operation can be conducted, even on grounds of a clear medico-social indication, such as the patient's being particularly dangerous as a potential sexual offender. Above all, he must be least 25 years of age.[236] In cases of a sterilisation not indicated medically, but solely for contraceptive purposes, the physician is required to give detailed information on the possible psychological consequences of the intervention. He or she must also go to the furthest possible lengths to ensure – if necessary with the help of a psychological or psychiatric expertise – that the patient clearly understands every individual element of this additional information. The elements a physician is required to explain are:

- The method, meaning, extent (gravity), and the immediate risks of the intervention;
- the extent of possible consequences;
- the possible irrevocability of those consequences;
- the meaning and practical importance of such consequences for the patient's life;
- the concrete probability (risk) of those consequences.

These elements may expand the duty of disclosure and information on the side of the physician considerably, as compared with those duties in clear-cut cases of treatment. Moreover, they may also expand the requirements for informed consent on the side of the patient or the consumer. However, if the latter sufficiently understands the meaning and importance of all of those points, she must be considered legally autonomous with regard to her final decision. The law's recognition of this autonomy is an all-or-nothing matter: the patient either has autonomy over her decision or she does not. There can be no middle ground or "partial legal autonomy". A general, paternalistic supervision of an individual's decisions, in cases where those decisions may have potentially harmful effects on the individual her-

[236] Cf. §§ 1–3 GermKastrG (i.e. German Sterilisation Act of 1969).

self, is clearly impermissible.[237] Hence, once consent is given, following the informational process detailed above, the intervention is legally allowed.

All of this holds true for the possibility of an enhancement of mental features as well. A general prohibition of such interventions by restricting the range of a consumer's autonomy would be impermissible under principles of constitutional law. Certainly, enhancements are normally only sought for certain, specific (mental or physical) characteristics; often only one single characteristic is targeted. On the other hand, the effects of the intervention procedure may be disadvantageous or even seriously harmful with regard to other of the individual's features. However, such trade-off calculations of risks and benefits are, in principle, the sole business of the autonomous person herself. They must not be scrutinised and possibly corrected according to "objective criteria" of reasonableness. As we have pointed out already, possible negative consequences that may reasonably be reckoned with must, however, fall short of constituting a "grave affronts to common ethical convictions". If they do not constitute such an affront, however, they are of no concern for the law. Even if the enhancement in question may lead to a radical change in the enhanced person's character, such a change would not fall within the scope of legal control[238] since, according to traditional legal rules, the said "grave affront" must arise specifically from a *physical* injury. Certainly, the relevant statutes could be adapted by the legislature, so as to include (minimal) neurophysiological changes with psychic consequences of a sufficient magnitude, if these latter consequences were judged gravely objectionable from the point of view of common ethical convictions. However, whether the law should contain such provisions or not, can only be decided after the clarification of the relevant moral concerns (which we will undertake later in this chapter).

Thus, "autonomy" in the legal sense is largely a black-box concept. As long as one remains within its legal limits, which coincide, by and large, with the legal boundaries protecting the liberty (legal autonomy) of others, the law does not take an interest in what is going on inside those limits. Motives, desires, emotions, life-plans, individual value-systems and any other merely subjective states of mind that might accompany legally correct behaviour remain within the sphere of mental privacy, regardless of whether they

---

[237] The state is not even entitled to refuse the recognition of the consequences of such a medical intervention in order, for instance, to create a negative incentive for future interventions of that kind. The German Constitutional Court (Bundesverfassungsgericht) ruled in 1978 that the refusal of the state to officially acknowledge the conversion of gender of a (former) transsexual man is unconstitutional (BVerfGE 49 1979:286).

[238] Unless, of course, if a "new character," of a particularly dangerous kind, were created that way. However, the law's concern would still not be with the "enhancement" itself (if one wants to label this sort of change an "enhancement") but with the – quite ordinary – fact that a new danger to the legal order may have arisen.

appear misguided, erroneous, or even gravely objectionable from a moral point of view.

However, the above does not address the problem of possible harms done to others or to society as a whole through measures of self-enhancements. (We will return to this point later.) Nor does it answer any *ethical* questions concerning autonomy that might be raised by such enhancements. It is to these ethical issues that we now turn.

6.4.3.2 Ethical Considerations and "Duties to Oneself"

In engaging with the issue of imposing moral limits to the reach of personal autonomy, one is immediately presented with the Kantian theory of certain ("imperfect") duties that every reasonable subject has to him- or herself (Kant 1907/14 [AA VI]:417–447).[239] We should point out from the start that duties to oneself cannot, according to Kant, be duties of law. For the law only regulates the scope of individual liberty amongst equal persons in a strictly legal sense. This means that it only deals with the "outer" relations between those persons, not with whatever normative relations a person might have to herself. Furthermore, the law, according to Kant, differs from morality, in that it imposes only "perfect" (i.e. completely determined) or "negative" duties (prohibitions).[240] There is, it should be added, some dispute in the philosophical literature about whether or not the absolute prohibition of suicide that Kant postulates was meant by him to be a *legal* duty to self. This debate has arisen since the prohibition of suicide is also a "perfect" (viz completely determinate) duty, as all legal duties are. However, such an assumption hardly fits into Kant's general conception of law and it is, regardless of what Kant himself thought, quite implausible anyway.

Moral duties to oneself seem, to raise a logical problem right from the outset. The problem arises from the fact that the person who is obliged is identical with the person he or she is obliged to. Or, put somewhat metaphorically, the "creditor" and the "debtor" of a particular duty are one and the same. From a strict normo-logical point of view this is impossible. Nobody can really be obligated to him- or herself.[241] Kant saw this problem and he notoriously tried to solve it by introducing a principal dualism of the

[239] Almost all of those duties are, in Kantian terms, "imperfect" (with the prohibition of suicide and of self-maiming acts as exceptions) because the concrete demands they make on individuals are not completely determinable. This is because the direction in which a person wishes to develop her natural dispositions is exclusively a matter of her own autonomous decision, hence indeterminate.

[240] We do not find this strict confinement of legal duties to negative ones at all convincing. Moreover, it does not coincide with most modern positive legal orders. This whole point obviously lies outside our present analysis though.

[241] To most developed codes of civil law this problem is well-known. Usually it occurs in the law of succession. The typical case is the heir of a deceased person who was the testator's debtor before the latter's death. The debt then immediately lapses by law (or, rather, by the sheer logic of the legal concepts of creditor and debtor).

human person: a division of the mode of existing of persons into a *homo noumenon* and a *homo phaenomenon.* As beings capable of reason and autonomy (i.e. possessing free will), human beings participate in the "essence of reason" ("Vernunftwesen") of all of humankind. Their "nature of reason" obliges them in a particular way. The ground for this duty is, in principle, no different to that which obligates a human person towards other persons. As far as she is a "being of reason" herself, she obviously belongs to "all humankind", meaning that she is one of the creditors of the respective duty herself. Kant states that the *homo noumenon,* endowed with freedom of the will, owes this duty to himself insofar as he "also embodies humankind in his own person" and that he, as an empirical human being, a *homo phaenomenon,* was "entrusted" to himself as a *homo noumenon* "under the duty of maintenance" (Kant 1907/14 [AA VI]:422). Hence, Kant solves the problem of the logical impossibility of the "debtor" and "creditor" of a duty by the same person by making humankind itself (embodied in the individual person) the creditor of that duty.[242]

One may, of course, debate the plausibility of such a conception. In particular, the rather curious applications of this conception by Kant in the appendices ("Casuistic Questions") which he attaches to the theoretical chapters in his "Metaphysical Principles of Virtue" are simply unconvincing. These applications are much more rooted in and limited by the particular views of his times than are his philosophical doctrines. However, this need not concern us here, for it is certainly not too far-fetched to assume that *some* moral duties should originate specifically from one's status as a rational and, at least in some sense, autonomous being. What we do not endorse in Kant's conception, though, is the more or less literal way in which he identifies the true object (and thus the true "creditor", of the respect a person allegedly owes to herself) as being something other than that person herself (i.e. all of humanity). Conceptually speaking, this seems to transgress the bounds of a "duty to self", since the duty in question is really owed to a third party or an external authority. This criticism is, in itself, of no particular normative importance. However, the following objection certainly is. The Kantian conception personifies, and thus exaggerates, the independent status of that alien authority, present within an actor, to which the duty of care is truly owed. Hence, such a conception is bound to exaggerate the demands on the person that is the "debtor" of this respect as well. Any trade-offs of interests, for instance, reasonable as they might be *within* the sphere of interests of one

[242] Kant's further distinctions within his conception of duties to the self are considerably more nuanced than we present them to be here. He distinguishes between perfect and imperfect duties to the self (depending on the logical space they leave for an individual's decisions on how to discharge them, with "perfect duties" not leaving any such space). Amongst the former, he differentiates between duties to oneself "only as a moral being", and to oneself as an "animal (physical) and a moral being" (Kant 1907/14 [AA VI]:419–420).

and the same person, are, in principle, not acceptable if they cross the protected boundaries of others, and infringe upon their rights.[243] If such duties "to oneself" were really nothing but *rights* of another (i.e. of all humankind), they would impose far too strict a burden on the obligated individual.[244]

Thus, if there are moral duties to the self, they should not be identified with the rights of some overwhelming alien authority, even if the self is, in a certain sense, also a constituent part of this external authority. What then might these duties consist in? To what extent might they limit one's moral competence of self-disposition?

As far as our problem of *mental* self-enhancement is concerned, even Kant himself does not provide us with an answer. As perfect duties to oneself he states, *inter alia*, the absolute prohibition of suicide and also of acts of "self-mutilation". The latter he calls "partial suicide" and among them he counts such deeds as donating an organ or a tooth or having oneself castrated in order to maintain a high pitched singing voice (Kant 1907/14 [AA VI]:423). This may appear to point in the direction of a strict prohibition of having one's body substantially altered in an irrevocable way. To the extent that a psychic enhancement would consist in some irreversible intervention into one's own brain, one might be inclined to drawing the (possibly) Kantian conclusion that such an enhancement cannot be morally permissible. However unconvincing most of these Kantian suggestions are, their bearing upon our problem becomes all the more ambiguous when we take into account that Kant also postulated an "imperfect duty" to oneself of developing one's human (i.e. physical and mental) capabilities to their fullest flourishing (Kant 1907/14 [AA VI]:386, 444–447; cf. also Kant 1907/17 [AA VII]:321–322).[245] Taking this into account, one must not overlook the fact that mental enhancements cannot work by creating particular capabilities out of nothing and installing them somehow in their users' mind or brains. Rather, they raise the user's level of favourable subjective preconditions for acquiring such capabilities. They

---

[243] This, of course, invokes the notorious basic problem of utilitarian accounts of ethics. We cannot elaborate on this here. Suffice it to point out that we reject the basic idea of utilitarianism exactly for its inability to take seriously enough the "distinction between persons" (Rawls 1971:27). If it is prudent for an individual to make painful short-term sacrifices for much weightier long-term goods (for example, to go to a dentist now instead of delaying the necessary treatment and making it much more painful later), this cannot morally require anybody to make equally painful sacrifices for equally weighty goods of *others* (not beyond the narrow limits of required solidarity, anyway). However, utilitarian accounts of ethics are, in principle, committed to demanding just that.

[244] Consider Kant's absolute verdict on suicide. It is certainly consequent. For if committing suicide is really violating the right of "someone else", namely humankind, it must, in principle, be no less strictly forbidden than murder. However, we do not find this conception at all convincing.

[245] Recall that "imperfect" does not relate to some relative moral weight of a duty but only to the relative exactness of its imperative content.

do not spare the individual her own endeavours to reach her desired goals. They either make it easier to get there, or make goals attainable that lie beyond the "natural" limits of the unenhanced user. Thus an enhanced mind, as it were, is still subject to the very same Kantian postulate to develop its capabilities "to their fullest flourishing" as it was before. Just as before it is equally capable of meeting the requirements of this postulate or failing to do so. If it meets them, the difference will consist only in its performing on a higher level in certain respects than it would otherwise have been able to.

Thus, from a purely orthodox Kantian perspective, a neuro-physiological enhancement of one's cognitive or emotional capacities may not interfere with the "imperfect duty to oneself" to develop one's personal capabilities. The question must, at least, be left open whether such an intervention could be morally justified. This we are even more inclined to do since we do not believe that solutions to such problems should simply (or even primarily) be derived from an exegesis of a classical philosophical text, whether it be the thoughts of Kant or of any other philosopher. It goes without saying that this reasoning excludes any possibility of justifying a legal prohibition founded exclusively on whatever interpretation of the Kantian conception one might prefer. [246] (And to this even Kant himself would certainly agree.)

Following Joel Feinberg, we have distinguished four different conceptions of autonomy. Within the second – the "autonomy as a set of factual preconditions of self-government" – Feinberg quite plausibly differentiates between twelve personal (or at least *prima-facie)* virtues, that appear to be constitutive elements of this particular conception of autonomy. Most of them he takes up again in the subsequent chapter on "autonomy as an ideal" and reshapes them from the factual to the normative, i.e. to something like "an ideal complex of character traits" which, taken together, might form what we may call a truly autonomous person or character. (Recall that both these conceptions of "autonomy" belong exclusively to the *ethical* sphere of the concept.) Not all of the elements identified by Feinberg are of equal weight, most of them are not such "that the more one has the better" and actually, only three of them seem to be of specific relevance to our purposes here. These are the concepts of:

- authenticity – in the sense of "self-selection";
- moral authenticity – in the sense of having one's character rooted in one's own moral convictions;
- integrity or self-fidelity – in the sense of being faithful to one's own principles. (cf. Feinberg 1986:32, 36, 40)

[246] Some of Jürgen Habermas' reasoning on "The Future of Human Nature" also point in that Kantian direction. He speaks of the "inconspicuous normative interplay between the morally obligatory and legally guaranteed inviolability of persons and the indisposability of the natural mode of their physical embodiment" (Habermas 2001:41).

These concepts seem to be intertwined with one another in various aspects. Let us begin with that of authenticity. Whatever its exact content, the virtue it is supposed to characterise seems to be of a twofold relevance to the subject of enhancing one's own mental features. First, a person may wish for such an enhancement for "inauthentic" reasons, meaning that, in seeking such an enhancement, she does not follow her own inner values and preferences, but, instead, relies on some trend fashion or such like. Second, by substantially altering one's psychic features, one may, in some sense, become somebody else, at least if judged primarily by the character traits one exhibits now as compared to those one had before. This switch of character, so to speak, may amount to becoming "inauthentic" in the sense of not being true to one's "real", "original" or "natural" self. That is to say the one before the enhancement intervention.

Let us begin with the problem of inauthentic motives for enhancements. Feinberg elucidates the meaning of the concept of authenticity through its negation. "The inauthentic person of this type is essentially the manipulated consumer." (ibid.:32). An "authentic" person, by contrast, is someone who, firstly, orientates her decisions and her actions towards her own values, preferences, and ideals, and, secondly, subjects these values etc. at due times to the scrutiny of reason. Thus, they are consciously adopted by the individual and are, therefore, truly her own.

A more in depth conception of authenticity may take two basic questions as its point of departure: (1) Who am I? (2) How do I conceive of myself? Since a person may have an erroneous or distorted self-conception, failing to take account of important objective features of who she really is, these are different questions (cf. Oshana 2005:78).[247] Various authors have suggested lists of necessary and/or sufficient characteristics that make up a person's "central identity traits" (Rorty and Wong 1990:20). Harry Frankfurt has developed three criteria by which to identify what the core character traits are that constitute a self as an agent, and that are essential to this person's self-conception: "the ineliminable, the intractable, and the unthinkable" (Frankfurt 1999:111–113). This is to point out that a person usually has certain very fundamental character traits that substantially govern her way of acting, that she could not willingly strip herself of ("ineliminable"), nor even attempt to get rid of ("intractable"), or even think about getting rid of ("unthinkable"). Whatever belongs to those traits,[248] most or perhaps all, may materialise in a rather wide range of different grades. Therefore,

[247] Even though one would have to account for the fact that having an erroneous self-image is, itself, an objective fact about a person.

[248] Frankfurt speaks of "volitional necessities", and elaborates on them a lot more, developing a host of further illuminating differentiations that we need not trace here. Frankfurt's conception, by the way, bridges the gap between the subjective self-conception and the objective "real" self of a person. What is subjectively "unthinkable" and "intractable" about someone's core characteristics is just what is objectively "ineliminable" for him as an agent.

authenticity, thus understood, is itself a matter of gradation. Summing up what these conceptions have in common, it seems fair to say that it is the presumption that the features necessary for the authenticity of a person's self-conception are also necessary for her being truly autonomous.[249]

Turning to our question of inauthentic motives for personal enhancements, there is certainly abundant reason for the assumption that psychic enhancements, presuming they were fairly safe and commonly available at reasonable prices, would find hundreds of thousands of interested parties who were just "manipulated consumers". However unpleasant that idea may be, it is certainly nothing unusual at all.[250] It is and, to some extent, has perhaps always been a normal part of the life of any society with sufficiently effective means of communication. To be sure, being motivated to certain decisions by current societal trends is not in itself morally suspect. One may have examined the reasons for and against adapting to the respective trend, and may have decided to follow it on good grounds of one's own. Certainly, one ought to try as best as one can to avoid being inauthentic in the sense explained above. But it appears rather unclear whether we should consider this sort of "ought" as delineating, or even substantially contributing to, a moral duty one has to oneself. One could, with good reason, opt for a more restricted use of the concept of duty, saving it for more weighty obligations (to oneself or to others) and thus avoid unduly inflated versions of the concept and its contamination with an air of triviality. Be that as it may, if one wishes to call the "ought" of authenticity of one's decisions a moral duty to oneself it certainly is a duty of comparatively little weight.[251] Furthermore, it confronts us with no problems that were specific to our subject of mental enhancement. So just their being "inauthentically motivated" in a large numbers of cases, would not count decisively against the ethical acceptability of such enhancements.

If one does not look at the motives, but rather at the possible results of a psychic enhancement, the difficulty of the emerging problems seems to increase. There are two main concerns which surface here. First, future methods of such enhancements may be effective enough to substantially alter a person's personality, thus perhaps alienating that person's character from her authentic (i.e. original) self. Second, character traits sufficiently profiled to form an authentic self may be of a kind that could not be created or shaped by technical means at all. For such character traits might belong to

[249] We do have some doubts as to that presumption. However, it is of no decisive relevance to our arguments so we accept this prevailing view on authenticity and autonomy.

[250] Somewhat cynically, one might even ask why not accept a person's inclination always to follow fashionable trends as his or her "true" or "authentic" self? Certainly, that would run counter to the whole enterprise of developing a normatively sensible concept of authenticity. However, this does not exclude the possibility to call such a character a person's *factually* "true" self.

[251] This is not saying, of course, that the "ought" would disappear.

some metaphysical realm that one has to work his way through, in order to truly earn and deserve the results.

The first concern presumes that changes of a person's psychic features might be radical enough to impair that person's authentic self-conception and thus her autonomy. A change of identity would, one might say, make the enhanced person, in some sense, depart from her own past, thus committing a kind of betrayal of her former being. The questions involved here largely center around the metaphysical problems and the normative implications of personal identity and its possible changes. We deal extensively with those problems in our chapter on personal identity so we just refer the reader to that chapter for further analysis of this specific question.

Suffice it here to say that conceptions of personal identity can be moulded on very different paradigms, depending on the metaphysical or practical ends one pursues. They may then generate widely varying conceptions, each (more or less) plausible under the specific criterion that principally guides its function. What we want to explore here are the *normative implications* of different conceptions of personal identity. For this purpose, a very basic distinction needs to be drawn between changes sufficiently radical to alter "numerical identity" (i.e. literally creating a different self), and mere modifications of someone's "narrative identity", leaving the original self intact (cf. DeGrazia 2005:Chaps. 2, 3, and 6). Perhaps more graphically, one might distinguish between changes of a person's core identity, and mere changes of her personality (see Chapter 5 of the present volume). All of us all have developed, and continue to develop, our personal traits, our character, intellect, emotions, and desires, over the course of time. That is to say, we have substantially altered parts of our personality and still keep doing so to some extent. Artificially enhancing some of the features that make up this personality, certainly differs in some, perhaps very important, respects from the ordinary (educational and self-educational) way of character development. However, they do not differ with regard to what is being changed, and not, at least not necessarily, with regard to the magnitude of this change. Therefore, if an artificial enhancement of cognitive abilities and emotional or motivational virtues remains within the scope of mere personality changes, it does not raise problems of impairing one's autonomy. These changes, be they objectionable for other reasons or not, are certainly not impermissible merely for their outcome and for whatever impact they may have on personal autonomy or authenticity. The quite different problems of "numerical" identity alterations, (i.e. the question of which changes would be radical enough to somehow extinguish the original person, replacing her with a new one) need not concern us here. Thus we also need not look into the related question of whether any realistic conception of mental enhancement, available within the foreseeable future, could possibly bring about such a radical personality change. Hence, we may also leave open here the normative conclusions that would have to be drawn from such a possibility (cf. Chapter 5 of the present volume).

Our second concern above was that it might be somehow objectionable *a priori* to create or shape desired character traits by using psycho-technical means. Perhaps one can only *really* own such traits if one truly deserves them. At least that's what the popular proverb "no pain no gain" seems to suggest. Thus, a true ownership of certain traits might only be possible if one has earned them by personal endeavour and discipline, not simply by purchasing them as the product of a pack of enhancement measures. One could even argue that for valuable personal traits to be "real," they must in some sense be grounded in and certified by a whole character. The latter, being more than just the sum of individual personal traits, may, in turn, only be achievable by a long, complex and strenuous process of self-formation. Thus, a person acquiring certain abilities by artificially enhancing her natural psychic capacities might strip them of their necessary foundation and thus, in a certain sense at least, deceive herself about the fruits of her endeavours since her way of acquiring them might radically devalue the fruits themselves.

Considering this objection, one should carefully distinguish between the two different questions it points to. First, if the above suspicion is true, the enhancing attempt might in the end prove useless and senseless for the person undertaking it. (Whether or not this senselessness would impair the person's autonomy or authenticity, thus perhaps making his attempt morally objectionable, is a different question still.) Second, the possible devaluation of commonly appreciated virtues by making them artificially available might finally impair the social value of those virtues themselves if such practices were to become widespread. It might turn them simply into commodities and thus trivialise them to such an extent that they would no longer be considered virtues.

Obviously, the latter question is not one of personal autonomy at all. It concerns the possible harm to society as a whole by the large-scale employment of psycho-technical enhancements. We will address this problem later.[252] As far as the former question is concerned, it certainly might point to problems of personal authenticity as part of one's autonomy. However, it is not easy to see in what way self-deception about the nature of one's desired ends could in a relevant sense impair one's autonomy or authenticity and thus make the whole procedure a violation of a moral duty to oneself. Perhaps the analogy of doping in sports may help to elucidate this point. Many people believe that even though taking steroids or using methods of blood doping to enhance one's athletic performance might enable an athlete to achieve a higher level of performance, that level is not really his or her accomplishment. Instead, what makes the decisive difference between the old and the new level of performance is brought about only by means "separate and external" to the person using them, thus alienating the person from

[252] Cf. infra 6.4.5.

what he or she achieves (cf. Simon 1984). If we grant that this alienation and, therefore, the devaluation presumption is correct – which is by no means beyond dispute[253] – there are certainly many good reasons to abstain from such an undertaking. The sort of self-deception sketched above certainly figures prominently among these.

Still, it does not seem plausible to assume that this specific aspect of self-deception, without any deception by, or of, others being involved, could be decisive for an unethical encroachment on one's autonomy. Why not accept the free decision of a person to technically enhance some of his personal properties as a part of his authentic self? Maybe his attempt to realise that decision is doomed to failure because in the end nobody, including himself, would really appreciate the newly acquired capacities as "sufficiently real" or "authentic". But why say that would make the person himself inauthentic, in a morally relevant sense, let alone deprive him in part of his autonomy? Let's draw another parallel. Take someone who enhanced her physical appearance (at least according to her own judgment) by a whole series of cosmetic surgery, and nobody amongst her personal acquaintances has any appreciation for the results. Of course, there were plenty of prudential reasons not to undertake such efforts. But would we really want to say that this person herself, rather than simply some of her physical features, has become "physically inauthentic" in an ethically relevant sense, rendering the whole venture a violation of a moral duty to herself?[254] What should be emphasised here is that moral duties to oneself, whatever scope one wishes to assign to them, must be grounded in stronger normative principles than just prudential reasons with respect to one's own interests. Not only in law but also in ethics it belongs to the core of a person's autonomy and does not transgress her normative limits to decide for and do things to herself that most other people consider wrong or even harmful to that person.

Finally, one should not overlook the fact that an enhancement of mental traits can only be effective through the complex interplay of several additional enabling conditions that fall entirely within the range of "natural" properties of the enhancer. Hypothetically speaking, even assuming that somebody managed to enhance all of his cognitive abilities by psycho-technical interventions, that in itself, would not get him anywhere near to being a respected scientist.

What all of this leaves us with is the contention that none of the objections considered above is sufficient to make an artificial enhancement of mental features, be they of a cognitive, an emotional, or a motivational nature, an immoral attack on one's personal autonomy, and thus a violation of a duty to oneself. That does not mean that there are no well-founded objections against such enhancements. It does mean, however, that any such

---

[253] See our attempt to clarify this, infra 4.5; see also Fost (1986).

[254] Of course, the analogue suffers from several flaws, since the predicate "authentic" seems to be linked to mental capacities in a stronger and more poignant way than to physical features. Still, the parallel is plausible enough to elucidate our point here.

objections must be rooted in *other* normative grounds. Above all, what our considerations about personal autonomy certainly have not established, is a legitimate basis for an outright legal prohibition of mental enhancements. Such prohibitive measures would have to be rooted in other normative grounds as well.

6.4.4 Concerns about the Corruption of the True Nature of Human Beings

In bioethical debates of the last two decades, the concept of "human nature" has drawn considerable suspicion of being a misused and ideological topic, aimed only at a blocking rational argument. The charge has been made against those who simply speak out "in defense of human nature" that they are not really willing to engage in sensible discussion, but instead rejecting all high-tech developments in medicine and medical research out of hand simply for the fact that they involve an advancement in technology and, consequently, are considered to be "unnatural". Much of this suspicion about this type of human-nature argument has certainly been justified. There is no logical, or otherwise rationally certified way of deriving normative principles for human conduct from whatever facts of human (or nonhuman) nature one wishes to take into account. Moreover, it can be argued that an element of permanent self-modification – an endless process of transcending previously insurmountable limits of humanity –, is an integral part of human nature itself. Furthermore, in developing their mental capabilities, humans have always employed artificial means of different sorts by coupling them, as it were, with their "natural" brain functions. Such activity is part of an ongoing process, which began with developments such as the use of pen and paper in arithmetic calculations and that has led to the use today of the most advanced super-computers to conduct complex calculations, far beyond natural human abilities. Some philosophers have recently come to characterise this "brain-artefact interface" (which has always been part of the development of human mental capabilities) by employing the concept of an ever-more artificially "extended human mind" as a regular phenomenon of human thinking (see e.g. Clark and Chalmers 1998; Adams and Aizawa 2001; Clark 2005). From the perspective of "naturalness" (and "unnaturalness" respectively), what is the a-priori normative difference between coupling one's natural mental abilities with the functions of a computer, by using one's hands on the computer keyboard, and having one's brain functions directly linked with that computer, with no more manual bridging necessary in between?[255] It would not appear easy to give a well-founded answer

[255] The risks of the implantation of the computer device into one's body aside, of course. They belong to the realm of problematic side effects. For our present purpose, we (counterfactually) presuppose the complete safety of that brain-machine interface in order to clarify whether there are *other* objections against such a procedure.

to this question. On the contrary, one conclusion that we would seem able to draw at this stage is that there appear to be sound reasons to assume that a principled difference between these two types of activity resting simply on the "unnaturalness" of the latter does not exist.

On the other hand, there might be better, theoretically more appropriate ways of deploying the term "human nature" in normative discourse. First, as indicated above, one must distinguish between the various descriptive contents and the alleged normative implications one wishes to base on certain facts these descriptions might contain or depict. And second, since there is no rational way to derive such normative implications *directly* from the facts, one must demonstrate or stipulate some background norm as a plausible premise to be applied to the factual situation, thus yielding the alleged normative consequences. Following philosopher Neil Roughley (who in some respects refers to a much older conception by Aristotle), we suggest three basic distinctions within the semantic realm of "human nature" (cf. Roughley 2005:137):

- species membership,
- the characteristically human form of life,
- "interventionless" human features, i.e. objects and states of affairs belonging to human existence, and emerging or developing without any causal or otherwise intervening human conduct.

For reasons of convenience, we will follow Roughley in labeling these three concepts of human nature "HN 1", "HN 2", and "HN 3". In this way, they are merely descriptive concepts, devoid of any normative content. As we have pointed out, making each of them normatively relevant requires their affiliation with a valid norm, containing a so-called normative operator ("prohibited", "obligatory", "permissible"), which determines what should be the case with regard to the factual elements depicted by the descriptive concepts. We presuppose that only HN 2 and HN 3 can plausibly be taken as points of departure to effectuate normative prescriptions alongside their descriptive content. Possible norms to be invoked by such a theoretical operation lie readily at hand. For HN 2, the required norm could read as follows: "Certain basic features that constitute the particular human form of life are valuable for human individuals and society. Therefore, they should be preserved to the greatest extent possible (alternatively: to the extent most reasonable)." As for HN 3, a relevant normative prescription could read:

> Naturally developed human features, i.e. features not (at least not primarily) brought about by the external interventions of other human actors, are to be judged as being more valuable than human features that are artificially arranged or induced. Therefore, human development without intervention should be pursued to the greatest extent possible (alternatively: to the extent most reasonable).

Obviously, the latter sentence must be qualified in some sense to make it an object of serious deliberation. Since very much, or even most, of what is crucial to the development of an autonomous person from infancy to adulthood must somehow be caused or influenced by the conscious interventions of other people (parents, teachers, peer groups, etc.), the norm invoked could not seriously stipulate that individual human development should, to the greatest extent possible, be free from formative interventions by others. One might accept such a qualified version of this stipulation and select only a few particular features of the typical natural make-up of a human person, such as "the anthropological state of imperfectness, vulnerability, and neediness" (Siep 2002:114). Then one might consider these features valuable *per se*, perhaps based on the important role they play for the development of certain virtues in human society (such as solidarity or compassion). However, the identification of such an important role neither makes these features valuable in themselves (i.e. a good thing to have), nor can it imply that we should not try to help people to minimise their "imperfectness, vulnerability, and neediness" as best they can. This becomes obvious if we follow the implications of this position to its normative conclusion. One could then put the above argument as follows: See to it that there are always helpless, needy, vulnerable people (even if you could prevent them from being so), so that enough others will have an opportunity to develop virtues like solidarity, compassion, and the like. It is ethically wrong to intentionally preserve certain states of affairs in order to grant some people opportunities to exhibit socially valuable attitudes at the expense of others' misery.

However, it is one thing to reject such sweeping claims as unpersuasive, but quite another to say that humans, nevertheless, have good reasons to observe some limits of "natural" normality (in the sense of HN 3) in their individual physical and mental development, which should not be crossed by intentional bio-medical interventions. Of course, individual human development is always driven and shaped by a complex interplay of natural and cultural (artificial) forces. Hence this "limit of normality" is anything but a clear-cut demarcation that could be defined scientifically or philosophically. Instead, it is a complex, vague, value-laden, gradable and, in many of its facets, disputable concept. Similarly, the corresponding concept of "human nature" (HN 3), in the sense of a *condicio humana*, that remains within the boundaries thus defined is equally complex and, to some extent, elusive. Up to the present time, however, there has been no great need to clarify these concepts with respect to anything like their practical applicability on human action. Of course, there have always been individual shifts of emphasis between nature and nurture as (traditional) sources of human flourishing, but they have usually been considered a matter of private liberty and not been subject to any great ethical concern.

However, this may presently be about to change with the development of procedures capable of genetically altering basic human features in order to substantially enhance certain physical or mental capacities. We are now, or at least may soon be, confronted with the question of where to draw the line between ethically permissible interventions into natural human conditions, and other interventions that we should avoid or prevent.[256] Such reasons might be concerned with two different types of risks. On the one hand, certain risks will be associated with the possible emergence of features that humans do not naturally possess and that, for various reasons, we would not want them to be endowed with. On the other hand, risks may also be associated with the danger that the very complex interplay of biological features, especially in the human brain, might be profoundly distorted by the "unnatural" enhancement of one set of features at the expense of others.

Turning to the first set of risks, one might think of physical capacities such as a bat-like "radar vision" or a plant-like ability to photosynthesise (each affiliated with a host of incalculable consequences), or mental capacities, such as the ability to block out from one's consciousness any vestige of empathy towards fellow humans.[257] We certainly have reason to pause and think – and probably to intervene – before we allow such developments to occur. In addition, it is clear that the occurrence of sufficiently large numbers of individuals exhibiting such non-natural traits would also exert an almost incalculable distorting influence on HN 2, i.e. on the fundamental characteristics of the specifically human form of social life. However, for all we presently know, this possibility of intentionally introducing completely new human traits by transgressing the biological boundaries of "human nature" (as explicated above in HN 3) will, in the foreseeable future, if ever, only be possible through such deep-running interventions as germ-line alterations of the human genome. The means and methods that we address in our inquiry do not, at least not yet, hold such potential. Intervening in the human brain by employing such methods may certainly pose serious risks of grave side effects. However, side effects are not what we are talking about when expressing concerns about "human nature". On the other hand, interventions that *aim* at the enhancement of specific mental capacities always need to draw on something that is already there, a minimum stock, as it were, of the capacities to be enhanced. Even if the results of such an enhancement were to reach a "superhuman" quality (e.g. of intelligence, memory, alertness, etc.) that some might find repulsive for whatever reasons, it could not bring about completely new traits previously unknown in human beings (as some genetic enhancements certainly could).

Hence, we do not feel compelled to embark on the difficult task of delineating legal and ethical limits to future enhancements that would be equiva-

[256] Note that we do not have to possess a clear definition of the "permissible" in the above sense, or anything like certainty of where to draw the line, to nevertheless be completely safe in judging that some instances are doubtlessly beyond that limit.

[257] To be sure, such individuals might actually exist; but this does not mean that we could reasonably blame their being thus on "nature", nor that we would accept, let alone endorse, their having that trait, nor that we would seriously deliberate on intentionally bringing it about.

lent to enhancements altering the human genome. Suffice it to say that the future development of the techniques of intervening in the brain should be monitored closely. The development and use of techniques, comparable to those which germ-line genetic interventions might soon possess (viz a potential to transgress norm-sensitive borderlines of HN 3, wherever they be drawn) should not be allowed to be developed and utilised, not, at least, until the far-reaching implications of such a development have been sufficiently clarified and found to be normatively acceptable.

Much more realistic are concerns that enhancements through interventions in the brain could massively distort a very delicate equilibrium in the most complex piece of matter in the human body, perhaps even in the entire universe. This points, first of all, to problems of undesired side effects which are not our present concern. However, it also attempts to identify a certain standard, derived from a criterion of "naturalness" which, if deviated from, will supposedly cause such effects. This standard might be labeled "the wisdom of billions of years of evolutionary history" whose physiological product is the human brain (cf. a similar remark in Marcus 2002:174). To interfere with such an immensely complex structure, still far from being sufficiently understood, by disturbing the fine-tuned balance between its various functions is bound (so the argument goes) to open up a Pandora's Box of unforeseeable and potentially dangerous consequences.

This does certainly not provide us with anything like a clear, applicable criterion by which to judge right from wrong in the present context. However, it does not simply testify to an irrational or ideological view. It rightly reminds us of our continuing and profound ignorance of the hyper-complex system of interdependencies between processes and functions that are realised on the cellular level of the human brain. This ignorance increases considerably with respect to unwelcome consequences which might result from risky interferences in those processes. Thus, it certainly warrants a strong principle of caution, which should apply to all attempts to isolate and amplify (enhance) particular brain functions by directly targeting them on the cellular level and thus possibly disturbing their systemic interconnectivity with other important functions. This maxim of caution might be confirmed by the rather irritating observation that so-called "savant idiots", individuals who exhibit one specific mental ability (e.g. memory) to an extent far beyond anything that could be called "normal" or even "extraordinary". Quite often, though, this "super-human" strength of the one skill or function goes along with a significant impairment of others and, hence, usually with an overall intellectual disability (cf. Hermelin et al. 1999; Treffert 2006).

Thus the initial insistence on an allegedly "true nature of human beings," with which we started out, turned out to be not so much a concern for human nature, but for human well-being. The latter, of course, is central to ethical debates in general. Human nature (or at least a critically refined conception of it) is not so much the object to be defended *for its own sake*, but is a reasonable measure of pursuing moral goals, i.e. in the service of human needs and interests. The precautionary principle we wish to advocate in this respect is, as all such principles are, not a strict but a "soft norm" (to invoke an illustrative analogy to the concept of "soft law" in public international law). This means that it should not be handled as a prohibitive blockade, but as a flexible instrument of scepticism. There should be a shift of the burden of proof from the sceptics to those who wish to transgress sensible boundaries of "natural" human biology through the introduction of new procedures to enhance mental traits through intervention in the brain.

6.4.5 Concerns about the Corruption of the Desired Goals Themselves

6.4.5.1 "Win Races and Lose Racing"? – The Example of Physical Enhancements

The type of concern referred to in the above subtitle is nicely illustrated by a short passage in Bill McKibben's 2003 book "Enough". The enhancements McKibben talks about are of a genetic origin, and they refer only to physical abilities. However, he clearly takes the normative problems he wants to elucidate in his paradigm case to be common to all types of artificial enhancement. Thus, his argument would also seem to encompass the problem of mental enhancements that are the topic of the current inquiry:

> As we move into this new world of genetic engineering, we won't simply lose races, we'll lose racing: We'll lose the possibility of the test, the challenge, the celebration that athletics represents. [...] Say you've reached Mile 23, and you're feeling strong. Is it because of your hard training and your character, or because the gene pack inside you is pumping out more red blood cells than your body knows what to do with? Will anyone be impressed with your dedication? More to the point, will you be impressed with your dedication? Will you know what part of it is you, and what part is your upgrade? (McKibben 2003:6)

The basic idea behind this worry seems to be that we view and appreciate ourselves and others not just in the light of what we (or they) are factually able to do, but also in the light of what we (they) deserve praise or reproach for. That is, we usually judge a person in terms of what she has achieved or made of herself. Seen in that light, even interventions into the brain that aim only at eliminating real psychic diseases by using purely medical means may sometimes draw some suspicion. To illustrate the point further, serious emotional suffering, say in the course of a major depression (as an example of a genuine disease) seems to be different in important respects from physical pain. It usually has its roots, or at least some of them, in deep structures of the individual psyche which are often the results of particular features of an individual biography. If psychotherapy takes as its normative ground the idea of maintaining or restoring a personal *self*, it might be committed not just to abolishing suffering, but to doing this in a way that involves the whole personal background of that suffering, in which the individual is made to understand the roots of his or her suffering, and is helped to work through the problematic issues. Thereby the patient is helped, through reason and understanding to regain a full and adequate picture of herself and her personal history. In short, the condition is alleviated on the grounds of personal autonomy, rather than by giving and taking "aspirin for the mind" (cf. Freedman 1998:135, 140).

If we try to pursue this line of reasoning on a more general level beyond that of pure treatment or disease, we may perhaps say the following. There seem to be at least some, perhaps even many, human capabilities, which we admire or desire for ourselves, whose achievement is somehow connected with the traditional ways of investing certain amounts of personal endeavour to developing those capabilities. To admire somebody who has reached one of those aims, then, does not simply mean admiration for the final result or product, but encompasses at least en element of admiration for the sacrifices and the efforts that person made *on the way* to achieving that goal. If we learn that there is a convenient shortcut to reach this aim, enabling in principle anybody to get there without any significant investment in terms of personal endeavour, we might lose our respect for the result itself. Projected onto the horizon of a common societal practice, this might in the long run lead to a profound devaluation of these previously admired goals. Consequently, this might lead to a gradual loss or "thinning out" of the values commonly associated with certain goals and held in esteem by society.

The following example from the field of athletics illustrates this point exactly. Our admiration of a person's ability, say, to run 100 metres in less than ten seconds would practically vanish if we learned that this result was brought about almost entirely by a (physical) medical intervention which could, in principle, enable any healthy young person to run that fast. After all, simply the ability of a living being to run 100 metres in, say, eight seconds or to swim 100 metres in, say, forty seconds is, in itself, nothing to be admired. Many animals are capable of doing either of these activities more quickly and more efficiently. Thus, the effort required for humans to reach that level of performance in the "normal" way seems to be an integral part of the preconditions for our admiration. To the degree that this "normality" can be circumvented by medical interventions, our interest in, and excitement about, the entire event would perhaps vanish. So whatever social or cultural value one wishes to assign to the present enterprise of competitive sports, that value might, at least to a large extent, be corrupted, and thus disappear, if the complete legalisation of all performance enhancing drugs were to take place. We might then, as McKibben puts it, not only lose a race or races of whatever sort, but racing itself. Of course, it is always us, human beings and the societies we form, who invest such things as events and performances with meaning. Thus it is not unlikely that a new form of appreciation for this new type of athletics would evolve, perhaps, in some sense, it would resemble the sensational interests that citizens of ancient Rome took in the circus and gladiatorial games. However, something more profound would be lost. Something that characterises sport in its present form and that many people value in that particular respect.

This perspective on human performance with regard to athletics has been developed eloquently, and at great length, in The President's Council's 2003 Report "Beyond Therapy". The following excerpt summarises succinctly the issues at hand:

> What is a human performance and what is an excellent one? And what makes it excellent as a human performance? For it seems that some performance-enhancing agents, from stimulants to blood doping to genetic engineering of muscles, call into question the dignity of the performance of those who use them. The performance seems less real, less one's own, less worthy of our admiration. Not only do such enhancing agents distort or damage other dimensions of human life – for example, by causing early death or sexual impotence – they also seem to distort the athletic activity itself. [...] What is at stake here is the very meaning of human agency, the meaning of being at-work in the world, being at-work as myself, and being at-work in a humanly excellent way. (President's Council on Bioethics 2003:140–141)

The Council expressly confines its analysis to the particular area of "human sport" (ibid.:105). However, the last sentence quoted above demonstrates the Council's unmistakable tendency, manifested in several other parts of the report as well, to generalise its view on athletics over a broad (perhaps even the entire) spectrum of positively valued human activity. The question is whether such a generalisation stands on firm argumentative ground.

6.4.5.2 Mental Performance: Output-oriented versus Engagement-oriented

To clarify this point, let's test our criterion of means-sensitivity of certain human achievements by applying it to performances of a mainly mental or intellectual origin. What springs to mind here is the example of a competitive performance which combines sporting and intellectual elements, namely chess. When years ago the first chess computer, the IBM-model "Big Blue", beat the then world champion Gary Kasparov, it marked a great advance in the skills and techniques of computer programming and perhaps even in computer science in general. However, it would almost certainly not have induced anybody to admire the performance of Big Blue. And as far as the engineer who designed its programme is concerned, nobody would have seriously suggested that he or she should be declared the new or "real" chess world champion.[258] For all the reasons there were to admire various aspects associated with this event, the chess skills and the level of performance of the IBM computer were not due our admiration at all.[259] These purely technical

[258] I borrow this illustrative example from Brock (2003:364).

[259] This remark about the absence of admiration for the chess performance is not to be confused with a remark about admiration for the computer itself. This is also certainly nothing to be admired in and for itself.

processes had in itself no value whatsoever. On the other hand, if we envisage that very same chess performance carried out move by move by a human player, we certainly arrive at the best of all reasons to admire that player's achievement. The only difference between both performances obviously lies in their respective causal sources, one being artificial and technical, the other being human. Thus it seems perfectly plausible to assume that in cases of mixed causal sources of a chess performance, say of a player employing a brain-computer interface that greatly enhances her ability to play, the machine would not only contribute to the enhancement but also, and to the very same extent, to the gradual devaluing of that performance.

There appears to be at least one further area of human achievements where the criterion of means-sensitivity that we derived from the paradigm case of sports (including chess) seems to hold as well: the field of art. A simple thought experiment, although empirically absurd, may nevertheless serve to outline the idea. If we learned that all the (otherwise untalented) composer Ludwig van Beethoven had to do to compose his Ninth Symphony was to take a pill or connect his brain with a technical device that enabled him to do so, this would probably not only dramatically reduce our admiration for Beethoven, but would, for many people, also contaminate (or perhaps even destroy) the pleasure they derive from listening to that symphony.

This latter point may certainly be doubted. After all, the sound of the music itself, loved by so many before the disclosure of its artificial origin, would not be altered in the least by that new knowledge. However, one may probe this counter claim by a more realistic thought experiment. Imagine a fascinating new symphonic composition (or a highly acclaimed sonett) that emerged from some remote archive and was quickly classified by all music (literature) experts in the world as "almost certainly written by Ludwig van Beethoven" (or, respectively, William Shakespeare). Imagine, furthermore, that most lovers of these fine arts became highly enthusiastic while hearing (or reading) the newly found masterpiece. Imagine then it turned out that the whole thing was merely a fraud, initiated by an international gang of organised criminals, and that the "piece of art" was entirely the product of a computer and some new and highly complex software. It is certainly not too speculative a guess that all or most of the former excitement in listening to that music or reading the poetry would vanish at once and that the admiration for it would be reduced to the interest in a curiosity (and perhaps to a completely different sort of admiration for the engineer who developed the software).

So it seems that the common admiration for at least some "mental" achievements, namely those that enable artists to produce their creations, is also somehow connected with the usual labour involved in realising those exceptional capabilities. Our appreciation for artistic performances seems to rely to a great extent on what they express about human abilities and not just on the product itself. Put differently, focusing our admiration exclusively on the product, regardless of its origin, would somehow miss the real value that we invest this product with by tacitly including a complex interplay of commitment, engagement and achievement into our judgment. Ignoring the latter would amount to a quite a different sort of appreciation, one that might perhaps be labeled "efficiency" or "output-oriented", as opposed to, say, "engagement-oriented", or (a bit weaker) "engagement-related".[260] And this just does not seem to do justice to the way we actually value important cultural achievements.

6.4.5.3 Some Reservations

However, this insight and our tentative generalisation so far, is certainly not the whole story. First, it is subject to some considerable reservations, even with regard to artistic achievements alone. Second, if projected onto other areas of intellectual performances, its plausibility largely vanishes.

Let us turn to the first proviso. In areas other than athletics, we accept to a considerable extent that artists may use specific forms of "mind altering" procedures or artificial enhancers of their creativity, without in the least lowering our admiration for the works they produce. For example, the fact that Charles Baudelaire took cocaine before writing some of the poems from the "Fleurs du Mal", leaving more or less obvious vestiges of this enhancing substance in the poems themselves, does not diminish their artistic value (although some people with a faint puritan inclination may find that it diminishes their respect for Baudelaire as a poet and a person). Contrasting that real-life example with our Beethoven thought experiment above, the following supposition seems fairly plausible. Artificial means *intentionally* applied for the purpose of enhancement in a creative process of art, would probably have to cover an overwhelming share of the entire range of preconditions of that process, before we would consider them having a substantial devaluing effect on the final piece of art. Certainly, beyond a certain borderline we would be inclined to assign the entire result largely to the enhancing means rather than to the artist herself and this would certainly affect the worth of the result in a negative sense. (Imagine, at some point in the future, the possibility of a brain-computer interface where most of the productive part in the creational process was simply and independently taken over by the machine.) However, before the transgression of that line, we would not lower our appreciation of the artistic work (nor of its creator), regardless of our knowledge of some artificially enhancing method having been involved in its origins.

So the insights or presumptions that the President's Council developed and derived from the paradigm of competitive athletics do not seem to allow

---

[260] Erik Parens speaks of "expressing the value of efficiency" by preferring the short-cut of a "smart pill" to good results in college exams, rather than taking the laborious ways of studying hard and (on the part of the school) improving the teacher-student ratio. Both of these traditional ways he sees to be standing for a different value than (just) that of efficiency; cf. Parens (2002:156).

for sweeping generalisations over the area of psychic enhancements. (And reconsidering competitive sports with a cursory second thought for a moment, we might even have reason for a pausing *caveat* there: If we discovered that some outstanding athletic performance was to a large extent simply due to the extraordinary natural talent of the performing individual, say, some exceptional genetic disposition, other than ordinary personal efforts, we would probably not in the least diminish our admiration for the person or for his achievement.[261] What then exactly explains the difference if we substitute "artificial medical enhancement" for "genetic giftedness"? After all, in neither case the respective athlete truly merits *all* the credit for his achievement, and in each case he might merit it to exactly the same degree.

The scepticism that arises out of these considerations is strengthened when we examine our second proviso above. In so doing, we leave the sphere of arts altogether and attempt instead to apply the President's Council's concerns about devaluating effects of enhancement practices to other fields of intellectual performances. Let's begin with the rather trivial (though useful and sometimes very challenging) example of learning a foreign language. Let us assume, at some remote point in the future, it became possible to have a chip implanted in one's brain that would enable the recipient instantly to be able to speak and understand, say, Chinese (without any considerable risks or negative side effects). Would we have any normative objections to applying that method of "learning" Chinese, instead of subjecting oneself to the traditional, arduous task of years of studying that language? Would the resulting capability be downgraded in any sense by the new and easy way of achieving it? Would we, in McKibbens words, "lose racing," or in this case, the empathetic virtue of being able to communicate with foreign people in their own language? Would the trivial technical route to that ability amount to a form of cheating ourselves?

The most plausible answer to all of these questions seems to be a firm "no". In the terminology we suggested above, acquiring the ability to speak a foreign language seems to be an output- or efficiency-oriented intellectual endeavour. What counts, are the results, not the ways of achieving them.

The same seems to be true as well for most other intellectual performances beyond the sphere of art. Take, for example, important scientific achievements and discoveries (and allow us one more empirically absurd

[261] This scenario (unlike others in our analysis) has no aura of science-fiction at all. There is such a genetic disposition, causing a considerably higher capacity of red blood cells to transport oxygen by increasing the level of a hormone called erythropoietin (EPO). That was, for example, the case with Eero Mäntyranta, a Finnish Olympic gold medalist in cross-country skiing in 1964 and 1968. With his benign genetic mutation he had a natural advantage over his co-competitors which practically equated to that of manifest doping. He was, of course, not disqualified and nobody seriously thought about downgrading his success in any respect after the true cause of the increased level of his red blood cells was detected.

thought experiment). If we learned that the ingenious insights of Albert Einstein's general theory of relativity were the product not of his genius and of years of hard work, but of some supernatural inspiration that could, in principle, have been given or dictated to any non-physicist as well, we would certainly not come to the conclusion that this superhuman origin downgraded the value of the theory and its impressive beauty, testified to by physicists (and unfortunately only accessible to them). Of course, we would not credit Einstein anymore for the great scientific achievement. But not because we would accuse him of having done something morally objectionable (as we certainly would an Olympic gold medalist after discovering that he had used a means of performance enhancement like blood doping). Rather, we would just cease to consider him the true author of the general theory of relativity. The scientific value of the theory itself would remain untouched by the withdrawal of, or, at very least, alteration in our admiration for its origin.

As a matter of fact, it seems rather difficult to identify *any* other area of human performance, besides those of athletics (including chess) and (with some qualifications) of art, where an artificial (medical) enhancement of the performing persons would, with a rational degree of probability, have corrupting effects on the results. That does not mean that there are no normative objections against medical techniques of psychological enhancements! What we have been concerned with in the current chapter is only the question of possible destructive effects on desired ends that might be exerted by certain artificial means of mental enhancements.[262] There might, of course, be other normative reasons to resist the introduction and development of psychological enhancement techniques in our societies (and we will examine some further candidates in the following passages of this chapter). Furthermore, we found that, at least in some areas of human activity, such as athletics and art, there could be a real danger of such corrupting effects, at least if the underlying enhancing methods were to become mass phenomena. That insight should be enough for raising a moral warning flag if it comes to the question of really introducing such enhancement techniques on a society-wide level, or letting them develop to that extent. That warning's function consists in proposing to legislators and other competent institutions a close monitoring of social developments that might be associated with such an introduction, such as the possible metamorphosis that some of our socially appreciated values might undergo.

At present, it could hardly be more than that. As far as potential legal measures of intervening in such developments of science and/or society are concerned (including perhaps even an outright prohibition of psychologi-

[262] The analysis in the present chapter has largely, if not exclusively, referred to enhancements of cognitive capacities in a broad sense (including features of artistic creativity). It does not seem to make much sense to ask whether an enhancement of emotional or motivational states could corrupt the results thereby brought about.

cally enhancing techniques), legislators would, at the present time, be ill-advised to resort to such measures simply in an attempt to protect our social values. In most countries with a liberal constitutional order, such legislation would, most probably, amount to a violation of constitutional rights which themselves belong to our most important social values. These include the right to privacy, the general right to freedom of action and the right to the particular professional liberties of physicians.

6.4.6 Concerns about the Expanding Medicalisation of Human Behaviour

"Medicalisation" is commonly understood as "the process by which a phenomenon or issue not usually seen as a medical problem comes to be regarded as susceptible to medical analysis and response" (Wachbroit 2001:229). In the current context, "medicalisation" means a gradual shift of the demarcation line between treatment and enhancement, expanding the sphere of the former while diminishing that of the latter. A growing number of what used to be (at most) mild indispositions is being re-defined "disorder" or manifest "disease" and thus being absorbed into the system of medicine.

This phenomenon manifests itself, first of all, in a dramatic increase in the use of certain stimulating drugs, aimed at enhancing mental capacities, in western societies, above all in the U.S. This increase is mirrored in the escalating figures of the production of such drugs, above all Methylphenidate and Fluoxetine. According to a testimony of the Deputy Director of the U.S. American Drug Enforcement Administration (DEA) before the House Subcommittee on Early Childhood, Youth and Families, the Methylphenidate quota in the US increased from 1768 kilograms in 1990 to 14,957 kilograms in 2000 (Woodworth 2000). Much of this increased use is due to an expanding diversion of the drug and to other illicit practices. However, a significant portion of this escalating figure has to do with the practice of physicians prescribing the drug for a growing multitude of minor indispositions or insignificant (if undesired) behaviour variants, especially in children, that would formerly not have been considered "disease" or "disorder". As Charles Krauthammer, a member of the US President's Council on Bioethics, put it at one of the Council's meetings in 2003:

> [...] this explosion, this doubling or tripling of the use of drugs in adolescents and in children is clearly a result of the fact that it has all been opened wide by the vagueness and the often arbitrariness of psychiatric diagnosis. It's as if a psychiatric diagnosis is sort of the wild West. There is no law, and anybody can come in and stake his claim and claim that they're treating an illness when we're not even sure what that illness really is. [...] The fact is that we have what, almost six percent of our kids being medicated... (President's Council on Bioethics 2003)

In a similar manner, Richard DeGrandpre points out that this process is massively promoted by the fact that, as to ADHD (the regular target of methyphenidate), there is no conclusive way "to draw a sharp boundary between those who are considered 'normal' and those [considered] to be ill". (DeGrandpere 1999:133)

This certainly describes a serious problem, and one that is escalating not only in the US, but in European countries as well. However, in the context of our inquiry, it is not a problem in its own theoretical right. Rather, it belongs to the debate on the distinction between treatment and enhancement, which is itself closely affiliated with questions of distributive justice. Of course, this process of medicalisation might, to some extent, reflect a social demand for the re-definition of the treatment-enhancement distinction. Yet such a re-definition must not be left to free-market forces, but be based on conscious decisions by the competent institutions of democracy, since any such decision concerns a particularly sensitive area of social justice, As we have pointed out, legislators have a "robust" competence in this respect, the fact notwithstanding that there is no objectively provable criterion as to where the concrete borderline should run. However, by far the larger part of the said medicalisation process is nothing but the aggregate result of a massively spreading practice of misnaming: What is really a desire of people for enhancement is tacitly accepted and treated as "disease" by thousands of individual physicians in individual prescriptions. This yields no sufficient normative basis for the social distribution of scarce; costly, and potentially life-saving resources.

Hence. above all legislators and politicians, but also the associations of the medical professions, are called for to stop this privately induced and uncontrolled process of extensive medicalisation. This is certainly a weighty political postulate, but it denotes only a secondary, pragmatic, not a primary normative concern (or put differently: a concern of the enforcement, not of the establishment of a normative principle). The question it addresses might inevitably surface in the wake of whatever solution a society establishes to the normative problem of line-drawing. However, it is not itself a part of this problem. Thus we shall not address it separately here. Instead we refer the reader to the discussion of the treatment-enhancement distinction above, and to that of the problems of justice in the subsequent chapter below.

6.4.7 Concerns of Justice

6.4.7.1 The Concept of Justice: Forms, Subjects, Objects, and Basic Distinctions

"Justice" is a notoriously complex and multi-faceted concept. Famously, Aristotle was the first thinker to distinguish between two basic forms or divisions of justice in his "Nicomachean Ethics": distributive justice *(iustitia distributiva)*, and "commutative" justice *(iustitia commutativa)*, the latter being further differentiated into (i) justice of fair exchanges, (ii) restitutive justice (justice of fair compensation), and (iii) corrective or retributive justice (cf.

Aristotle 1951:book V, 1129a–1135a). Furthermore, from these basic forms on the interpersonal level, which he called "particular justice" *(iustitia particularis)*, Aristotle already distinguished a form of "collective justice" *(iustitia universalis)*, even though he did not really, or at least not very clearly, project that notion onto the subjects of whole political systems or their institutions. Aristotle's conceptions have remained influential up to the present day.

In contemporary theories, most suggestions to differentiate between divisions of justice encompass the notions of (i) distributive, (ii) exchange (viz commutative), (iii) corrective and (iv) political justice. Within these four divisions, several additional distinctions are usually suggested, most of them draw rough conceptual and normative lines between:

- the subjects that are possible addressees or debtors of the duties of justice (e.g. individuals, political systems, states, etc.), or possible bearers of the predicate "just" (e.g. individual character, social institutions, laws and legal orders, court decisions etc.);
- the subjects that are possible addressees or recipients of the benefits of justice (individual persons, groups, social classes, states etc.);
- the basic principles upon which procedures of justice, especially just distributions, are to be grounded (e.g. equality, needs, desert, free-market rules, etc.);
- the objects or goods that are subject to procedures of just distributions (e.g. income, wealth, opportunities, well-being, etc.).

For the purposes of our present study, we may restrict that multiplicity of notions in various ways. First, as far as the divisions of justice are concerned, we have to deal primarily with matters of distributive justice. For this is the only type of justice whose principles might be required in evaluating the potential ramifications of psychic enhancements. Above and beyond that, we must only concern ourselves with certain aspects of political justice: with social effects that a widespread use of techniques of psychic enhancements might produce and that might call for regulations, according to principles of justice, in a well-ordered society.

6.4.7.2 Enhancement Techniques and Distributive Justice

Generally speaking, theories of distributive justice aim at establishing principles of fair distribution of certain benefits and burdens ensuing from interactions between members of cooperative societies. A host of such principles have been proposed in moral, legal and political philosophy, varying in numerous aspects, such as what benefits should be subject to distribution (e.g. income, opportunities, well-being), or what primary criterion or mechanism the process of allocating such benefits should be governed by (e.g. equality, desert, need, free market transactions). Divergent opinions on all of these matters notwithstanding, there is a consensus that not all objects, merely by virtue of having value, are also possible objects of concern for principles of justice. Only "primary social goods", to employ John Rawls' famous term, are proper objects of distributive justice, i.e. goods that are (1) not merely natural endowments and are (2) valuable for every rational member of society, irrespective of his or her individual preferences and personal life plan (cf. Rawls 1971:§ 11:62; § 15:90).

Health care services surely belong among those primary goods. They are socially distributed (and hence are social goods) and they are destined to preserve or restore health, which is an "enabling" (or "all-purpose") precondition for any reasonable life plan of any rational person (and hence are primary goods as well). Rawls, though, did not originally mention them in the index of primary social goods that he provides in his "Theory of Justice". However, in a later reply to objections raised by Amartya Sen, he adjusted this index by pointing out that, on the level of concrete political decisions, it adopts a much greater flexibility than on the level of an abstract theory. On this level, he says, a system of public health care must be included in an enlarged index of primary goods. (cf. Rawls 2001:§ 51.5.–51.7.,171–176).

In contrast, "political justice," as we shall employ the term for purposes of our analysis,[263] encompasses all other tasks of surveying, controlling and, if necessary, correcting social developments in the realm of medicine which actually, or potentially, concern the rights or interests of each individual and of society as a whole.

With regard to questions of distributive justice, i.e. to the just allocation of social primary goods, there does not appear to be any particular normative problems that are specific to the distribution of medical resources in any of the three genuine spheres of medicine, namely treatment (as delineated above), prevention and research. Some of the uncommon intricacies of the new methods of brain intervention may raise the question whether their inclusion in the basic package of medical care that any public health system should provide accords with an appropriate ratio of costs and benefits. In some cases, the wisdom of recognising such interventions as medical treatments may appear doubtful and the matter may certainly be handled differently in different jurisdictions without necessarily raising concerns of justice. However, such problems are common to most, or even all, innovative and technologically complex, (and therefore expensive) medical means. They do not genuinely concern principles of justice but, rather, definitional questions and matters of political and economic prudence. Hence, we shall not address them here.

Difficult problems of justice, however, do arise with respect to enhancements. Two different types might be distinguished. Roughly, they could be labelled the "inequality-exacerbating effect" and the "resource-squandering effect". The problem of the former effect ensues if one, strictly excludes, as we

[263] Note that this use of the term is consistent with its wide-spread use in philosophical discourse, but not with the meaning it bears in Rawls (1971). He uses it as an umbrella concept covering the entire realm of social justice that he concerns himself with, including, above all, the whole range of problems of distributive justice.

suggest one should (cf. 6.3 above), mere enhancements from the publicly funded systems of medicine. In this case only those who can afford to pay for such services will be in a position to benefit from their positive, "mind enhancing" effects. Since most of these services are, and will certainly continue to be, very costly, only well-off people will be able to obtain these benefits. This might exacerbate existing social inequalities. Wealthy people, privileged as they are anyway, are the only ones able to buy these services for themselves or their next of kin, thereby acquiring yet more advantages in many areas of social competition.

If this prospect became reality, it would surely raise serious concerns about distributive justice (cf. Selgelid 2003, for genetic enhancements). Most mental capacities that are positively valued in public or professional life, such as alertness, promptness, accuracy in thinking or (to employ an all-inclusive concept) intelligence, are what economists call "positional goods". This is to say that they confer substantial advantages on their possessors relative to others within the context of social competition for scarce and valued positions and other desired goods. To the extent that basic mental capacities or talents that used to be purely natural assets lose this status and become the objectives of human intervention, the means of obtaining these interventions themselves gradually gain the status of purchasable positional goods. Consequently, they must be given the status of genuine objects of distributive social justice.

This could initiate a spiralling effect. If (1) means of mental enhancements are available only to the wealthy and (2) making use of such means confers substantial competitive advantages for the acquisition of additional advantages, including wealth, and (3) a grossly unequal distribution of wealth is a matter of concern for distributive justice, then the exacerbating effect of artificial mental enhancements on problematic patterns of social distribution is obvious.

As is well known, premise (3) has been subject to controversial philosophical debate for centuries. We could not fruitfully attempt to embark on that discussion here. For the purposes of our inquiry, it should suffice to say the following. Western liberal societies have always experienced unequal distribution of wealth and opportunities. The majority of the population in these societies has come to accept this distributive mechanism as, at least, not completely inconsistent with principles of justice. However, there is little doubt that legislatures even of decidedly liberal states are justified in acting to counterbalance the social effects of dramatically increasing inequalities in wealth amongst their citizens.[264] This is especially true when the driving force behind such tendencies is not grounded in anything like desert on the part of the privileged. This would be the case, by and large, for the positional

[264] Even though some philosophers are very sceptical about that, most prominently so perhaps Nozick (1974).

advantages of artificial mental enhancements, should the social development described above occur in substantial measure. We do not overlook the fact that such enhancements will usually confer the said advantages only in an indirect way which does not exempt the person thus enhanced from the necessity to expend considerable endeavour in order to achieve the desired effect. Yet the positional advantages thus achieved would suffice to make the underlying enhancements problematic under criteria of justice, since the very same amount of endeavour by unenhanced individuals, whose natural intellectual capacities were not originally inferior to those of their now enhanced fellow citizens, could not yield comparably good results.

It is difficult to assess these problems. Much of what a reasonable (and legitimate) strategy for preventing such a social development would have to consider hinges on the empirical probability of the above envisaged undesirable scenario. Regarding this question, we do not have any clear indications yet. However, apart from the lack of current empirical evidence, it does not appear totally improbable that some inequality-exacerbating effect of the kind described above might occur in the future. This is reason enough to invoke a principle of caution again or to raise a moral warning flag. Potential developments such as those described in the preceding paragraphs should be monitored closely by the competent political, scientific and societal institutions. Clear indications that an increasing availability of purchasable mental enhancements might lead to a starkly unequal distribution of wealth and social opportunities, should be counteracted by political and legislative measures (cf. Brock 2003:366; Buchanan et al. 2000:319, both for genetic enhancements). Such measures would, of course, have to meet common criteria of proportionality. Hence their concrete embodiments could be manifold, spreading across a wide spectrum of legal instruments – from tax policies, restrictive licensing practices vis-à-vis medical enhancements, up to the *ultima ratio* of legal prohibition, possibly backed up by a threat of punishment.

It is important to notice that it would not sufficiently satisfy the demands of distributive justice to counteract the above scenario, should it ever occur, through a (partial) redistribution of the unequally accumulated wealth via means of general taxation. A grossly unequal distribution of social opportunities, be they for desired professional positions or other goods relevant to the quality of individual life, usually has additional negative consequences beyond the narrow economic sphere. It also favours an unequal distribution of basic conditions of self-esteem, at least with regard to those who are pushed out of the labour market completely for reasons of not being able to keep up with their artificially enhanced competitors. Such conditions of self-esteem, whatever the exact list of their necessary and sufficient elements, may well constitute, as John Rawls has argued, the most important of all primary goods (cf. Rawls 1971:§ 67:440–446). One of these conditions is, according to all empirical psychological evidence, rooted in the personal experience of serving a social function that is somehow valuable for, and needed by, one's fellow citizens or society as a whole. For most people the possibility of this experience is simply associated with having a job, that is, with the opportunity to earn their living through their own work. This is why the kind of exacerbated inequality that might occur in the wake of a grossly unequal distribution of mental enhancements cannot sufficiently be compensated for by mere financial measures. The often invoked "scandal of liberal economies" – that they usually exclude a significant portion of the population from the labour market – must, to all our present knowledge, be accepted for an as yet indefinite period of time. However, it should not be intensified by avoidable social developments.

The same considerations hold for the question of research into brain-invasive measures exclusively designed to further purposes of mental enhancement. Such research should not be supported through public funding. This would constitute just as great a misallocation of scarce resources, and thus a violation of principles of distributive justice, as would the decision by a publicly funded health insurance system to cover the cost of an actual enhancement procedure. A different matter, though, is basic research destined to clarify the conditions of effectiveness or the pathogenic functions of such enhancement methods. To elucidate this point, one may invoke an analogy from the realm of purely *physical* enhancements. No research aiming at new methods of illegal performance enhancement in sports should be publicly sponsored. However, basic research into the functional and pathogenic mechanisms of such enhancement methods certainly should. None of this suggests a moral verdict on, let alone a call for an outright legal prohibition of, such research. What we wish to emphasise, though, is that it should be left entirely to private enterprise.

Having expounded all of the preceding considerations, however, we now wish to add a twofold *caveat* against adopting interventionist policies too rashly at the present time.

(1) As we said above, whether or not the potential negative developments will become manifest is an empirical question. It cannot be answered by mere theoretical speculations, plausible as they may appear, but must be proven by observable facts. Up to now, such facts have not been established. Even technologically advanced societies with strong inclinations towards science and technological innovations seem, as yet, pretty far from experiencing such detrimental effects on distributive justice. Of course, legitimate policies can, and should, aim at preventing potential undesired developments. However, that requires a complex process of weighing protection against concerns about the possible infringement of civil liberties. This process, in turn, must be based on sufficient information about impending risks. Without such knowledge, rational and proportionate countermeasures are hardly conceivable. The information available for leg-

islators and other political decision makers is clearly insufficient for a sensible assessment of the issue at the present time (cf. Lindsay, 2005, for genetic enhancements). Since political impediments, let alone legal prohibitions, always come at a price for individual and societal liberty, we propose that governments and legislatures currently confine their policies to the procedures of attentive observation that we pointed at above (similarly Mehlman 2004).

(2) This call for political restraint is strengthened by a further thought. As we said in the previous section, certain mental capacities are positional goods, i.e. they confer competitive advantages in numerous contexts of social life. But that is not the whole story. These capacities also have what can be called independent value, i.e. value for the individual life and well-being of their possessor alone (Lindsay 2005). Particularly well-developed cognitive abilities may enable the person endowed with them to successfully participate in competitive enterprises. Yet they can also lay the ground for the development and satisfaction of elaborate intellectual preferences, which serve the wishes for personal enjoyment or favour the fruition of individual inclinations in art, literature or science, with no intent of these being used for economic gain. The freedom of developing one's subjective capacities for a more fulfilling mental life should not be ignored or underestimated. It is, to a large extent, constitutive for the process of building up one's own personal character. The basic preconditions of this process, such as alertness, memory or the ability to concentrate over sufficiently long periods of time, are all-purpose mental capabilities and, as such, are what we have labelled above "output-oriented". This is to say that whatever concrete intellectual or artistic ability one might acquire (at least partly) through artificial enhancement, these all-purpose capabilities are not devalued in the least by such a procedure (cf. our discussion Section 6.4.5 *supra)*.

Both these considerations corroborate the above proposal to refrain at the current time from strictly prohibitive interferences with the development and applications of brain-invasive techniques of mental enhancement. Current policy should be restricted to the role of the keen observer of the social consequences that might ensue from these developing techniques (similarly Buchanan et al. 2000:318–321; Lindsay 2005, both for genetic enhancements[265]).

The second main concern that we formulated above, besides the "inequality exacerbating effect", we called the "resource-squandering" effect. It purports that the utilisation of medical means for mere enhancement purposes amounts to a wastage of scarce life-saving resources in areas beyond therapy or prevention. Note that the justifiability of this reproach does not depend on the question of who pays for the (mis)application of such means.

[265] See also Mehlman 2005, opting *against* the permissibility of genetic enhancements, while opting *for* the permissibility of drug-based enhancement in 2004.

Hence, it is of no relevance that, according to our argument above, it must always be the private recipient of the enhancement, not the socially financed system of health care, who has to bear the immediate cost. Rather, the critique of the research-squandering effect points to the limitation of medical resources in absolute terms. That is to say, it refers to the fact that medical means, including expert manpower, used up for one particular purpose are necessarily unavailable for any other potential application. If they are used for enhancement purposes, the resources thus deployed are not available for use in the much more important area of treatment, where they function as potentially life-saving or health-restoring means. There may not be a concrete link between the particular usage of means in one context, and their abscence from another functional context. Nevertheless, if we take the system of health care as a whole, the said interdependence is inevitable. Or so the argument goes.

This reproach appears conclusive under either of two empirical premises. First, it could rest on the assumption that the entirety of medical resources in a given society is always, or at least normally, subject to a more or less exhaustive demand by that society's members. Consequently, at any given time resources are being utilised to somewhere near their full capacity. The scarcity of medical resources in certain areas notwithstanding, this does not appear to be a very plausible empirical assumption. Another, somewhat weaker premise might claim that the widespread use of medical resources for purposes of mental enhancements actually exerts a noticeable compromising influence on their availability for treatments. In this case too their application for mere enhancements would be, to some extent, parasitic on their primary purpose. This might also be criticised as a violation of principles of distributive justice. After all, not only the application, but also the production of medical resources, is a huge and permanent drain on society's financial resources. Hence, any use of these resources for purposes other than the treatment or prevention of ill-health – the *raison d'être* of the whole system of health care and the principal justification for its maintenance by large public funds – is a misuse of these funds.

This reproach appears plausible, at least to some extent, provided that it rests on a sound empirical basis. Whether or not this is the case, is quite unclear at present. One must not overlook the fact that exactly the same type of resource-squandering effect can be seen in the current practice of cosmetic surgery, which is widely approved of by the public and by the legal systems in western societies. However, this lack of clarity with regard to the empirical premises of the argument is reason enough to raise a moral warning flag once more and to urge close observation of future social developments in this area. It does not, however, presently render sufficient ground for an outright legal prohibition of possible applications of brain interventions for mental enhancement.

6.4.7.3 Mass Enhancements and Political Justice

On several occasions (cf. e.g. Section 6.4.3.2 *supra*), we have already alluded to the risk that a widespread use of brain-invasive mental enhancements might transcend the entire sphere of normative problems associated with their purely individual use. If interventions aimed at an enhancement of certain cognitive capabilities became a social practice undertaken by large numbers of people, this practice might begin to exert a growing pressure on others who are unwilling to undergo such a procedure. For if these dissenters are also disinclined to accept substantial competitive disadvantages in social and professional life, which might be associated with their refusal to undergo enhancement procedures, they are faced with a serious dilemma that is forced on them by the aggregate will of others.

As we argued above, this type of social pressure would not infringe on the dissenters' legal autonomy, even though its origins are not of a natural, but of a man-made kind. Forms of social life that evolve (legally[266]) in a society are simply part of the objective environment of an individual, just as his or her natural surroundings are. The former do not affect someone's legal autonomy any more than the latter, regardless of how irresistible their influence on the individual's decisions might be.[267] Hence, the social pressure placed on some people in the wake of a widespread practice of self-enhancements in others, would not touch upon the validity of their (albeit unwillingly given) consent, should they in the end concede and undergo such a brain-invasive procedure themselves.

However, the legal rules structuring interpersonal relations are only part of the story. The state's (viz the legislature's) undeniable right – even its *prima facie* duty (within certain limits set by the constraints of its own discretionary power) – to interfere in such social developments in order to shield its citizens from coercive societal demands is also of relevance in this instance. A collective pressure to undergo physically invasive procedures bears considerably more weight than, say, the coercive effect of a largely motorised society on its members to obtain a drivers license and use a car in order to remain competitive in one's professional life. Given the primary importance of the state's duty to protect the life and health of its citizens, even an indirect and mediated danger to physical integrity of the kind we are currently assessing demands careful scrutiny. The state must take on that challenge and address the question of whether or not to block the (albeit indirect) danger to people's physical integrity by means of legal prohibitions.

Again, the plausibility of postulating a more or less immediate prohibition of such interventions by the state hinges upon the empirical question of

[266] Criminal subcultures (e.g. the Mafia), even though they operate on a mass scale, always act beyond the normative boundaries of society. The influence they might exert on others to act contrary to the law remains, of course, criminal duress.

[267] A brief glance at the phenomenon of fashion trends may serve to illustrate the point. Decisive as their influence on many people's decisions may be, it does not in any way affect the status of these decisions as being legally autonomous.

whether the said social pressure for mental enhancement is actually going to emerge. This again cannot presently be predicted with anything approaching certainty. However, nor can it be excluded with any great deal of certainty either. This is reason enough for a final, and particularly important, warning flag in the realm of social justice. The possibility of an impending threat on people's liberty to abstain from brain-invasive enhancements should be subject to especially vigilant monitoring by competent political authorities and scientific institutions. Should clear indications of such a development in sufficiently large social dimensions emerge, then intervention by the state to protect those citizens who decide against undergoing brain-invasive enhancements seems imperative.[268]

However, unless there is evidence of this kind of development, outright prohibitions should be withheld. A completely abstract risk provision by legal measures against unwanted but uncertain social threats, the possible effects of which could still be blocked effectively if or when they occur, is not justified in constitutional liberal states. Even the most plausible aspiration to protect the liberty of individuals to abstain from mental enhancements must not lead the state to ignore the associated costs in terms of the individual liberty of others, namely those who would seek such an enhancement and who would claim their (undisputed) constitutional right to dispose of their own physical and mental matters in the way they themselves choose to. Thus, if the envisaged negative development should occur, it will still pose difficult problems of weighing conflicting interests for the legislators. How these problems are to be solved, cannot be debated on the general level of the present analysis. As always, it will be a matter of prudently weighing up the potential positive and negative effects of any concrete solution proposed.

At least a passing mention should be made of one final problem of political justice that might ensue from the prospective practice of mental enhancements: a particular form of misallocation of costly medical resources. Granted (counterfactually) that no significant opposition against that practice would arise and granted, furthermore (counterfactually again), that it was possible to safeguard equal access for all citizens to the new enhancement methods, this might yet be prone to create a new and specific problem of wasting medical resources. It would possibly establish a tendency for those enhancing measures to be self-defeating. As we said above, enhanced mental features are primarily, albeit not exclusively, positional advantages. Thus, if everyone has them, they lose their character as advantages. This might not be bad in itself. However, the misallocation of expensive medical and research resources that this entails is fairly obvious. One

[268] Decidedly so Selgelid (2003) and Mehlman (2003), both, however, debating such a social pressure originating from a widespread practice of *genetic* enhancements, which would certainly amount to a much more profound threat to people's liberty and physical integrity than mental enhancements through brain interventions.

could, perhaps, counter this concern with the overall positive effect on society's well-being that might result from a mass enhancement of mental capabilities of its citizens, even if it conferred no positional advantage on any individual person anymore. However, a new form of positional advantage might even ensue from such a practice. Whilst no advantage would be gained by individuals competing against others within their society, there would be a potential advantage gained by that society as a whole in terms of its ability to compete with other societies in foreign states. The argument, somewhat crudely stated, is that a considerable lift of the average I.Q. of an entire population could certainly confer a positional advantage on that state in the arena of international affairs.

However, most of this is still mere speculation (although by no means implausible). This supports our general proposal to monitor current developments closely, and to be prepared to act prudently, and in good time, should any of these undesired consequences occur.

6.5 Enhancing the Mental Features in Others

Such enhancements raise particular problems if and when exerted on people not in a position to give informed consent. The paradigm group that comes to mind is, of course, children. The basic question then is whether parents should be allowed to have their offspring mentally enhanced by artificial interventions and whether such decisions should be dictated by the parents alone?

However, children are not the only group of people to fall under the above heading. As far as mentally disabled or otherwise ill persons are concerned, one would normally consider interventions destined to improve their situation treatments, not just enhancements, the gliding spectrum between these two concepts notwithstanding (cf. 6.3 *supra*). For this reason, we will not specifically deal with problems concerning this group here.[269] However, there is a third group of interest to us here, namely detainees in prison. Consider, for example, the following scenario: Someone who committed a severe crime does not only have to serve his sentence, but is confronted with the bleak possibility of remaining detained indefinitely because he has been deemed a threat to society.[270] Psychiatrists describe the source of

[269] Of course, one could think of far fetched examples such as enhancing certain psychic features of a mentally disabled person that are not connected with her disability. However, these are rather artificial thought experiments, far removed from real-life problems, so we will not deal with them here.

[270] Most developed systems of criminal law today differentiate between imprisonment as punishment, imposed for a culpably committed crime, and detention, as a preventive measure, possibly imposed for the time after a completed sentence, simply for the fact that someone continues to pose a danger and without any (further) culpable deed on his part as a necessary normative ground for this detention. This is sometimes referred to as the "two-tracked structure" of the criminal law (cf. in the German Criminal Code §§ 61 et sequ.).

his dangerousness as a manifest sociopathy, rooted in various character traits that can be identified individually. Mental enhancement techniques of various kinds have developed tremendously over the preceding years. The experts say that there is a very good prospect of treating the detainee's sociopathy successfully by giving him a range of powerful new psychotropic drugs and/or intervening into his brain by using other, more direct measures.

The scenario raises a host of different questions. Isn't what the psychiatrists suggest just treatment of an illness ("sociopathy")? Are there any differences between interventions of the suggested kind and ordinary, traditional treatments of prison inmates? What if the detainee refuses to give consent? Could he, under any circumstances, be subjected to forced treatment (or enhancement depending on how it is to be defined)? What if he does not refuse consent? Could his consent, under the specific circumstances, be considered to be "freely given", where the only alternative he had was to remain in detention indefinitely? Is it legitimate for the state to make offers that are, in the above sense, necessarily coercive to some extent? Finally, considering this coercion, what about possibly grave side effects that might occur after such an intervention? Would responsibility for them fall on the coercer?

6.5.1 The Mental Enhancement of Children

We restrict the following analysis to the paradigm case of personal relationships where decisions to intervene in a child's physical or psychic integrity may occur, namely the relationship between children and their parents.[271] There are, of course, other personal or institutional settings where such decisions may also be taken. However, these do not seem to pose any additional normative problems; so we can safely disregard them here. We will also not take up again the problem of possible normative objections against the new means of mental enhancement (or their alleged consequences) *just in themselves,* for instance the feared social devaluation of the desired ends for which those means might be employed. The questions involved here do not appear to differ in any important respect when those means are applied to children instead of adults. So in the case of these problems, we may just simply refer the reader to our analysis above. On the other hand, what is certainly very different from the case of adults is the question of the possible side effects of such enhancement strategies. Consequently, we will deal briefly with that problem once more in our present context.

A few preliminary distinctions seem in place to provide us with an initial overview of the range of problems that we encounter here. First, we must recall and re-emphasise our basic normative distinction: that between law and ethics. What might be morally objectionable or, at least, undesirable as

[271] The latter may be genetic, biological, adoptive or foster parents. For the purpose of our enquiry there is no normative difference between these types of parenthood.

an educational measure might still be legally allowed or perhaps granted as a parental right.[272] Furthermore, within both normative spheres we want to distinguish four abstract levels and, on each of them, contrast two concrete types of problem:

- First, on the level of the parent-child relationship, the right of parents to define which goals, values and orientations they want to guide their children's lives, and their complementary right to decide on and implement the educational measures they consider necessary or useful to achieve those goals, must be weighed against the protected rights of children that parents have a duty not to infringe upon.
- Second, on the level of the methods of intervention to be employed, enhancement measures that aim at improving specific mental features (like, for instance, musical talent), correlated with only particular goals of human acting (a career as a musician)[273], versus "general-purpose means" (Buchanan et al. 2000:167), destined to improve basic, abstract capabilities underlying most or all specific cognitive performances, and thus being valuable for any life plan (for instance, memory, alertness, the ability to concentrate and the like).
- Third, on the level of possible consequences, interventions with effects that are limited in time, or at least reversible in principle, versus interventions with expectedly permanent and irreversible consequences.
- And fourth, on the level of possible targets of an intervention, enhancements of a child's cognitive abilities, versus enhancements of his or her mood or motivational states. It is not clear from the outset that normative questions possibly raised by these types of intervention should be the same for all of them.

6.5.1.1 Questions of Law and Legal Principles

Normatively speaking, in modern liberal democracies the parent-child relationship is basically constituted by three components (cf. Noggle 2002:97):

(1) A parental *duty* to observe and protect their children's rights and to promote their children's perspectives for positive personal development.
(2) A parental *right* to decide on and choose their own preferred ways of raising and educating their offspring, thereby shaping the physical and mental "being" of their children in many important respects.
(3) A corresponding parental *authority* to enforce those decisions vis-à-vis their children and to exercise (moderate) coercive measures on them for that purpose.

[272] Even the reverse may be true: what is legally forbidden might not raise objections from a moral point of view.
[273] Notwithstanding the fact, of course, that presently there are very few (if any) enhancement methods available that can specifically target particular features like artistic or mathematical talent.

As far as right (2) is concerned, the law in most well-ordered, modern societies grants great discretion to parents to choose and prescribe the course of education for their children. Usually the respective basic choices are taken by selecting, modifying or else banning numerous environmental contexts and factors that children are engaged in or come in contact with, which could exert relevant influences on them. In numerous liberal legal orders, such as in Germany, this broad authority to decide on such factors is a fundamental constitutional right of parents. It is, of course, subject to certain constraints. These are marked by the protective boundaries of the children's own constitutional rights which parents have a duty to observe (listed in point 1 above) and the state is obliged to safeguard or, if necessary, to enforce.

The last sentence may give the somewhat misleading impression of a primarily confrontational relationship between these two domains of rights. However, one very important idea in the normative underpinnings of these parental rights is the assumption that, at least in well functioning families, children also benefit enormously from their parents' having the above rights. Besides the basic experience of love and trust, children need guidance and orientation in various important respects in order to be able to develop their own personalities and the capacity to lead their own, autonomous lives in society later on. It is probably undisputed that (at least under relatively normal familial circumstances) it is those towards whom children usually display their most fundamental natural experience, that of love and trust, who are best-suited to provide the guidance that is necessary for a child to flourish physically and mentally. In that respect, parent's and children's rights simply coincide. The setting in which this process takes place must, for obvious reasons, be granted a considerable amount of protection from any external control over the relevant parental decisions.

However, there must also be limits. In taking decisions about their children's welfare, parents are not allowed to foreseeably cause considerable harm to their children's present well-being and future perspectives. As far as this prohibition is concerned, though, one needs to distinguish between two types of harm: physical and mental harm. Legally, parents do not have the right to cause any physical harm to their children, whether it be actively brought about or passively allowed to occur.[274] However, they certainly do have the legal authority to intentionally direct their children's mental devel-

[274] To be sure, parents certainly do have the right to expose their children to moderate *risks* associated with the normal course of a child's development and education, which could possibly lead to minor injuries or illnesses like small lesions caused by a fall from the bicycle or a cold resulting from a skiing or an ice-skating trip. However, stated more precisely, what are permitted are not the injuries themselves but only the risks that may eventually lead to them. Consequently, the parents are "distanced" from the harmful results, i.e. the latter are not legally attributed to the parents' behaviour.

opment in a direction that most reasonable observers would deem psychologically harmful.

The famous American case of the community of the so-called Old Amish Order may serve to illustrate this point. The Amish sect, for religious reasons, claimed the right to restrict schooling for their children to 14 years of age, two years less than was required by state law. The motive behind this claim was to ensure the prospect of a modest agrarian life for their children, "aloof from the world and its values", as the Supreme Court of the United States formulated it in its 1972 ruling on the case (Wisconsin v. Yoder 406 U.S. 205 [1972]:210). The deliberate aim of the Amish was to close off any other future option beyond that agrarian life for their offspring. After having been denied such a right by the Kansas Supreme Court, "they won a resounding victory in the Supreme Court" six years later (Feinberg 1992:76, 83). It is certainly not too malicious a formulation to call this the granting of a parental right to inflict some (largely "mental") kind of harm onto their children by substantially curtailing their future chance of an autonomous choice about how to lead their own lives. We do not want to suggest that the decision was wrong.[275] Maybe it was not. What we want to point out is the width of the scope of parental discretionary authority. Even the deliberate shaping of one's children's character in ways that most reasonable people would consider seriously harmful for their own children does not necessarily exclude such actions from the realm of legitimate parental behaviour. The legal problem for the respective state institutions to draw a reasonable line between the protection of children from harm and protection of their parents' freedom to implement choices about the most fundamental impacts on the "bodies and souls" of their children can pose very difficult questions. As the Amish case demonstrates, that is, of course, a general problem. So we need not go into any further detail here.

Taken as an illustration for the point we want to make here, the Amish example suffers from one particular, if minor, flaw. The right of the Amish to raise their children according to their own values is not only an individual right of parents. Rather, in this particular case the parental rights are, or were, supported by the rights of the entire group to their cultural and religious identity. These rights certainly entitle the Amish to reasonable measures of securing their continued existence as a group. Perhaps such considerations were even part of the decisive aspects of the Supreme Court's decision in "Yoder". Now, questions of group rights would certainly not normally be involved in individual decisions of parents to enhance the mental capacities of their children (though they might be involved in individual Amish parents' decisions to do the opposite to their children). However, this particular weakness of our analogy does not render it useless or implausible for our purpose. Though the contribution of the group-rights dimension to the

[275] Joel Feinberg thought it was; cf. Feinberg o. cit., 84–87.

field of individual rights of parents who belong to a cultural minority must not be discounted, its significance should not be overstated either. What group rights add to the process of weighing parental rights to educate their children against the children's own rights not to be seriously harmed are typical utilitarian considerations to the effect of somewhat increasing the weight of rights on the side of the parents. From a legal perspective, sheer utility based concerns or interests can usually not outweigh basic individual rights. Since what is at stake on the other side of the weighing process are the constitutional, individual rights of children, the extraweight of the utilitarian argument brought to bear on the side of the parents might suffice to tip the scales in cases of otherwise nearly equal positions. However, it could certainly not make the decisive difference to overturn children's rights that can otherwise claim clear pre-eminence over those of their parents. Thus, utility based arguments could not have played that sort of decisive role in "Yoder" either. There are certainly no such group rights which can infringe upon basic rights of the group's individual members simply for the purpose of securing the continuity of some cultural trait of the group that the respective individuals wish to ignore or escape from. So the Supreme Court's decision in "Yoder", yielding to the Amish parents' rights, serves as an apt example to demonstrate the far-reaching discretionary powers that parents also have in normal cases of educating their children according to their own preferences, even where there are no group-rights aspects involved.

The most obvious question that arises for our analysis out of these considerations is whether the right of parents to choose what they consider "best" for their children's development encompasses the competence to apply intrusive medical means for the sole purpose of enhancing their children's mental capacities? If it does in principle, where are the limits to such a competence? It should be born in mind that we are currently considering these questions from the perspective of the principles of law and not from the standpoint of ethics. Consequently, it is difficult to imagine any even halfway realistic case where a parental decision to have a particular mental capacity of their child enhanced, could transgress the legal boundaries of parental authority and infringe upon the child's right to be free from the infliction of serious mental "harm" simply (and only) as a result of bringing about of this enhanced feature. (The issue of the potential physical side effects of such a procedure is a different matter and we will come to it shortly.)

Certainly, if evaluated as improvements, enhancements of mental capacities are relative in at least a twofold sense. First, they are relative to a set of basic values which allow for the identification of the respective enhanced capacity as desirable, i.e. as an improvement. Second, they are relative to other mental features, in the sense that the enhancement of a desired property x may only be possible at the expense of some other property y which, in itself, is also judged favourably by reasonable standards. However, in both respects parents have a wide discretionary power to decide on the principal orientation of their children's development. We will illustrate this point with a scientifically unrealistic, but very graphic, example. If, for example, parents of an Amish background desire the features of humbleness and modesty for their children, they are in principle entitled to take a course of action designed to bring those features about and to accept the associated trade-offs with other capacities. (As far as they were to employ only traditional educational measures, nobody would seriously doubt that they were acting within their rights.) However, if the most effective way to bring about this desired result is a pharmacologic intervention in the CNS, parents are also entitled – assuming there to be no physical side effects for the time being – to authorise that intervention, even if it were irrevocable in its psychological effect. This parental authority is not restricted by the foreseeable consequence that this intervention (let us assume for arguments sake) will foreclose the development of other mental features which, judged on the ground of different values, are also favourable properties to have, such as intellectual alertness, artistic creativity and professional competitiveness. One should not overlook that these closed-off consequence might just as well occur if the parents only employ traditional means of education, which they are undisputedly allowed to do.

From a moral point of view, such a parental course of shaping, or rather curtailing, a child's future raises more serious concerns. We will deal with them later in the current chapter. However, the law's tolerance towards parental rights is wide enough to enclose such a far-reaching authority.

A different matter, as we already mentioned in passing, is the question of physical side effects of this type of enhancing strategy. Parents are, in principle, only allowed to authorise medical interventions to the advantage of their children. In cases of treatment of diseases this encompasses the acceptance of a reasonable risk-benefit ratio of medically directed measures. It may, therefore, justify even serious risks of grave physical harm in respectively serious cases of illness.

In the case of the Amish people, detailed above, this means that the mere modification of certain neurostructures in the child's brain, that are directly correlated with a desired characteristic, cannot be considered a disadvantageous physical intrusion. Thus, it cannot be prohibited as long as the associated feature is not itself harmful to the child. Other physical side effects must also satisfy the criteria of a reasonable risk-benefit ratio. It is important to mark clearly the three main features of this particular risk-benefit ratio of enhancement interventions:

- First, it obviously cannot be the same as in treatment cases.
- Second, the benefit to be taken into account is not the final end of the intervention, i.e. not the psychic trait desired by the parents for their child (in our Amish-like example: humbleness and modesty). The law neutrally

tolerates this end, but without judging, let alone endorsing it from a normative point of view.[276]

– Third, the value to be inserted into the risk-benefit calculation is, therefore, solely the parental freedom to make choices of the said kind for their children.

This freedom does not justify the deliberate infliction of physical harm of any considerable weight. It does, though, encompass the acceptance of certain serious risks of very moderate harms (as well as very moderate risks of more serious harms) associated with the course of normal or universally acceptable measures of education. A mother determined to fostering a sense of altruism in her ten year old son may, for example, make him crawl into a narrow hole in the ground to rescue the neighbour's daughter's kitten, even though she knows with near certainty that this will lead to her son receiving scratches and bruises in following her command.

This example, trivial as it is, may serve as a paradigm for shedding some light on what a justified risk-benefit ratio in educational measures with foreseeable consequences of physical harm might look like. Note that there is a sliding scale of mutual interdependence between risk on the one hand and educational benefit on the other. The acceptable potential harm may be somewhat greater if the risk of its coming about is vague and small. It is important, though, that this mutual interdependence is only acceptable within a relatively small part of the range of overall possibilities. Real risks of serious physical harm as foreseeable consequences of educational measures cannot be justified at all, regardless of where exactly one wants to draw the line where such "seriousness" begins. Of course, there is always a risk of serious harm, even death, arising accidentally out of even the most mundane everyday practices of normal parenthood. As long as these practices remain within the limits of "normality" – like, for instance, letting one's twelve year old ride his bike in public traffic – they are part of the ubiquitous "permissible risk" of living and acting in a complex and therefore dangerous world. Catastrophic results of that normality are misfortunes, not matters of the legal responsibility of parents.

Now we have laid out the basic normative framework to deal with the problem of physical side effects foreseeably associated with mental enhancement measures. Again, there is no clear-cut formal apparatus to deliver solutions for concrete cases. However, two consequences of our analysis should have become sufficiently clear. First, that mere enhancement measures are to be considered parental idiosyncrasies, neutrally accepted by the law as part of parental discretional authority, but not, in themselves, legally valued (even if they were doubtlessly valuable from an ethical point of view). Second, exactly for this reason, risks of physical side effects are, in principle, only tolerable

[276] It only judges whether or not the limits of parental discretionary power have been transgressed.

within the very narrow limits that regularly confine the acceptability of negative physical consequences of educational measures. A somewhat futuristic example can help to illustrate this point. A major surgery to implant some cognition enhancing device in the brain of a normal child would not be acceptable on current legal principles, even if it caused no significant further risk beyond the immediate injury associated with the intrusive operation itself. The latter alone suffices to make the intervention illegitimate.

These are the substantive rules and principles which a physician should observe when confronted with the urge of parents to help them in enhancing some mental feature of their child. If those rules are neglected, the "informed consent" given by the parents will not exonerate the physician from her own responsibility. For only within their own normative limits of parental discretionary authority are parents in a position to give a valid proxy consent for their children.[277]

All of this does not yield any easy decisions for concrete cases. Our framework contains more than one concept falling across a rather wide spectrum of different possible meanings. This is especially true for the basic concepts of treatment and enhancement themselves. If applied to mental features, they exhibit a range of gradual transitions of one into the other on a rather wide scale of possibilities. Furthermore, in real-life cases all of those notions, so to speak, interact normatively. So what they may require is a very complex process of integrating a set of different, but interdependent, judgments each of which must be pinned down to a conceptual scale which allows for numerous gradations. One may justly say that quite a bit of Kantian "Urteilskraft" ("power of judgment") is again called for to come to reasonable solutions in concrete cases.

6.5.1.2 Ethical Questions

Unlike our legal reasoning, the ethical analysis is not primarily concerned with the normative authority of parents to shape their children's mental development. Rather, it tries to clarify the criteria of a morally good, or at least morally acceptable, decision within that scope of parental authority. The main ethical question, therefore, does not concern the limits of the permissible – as judged from the outside, according to confining norms of the law. Rather, it concerns the preconditions of the good – as judged from the inside, according to guiding moral norms for the individual actor. Loosely stated, the emphasis on the educational maxims for parents shifts, to a certain extent, from the *negative* – "don't transgress your limits in child rearing!" – to the *positive* – "do the (morally) right thing in shaping your children's future!" Of course, this also encompasses a negative duty to observe and not transgress the moral limits of parents' discretionary power. As far as this is concerned, it is rather obvious that the moral limits of what *ought* to

[277] This question must not be confused with the quite different question of which harmful deeds are prohibited despite a valid, informed consent by the *addressee* of the respective action. See the above analysis.

be done are considerably narrower than the legal limits of what *can* be done without interference by the state. Therefore, some educational measures to direct – and foreclose – one's children's future (such as those in the Amish community) might still be perfectly legal while at the same time clearly constituting a serious moral wrong.

Normally, parents' endeavours to do "the best" for their offspring are not only permissible but laudable.[278] This "best" includes all kinds of reasonable support for the development of their children's physical and mental capacities. This goes without saying for parental attempts to ensure environmental conditions that are most favourable to the enhancement of the said capacities. In his book *Clones, Genes, and Immortality,* John Harris sets forth the following scenario:

Suppose a school were to set out deliberately to improve the mental and physical capacities of its students, suppose its stated aims were to ensure that the pupils left the school not only more intelligent and more physically fit than when they arrived, but more intelligent and more physically fit than they would be at any other school. (Harris 1998:171)

Is there anything wrong with that project? One might, as Harris points out, wonder what sacrifices the children are expected to make to achieve those ambitious goals. However, that does not cast any doubt on the value of the goals themselves. Assume that the school manages to establish and safeguard a well-balanced ratio of sacrifices and achievements in the curriculum of all of its students. It appears, then, that the whole enterprise would be highly laudable, not only from a pragmatic, but also from an ethical, point of view. Would we reverse our judgment on the laudability of these goals if we learned that their supremacy (over an otherwise quite normal educational program) was only achieved by medical, or pharmacologic, interventions into the students' bodies and brains?

We have already dealt with the major implications of this question including the. possible objections against such practices (concerns of safety, autonomy, corruption, fairness, and numerous society interests). We found that, apart from athletic and artistic capacities, there are no convincing legal or ethical arguments to rule out such enhancement strategies *in principle* or even to vote for them being legally banned, even though quite a few normative warning flags should certainly be raised at certain points,. Our analysis

[278] Notwithstanding the fact that parents are not morally *obliged* to aim at "the best" (whatever that might be) for their children, but only to provide for as good an education and as decent a perspective of development as is reasonably compatible with their own legitimate interests. This seems in fact to be contradicted by Art. 6 (2) of the "UN Convention on the Right of the Child" (1990), which demands from state parties that they not only ensure "the survival", but also the "development" of every child "to the maximum extent possible". However, on a literal reading this cannot not be taken seriously as it amounts to a patent impossibility and has nothing to do with fundamental legal principles of the state. Consequently, it must be seen as little more than a useless piece of political rhetoric.

dealt with the typical case of a normal adult consumer of such enhancement practices. Now we want to clarify the ethical problems raised by enhancements of children according to parental decisions.[279]

Note that in the present context we are no longer concerned with the principled questions listed in the above paragraph and elsewhere, even though all of them certainly arise in the parent-children perspective as well. To the extent we have been able to answer these questions, we now rely simply on our results. In particular, let us briefly recall that, as far as parent's pursuits of their children's well-being are concerned, we do not acknowledge any a priori normative difference between (allegedly) purely environmental modifications, such as providing for the resources of a good education, and direct physical or mental interventions destined to further the same objective. Many parental decisions to develop their children's capacities by modifying environmental factors, such as nutrition, athletic education, etc., actually amount to modifying the phenotype of their offspring as well (cf. Buchanan et al. 2000:159). Furthermore, neuroscientists assure us that every environment based influence on a child's mental states is associated with a modification of her brain states. Hence, influencing such a brain state directly by a medical intervention cannot plausibly be rejected solely in virtue of its being a modification of the child's body instead of her environment.

We conclude that there are, in principle, conceivable methods of a medical enhancement of mental capacities that meet all the required normative constraints on such methods: safety, fairness, societal concerns, etc. No principled objections, therefore, appear to stand in the way of parents' decisions to apply such measures to their offspring. What we want to explore now in more detail are the ethical criteria by which parents should make their choices. Stated from a different perspective, we turn now to the moral preconditions which such enhancement methods have to meet in order to be ethically acceptable.

Joel Feinberg, commenting on the above-mentioned Amish case more than 25 years ago, coined the phrase "the child's right to an open future" (Feinberg 1992:76–97). This phrase aptly, though somewhat abstractly, catches a very basic idea. In some sense it seems to underlie the whole range of specifically educational obligations that parents have towards their children. Parents are certainly not morally required to always pursue what is "best" for their children.[280] They have legitimate interests of their own and

[279] One could, of course, widen the scope of the present inquiry by posing the further question whether parents could even be morally *required* to employ enhancement techniques for their offspring. We will, however, omit this question from our discussion. We do not believe, though, that, for the typical parent-child relationship, there are good arguments for an affirmative answer.

[280] Apart from the very difficult questions of what "the best" would be in a complex world, full of possible options for a child's development and who should (and by which substantive criteria) decide about that.

these might now and then collide with and sometimes outweigh their children's interests. They usually have moral obligations and commitments towards other people too and they may certainly claim respect for their attempts to meet those additional duties. However, what remains constant throughout all the imaginable conflicts of interests between parents and their offspring is the fundamental moral obligation of the former to safeguard their children's development towards a future of their own choosing. This future will only be "open" if it holds the chance for their children to develop their own authentic, autonomous self. And this can only be the case if their education does not foreclose too many options for them to make life- and character-forming choices of their own. Put in these abstract terms, this may well yield the most fundamental moral maxim that ought to guide parents' educational decisions.

However, it is clearly very difficult to flesh this abstract principle out in any detail. Let's take the Amish case as our example once again. Legally, Amish parents were granted the right to direct their children's futures in the way we described above. However, that only delineated the scope of parental rights, it did not speak to the question of moral claims of children against their parents. There are good reasons to assume that, within the scope of those legal rights, the educational practices of Amish parents violate the justified moral claims of their children. Feinberg thinks, as we noted above, that these practices violated the children's legally protected rights and that the Supreme Court's decision, therefore, violated those rights too. We are uncertain about that. However, we do agree with Feinberg that the said Amish education is or, at any rate was[281], a violation of their offspring's ethical rights to an open future. The main reason for this conclusion is that the said practice of education not only forces the development of the children onto a rigid and extremely narrow path, it also largely excludes them from receiving the necessary capabilities to reflect on their own biographical past, their future perspectives, their life plans, their underlying values and to take a critical stance towards them.

If we project this onto the question of enhancing children's mental features, it suggests an important distinction between specified capacities for particular psychic traits and capacities for "general-purpose means".[282] For the precondition of a person's ability to become autonomous in a sense deserving of that label, i.e. of her ability to make use of her "open future" and to lead her own life, is a sufficient amount of such general-purpose means. These are basic human capacities, useful, and to some extent necessary, for nearly every conceivable life plan that human beings might want to pursue. The presence of general-purpose means, or of a sufficient part of them, thus

[281] We do not know whether the said educational practices are still present in the Amish community.

[282] This is our second distinction (cf. 6.5.1 supra) following Buchanan et al. 2000:167.

belongs to the "enabling conditions" of health, specifying its status as a "transcendental good" in the life of practically all human beings.[283] The complete or, at any rate, inadequate absence of such enabling conditions is, therefore, usually and uncontroversially taken to be a disease or a disability. Typical examples at hand are the physical ability of moving one's limbs or the sensory capacities of hearing and of seeing.[284]

As far as mental capacities are concerned, one would certainly include basic cognitive capacities in that list. A certain minimum level of understanding, of memory, of reasonable adaptation to the everyday challenges of the social world, of the ability to engage in communicative interactions with others by using language or other symbols with semantic meaning and the like. Such capacities are general-purpose means in the obvious sense that being in the possession of a sufficient amount of them is a precondition of mental health for every human being, while lacking certain basic capacities is, consequently, considered a disease or a disability. If we think now of a specific mental ability like, for instance, musical or poetic or mathematical talent, even the complete absence of any vestige of a level of ability that could justly be called a "talent" of that kind would *not* be considered a disability.[285] Thus, having such a particular mental feature is not a "transcendental" good of human life. To put this in perspective with our present reasoning, it is not a condition of the "openness" of a child's future.

Here we find the link to our enhancement debate. Since possessing general-purpose mental capacities is a condition of mental health and, therefore, of one's present or future autonomy in the full sense of the term, the enhancement of such features, far from being a threat to a child's open future, rather seems to contribute to that openness. "Transcendental" capacities in the said sense do not foreclose the pursuit of any particular life plan, whatever specific mental features it might presuppose. For such capacities are, as we have pointed out, enabling conditions, underlying all conceivable life plans. So there is, in principle, no objection to the permissibility of such enhancements.[286]

---

[283] For this terminology see the above discussion in Section 6.3.4.

[284] We disregard here the (otherwise important) debate as to what extent the absence of certain physical or mental abilities really is a kind of natural phenomenon of impairment, rather than a *socially induced* form of disability. The complete absence of basic human capacities like those listed above is, undoubtedly, a disabling condition in any conceivable form of social life, notwithstanding the fact that societies can significantly enlarge or diminish the extent of its disabling function for the lives of afflicted persons.

[285] Provided, of course, that it is not due to a complete lack of general-purpose capacities in the said sense. In that case, the lack of the respective general-purpose abilities would be the real disease or disability.

[286] Recall that, in the present context, we only deal with the plausibility of such principled objections, ignoring all possible "secondary" objections like safety or society concerns and such like.

This might be different with enhancements of specific mental capacities like the above-mentioned particular talents. Since the human mind (or, in any case, an individual human life) provides only limited scope for the range of options one can reasonably choose to develop, any particular development of a specific mental feature comes at some, albeit often minimal, expense of alternative possibilities. The more such a specific trait is cultivated, and the greater the share it claims of one's mind and lifetime, the smaller the remaining space becomes for alternative options. If one pursues a career as a (possibly world-famous) pianist, committing oneself to decades of practicing the piano six to eight hours a day, one certainly closes off most, if not all, possibilities of an alternative self-realisation or fulfillment in one's professional life.

It goes without saying that the above is not meant as a criticism. On the contrary, it belongs to the core content of any reasonable conception of autonomy that one be able to develop and shape the features of one's own personality and to make substantial commitments to realise one's life plans. What we want to point out, instead, is that if a specific mental property that steers a person's life in one particular direction, rather than another, is firmly implanted into that person's mind very early in childhood, then the possibility of choosing a different path later in life might be foreclosed long before her mental development has reached anywhere near the level of development required for autonomous decision making. (It is precisely this fact that the Amish people rely on when dictating the length of schooling of their children). Thus, if parents try to establish narrow and irrevocable tracks for their later development very early in their children's lives, they at the same time objectively pursue a course of closing off future options for their children. This is in principle inconsistent with an ethic of respect for the persons their children are or will become. This conclusion does not rest upon any consideration of whether the established, irreversible track chosen by the parents is one that many people might judge trivial or narrow-minded (as many people would perhaps find the Amish way of life to be) or, in contrast, one that many people would find highly admirable (like the career of the concert pianist). All that matters is that the child develops the basic ability, in her adult life, to autonomously accept, modify or reject the original parental preferences of what her life should be like.

Of course, this is not to say that parents should not try to direct their children's lives onto particular paths. Rather, the contrary is true. What it does mean, though, is that parents should, along with their own ideas about their children's future, try to promote at the same time their children's basic capacities to either autonomously endorse the original parental arrangements or take a critical stance towards them in their later lives.

All of this has a bearing on our normative analysis of the enhancement problem. The more clearly a mental feature belongs to the range of enabling conditions of autonomy, or of general-purpose psychic capacities of persons, the less problematic is the decision to have this capacity enhanced in one's child by a medical intervention.[287] For such a capacity strengthens rather than counteracts the child's moral right to an open future. Seen the other way around, the more specified a mental feature is, thereby setting a firm course for the child's entire future, the more a moral warning flag must be raised regarding any decision to have that feature enhanced by artificial means.

A final but, nevertheless, crucial *caveat* is in order here. All substantive processes of a child's development and education take place within a very complex interplay of numerous circumstances, be they material or metaphysical in nature. Thus, our normative framework above must, at least to some extent, be capable of absorbing and reflecting that complexity. Furthermore, most or all of the basic elements constituting this complex setting fall across a wide range of degrees. All of this renders the idea of an exact calculation of the "good" or "right" educational measures at any given time in a child's development, and thus an ethic of child-rearing, completely illusory. What we have tried to develop, instead, is a basic normative conceptional framework, whose basic function is not so much to deliver answers, but to help generate them for any particular moral question that might arise in the context of enhancing mental traits in children.

6.5.2 The Mental Enhancement of Detainees in Prison

Therapeutic brain intervention undertaken on an (otherwise competent) person, who is presently detained in prison or subjected to another form of legally justified custody, are prone to raise doubts about that person's ability to consent freely to the measure. Given the particular circumstances, can this consent be truly autonomous, and thus legally valid? Before attempting to give an answer, we should define the question more precisely. The first scenario to envisage is the standard situation of an illness manifesting itself during a legal term of imprisonment and treatable by a brain intervention. This poses no particular problem. There is, as we said, no legitimate way of forcing treatment on competent persons. This pertains no less to prisoners than to any other people. However, problems do arise in other settings. If and when (1) the detained person has served his full term of legal punishment but (2) remains in custody (so-called preventive detention) because (3) he exhibits a severe form of sociopathy, which renders him a permanent danger to his fellow citizens, but (4) which could possibly be treated by a novel method of brain intervention.

We are quite aware that the current projection of such a medical possibility has an air of science fiction about it. However, this may very well change in the not too distant future. Thus we shall attempt to explore the normative problems it raises. Do the alternatives presented to such a sociopath, to undergo the said brain intervention or remain detained indefinitely, leave

[287] Only, of course, within the boundaries developed in our legal analysis above.

room on his part to make an autonomous decision and to give valid consent to such an intervention?

The answer is clearly yes. The mere weight of the pressure, under which consent may be given, does not necessarily inhibit its autonomy and legal validity. If that pressure is not exerted, or wilfully controlled, by other people but only by naturally given circumstances, it may be as high as one pleases, it may even, for any reasonable person, come close to being completely determinative of the ensuing decision, yet it does not touch upon the autonomy and validity of that decision in the least. Hypothetically speaking, a patient diagnosed with kidney cancer and confronted with the choice of either consenting to a removal of the diseased kidney or to face certain death within a few months, will most probably choose the former. Her consent to the surgery is doubtlessly autonomous and valid, even though she may feel quite intensely that she has no reasonable alternative. By contrast, that same person, confronted with the threat exerted on her by somebody else that she be killed if she refused to consent to a removal of her kidney for transplantation purposes, would not be said to consent autonomously or validly if she agreed to the procedure.

The reason why the law treats these two instances of consent completely differently, despite their apparent similarities, is not difficult to see. The law aims at regulating the interaction of persons. It is not its duty to shield people from the risks of their natural environment. Hence, the autonomy of a decision made under whatever natural circumstances is not affected at all by the psychological influence these circumstances might exert on the decision. From a legal perspective, it is solely a person's own concern how she deals with compelling, constraining or necessitating forces arising out of whatever natural circumstances she may encounter. The situation changes completely, however, if such forces are exerted by one person on another. In this case, the decision to yield to this sort of "man-made" pressure has its true origin in the coercers mind and, hence, is really *his* decision. This fact, not the weight of the pressure exerted, leads us to attribute responsibility for the decision (and, thus, the ensuing action) not to the person called upon to undergo a certain procedure, but to the coercer. Consequently, we cannot consider any person thus coerced to be autonomous when making that decision.

Projected onto the problem of the detained sociopath this implies the following. The pressure placed on a person by others who are legally entitled, perhaps even obliged, to exert that force is really nothing other than pressure exerted by the norms of law themselves. As far as the autonomy of somebody confronted with that pressure is concerned, the force of the legal order (as part of the social environment) is on a par with the force of the natural order (the natural environment).[288] Hence, decisions of persons taken under com-

[288] We presuppose here the normal case of a legal system that is, in principle, ethically legitimate. Terrorist or totalitarian regimes and their freedom restricting suppressive measures are a different matter; an enhancement offer under such circumstances would indeed amount to illegitimate blackmailing.

pulsion of legal norms are no less autonomous than decisions under the compelling force of natural circumstances. Whether that compulsion is the result of a direct effect of those norms on the deciding person, or else the result of enforcement measures by intermediaries acting within their legal competence, does not make a difference.

Therefore, we hold the following position. Should a brain-invasive treatment for severe psychopathy ever become available, subject to common criteria for weighing the potential risks against the potential benefits of this procedure, then nothing stands in the way of offering such a treatment to people in preventive detention if that is the only alternative to their being kept in custody indefinitely. The sheer force of pressure exerted on the detainee by those circumstances would neither infringe the autonomy, nor the legal validity, of his or her decision. We hold that, in such a situation, the state would be not only entitled but even obliged to make the respective offer for the following reasons. Having a brain-invasive treatment for psycho-/sociopathy in order to regain one's status as a free person might be less burdensome to that person than an indefinite detention and yet might still be capable to accomplish the same effect, namely the protection of the general public from a dangerous individual. Since all of the state's coercive measures towards its citizens are subject to the principle of proportionality, this obliges it to offer the prisoner the opportunity of mental enhancement. Whether or not such an intervention really is a lesser burden than the prospect of a continued detention, is to be left solely to the decision of the person affected, i.e. the detainee.

We add that this reasoning would not be altered even if one rejects the idea of calling a violent and dangerous disposition a disorder and, consequently, its abolishment by an intervention in the brain a form of treatment. This is certainly a defensible view. One might prefer to consider such an intervention, at best, an enhancement. However, in this case too the principle of proportionality urges the state to offer a choice of the lesser of two burdens, if both are equally suited to safeguard the legally required effect. The question of who has to pay for such an enhancement is a different matter. It would be fair, and certainly legitimate, to have the detainee pay for himself. However, if he or she does not have sufficient funds to pay for this treatment, a kind of fiduciary duty of the state to take over the costs might ensue. This question, though, clearly draws us away from the subject matter of the present inquiry and into more mundane, everyday questions of the law. This is where we shall leave it for the time being.

7 Conclusions and Recommendations

7.1 Conceptual Clarifications ... 386
7.1.1 Concerns about the Integrity of Persons ... 386
7.1.2 The Proper Limits of Medicine: Treatment – Enhancement – Prevention ... 387
7.1.2.1 The Legitimacy of Medicine Proper ... 387
7.1.2.2 Enhancement versus Treatment ... 388
7.1.2.3 The Purpose of Medicine: Fighting Disease ... 388
7.1.2.4 Enhancement Does Not Serve the Purpose of Medicine ... 389
7.1.2.5 Self-Enhancement versus Enhancement of Others ... 390
7.2 Normative Foundations ... 391
7.2.1 Nonmaleficence: Avoiding Harm in Intervening in the Brain ... 391
7.2.1.1 Dealing with Side Effects in Research and Medical Practice ... 392
Monitoring for Subtle Mental Side Effects ... 392
The Subtlety of Personality Changes ... 393
7.2.1.2 Minimising Harm by Careful Study Design ... 394
7.2.1.3 The Possible Harm of Enhancement ... 395
Are There Illegitimate Goals of Enhancements? ... 395
Dealing with Side Effects of Enhancements ... 398
7.2.2 Beneficence: The Limits of Doing Good to Others ... 399
7.2.2.1 Treatment and Prevention ... 399
7.2.2.2 Responsibility and Liability Regarding Enhancement ... 399
7.2.2.3 Public Funding for Research ... 400
7.2.3 Autonomy: Issues of Informed Consent and Coercion ... 402
7.2.3.1 Treatment, Prevention and Research ... 402
The Incomprehensibility of Mental Harm as an Obstacle to Informed Consent ... 402
Exercising Autonomy under Coercion ... 403
7.2.3.2 Enhancement and the Limits of Autonomy ... 405
Enhancement and the "Grave Affront" Principle ... 405
Enhancing Children: The Scope of Parental Discretion ... 406
Concerns about Authenticity ... 408

7.2.4 Justice: Inequality, Fair Distribution, Political Justice 410
7.2.4.1 Problems of Distributive Justice 411
Does Enhancement Exacerbate Existing Social Inequality? 411
Does Enhancement Entail Wastage of Medical Resources? 413
7.2.4.2 Problems of Political Justice in General 414

7 Conclusions and Recommendations[289]

The history of therapeutic interventions in the psyche is as old as the history of medicine. Ancient Egyptian, Chinese and Greek medicine already included prescriptions for the treatment of what would nowadays be called "mental illness" (Millon 2004). Similarly, beyond the realm of therapy mankind has always sought means to enhance and develop features of the mind, as is evidenced by varied traditions of religious and spiritual practices. It is important to bear this historical perspective in mind when commenting on the concerns raised by recent methods of intervention in the central nervous system (CNS) which, in addition to providing new opportunities for treating and enhancing the psyche, may have inadvertent effects on the mental level as well.

➔ Having studied these new methods in psychopharmacology, neurotransplantation, gene transfer, neural prosthetics and electrical brain stimulation, the authors of this book acknowledge and endorse their potential to benefit the individual, as well as society, by yielding innovative therapeutic applications. Of course, since these interventions operate directly on the brain, it is obligatory to handle them with appropriate caution, even if they are used for treatment purposes only.

Due to the integrated structure of brain functions, the possibility of a therapeutic intervention in the brain having unwanted side effects on the mental level can hardly ever be ruled out, regardless of whether it is intended to have an effect on the psyche or not. The task of dealing with risks of this kind in an ethically acceptable manner is certainly not new. On the contrary, ever since therapeutic goals have been pursued by deliberately introducing physiological or structural changes in the CNS, there has been the need to cope with unanticipated side effects occurring not only on the mental level, but on all levels of human functioning. Moreover, the general challenge of how to balance the likely benefits of a treatment option with the probability, and the potential severity, of associated mental harm is not unique to interventions in

[289] This final chapter contains important results from the entire study. However, since the main aim of this chapter is to draw practical conclusions addressing decision makers in politics and medicine, many results pertaining to specific techniques of intervention have not been included in this résumé. We refer readers interested in these results to the concluding sections of each chapter in the first part of this study. Also Chapter 5 contains a more detailed summary in its final section (5.5).

the *brain.* Other types of medical procedures must be subject to similar risk assessments before they are undertaken. For instance, mastectomy has long been associated with a wide array of "mental" side effects, ranging from transient depression to lasting changes in a woman's self-concept.

7.1 Conceptual Clarifications

7.1.1 Concerns about the Integrity of Persons

Those who consider even therapeutic applications of new techniques for intervening in the brain ethically dubious usually do not base their arguments solely on the possibility of mental side effects as such. Rather, new treatment options in this field are typically challenged on the grounds that they may transform patients in more radical or profound ways than more established techniques of intervention. The most common way to express these concerns is to argue that new interventions in the brain may threaten personal identity. The suggestion that such interventions are equivalent to turning someone into someone else by "messing with his brain" could mobilise public opinion against promising areas of research and frustrate the development of new, and urgently required, treatments. Furthermore, the vague fear that due to the treatment they may no longer be "the one I used to be" could prevent individual patients from undergoing such medical procedures. In this study, therefore, we took efforts to dispel fears that new options for treatment in the areas of psychopharmacology, molecular and cellular interventions, neural prosthetics and electrical brain stimulation may threaten the identity of patients who undergo them. However, because the precise nature of the threat is so hard to define, it is also difficult to refute. In trying to make sense of this threat, we eventually came to the conclusion that a change of personal identity evoked by an intervention in the brain would have to manifest itself as a dissociative disorder, e.g. retrograde amnesia or dissociative identity disorder (Section 5.4.5). Of course, once the harm of identity change is described in this way, it becomes apparent that it does not represent a hitherto unknown kind of mental side effect which could not be caused by, for instance, clinically established lesioning procedures in brain surgery.

With respect to the types of intervention examined in this study, there is, in fact, no evidence yet that any of them are associated with a significant probability of causing dissociative disorders or other comparably grave mental side effects which might come close to a threat on personal identity. However, even if a certain type of therapeutic intervention in the brain is known to occasionally bring about severe mental harm, it must still be decided on a case-by-case basis whether it is acceptable – or, in some instances, even *advisable* – to take this risk. It is common practice to arrive at treatment decisions of this kind by taking into account the availability, effectiveness and safety of alternative therapeutic options on the one hand, and the dangers in leaving a patient untreated on the other hand. Again it deserves emphasis that the difficult ethical dilemmas one inevitably has to face in medical risk-benefit assessments are by no means peculiar to therapeutic applications of new methods for intervening in the brain.

→ The public preoccupation with the possibility of patients being transformed in radical and obvious ways might detract attention from those side effects which actually give more reason for concern, namely *subtle* changes of the psyche in general, and of personality in particular, which may easily go unnoticed.

In Section 7.2.1.1 we offer some concrete suggestions on how to adjust existing research and treatment guidelines so as to account for subtle forms of mental side effect.

7.1.2 The Proper Limits of Medicine: Treatment – Enhancement – Prevention

New social challenges arise with respect to non-therapeutic applications of new techniques for intervening in the brain. This is particularly the case when they are applied for enhancement purposes and perhaps also when they are designed as preventive measures. Stating this, it is essential to elucidate the meanings of, and the relations between, the concepts of therapy, prevention and enhancement. We start out with a common-sense notion of "enhancement" and explain it as a *prima facie* negative boundary concept in that it delineates those procedures which can neither be considered part of conventional medicine, nor be defined as a form of "treatment" as the term is generally applied. This conceptual strategy confronts us with two basic questions: (1) what is "proper medicine"? and (2), what is "treatment"?

7.1.2.1 The Legitimacy of Medicine Proper

In dealing with (1), we take as a premise that "proper medicine" is, at least in one respect, a normative concept. For the whole plethora of medical practices have one normative feature in common: that of being legitimate in their respective contexts. In further clarifying the concept, we draw a distinction between medicine as a social (and in some way publicly financed) system, and medicine as an interpersonal or intrapersonal practice. Possible answers to the question about the purview of "proper medicine" may take quite different routes, depending on whether one seeks to define the limits of medicine in terms of the former (i.e. of what a system of public health ought to provide), or of the latter (i.e. of what one person may legitimately do to herself, or to another person, by using medical means). Of course, those activities that are beyond the limits of what a person may justifiably do to herself or to another person cannot be legitimately included in any well-ordered system of public health. However, this does not hold the other way around: Many medical procedures that might rightly be banned from the system of public health (viz., from the package of basic care that such a system should provide for all members of society) may yet be perfectly justified if performed on a consenting person by a medical doctor or by that person themselves. Medical interventions for purely cosmetic reasons may serve to illustrate that point.

7.1.2.2 Enhancement versus Treatment

As far as medicine as a social system of healthcare is concerned, we consider the treatment-enhancement distinction to be a useful conceptual tool in delineating the proper boundaries of this system or, rather, one of its proper boundaries, the other one being drawn by prevention (to which we will turn shortly). Obviously, the conceptual opposition between treatment and enhancement alone does not tell us where exactly to draw the line in practice. This leads us to question (2) above. We suggest that this line ought to be drawn not by defining "enhancement", but rather by defining "disease" or "illness" (including "disability"), i.e. the conceptual counterpart and the practical target of "treatment" (thus rendering "enhancement" the "negatively defined boundary concept" we characterised it to be above). The concept of disease has been subject to intense debate in the philosophy of medicine, and a host of widely differing conceptions have been developed. We agree, by and large, with philosopher Norman Daniels in defining disease as a significant deviation from the species-typical functioning of physical and/or mental human systems, features, and qualities. But we do not think, as Daniels seems to, that this renders "disease" a purely descriptive, or naturalistic, concept. For, what comes to lie on this side of the boundary of species-typicality, or else what is a significant deviation from it, is not simply a matter of scientific fact. Rather, in any complex borderline case, it is inevitably subject to a *decision,* containing an irreducible normative element that lies beyond proof or refutation by natural, biological science. Against this conceptual background, any technical intervention aimed at improving some physical or psychological aspect of an individual, but which cannot be categorised as "treatment", is to count as "enhancement".

7.1.2.3 The Purpose of Medicine: Fighting Disease

For the demarcation of the proper sphere of medicine as a social system, the treatment-enhancement distinction is not sufficient. It fails to do justice to the concept and the role of prevention. We take "prevention" to have a twofold affinity to the treatment-enhancement dichotomy. Normatively speaking, prevention evidently participates in the *a limine* justification of measures of treatment. Just like treatment, prevention is an instrument to fight off disease and, with respect to this goal, it is justified to include all measures of prevention along with all kinds of treatment in the realm of proper medicine. Descriptively speaking, certain exemplary (although obviously not all) types of prevention, notably vaccinations, are also a form of enhancement. Vaccination is meant to amplify (or enhance) natural physical capabilities in order to (potentially) neutralise pathogenic microorganisms and other disease-causing agents to which the physical system might become exposed. Thus, we believe that prevention is conceptually distinct from enhancement and treatment. Hence, we extend our dichotomy "treatment – enhancement" to become a trichotomy of "treatment – prevention – enhancement".

With regard to the question of the proper limits of medicine as a social system, the introduction of this trichotomy creates no additional problems. As we already indicated, any activity intended to, and potentially capable of preventing a state of affairs that would rightly be considered a "disease" is equally justified in being assigned to the realm of "proper medicine" as are measures of treatment against that disease in the case where it is already present.[290] In this respect, there is no difference in principle concerning treatment or prevention of mental diseases by new methods of intervening in the brain.

7.1.2.4 Enhancement Does Not Serve the Purpose of Medicine

Having thus clarified our basic concepts, we stipulate:

➔ Enhancements which cannot at least count as prevention of disease/disability ("mere" enhancements) should not be included in the sphere of "proper medicine" as a social system.

We acknowledge and emphasise that, in certain cases, this recommendation may create tensions with respect to individual justice. But no theoretical strategy to demarcate the limits of medicine could avoid such problems altogether. The strategy we endorse and develop locates these problems on the most plausible conceptual and normative level. All of this does not exclude, of course, that the same medico-technical measure can be an enhancement in one case and a treatment in another. If, for instance, a person *A* falls short of the species typical standard for a certain cognitive function *x* without thereby fulfilling diagnostic criteria for intellectual disability, then an intervention that improves *x* in that person can be considered an enhancement. The same intervention, however, could correctly be classified as treatment in a person *B* who is so impaired with respect to *x* as to be considered mentally disabled in a clinical sense.

Finally, we assign what we call a "robust discretionary power" to legislators and other "gatekeepers" of the social system of medicine such as courts, health insurance organisations and others to decide, within their respective functional remit, which concrete medical measure to include within that system, and which to exclude. Such decisions are never obligated to the criteria of individual justice alone, but rather to the requirement of generalisability over the whole range of sufficiently similar cases, present and future, within

[290] Differences, of course, arise with respect to the question of whether such measures are not only justified, but also *obligatory* for a system of public health. This is largely a problem of a just and prudential distribution of scarce and costly resources. It obviously need not concern us here.

the entire system. Hence, they must also make allowance for the constraints imposed by the scarcity of costly life-saving resources. In so doing, the aforementioned discretionary power is required. So it may very well occur that a specific medical measure is classified as "treatment" in one jurisdiction, whilst being viewed as "enhancement" in another, and thus being excluded from the sphere of "proper medicine".

7.1.2.5 Self-Enhancement versus Enhancement of Others

As far as the limits of proper medicine as an interpersonal and intrapersonal practice is concerned, we take the treatment/prevention – enhancement distinction as only a provisional point of departure for further analysis. On the one hand, it is clear from the outset that whatever is rightly considered treatment is *ipso facto* justified when applied by one person, say a medical doctor, onto another, the patient, as a medical measure in accordance with the common criteria of respect for autonomy and of weighing intended therapeutic benefits against potential adverse side effects. In this limited sense, our conceptual trichotomy once more serves as a useful normative tool to begin with. However, in marked contrast to what we pointed out above in our discussion of medicine as a social system, it is by no means clear that every physical or mental improvement that extends beyond the sphere of treatment and prevention (i.e. enhancement) should, for that reason alone, be treated with suspicion, let alone be considered illegitimate. On the contrary, many enhancing medical interventions that are possible today, or could be conceived as being possible in the future, do not seem to violate any inter- or intrapersonal ethical or legal norms.

However, there remain some normative limits. To clarify them, we distinguish cases of self-enhancement from cases of applying enhancing measures to other persons. Within the former category we differentiate between "one-party cases" and "two-party cases". The former comprise all forms of a competent person administering enhancing means to themselves. The latter, by contrast, refers to one person administering an enhancement measure to another one. In standard two-party cases, a medical doctor administers a method of enhancement to another person after having obtained informed consent. From this basic scenario an array of normative problems ensue, ranging from specific questions of side effects to problems of justice. We expound the results of our systematic analysis of those problems below.

Different normative problems arise when we turn from self-enhancement to the enhancement of others. What characterises the latter is the fact that typical cases in this category have a structure that could be labelled a "three-party case": Usually, there is a person *X* deciding on, or wishing for, an enhancement to be performed on another person *Y* by a third person *Z* (the latter normally being a medical expert). We analyse the particular problems ensuing from that structure in two paradigmatic settings: that of parents who ask for an enhancement of their minor children, and that of detainees in prison who give the state particular reasons to consider the possibility of having them mentally enhanced in certain respects. The results of our analysis, along with our recommendations, will also be expounded below.

7.2 Normative Foundations

We do not recognise a need for introducing new basic normative principles in order to cope with the social challenges raised by the new developments we deal with. Rather, most of the normative issues we address in this study can be adequately dealt with by making use of four widely accepted general principles of medical ethics: nonmaleficence (prohibition of harm), beneficence (duty to assist), respect for autonomy, and justice.[291] These four principles offer a convenient structure for the remainder of this section in which we will draw some action-oriented conclusions in order to further interdisciplinary debate, enrich the public discussion, and support political decision makers and other stakeholders.

7.2.1 Nonmaleficence: Avoiding Harm in Intervening in the Brain

The general obligation not to inflict harm on others may justly be considered the most basic moral principle of all known cultures throughout history. Accordingly, it is also the most important principle in healthcare and in medical research, and is often expressed in the maxim *primum non nocere*. It states that acts of harming are *prima facie* wrong, i.e. that they are subject to prohibition on an abstract normative level. However, such generally forbidden acts may yet be legitimate in concrete individual cases, provided that certain justifying circumstances are present. Besides being in accordance with the affected person's autonomy (i.e. having obtained his/her informed consent), the harm done to a human being by a particular medical intervention must be outweighed by the benefit which can be reasonably expected to be brought about by that action. We restrict our analysis of such balancing considerations to trade-offs within the sphere of interests of the affected subject themselves, for we do not, in principle, endorse utilitarian justifications of doing harm to someone in order to benefit others.[292]

---

[291] This particular set of four principles was introduced by Tom L. Beauchamp and James F. Childress in their influential Principles of Medical Ethics (2001). In deliberate deviation from their textbook presentation we start our discussion with nonmaleficence thereby reflecting the particular importance of this principle for the issues at hand.

[292] Most deontological and other non-utilitarian ethics also do know and rightly accept, if only within narrow limits, the possibility of certain trade-offs between benefits and harms across the boundaries that separate persons from each other. They accept (comparably weak) duties of solidarity in cases of danger to one person (*X*), allowing the infliction of very minor harm on another person (*Y*) not involved in the causation of that danger, if this act benefits *X* to a much larger extent than it harms *Y*. Even though this principle has a certain role in medical research on persons not able to give informed consent, we may safely neglect it here as of no particular importance to the subject of our study.

7.2.1.1 Dealing with Side Effects in Research and Medical Practice

In the context of decisions about the permissibility of interventions in the brain, the principle of nonmaleficence pertains, by and large, to the issue of side effects only. The intended primary effects of treatment or preventive measures are, *by definition,* no harm. Our concept of enhancement assumes that the person undergoing this intervention, at least, considers its intended effect to be an improvement. Thus, with regard to their intended primary effects, enhancing interventions are, albeit subject to certain qualifications which will be addressed sub 7.2.1.2, not meant to cause harm.

Monitoring for Subtle Mental Side Effects

In the introductory remarks to this chapter we argued that it is, first and foremost, the more subtle mental side effects that give us reason to scrutinise recently developed methods for intervening in the CNS. By *subtle* mental harm we mean those adverse side effects that may easily go unnoticed, and affect either personality or mental functions which are constitutive of personhood[293]. Although the possibility of bringing about this kind of mental harm is by no means limited to interventions in the brain, due to the brain's central function in determining the mental state of an individual, such interventions present unique risks in this regard. Furthermore, it is plausible that any brain intervention which is *meant* to exert an influence on the psyche is more prone to cause subtle side effects of the kind detailed above. Hence, the following recommendations are in order:

- ➔ During the research phase, any new method of intervening in the brain should be monitored systematically for subtle side effects pertaining to personality and those mental capacities related to personhood.
- ➔ If a particular type of brain intervention with known possible subtle side effects pertaining to personality or mental capacities related to personhood is approved for certain therapeutic or preventive applications, then every person undergoing that procedure should be carefully monitored for the occurrence of such side effects after the procedure is conducted so that they can receive appropriate treatment if necessary.

For most methods of brain interventions developed recently, including the ones reviewed in this study, some efforts were made to meet these requirements. On the whole, however, we think that there is a need for more rigorous testing in accordance with improved methodical procedures. Rather than going into detailed suggestions, it will suffice here to indicate some aspects of the monitoring procedure deserving closer atten-

[293] In particular, this means discriminative abilities (perception and recognition), episodic memory, learning abilities, abilities of language and deliberation, the ability to entertain purposes, the disposition to satisfy natural needs, and the capacity to feel sensations of like and dislike. See Section 5.3 for details.

tion and to highlight a number of obstacles one may face in attempting to do so.

First, the very "subtlety" of potential side effects on the level of the psyche can mean that they become apparent only in the long term. This is particularly pertinent for interventions in the developing brain since, during this stage (in humans ranging from the intrauterine stage up to the post-pubescence), it is especially difficult to identify induced changes against the complex backdrop of "naturally" occurring changes. Paying due attention to the issue of long-term side effects obviously raises the problem of safety trials for new brain interventions becoming more time-consuming and costly. One way to keep the costs for new types of intervention within manageable limits might be to require extensive post-marketing safety surveillance in addition to clinical testing prior to its release on the market. Depending on national data protection law, the implementation of this kind of surveillance strategy can be frustrated by restrictions on access to the relevant data. Perhaps the easiest way to resolve this normative conflict would be a provision for patients to waive their right to protection of personal data in view of their own vested interest in the conduct of appropriate long-term safety testing.

Even though we did not enter the methodological debate on assessment tools for personality changes in this study, the narrative approach to personality expounded in Chapter 5 has some obvious implications for methodological issues. Since the self-concept is an essential part of a person's character, it must be taken into account in any comprehensive assessment of personality changes which may result from interventions in the brain. While this requires paying attention to the testimony an individual provides about who she is, a reliable account of personality changes cannot be gained by merely asking people before and after an intervention whether their personalities have changed or not. Rather, efforts should be taken to screen for differences between a subject's self assessment and the way others describe the impact an intervention may have had on her personality. If such differences are identified which, moreover, seem to be of importance for the assessment of an intervention's outcome, then it is advisable to think about more objective ways to describe contested personality traits, for instance by applying behavioural criteria. Rather than merely assigning values (of magnitude) to personality attributes, their relative importance for the integrated whole of a person's character should also be considered. In so doing, the possibility of differing judgements emerging from first- and third-person perspectives must be taken into account once again.

The Subtlety of Personality Changes

One particular reason why – without further checking – personality changes introduced through an intervention could go unnoticed is that persons are (fortunately) very adaptive. Consequently, rather than sticking out like sore thumbs, personality changes are, in many cases, incorporated into one's self-concept. In particular, one's individual value system, which represents an important part of a person's self-concept, often reacts in a very dynamic way to personality changes. Somewhat provocatively, one could argue that no matter how a person's character may be changed by an intervention in her brain, she will quite likely adapt to and come to appreciate her changed personality, so that, ultimately, no *harm* can be said to have been done to her. However, while the "positive" outcome of the adaptation process is far less certain than this statement suggests, its conclusion, at least, is blatantly wrong. Even if a person approves of a particular change to her personality considered in isolation, the further consequences of having been changed in this way may still amount to great harm. Regardless of whether the affected person herself is happy with the changes to her personality, this is no guarantee that others will be so readily accepting of these changes. They may result in anti-social character traits, which lead other people to shun her. The resultant isolation will most likely cause great harm to that person. However, even if the changes in her personality are socially acceptable, or even appreciated by society, this would not necessarily mean that no harm has been done. This appears to be the case only if all that we take into account is the perspective of persons assessing their situation *after* their personality has already been altered by an intervention. Against this we maintain:

➔ Whether the prospect of an intervention in the brain having a certain personality change as a side effect is acceptable, or even desirable, can only be decided by the affected persons themselves *before* they undergo that intervention.

This also implies that the question of whether anyone else welcomes the prospect of someone's personality being changed in a certain way due to an intervention is irrelevant for deciding whether a side effect represents harm, or not. In the same vein, provided an affected person considers a possible effect on her personality as a harm, nobody except that person herself can decide whether it is acceptable to take that risk. Of course, the precise nature of any potential personality change and the likelihood of these changes occurring are of great relevance to anyone considering whether or not to undergo a certain intervention. At any rate, informing a person about these risks should involve an explicit warning that any unintended effect on personality may be accompanied by changes in the perception of the obtained effects themselves. If the patient consents to that risk (and the intervention is carried out), the subsequent change of his or her subjective criteria for evaluating the outcome of this intervention must be accepted, with the new criteria now providing the yardstick for measuring the patient's well-being.

7.2.1.2 Minimising Harm by Careful Study Design

Clinical research is subject to legislation in which informed consent (see below 7.2.3) and the evaluation by a medical ethics committee play critical roles in establishing which procedures may be undertaken. This is no different for the new types of brain intervention that were reviewed in this study. However, the particular risk of them causing subtle mental side effects means that special care must be taken in designing studies. Not only should clinical trials not be performed when interpretable and meaningful results cannot be obtained (such trials would, in fact, be unethical). In addition, the significance of obtained data will be higher if a standard protocol for the essential symptom measures of brain anomalies is used. The number of patients subjected to experimental interventions in the CNS could be minimised if such standard or core evaluation protocols were available. This leads us to the following recommendation:

➔ For experimental interventions in patients with neurological and psychiatric disorders, time-scheduled and disease-specific core assessment protocols (CAPs) should be established in order to (1) obtain meaningful results and (2) enable comparisons between different treatment approaches.

As for every neurological or psychiatric brain disorder a specific CAP will be needed, these protocols are themselves subject to research and agreement amongst the scientists and clinicians who specialise on a particular brain syndrome. Thus, this recommendation is addressed above all at researchers, rather than legislators. It favours, however, multi-centre collaborations in clinical studies on specific interventions as is currently the case in the field of pharmacology.

7.2.1.3 The Possible Harm of Enhancement

As stated above, the intended primary effects of enhancing interventions cannot normally be considered as harms. If they are enhancements, then they must constitute an improvement – at least from the point of view of the person undergoing the intervention – in terms of bringing about the particular effects they are designed to produce. Improvements are not harms. Furthermore, since their intended effects are realised only in the person requesting them, it is this person's judgment alone (as idiosyncratic as it may be) which can decide whether these effects constitute harms or improvements.[294]

Are There Illegitimate Goals of Enhancements?

This purely subjective means of assessing the intended outcomes of an enhancement solely in terms of the individual preferences of the person involved, certainly concurs, in principle, with basic ethical norms. It holds without exception in "one-party cases": What a person of (otherwise) sound mind does exclusively to herself is, in principle, a matter of her own protected privacy, regardless of what other people might think about the self-inflicted intervention.[295] In "two-party cases," however, this principle is sub-

[294] Possible negative effects of mass enhancements of the respective type *on society* are a different matter. We deal with it under the heading of "Justice".

[295] We ignore here specific constellations characterised by particular moral obligations of one person towards another that possibly include a duty not to profoundly change her personality (e.g. a mother's obligations towards her minor child).

ject to specific limitations. Most developed legal orders curtail the permissible justifications for *physical* intrusions into another person's body, even where that person's informed consent has been obtained. This limit is usually drawn where the particular intervention constitutes a "grave affront to common ethical convictions and rules".[296] This confining legal principle may, and in some legal orders does, take into account not only the immediate physical effect of the intervention, but any further intended effects associated with it as well. The physical intervention itself might be judged to be an unjustified harm by objective normative criteria (a "grave affront" in the above sense) due only to its associated secondary effects. This judgment would be made regardless of the fact that the affected person herself considers it an enhancement.

Two different types of cases can be distinguished here. First, there are cases in which an enhancement is desired only in order to pursue an illegitimate goal. Second, there are cases in which interventions are defined as enhancements by the respective person who wishes to obtain them, but which would be considered gravely harmful by any reasonable observer. An example of the first type of case would be if a person wanted to evade responsibility for a murder he committed and, therefore, sought an alteration of his mind to erase his memory of the crime. Whilst he certainly had understandable reasons to consider that change advantageous, and thus an enhancement, the law could well refuse to accept such a subjective definition of "enhancement" as legally relevant. Consequently, such an intervention would be deemed unjustified on the part of the physician who performs it in full knowledge of the murderer's intent. Further examples of mental enhancements with illegitimate goals (e.g. fraudulent ones) are not hard to imagine and should be considered realistic future possibilities.

Examples of the second type of case present themselves less readily. One possible example, however, would be a person wishing to seriously curtail his or her cognitive abilities while defining this as an enhancement for him- or herself. This scenario may appear completely unrealistic, but a similar case in the sphere of physical interventions may caution against a premature dismissal of the idea. Surgeons in various countries have been urged by otherwise normal, competent persons to amputate perfectly healthy limbs.[297] To our knowledge, there are no documented instances of comparable cases involving mental features. Nevertheless, the possibility of such cases should not be dismissed out of hand. Two ways of dealing with them can be distinguished: On the one hand, the desire for such an "amputation", or at least the suffering (which may amount to manifest depression) that goes along with that desire not being satisfied, may be considered a mental disease. If this is

[296] For reasons of convenience, we use this formula of § 228 of the German Criminal Code; most other legal orders contain similar norms with more or less comparable formulas.

[297] So-called "amputees-by-choice" cases (Bayne and Levy 2005).

the case, such a disabling intervention could, under certain circumstances, even count as a justified treatment.[298] On the other hand, the idea of justifying such an intervention may be rejected unconditionally on the grounds that it amounted to a "grave affront to common, basic moral convictions" under all conceivable circumstances. In the meantime, this entire problem may be left open to further debate. Examples like these have an exotic and futuristic flavour and they represent only rare and exceptional cases. However, their rarity is no reason to ignore them completely. There is currently no legislative need to draft new legal norms for this type of hypothetical scenario, but future developments in brain interventions might open up new ways of altering the mind. Therefore, research into these matters should also be undertaken, in order to provide the empirical grounds for normative solutions that might become necessary in the future.

Related to the above problem is the question whether techniques of mental enhancement should ever be developed and/or employed for purely military purposes, i.e. to improve the cognitive, emotional or motivational capacities of soldiers in order to make them better combatants. Any answer oriented by normative criteria would necessarily transgress the realm of bio- or neuroethics and enter the sphere of political ethics, especially the legal and moral philosophy of war and peace. For obvious reasons, we do not want to embark on that debate in the present context. However, we offer the following general remarks: As long as one accepts the right of states to wage armed conflict in accordance with the strictly confining criteria of contemporary international law (as the current authors do), objections to the idea of an enhancement for military purposes based *solely* on the fact that they are belligerent in nature are unfounded. Quite a different matter is the question of whether the risks of those techniques being misused in armed conflicts, or being used for illegitimate wars, should be regarded as being too great to justify a participation of scientists in military enterprises. However, trying to answer this would transgress the boundaries of our current inquiry, and we do not want to take a stance on it beyond a general assertion of the need for extreme caution with regard to the use of science for establishing techniques designed to kill (or that take in stride the potential killing of) other human beings. As a last concern, we mention here the question of whether the use of those techniques could lead to a situation where soldiers (or people considering becoming soldiers) would be put under pressure to consent to enhancements, and whether such pressure would infringe their personal autonomy or be politically unjust. This issue will, therefore, be discussed (in a more general way) in the sections about authenticity and political justice below.

[298] Of course, the justification for such a grave intervention would presuppose a sufficiently grave suffering associated with the disease. But this can probably not be excluded either. In some of the amputees-by-choice cases, the affected persons seriously considered committing suicide when turned down with their requests.

Dealing with Side Effects of Enhancements

In contrast to treatments, interventions aimed at mental enhancements are not subject to a *prima facie* moral *obligation* on physicians (and the health care system) but, on the contrary, require moral *permission*. This is why the adverse side effects of pure enhancements gain, in general, greater prominence in the overall risk-assessment process. Hence, the same foreseeable, negative outcome might be acceptable as a side effect in treatments, but unacceptable in enhancements.

Not only is the significance of possible side effects increased, but the scope of side effects relevant to the risk assessment is also greatly enlarged in enhancement cases. On the side of the intervening physician, this leads to an expansion of her informational duties in two ways. First, she must inform herself about possible mental peculiarities of her client more thoroughly than she would have to in treatment cases. Second, she must also inform her client more comprehensively about the possibility of even the most subtle unwanted adverse effects. These maxims do not, of course, deviate from common basic principles in medical ethics. But in their application to mental enhancement cases, they are specific enough to deserve particular emphasis.

Concluding the foregoing discussion we offer the following summary of our position:

➔ We do not endorse a principled ethical rejection, let alone an outright legal prohibition, of interventions in the human brain aimed at mental enhancements solely on grounds of their physical or mental risks for the affected individual. It must be underlined, however, that potential negative side effects of mere enhancements weigh more heavily against intended positive effects than they would in treatment cases. Physicians intervening for enhancement purposes alone have enlarged informational duties towards their clients. To the extent that their duties to patients are increased, they are also obliged to acquire pertinent additional information for themselves.

For constitutional reasons, the law in liberal, democratic societies is not to be used as a tool for paternalistic control of individual preferences or the actions of autonomous citizens towards their own person. The same holds true, if only to a limited extent, for the secular conception of ethics to which the authors of this study, by and large, adhere, although with varying opinions in some particular aspects. Religious ethics may arrive at a different conclusion. Whilst we respect such positions, we wish to emphasise that, in a secular society endorsing widely differing ethical conceptions and governed by the rule of law, they cannot claim any general validity, and thus *a fortiori* no prominent role in shaping the legal order.

7.2.2 Beneficence: The Limits of Doing Good to Others

7.2.2.1 Treatment and Prevention

The principle of beneficence imposes a positive obligation on persons to contribute to the welfare of others. The extent to which ordinary people are morally obliged to not only refrain from inflicting harm on others but also to provide them with benefits is debatable. In certain situations and relationships, however, ordinary people are undoubtedly obliged to do so. Healthcare professionals, in virtue of their social role, have a clearly defined duty of care towards their patients. The provision of healthcare, and the legally safeguarded access to medical treatment for every citizen, count amongst the most fundamental positive duties of the modern state. On both the level of the individual physician as well as that of the public healthcare system, it is inevitable that there are limits to the scope of the respective obligations. Within this scope, however, legitimate treatments consisting in new types of brain interventions are equally subject to the general principle of beneficence – and to its limitations – as any other form of treatment for human disease. For, once a brain intervention of whatever type and magnitude has been deemed a legitimate (non-harmful) treatment by assessing the intended primary effects against potential adverse side effects, it is by definition beneficial. (Whether the ever widening scope of treatment options available requires a new and stricter regime of rationing such newly developed methods is a different matter, which does not fit under the present heading of beneficence, but under that of justice.)

7.2.2.2 Responsibility and Liability Regarding Enhancement

→ Enhancing healthy human beings is not a genuine part of the responsibility of health care professionals, which is to treat and prevent diseases. Hence, brain interventions aiming only at enhancement do not fall under the obligatory force of the principle of beneficence in medicine, notwithstanding the fact that there are borderline cases which are difficult to delineate from treatment.

As we stated above, mere enhancements should be excluded from the services of proper medicine as a public and publicly financed system. By implication, they also do not fall within the scope of an individual physician's general obligation to beneficence. There is not even a *prima facie* obligation for him or her to perform an enhancing intervention on anybody. This holds no less for mental interventions than it does for purely physical ("cosmetic") enhancements.

However, if an enhancing medical intervention is performed by either a competent person on herself or by a (medical or non-medical) actor on a consenting recipient, any potential side effects, such as addiction, may amount to diseases and thus become a legitimate object of treatment by specialised health care personnel. Those treatments themselves undoubtedly fall under the principle of beneficence. However, since their original cause did not, the question arises whether the financial costs for treating those side effects should be compensated for by a public insurance system for healthcare. There is no general and normatively cogent answer to this question. If the financial resources of a particular national healthcare system allow the inclusion of the costs of the treatment of such diseases arising as the result of enhancement procedures, they may well be covered by that system. However, neither the principle of beneficence, nor that of social justice commands such an inclusion. Hence, whether such costs are to be assigned to the individual who sought the enhancing procedure in the first place, and thus undertook the risk of causing the subsequent disease, is subject to a wide discretionary power of the respective national legislature. To avoid misunderstanding, we wish to underline that this holds only for the *costs* of treatment and not for the provision of treatment itself. The inclusion of such treatment into the system of proper healthcare is mandated by the principle of beneficence. From this, it follows that any person suffering from a disease brought on by a brain enhancement intervention, who is now *unable* to pay for the necessary treatment of this disease, must nevertheless be treated, and the costs for such treatment must be met by the social security system in accordance with the respective national law.

7.2.2.3 Public Funding for Research

States are under a positive *prima facie* obligation to further research into medical progress, this obligation being subject, of course, to a host of restraining criteria and to wide discretionary powers on the part of the state as to how to discharge this responsibility. This general principle of medical ethics also holds, with no particular modifications, for research into methods of brain intervention as long as it aims at new possibilities for treatment and prevention. While this kind of research does not, in principle, raise any specific normative questions, one certainly may ask whether the actual amount of public funding expended on it adequately corresponds to the clinical needs in this area.

In order to see that there is good reason to raise this question, it is important to understand the far-reaching consequences which brain diseases, brain injury, psychiatric disorders such as depression and schizophrenia, the sequelae of aging, and stress-related afflictions have for the functioning of human beings in society. In 2004, in the European Union alone, over 127 million individuals suffered from a brain disorder, which amounts to 27% of the total population. A large part of current health care expenditure is related to the treatment of brain disorders. For 2004, these expenses were estimated at € 386 billion. This is just the cost of health care. The indirect social costs are not included in this amount. Brain diseases (neurological, neurodegenerative, neurotraumatic and psychiatric) constitute an estimated

35% of the total burden of all diseases in Europe, which is much more than diseases such as cancer or heart disease. These figures[299] are likely to rise further, along with increasing life expectancy. It is argued that, as life expectancy grows, the body will increasingly come to outlive the brain. Improvements in clinical approaches to brain disorders will require adequate scientific research. Only as our *understanding* of the brain grows, the possibilities to *intervene* will increase. Every breakthrough in neuroscience has been brought about by close collaboration of scientists working in the field of pure and applied (clinical) research. The novel techniques of intervening in the brain for therapeutic purposes are, by and large, not fully explored to maximise putative beneficence in any of the brain disorders mentioned.

Despite the above-mentioned burden on individuals and on society, only a fraction of the total costs of brain diseases is spent on neuroscience research. On a European level, the 5th Research Framework Programme allocated a mere 0.01% of the estimated medical cost of brain diseases in Europe. Unless sufficient energy and financial investments are put into research in the brain, society soon will have every reason to blame politicians as well as scientists for having failed to improve the situation.

The normative situation is strikingly different when it comes to research aiming exclusively at the development of *purely* enhancing techniques of brain intervention. One may, of course, doubt that such research is even possible, or could sensibly be conceived of at all. This being as it may, if it is possible, it clearly falls outside the normative scope of the principle of beneficence. Thus:

➔ Research exclusively geared towards the development of means for mental enhancement by intervening in the brain should not be subsidised by public funds devoted to the social system of healthcare. Furthermore, the application of the products of such research to achieve mental enhancement should also not be funded by the healthcare system.

However, this principle does not relate to basic research into conditions of effectiveness or pathogenic functions of such enhancing methods. An analogy from the field of *physical* enhancements helps to elucidate this point: No research aimed at producing new methods of illegal performance enhancement in sports should be publicly sponsored. However, basic research into the functional and pathogenic mechanisms of such performance enhancing techniques should be. Finally, none of this is supposed to suggest anything like a moral judgement on, let alone a call for legal prohibition of, such research. It means rather that it should be left entirely to the private sector.

[299] All data mentioned are taken from a study by the European Brain Council (EBC) "The cost of disorders of the brain in Europe," which was published in a special issue of the European Journal of Neurology (Andlin-Sobocki et al. 2005).

7.2.3 Autonomy: Issues of Informed Consent and Coercion

Autonomy is a notoriously complex, multi-faceted concept. We distinguish broadly between autonomy as sovereignty (i.e. self-government) and autonomy as authenticity (i.e. being true to one's individual nature). Into this basic scheme, we insert a few more conceptual distinctions. Subsequently, we analyse the ensuing problems, first, in a legal perspective pertaining exclusively to "autonomy as sovereignty" and, second, in the perspective of ethics, encompassing aspects of both sovereignty and authenticity. It should be noted that questions pertaining to the latter can only arise in the context of intended *enhancements*. Whilst treatment or prevention can hardly be suspected of being based on "inauthentic" decisions, some forms of enhancement certainly can.

7.2.3.1 Treatment, Prevention and Research

If the aim of fighting disease through treatment or prevention is pursued by direct interventions in the brain, then this does not in itself raise specific normative problems with regard to autonomy. However, some of the common principles governing medical interventions in general acquire a particular importance in the context of therapeutic brain interventions.

The Incomprehensibility of Mental Harm as an Obstacle to Informed Consent

Respecting the autonomy of a patient (or research subject) mandates obtaining that patient's (or subject's) informed consent in advance. Sufficient knowledge of the nature, method, benefits and possible side effects of a planned medical intervention on the side of the patient is not only normatively, but also conceptually, necessary for them practicing their autonomy. For the act of giving consent can only be considered an expression of someone's autonomy in as much as they *know* what they are consenting to. Conveying that knowledge to the patients by informing them about all available facts that can be justly considered relevant to the decision process is, therefore, just as much an autonomy-related duty on the part of the physician as is the prohibition of curative interventions without any consent at all. There is no justification for forcing treatment on a competent patient, or for obtaining consent by concealing significant information, not even if the patient would otherwise face a severe risk of death. We emphasise that there is no reason to deviate from this well-founded principle of medical law and ethics with regard to the particular features of interventions in the brain.

A peculiarity of some of the possible effects of such interventions, though, lies in the fact that their full significance is sometimes very difficult to grasp. This may be true even for the intervening physician, and all the more so for the patient. For instance, our study shows that it is not obvious from the outset just what it means to say that a change of personal identity occurs. If a certain type of brain intervention is associated with a risk of identity change, then it can be difficult to convey that, in a certain important sense, this side effect is of a terminal nature. This difficulty may be compounded by the fact that a patient suffering from a serious medical condition is ready to grasp at any straw if it offers the chance possibility of a cure. In order to highlight the severity of such harm, it might be helpful to adopt the metaphor of "psychological death" which we introduced in Chapter 5. However, there is an obvious risk of a misleading overstatement in that expression, too. In our discussion above, we mention that there is usually a chance of overcoming even grave dissociative disorders which are the clearest manifestations of changes of personal identity. On the other hand, there is no guarantee of such a recovery. In this regard, it is plausible to draw the comparison with a state of coma in order to painstakingly point out to the patient that in a significant sense her personal self, primarily constituted by her present subjective consciousness, will possibly be non-existent for however long the dissociative state persists. This may indeed be forever.

Though representing a less drastic kind of mental harm, mere personality changes may also likely be underestimated as possible side effects. Concerning such side effects, it is crucial to describe their potential manifestations in as much detail as possible to a person reasoning about whether to undergo a certain intervention. However, it will be just as important to convey the principled prognostic limitations regarding personality changes, which result from the fact that any change in the narratively structured whole of a self-concept may give rise to an unforeseeable chain of reactions.

Exercising Autonomy under Coercive Circumstances

Doubts about the possibility of a truly autonomous consent may arise when a therapeutic brain intervention is to be undertaken on an (otherwise competent) person who is presently detained in prison or subjected to another form of legally justified custody. The standard situation of an illness manifesting itself during a legal term of imprisonment, and treatable by a brain intervention, poses no particular problem. There is, as we said, no legitimate way of forcing treatment on competent persons, and this pertains to prisoners no less than to other people. But problems do arise in a different setting: If and when (1) the detained person has served his full term of legal punishment, but (2), remains in custody (so-called preventive detention) because (3) he exhibits a severe form of sociopathy which renders him a permanent danger to his fellow citizens, but (4) which could possibly be treated by a novel method of brain intervention. (We are quite aware that presently the projection of such a medical possibility still has an air of science fiction to it. However, this may very well change in the not too distant future.) This gives rise to the following normative question: Does the only alternative that could be offered to such a sociopathic person (i.e. to either undergo the said brain intervention or remain detained indefinitely) leave enough leeway for an autonomous decision for viz. a valid consent to that intervention?

The answer is yes. The autonomy and thus the validity of a factual consent is not necessarily negated by the mere weight of the pressure under which it is given. If, for instance, that pressure is not exerted or wilfully controlled by other people but only by naturally given circumstances, it may be as high as one pleases, it may even, for any reasonable person, come close to being totally determinative of the ensuing decision, and yet not touch upon the autonomy and validity of that decision in the least. Hypothetically speaking, a patient diagnosed with kidney cancer, and confronted with the alternative of either consenting to a removal of the diseased kidney or certain death within a few months, will most probably choose the former. The person's consent to the surgery is doubtlessly autonomous and valid, even though she may feel that she has no reasonable alternative. In contrast, that same person, if threatened with death in case she refuses to consent to the removal of her kidney for transplantation purposes, could not be said to consent autonomously or validly to such a procedure. Projected onto our problem of the detained psychopath, the first thing to consider is that the pressure placed on a person by others who are legally entitled, or even obliged, to exert that force should be understood as really nothing other than the pressure exerted by the norms of law themselves. And as far as the autonomy of somebody confronted with that pressure is concerned, the force of the legal order (as part of the social environment) is on a par with the force of the natural order (the natural environment).[300] Hence, decisions of persons taken under compulsion of legal norms are no less autonomous than decisions under the compelling force of natural circumstances. Whether that compulsion is a direct effect of those norms on the deciding person or is the result of enforcement by intermediaries acting within their legal competence does not make a difference. Thus:

➔ If a brain-invasive treatment for severe psychopathy (that is in accord with the common criteria regarding the acceptability of associated risks) should ever become available, then nothing stands in the way of offering such a treatment to people in preventive detention if that is the only alternative to their being kept in custody indefinitely. The sheer force of pressure exerted on the detainee by those circumstances would infringe neither the autonomy nor the legal validity of his or her decision. We hold that, in such a situation, the state would be not only entitled but even obliged to make the respective offer.

---

[300] We presuppose here the normal case of legal systems that are, in principle, ethically legitimate. Terrorist or totalitarian regimes and their freedom restricting suppressive measures are a different matter; an enhancement offer under such circumstances would indeed amount to illegitimate blackmailing.

7.2.3.2 Enhancement and the Limits of Autonomy

Enhancement and the "Grave Affront" Principle

When considering issues of autonomy as they relate to measures of enhancement, legal considerations must be distinguished from purely ethical ones. As to the former, we refer to our above remarks on the limits of justifications for a physician to inflict physical harm on a consenting competent person. We marked the relevant boundary by using as the exemplary formula, derived from German criminal law, "grave affront to common ethical convictions and rules". Obviously, that limit of justification for the physician must be mirrored by a corresponding constraint on the side of the patient, viz. on his freedom of disposing of his physical integrity by prompting another person to carry out medico-technical interventions on him (i.e. in "two-party cases"). What the intervening physician is not justified in doing, the patient cannot legally permit by giving consent.

The "grave affront" boundary is certainly much lower in cases of mere enhancement than in cases of treatment.[301] However, the mere fact that an intervention in the brain for the sole purpose of enhancement may foreseeably result in significant alterations of a person's mental traits does not mean *ipso facto* that it transgresses that boundary. Hence, it does not *per se* exclude valid consent to such a measure.

➔ If an intervention in the brain is aimed at enhancement instead of treatment, this alone does not yet constitute a "grave affront" in the aforementioned sense. Regarding the question of whether individual enhancement can be justified, the individual liberty (autonomy as self-government) of a person wishing for such an enhancement provides a strong (though not yet decisive) argument in favour of it.

Still, the law can draw legitimate boundaries as to the scope of an individual's freedom of self-disposition. Most notably, it does so with regard to: i) the physical consequences of any procedure, if they consist in grave, disproportionate and irrevocable harm, and ii) the psychic consequences, if their manifestations can be considered comparably harmful or if they are clearly desired for fraudulent purposes alone.

It must be emphasised that these normative problems associated with the mental effects of enhancing brain interventions are only beginning to surface in legal scholarly debates. It is not at all clear yet where exactly the line that could be derived from the said "grave affront" standard should be

[301] As a matter of fact, treatments in accord with acknowledged medical standards can *never* transgress that boundary, since they not only presuppose an informed consent of the patient, but also an adequate weighing of risks and benefits of the intervention. Only treatments with a gravely disproportionate risk of bringing about severe and irrevocable harm as side effect could, in spite of the informed consent, amount to the "grave-affront" measure, e.g. in some, or most, of the "amputees-by-choice" cases (cf. note 297 supra).

drawn. Much further debate seems necessary. What we presently wish to warn against is the possible misuse of a legal standard formula (viz. the "grave affront" formula), developed for applications in a different normative area, by rashly employing it for an ideological struggle against all "artificial" methods of human self-development. Certainly, both of the limits of autonomy in two-party cases mentioned above are widely undisputed on the abstract semantic level of that formula, and this holds no less for interventions aiming at mental enhancements. However, it is not easy to solidify and illustrate that verbal abstraction with possible exemplary cases. We believe that this should caution legislators and courts against premature legal verdicts which always come at a social cost, even if only for personal liberties. There might be other grounds upon which the law can restrict the possibly unwelcome development of certain measures of mental enhancements than with recourse to the "grave affront" principle.

Enhancing Children: The Scope of Parental Discretion

A different matter, though, is that of enhancing brain interventions performed on children with their parents' "proxy consent". With regard to treatments, no specific normative problems appear to follow from brain-invasive methods as compared to other invasive medical procedures in children. By contrast, mere enhancements *do* pose specific problems. To clarify these, we emphasise an often overlooked insight which seems to gain special significance for such cases. Proxy consent must not be misunderstood as exercising a child's (or another incompetent person's) autonomy by a proxy. The very meaning of "autonomy" excludes such a possibility. Whatever else it may be, autonomy is, by its conceptual nature, something with respect to which one cannot be deputised by somebody else. The parental right to give or refuse proxy consent on behalf of their children encompasses two functions, neither of which has to do with the child's autonomy. First, proxy consent is intended to exercise control over what is done to their child for the sake of its well-being. Second, it is intended to realise the parents' own right to direct their child's upbringing within certain limits of the child's rights and well-being.

As far as brain-invasive procedures for purposes of mental enhancement are concerned, this double limitation of parental authority has two consequences (which, taken together, may be considered to establish a somewhat "paradoxical" legal situation). There exists nothing like an objective reasonable standard about what sort of "mind" is in a person's "best interest" (i.e. accords best to his or her well-being). Hence, on the one hand, the law rightly grants a wide discretional leeway to parents to shape their child's mental development according to what they themselves consider best. Thus, with regard to the development of a child's character traits in the widest sense, including its intellectual capacities, parents are legally entitled to instil their own value system in their offspring. They may even direct their child's mental development in ways that reasonable people would consider harmful to the child. This legal leeway certainly includes an abstract competence to decide in favour of furthering specific mental traits of the child, even at the cost of other developments, normally considered crucial for a child's future well-being. On the other hand, with regard to the physical condition of their child, parents do not possess such (potentially harmful) discretionary power. For in this instance, fairly clear objective standards of well-being exist and must not be violated by parents' decisions. According to present legal principles, physically invasive medical procedures on children can only be authorised by parental consent to the extent that they are necessary for the treatment of diseases. Parents have, for instance, no competence to authorise cosmetic surgery on their children, according to their own aesthetic preferences, unless, of course, such a surgery is deemed treatment, such as in the case of physical disfigurement. Thus:

➔ Although there is a legal parental right to modify a child's mental attributes according to the parents' own value-system by using traditional means of education, this right definitely ends where the physical integrity of the child begins. *A fortiori* brain-invasive procedures on a child solely for purposes of enhancement cannot, according to present legal standards, be validly consented to by the child's parents.

There is an obvious disparity between the wide leeway to instil even harmful mental developments by traditional means of education and the complete absence of any freedom to induce even useful mental enhancements by novel methods of brain intervention. Obviously, this creates a certain normative tension. This problem has as yet not been treated sufficiently by legal scholars and philosophers of law.

We urge the beginning of such a debate in both academia and society at large. It is especially necessary in light of the increasing exposure of children to cognition enhancing drugs, like Methylphenidate, which deeply influence the physical structure of the brain, as we are now well aware of. According to the legal standards sketched above, this current practice is, to a large extent, illicit. We believe that it is presently tolerated only on grounds of (1) collectively closing our eyes on the physical, viz. neuronal, effects of such drugs, and of (2) a tacitly growing medicalisation of heretofore normal, if undesired, variants of children's behaviour. The expansion of the concepts of both disease and treatment to include formerly normal mental features of children is problematic in various respects. It is reinforced by the conceptual vagueness of "mental disease", which considerably exceeds definitional ambiguities in the purely somatic sphere. Is a fidgety child a "milder case" of ADHD, or do they just present a minor, if undesired, deviation from parents' expectations, but remain well within the variants of normality? Much of the said tacit medicalisation takes place outside the normative control of legal institutions. Hence, it creates a host of social risks which society should address. This is not at all to say that all such brain-based enhancements on children should be fully and outrightly forbidden by law. It simply urges clarity, honesty and reasonable social control over a process that presently evolves on grounds of the *de facto* promotion of various interests, but is devoid of any normative justification. There will certainly be enhancement possibilities via brain interventions that are not acceptable for children, despite corresponding parental demands. However, just as certainly, other methods will be justifiable on grounds of legitimate parental wishes for the development of their offspring. This whole issue still awaits further clarification through social, scientific, and legal-ethical debate.

➔ Considering the many possible, but unexplored, long-term consequences of measures affecting the brain, we hold that presently a rather strict principle of caution is in order. In children, surgical interventions and electro-magnetic brain stimulations solely for enhancement purposes should, according to present legal rules, remain forbidden until a social consensus about the complex normative issues involved has been reached.

➔ With regard to the expansionist tendency of medicalisation, pharmaceutical interventions with possible long-term effects on the brain should be subject to more rigorous control, not only through financial instruments (for example through social security institutions), but also through an adequate enforcement of existing legal norms for the protection of children.

Concerns about Authenticity

Turning from issues of law to problems of ethics, we also turn to the second abstract meaning of autonomy, namely authenticity. Two questions arise around the enhancement of one's own mental capacities. The first concerns the *motive* for such an intervention whilst the second pertains to the *outcome* of the procedure. Roughly speaking, we must consider, first, whether the motive proffered for the proposed procedure is a "sufficiently authentic motive", and second, whether the mentally enhanced person will be a "sufficiently authentic self" in order for both to be truly autonomous. Both questions presuppose certain moral duties that autonomous persons have towards themselves, against which that sufficiency must be measured.

We do not elaborate on the philosophical problem of moral "duties to oneself" as stipulated by Kant and debated ever since, though we do accept the idea that some such duties can possibly be substantiated and defended on the grounds of a secular ethics. However, we may safely ignore this problem here. For there is obviously no moral duty to abstain from enhancing one's own mental capacities. Following Kant, many people would even claim the opposite: a moral duty to develop one's natural mental endowment. Whether one is merely permitted, or even obliged, to improve oneself, both possibilities entail the individual liberty to choose particular mental features for improvement, since not all of them could possibly be improved upon to the same degree. This freedom of choice extends, in principle, to the ways and means of self-improvement. That is to say, the mere fact that novel methods of brain interventions are in some way "unnatural" or "artificial" is no ground on which to doubt the basic moral entitlement to shape one's own mind, let alone to abolish and replace this entitlement with a moral duty to do the exact opposite. As we already saw, using such interventions for mental enhancement may give rise to various concerns about risks and side effects, or about their future use for fraudulent purposes. In "two-party cases" such concerns may certainly warrant not only a moral, but even a legal, prohibition. This is, however, a different problem. Such prohibitions are destined to prevent consensual harm amounting to a "grave affront" in the sense described above. However, they do certainly not aim at preserving one's "natural" (i.e. unenhanced) mental status.

A second concern about authenticity arises from fears that mass deployments of brain-invasive mental enhancements might create subtle, or even overt, pressure on everybody to participate in that new way of meeting the demands of social competition. Collective pressure of that kind would certainly give rise to a host of social concerns. Developments in this direction should be observed, and if sufficiently verified, counteracted by political and legal instruments. However, such a social pressure, unwelcome as it may be, would not infringe upon the authenticity (viz. autonomy) of individual decisions complying with it. After all, other kinds of social development like, for instance, new fashion trends or technical innovations (e.g. telephones or computers) do not compromise the autonomy of their adherents even though they certainly exert a massive influence on people's individual decisions. To be sure, there is a crucial moral difference between the social pressure to use a computer in order to meet one's daily professional demands, and the pressure to have one's mental capacities enhanced by a brain intervention for that very same purpose. But that difference does not concern the autonomy or authenticity of decisions yielding to such pressure. Rather, it concerns the inviolability of one's physical sphere, which is subject to a considerably stronger protection against invasions and, therefore, against external coercive forces urging such invasions, than is the "inviolability" of one's behaviour against coercive influences from societal developments. (We will return to that point *sub specie* "Justice", 7.2.4.2, below.)

Finally, we do not see a convincing reason to doubt that a person with artificially enhanced mental capacities is still an authentic self in the sense that her decisions can still be true to her nature.[302] One can surely be sceptical about the subjective value of such an enhancement for that person her-

[302] The assessment regarding her enhanced capacities may be different, especially if her "old nature" (her cognitive attributes and personality before the enhancement) is used as the yardstick.

self. As has been pointed out in Chapter 6, at least with respect to some human skills the means employed do matter for the assessment of the ends achieved. In these cases our admiration for other people's performance apparently hinges, to a great extent, on the personal effort by which those skills were acquired. The devaluation of athletic performances proven to have been enabled by performance enhancing drugs serves as a telling example. This may raise a warning flag against easy shortcuts to desired ends and it might even warrant a warning to completely abstain from, or at least not to enter too lightly into, artificial mental enhancements. While the possible devaluation of certain ends by the means employed to achieve them *can* be due to a lack of authenticity on the part of a person employing such means, this is not necessarily the case – no more so than any futile, or even detrimental modification of one's personality could be said to compromise one's authenticity simply by virtue of its worthlessness alone. We wish to highlight that judging this differently, i.e. considering an artificial mental enhancement to be a violation of a certain duty to oneself, would only mark a difference in ethical opinion. It would not, however, yield a sufficient normative ground for legal prohibition since modern constitutional states are *not* justified in legally enforcing every normative proposition just on account of it being a moral duty.

7.2.4 Justice: Inequality, Fair Distribution, Political Justice

"Justice" is at least as complex a concept as "autonomy". We distinguish, along common lines, four divisions of its meaning: distributive, commutative (viz. exchange), corrective, and political justice. Only the first and the last of these sub-concepts bear on the questions of our analysis.

Generally speaking, theories of distributive justice aim at establishing principles of fair distribution of certain benefits and burdens ensuing from interactions between members of cooperative societies. A host of such principles have been proposed in moral, legal, and political philosophy, which vary in numerous respects, e.g. in what benefits should be subject to distribution (e.g. income, opportunities, well-being), or what primary criterion or mechanism should be used to guide the process of allocating such benefits (e.g. equality, need, free market transactions). Divergent opinions on all of these matters notwithstanding, there is a general consensus that not all objects are subject to principles of distributive justice merely by virtue of their having value. Only "primary social goods", to employ John Rawls' famous term, are proper objects of distributive justice, i.e. goods that are (1) not merely natural endowments, and are (2) valuable for every rational member of society, irrespective of his or her individual preferences and personal life plan. Medical services surely belong among those primary goods. They are socially distributed and destined to preserve or restore health, which is an "enabling" (or "all-purpose") precondition for any reasonable life plan of any rational person. Less obvious, though, is the scope of human conditions medical services should be allocated to, ranging from life-threatening states to idiosyncratic personal preferences.

For the purpose of our analysis, we understand the term "political justice" to include all other tasks of surveying, controlling, and, if necessary, correcting social developments in the realm of medicine which actually or potentially concern the rights or interests of each individual, and of society as a whole.

7.2.4.1 Problems of Distributive Justice

With respect to the just allocation of resources, no normative problems arise which are specific to the subject of this study in any of the three genuine spheres of the medical profession: treatment (as delineated above), prevention and research. Some of the uncommon intricacies of the new methods of brain intervention may raise the question whether they yield a reasonable ratio of costs and benefits. In some cases the wisdom of recognising them as medical treatments may appear doubtful. For instance, loss of certain mental or physical functions can be alleviated with neural prosthesis. This would appear at first to be a clear example of a medical treatment. However, the less severe the functional loss which can be restored by such a neural prosthesis, the more likely health insurance companies and other financial providers will be to compare its implantation to cosmetic surgery and other such interventions which exist on the borderline between treatment and enhancement. However, such problems are common to most innovative, technologically complex, and hence expensive, medical procedures. These problems do not primarily concern principles of justice, but involve, rather, questions of definition and matters of political and economic prudence.

Difficult problems of justice, however, do arise with respect to enhancements. We distinguish two different types of problem, which might be roughly labelled the "inequality-exacerbating effect", and the "resource-squandering effect".

Does Enhancement Exacerbate Existing Social Inequality?

The problem of the inequality-exacerbating effect is connected with our recommendation for a strict exclusion of pure enhancement procedures from the publicly funded system of medicine. If the costs of enhancements are not taken over by *other* means of public funding, it then follows that only those who can afford to pay for such services will have a chance to benefit from their mind-enhancing effects. Most of these services are, and will continue to be, very costly. Thus only well-to-do people will be in a position to obtain such benefits for themselves or their families. This in turn could exacerbate existing social inequalities by granting those who are already privileged additional advantages in many areas of social competition.

If this prospect became reality, it would be bound to undermine distributive justice. Certain mental capacities, such as alertness or intelligence, are "positional goods", i.e. they confer substantial advantages on their possessors in relation to others in terms of their ability to compete for scarce positions or goods. If such capacities cease to be mere natural assets and become instead the potential result of human intervention, access to these intervention procedures may become a legitimate object of distributive justice. If (1) means of mental enhancements are available only to the wealthy, and (2) making use of such means confers substantial competitive advantages for the acquisition of wealth, and (3) a grossly unequal distribution of wealth is a matter of concern for distributive justice, then the exacerbating effect of artificial mental enhancements on problematic patterns of social distribution is obvious.

As is well known, premise (3) has been subject to longstanding and hotly contested philosophical debate. We could not seriously attempt to engage in that discussion here. Suffice it to say the following. There is no doubt that legislatures, even in the most liberal states, are justified in attempting to counteract the development of increasing inequalities in wealth amongst their citizens. This is especially true when the reason for such increased inequality is not in proportion with how deserving the privileged are of their increased relative prosperity. Broadly speaking, this would be the case for any social or financial advantages arising as a direct result of artificial mental enhancements, if they were to have the social effects described above. This, we hold, is reason enough to raise a moral warning flag. Thus, we wish to emphasise that potential developments such as those described above should be monitored closely by competent institutions in the fields of politics, science, and society in general:

➔ Clear indications that an increasing availability of purchasable mental enhancements fuels social inequality, in terms of the distribution of wealth and opportunities, should be counteracted.

The methods employed to counteract this must, of course, fulfil common criteria of proportionality. Hence, they fall across a wide spectrum of possible measures from tax policies, to restrictive licensing practices vis-à-vis medical enhancements, and even the *ultima ratio* of legal prohibition. We wish to underline that it would not be sufficient to counteract negative tendencies of the above kind by (partly) redistributing the unequally accumulated wealth via taxes. For a grossly unequal distribution of social opportunities, be they for professional positions or other goods relevant to the quality of individual life, also entails an unequal distribution of self-esteem, which may well constitute, as John Rawls has argued, the most important of all primary goods. That kind of inequality cannot sufficiently be compensated for by mere financial measures.

However, two *caveats* must be added at this juncture to ward against too readily adopting interventionist policies at the present time.

(1) Whether or not the sketched negative developments will become manifest is an empirical question. It cannot be answered by mere theoretical

speculations, no matter how plausible they may appear, but must be proven by observable facts. Up to now, such facts have not been established. Even technologically advanced societies with strong inclinations towards science and technological innovation seem, as yet, to be far from experiencing any such detrimental effects on distributive justice. Of course, legitimate policies may, and should, aim at preventing potential undesired developments. However, that requires a complex process of weighing the duty to protect individuals and society in terms of freedom and civil liberties. This process, in turn, must be based on sufficient information about impending risks. Without such knowledge, rational and proportionate countermeasures are hardly conceivable. We hold that the information presently available for legislators and other political decision makers is clearly insufficient for a sensible assessment of the issue. Since political impediments, let alone legal prohibitions, always come at a price for individual and societal liberty, we propose that governments and legislatures currently confine their policies to the procedures of attentive observation we mentioned above.

(2) Our call for political restraint is further strengthened by the following considerations. As argued above, certain mental capacities are positional goods, i.e. they confer competitive advantages in numerous contexts of social life. However, these capacities also have what can be called independent value, i.e. a value for the individual who possesses them alone. Well-developed cognitive abilities may, for example, enable the person endowed with them to successfully participate in competitive enterprises. Yet they can also lay the foundations for the development and satisfaction of certain intellectual preferences which relate only to personal enjoyment and will have little or no economic background. The freedom of developing one's subjective capacities for a more fulfilling mental life should not be ignored or underestimated. These considerations corroborate the above proposal to refrain at the current time from any prohibitive interference with the development and applications of brain-invasive techniques of mental enhancement.

Does Enhancement Entail Wastage of Medical Resources?

The use of medical resources for mere enhancement purposes could be criticised as a waste of the scarce resources otherwise available, and originally intended for, therapy or prevention. The justifiability of such a position would not depend upon who pays for the (mis)application of such means. Hence, it is of no relevance that, according to our recommendations so far, it should always be the individual recipient of an enhancement, as opposed to the public health care system, who has to bear the immediate cost. Rather, the critique hints at the *absolute limitation* of medical resources. In other words, regardless of who bears the costs of a medical procedure, medical resources (including individual expertise) which are used up for one particular purpose are, consequently, unavailable for any other potential application. Therefore, those resources deployed for enhancement purposes are unavailable for use for the purpose of treating serious, and even potentially life-threatening, medical conditions. There may not be a *direct* link between the use of a specific set of resources in one area and their lack in another functional context. Nevertheless, if we take the system of healthcare as a whole, a certain level of interdependence is inevitable.

This critique of enhancement procedures is based on two assumptions. First, that the entirety of medical resources in a given society is always, or at least normally, subject to a more or less exhaustive demand, or claim upon them, by that society's members. That is to say, available resources are, at any given time, being utilised at nearly full capacity. The scarcity of medical resources notwithstanding, this does not, however, appear to be a very plausible assumption. Second, a resource-squandering effect would be proven if the widespread use of medical resources for purposes of mental enhancements were actually to compromise significantly the availability of similar procedures for the purpose of medical treatment. In that case, their application for mere enhancements would be, to some extent, parasitic on their primary purpose as treatment. This could also be criticised as violating principles of distributive justice. After all, not only the application, but also the production, of medical resources is a huge and permanent drain on a society's financial resources.

We consider the critique based on the second assumption plausible to some extent, provided it turns out to rest on a sound empirical basis. Whether or not this is the case is quite unclear at present. (That type of resource-squandering effect could be just as well attested to the present, and widely accepted, practice of cosmetic surgery.) This is again reason enough to raise a moral warning flag, accompanied by an admonition to observe the various social effects of such practices. It does not, however, provide sufficient grounds, at the current time at least, for an outright legal prohibition of possible applications of brain interventions for mental enhancement.

7.2.4.2 Problems of Political Justice in General

When discussing authenticity, we already alluded to the risk that a widespread use of brain-invasive mental enhancements might begin to exert a growing pressure on people, otherwise unwilling to undergo such procedures, to do so for fear of suffering substantial competitive disadvantages. As argued above, this type of social pressure would not infringe on these people's legal autonomy. Hence, it would not invalidate their consent to such a brain-invasive procedure, should they yield to that pressure. However, the state surely has a right, and even – within certain limits set by its discretionary power – a *prima facie* duty to intervene to protect citizens from such coercive social demands. A social pressure to undergo physically invasive procedures bears considerably more weight than, say, the coercive effect of a largely motorised society on its members to obtain a drivers license and use a car to retain competitive ability. Given the primary importance of the state's duty to protect the physical integrity of its citizens, even an indirect and mediated danger to physical integrity requires careful consideration of whether to block potentially harmful developments by legal prohibitions.

The plausibility of calling for a more or less immediate prohibition depends on whether social pressure to undergo mental enhancement actually develops. This, in turn, cannot be predicted at present with any amount of accuracy. That gives us reason for a final, and particularly important, warning flag in the realm of social justice.

➔ The possibility of an impending threat on people's liberty to abstain from brain-invasive enhancements should be subject to especially vigilant monitoring by competent political authorities and scientific institutions. Should evidence of such a development emerge on a sufficiently large scale, it seems imperative for the state to intervene in order to protect those citizens averse to enhancement.

However, unless there is empirical evidence of this kind of development occurring, any prohibition on such enhancements should be withheld. Legislation against unwanted, but uncertain, social threats, whose effects could still potentially be blocked when, or if , they occur, is not justified in constitutional liberal states.

Main results

- Having studied new methods for intervening in the brain by means of psychopharmacology, neurotransplantation, gene transfer, neural prosthetics and electrical brain stimulation, the authors of this book acknowledge and endorse their potential to benefit the individual, as well as society, by yielding innovative therapeutic applications. Of course, since these interventions operate directly on the brain, it is obligatory to handle them with appropriate caution, even if they are used for treatment purposes only.
- There is a public preoccupation with the possibility of patients being transformed in radical and obvious ways by new techniques for intervening in the brain. This might detract attention from those side effects which actually give more reason for concern, namely subtle changes of the psyche in general, and of personality in particular, which may easily go unnoticed.
- During the research phase, any new method of intervening in the brain should be monitored systematically for subtle side effects pertaining to personality and those mental capacities related to personhood.
- If a particular type of brain intervention with known possible subtle side effects pertaining to personality or mental capacities related to personhood is approved for certain therapeutic or preventive applications, then every person undergoing that procedure should be carefully monitored for the occurrence of such side effects after the procedure is conducted so that they can receive appropriate treatment if necessary.
- Whether the prospect of an intervention in the brain having a certain personality change as a side effect is acceptable, or even desirable, can only be decided by the affected persons themselves *before* they undergo that intervention.
- For experimental interventions in patients with neurological and psychiatric disorders, time-scheduled and disease-specific core assessment protocols (CAPs) should be established in order to (1) obtain meaningful results and (2) enable comparisons between different treatment approaches.
- If an intervention in the brain is aimed at enhancement instead of treatment, this alone does not yet constitute a "grave affront to common ethical convictions and rules". Regarding the question of whether individual enhancement can be justified, the individual liberty (autonomy as self-government) of a person wishing for such an enhancement provides a strong (though not yet decisive) argument in favour of it.

- We do not endorse a principled ethical rejection, let alone an outright legal prohibition, of interventions in the human brain aimed at mental enhancements solely on grounds of their physical or mental risks for the affected individual. It must be underlined, however, that potential negative side effects of mere enhancements weigh more heavily against intended positive effects than they would in treatment cases. Physicians intervening for enhancement purposes alone have enlarged informational duties towards their clients. To the extent that their duties to patients are increased, they are also obliged to acquire pertinent additional information for themselves.
- Enhancing healthy human beings is not a genuine part of the responsibility of health care professionals, which is to treat and prevent diseases. Hence, brain interventions aiming only at enhancement do not fall under the obligatory force of the principle of beneficence in medicine, notwithstanding the fact that there are borderline cases which are difficult to delineate from treatment.
- Enhancements which cannot at least count as prevention of disease/disability ("mere" enhancements) should not be included in the sphere of "proper medicine" as a social system.
- Research exclusively geared towards the development of means for mental enhancement by intervening in the brain should not be subsidised by public funds devoted to the social system of healthcare. Furthermore, the application of the products of such research to achieve mental enhancement should also not be funded by the healthcare system.
- Although there is a legal parental right to modify a child's mental attributes according to the parents' own value-system by using traditional means of education, this right definitely ends where the physical integrity of the child begins. *A fortiori* brain-invasive procedures on a child solely for purposes of enhancement cannot, according to present legal standards, be validly consented to by the child's parents.
- Considering the many possible, but unexplored, long-term consequences of measures affecting the brain, we hold that presently a rather strict principle of caution is in order. In children, surgical interventions and electro-magnetic brain stimulations solely for enhancement purposes should, according to present legal rules, remain forbidden until a social consensus about the complex normative issues involved has been reached.

- With regard to the expansionist tendency of medicalisation, pharmaceutical interventions with possible long-term effects on the brain should be subject to more rigorous control, not only through financial instruments (for example through social security institutions), but also through an adequate enforcement of existing legal norms for the protection of children.
- If a brain-invasive treatment for severe psychopathy (that is in accord with the common criteria regarding the acceptability of associated risks) should ever become available, then nothing stands in the way of offering such a treatment to people in preventive detention if that is the only alternative to their being kept in custody indefinitely. The sheer force of pressure exerted on the detainee by those circumstances would infringe neither the autonomy nor the legal validity of his or her decision. We hold that, in such a situation, the state would be not only entitled but even obliged to make the respective offer.
- Clear indications that an increasing availability of purchasable mental enhancements fuels social inequality, in terms of the distribution of wealth and opportunities, should be counteracted.
- The possibility of an impending threat on people's liberty to abstain from brain-invasive enhancements should be subject to especially vigilant monitoring by competent political authorities and scientific institutions. Should evidence of such a development emerge on a sufficiently large scale, it seems imperative for the state to intervene in order to protect those citizens averse to enhancement.

Zusammenfassung

Zusammenfassung: Ergebnisse und Empfehlungen 421
1 Methoden zur Intervention am Gehirn 422
1.1 Psychopharmakanutzung bei Kindern und Jugendlichen 422
1.2 Neurotransplantation und Gentransfer 425
1.3 Neuroprothetik des zentralen Nervensystems 429
1.4 Elektrische Hirnstimulation bei psychiatrischen Störungen 432
2 Begriffliche Klärungen 433
2.1 Die Relevanz verschiedener Bedenken zur personalen Integrität .. 433
2.2 Grenzen des Sozialsystems Medizin: Behandlung – Enhancement – Prävention 435
2.2.1 Die Legitimität genuin medizinischer Verfahren 435
2.2.2 Enhancement versus Behandlung 436
2.2.3 Der Zweck der Medizin: Krankheiten bekämpfen 437
2.2.4 Enhancement dient nicht dem Zweck der Medizin 438
2.2.5 Selbst-Enhancement versus Enhancement anderer 438
3 Normative Grundlagen 440
3.1 Schädigungsverbot: Das Vermeiden von Schaden bei Eingriffen in das Gehirn 440
3.1.1 Zum Umgang mit Nebenwirkungen in Forschung und medizinischer Praxis 441
Die Überwachung subtiler psychischer Nebenwirkungen 441
Die Subtilität von Persönlichkeitsveränderungen 443
3.1.2 Möglichen Schaden durch sorgfältigen Studienentwurf minimieren 445
3.1.3 Mögliche Schädigungen durch Enhancement 445
Gibt es illegitime Ziele von Enhancements? 448
Zum Umgang mit möglichen Nebenwirkungen von Enhancements 449
3.2 Hilfe leisten („Wohltun"): Die Grenzen zwischenmenschlicher Wohltätigkeit 450
3.2.1 Behandlung und Prävention 450
3.2.2 Verantwortlichkeit und Haftung für Enhancement 450
3.2.3 Öffentliche Forschungsfinanzierung 451

3.3 Autonomie: Probleme der informierten Einwilligung und von Zwang 453
3.3.1 Behandlung, Prävention und Forschung 454
Die schwere Fassbarkeit psychischer Schäden als Hindernis für eine aufgeklärte Einwilligung 454
Das Ausüben von Autonomie unter äußerem Zwang 455
3.3.2 Enhancement und die Grenzen der Autonomie 457
Enhancement als möglicher „Verstoß gegen die guten Sitten" 457
Enhancement von Kindern: Der Umfang der elterlichen Entscheidungsgewalt 459
Die Authentizität betreffende Bedenken 461
3.4 Gerechtigkeit: Ungleichheit; gerechte Verteilung; politische Gerechtigkeit 464
3.4.1 Probleme der Verteilungsgerechtigkeit 465
Könnte Enhancement bestehende soziale Ungleichheiten verschärfen? 465
Bedeutet Enhancement eine Verschwendung medizinischer Ressourcen? 468
3.4.2 Allgemeine Probleme der politischen Gerechtigkeit 469

Zusammenfassung: Ergebnisse und Empfehlungen

Die Geschichte therapeutischer Eingriffe in die Psyche ist so alt wie die überlieferte Geschichte der Medizin selbst. Bereits die altägyptische, die traditionelle chinesische und die antike griechische Medizin enthielten Vorschriften zur Behandlung von Krankheiten, die heute als „psychische" aufgefasst werden (Millon 2004). Doch auch jenseits dessen, was als Therapie galt, hat die Menschheit schon immer nach Möglichkeiten gesucht, psychische Fähigkeiten und Zustände zu verbessern oder zu erweitern, was insbesondere durch die vielfältigen Traditionen religiöser und spiritueller Praktiken belegt wird. Diese historische Perspektive sollte nicht vergessen werden, wenn man sich mit einigen prinzipiellen Bedenken befasst, denen zufolge die neuartigen Methoden des Eingreifens in das zentrale Nervensystem nicht nur neue Möglichkeiten für Behandlung und *Enhancement*[303] der Psyche eröffnen, sondern auch unerwünschte Wirkungen auf mentaler Ebene haben können.

→ Die Autoren der hier zusammengefassten Studie haben wesentliche der besagten neuartigen Methoden aus den Bereichen Psychopharmarkologie, Neurotransplantation, Neuroprothetik und elektrische Hirnstimulation eingehend untersucht. Sie erkennen deren Potential zu therapeutischer Hilfe für den Einzelnen und zum Nutzen für die Gesellschaft an. Da solche Eingriffe unmittelbar auf das Gehirn einwirken, muss ihre Anwendung mit besonderer Sorgfalt erfolgen, auch wenn sie ausschließlich therapeutischen Zwecken zu dienen bestimmt sind.

Wegen der höchst komplexen, integrativen Funktionsweise des Gehirns lässt sich die Möglichkeit praktisch nicht ausschließen, dass bei therapeutischen Interventionen unerwünschte psychische Nebenwirkungen auftreten. Das gilt unbeschadet der Frage, ob der Eingriff Wirkungen auf psychischer Ebene herbeiführen soll oder nicht. Die Aufgabe, einen ethisch akzeptablen Umgang mit derartigen Risiken zu finden, ist gewiss nicht neu. Im Gegenteil, seitdem überhaupt therapeutische Eingriffe mittels physiologischer oder struktureller Veränderungen des zentralen Nervensystems unternommen werden, musste man mit dem Auftreten unvorhergesehener Effekte rechnen und das entsprechende Risiko rechtfertigen. Solche Effekte können nicht nur

[303] In etwa „Steigerung" oder „Verbesserung". Jedoch übernehmen wir den Ausdruck „Enhancement" im Folgenden als Terminus technicus, weil er sich als Lehnwort mit ganz eigenen Konnotationen mittlerweile auch in der deutschsprachigen Debatte durchgesetzt hat.

psychische, sondern auch andere Funktionen betreffen. Im Übrigen stellt sich die allgemeine Herausforderung, eine vernünftige Abwägung zwischen voraussichtlichem Nutzen einer therapeutischen Intervention und der Wahrscheinlichkeit sowie dem Gewicht möglicher psychischer Folgeschäden zu treffen, keineswegs nur für Eingriffe ins *Gehirn*. So können etwa – um nur ein Beispiel zu nennen – Mastektomien mit einer ganzen Reihe psychischer Nebenwirkungen verbunden sein, beginnend bei vorübergehenden Depressionen bis hin zu dauerhaften Veränderungen des weiblichen Selbstverständnisses betroffener Frauen.

Es folgt eine knappe Zusammenfassung wichtiger Resultate des ersten Teils dieser Studie (Kapitel 1–4), der eine Darstellung einzelner Methoden zur Intervention am Gehirn mit ihren gegenwärtigen Möglichkeiten und Entwicklungsperspektiven enthält. Anschließend werden die Empfehlungen der Autoren zum weiteren Umgang mit den hier untersuchten Interventionsmöglichkeiten vor dem Hintergrund der Ergebnisse des zweiten Teils dieser Studie (Kapitel 5 und 6) begründet.

1 Methoden zur Intervention am Gehirn

1.1 Psychopharmakanutzung bei Kindern und Jugendlichen

Innerhalb des Spektrums der in dieser Studie untersuchten Interventionsmöglichkeiten umfasst der Bereich der Psychopharmakologie die ältesten und am besten erforschten Methoden zur Einflussnahme auf psychische Zustände und psychiatrische Störungen. Das diesen Methoden gewidmete Kapitel 1 beschäftigt sich insbesondere mit der Psychopharmakologie des Kindes- und Jugendalters, weil sich anhand dieses Gebiets eine Reihe kritischer Themen herausarbeiten lässt, die auch für jüngst entwickelte Eingriffsmöglichkeiten in die Psyche von Belang ist. Das Kapitel bietet einen Überblick über die psychopharmakologischen Substanzklassen, die gegenwärtig bei der Behandlung von Kindern und Jugendlichen mit psychiatrischen Problemen zur Anwendung gelangen. Drei besonders wichtige Substanzklassen wurden ausgewählt, um den Leser in die ethischen Konflikte und technischen Schwierigkeiten einzuführen, die sich bezüglich Therapie und Forschung im Bereich der Psychopharmakologie des Kindes- und Jugendalters stellen:

1. Am Beispiel der Behandlung von Depressionen bei Kindern durch selektive Serotonin-Wiederaufnahmehemmer (SSRIs) lassen sich die vielfältigen Probleme der so genannten „off-label"-Verwendung von Medikamenten verdeutlichen. Allgemein gilt, dass mehr als 75% der an Kinder in psychiatrischen Einrichtungen verschriebenen Medikamente off-label, also ohne empirischen Nachweis der Sicherheit und Wirksamkeit durch

altersspezifische Studien, zur Anwendung gelangen. SSRIs sind in jüngerer Zeit in Verdacht geraten, bei depressiven Kindern und Jugendlichen zu erhöhter Suizidalität zu führen. Die bloße Möglichkeit eines solchen Risikos unterstreicht bereits das Erfordernis ausreichender Prüfungen der Medikamentensicherheit für verschiedene Altersgruppen. Ganz allgemein darf vermutet werden, dass das Auftreten von Spätfolgen durch therapeutische Interventionen am Gehirn umso wahrscheinlicher ist, je früher in der Individualentwicklung sie vorgenommen werden. Manche dieser Spätfolgen mögen sich als vorteilhaft erweisen, bei anderen kann es sich dagegen um spät auftretende Nebenwirkungen handeln. Weiterhin lässt sich aus dem SSRI-Skandal die Lehre ziehen, dass Forschungsergebnisse bisweilen unveröffentlicht bleiben, wenn Wissenschaftler in Interessenkonflikte mit Pharmaunternehmen geraten.

2. Dass psychopharmakologische Interventionen nicht nur für therapeutische, sondern auch für Zwecke des Enhancements genutzt werden können, zeigt das Beispiel der Behandlung der Aufmerksamkeitsdefizit-/Hyperaktivitätsstörung (ADHS) durch Stimulanzien. Es werden dringend zuverlässige diagnostische Verfahren benötigt, mit denen gesunde Personen, die ihre normal ausgeprägten kognitiven Fähigkeiten steigern wollen, unterschieden werden können von Patienten, die an einem kognitiven Defizit leiden oder allgemeiner eine psychiatrische Erkrankung bzw. Störung aufweisen.
3. Die letzte Fallstudie aus dem Bereich der Psychopharmakologie des Kindes- und Jugendalters betrifft die so genannten atypischen Neuroleptika. Deren Beispiel belegt die besondere Bedeutung, die Fragen der Entscheidungsfähigkeit und der informierten bzw. aufgeklärten Einwilligung im Kontext der Behandlung junger Patienten mit schweren psychiatrischen Erkrankungen zukommt. Die Ausführungen zu den atypischen Neuroleptika beginnen mit einem kritischen Überblick über Studien zur präventiven Behandlung von Jugendlichen in der prodromalen Phase der Schizophrenie. Dabei wird zunächst ein konsequentialistischer Standpunkt eingenommen und eine utilitaristische Analyse des Nutzens und der Risiken präventiver psychopharmakologischer Maßnahmen durchgeführt. Anschließend wird vor dem Hintergrund des Prinzips der Achtung vor fremder Autonomie dargestellt, wie der Wunsch junger Patienten nach Selbstbestimmung in Konflikt zu elterlichen Entscheidungen über Behandlungsmaßnahmen geraten kann.

Die Ergebnisse der genannten Fallstudien werden anschließend auf der Grundlage von vier weithin anerkannten Prinzipien der medizinischen Ethik kritisch reflektiert.[304] Im Zusammenhang der Psychopharmakologie

[304] In der hier gewählten Formulierung wurden die vier Prinzipien von Tom L. Beauchamp und James F. Childress in ihrem einflussreichen Werk „Principles of Biomedical Ethics“ (2001) eingeführt.

des Kindes- und Jugendalters lässt sich vom Schädigungsverbot *(nonmaleficence)* die Forderung nach größeren Anstrengungen zur Gewährleistung der langfristigen Sicherheit von pharmazeutischen Eingriffen während der Entwicklungsphase ableiten. Die komplementäre Forderung nach aussagekräftigen Belegen für die Wirksamkeit solcher Interventionen ergibt sich entsprechend aus dem Gebot zur Hilfeleistung *(beneficence)*. Das Prinzip der Achtung vor Autonomie *(respect for autonomy)* muss im gegebenen Kontext nicht nur im Verhältnis zwischen Arzt und Patient Berücksichtigung finden, sondern vielmehr bei der Vielzahl möglicher Interessenkonflikte im Beziehungsdreieck zwischen Eltern, Kind und Arzt. Das Paradigma der informierten Einwilligung, demzufolge die gültige Einwilligung zu einer medizinischen Maßnahme die umfassende Aufklärung über deren mögliche Folgen zur Voraussetzung hat, lässt sich nicht ohne weiteres auf diese Konstellation anwenden. Kinder haben besondere Informationsbedürfnisse und sollten psychiatrischen Interventionen zustimmen *(assent)*, auch wenn ihre Einwilligung *(consent)* nicht hinreicht, um deren Durchführung rechtlich zu legitimieren. Ein weiteres Problem der Selbstbestimmung, das in Kapitel 1 besprochen wird, betrifft den Gebrauch von Verfahren zur medikamentösen Ruhigstellung *(chemical restraint)* in der Psychiatrie. Zuletzt gibt auch das Prinzip der Gerechtigkeit *(justice)* Grund zu erheblichen Bedenken, wenn es um psychopharmakologische Interventionen bei Kindern und Jugendlichen geht. Kinder werden gelegentlich als „therapeutische Waisen" bezeichnet, weil so viele der ihnen verschriebenen Medikamente nur für Erwachsene zugelassen sind. Es müssen Regelungen eingeführt werden, um angemessene Prüfverfahren auch für solche Medikamente sicherzustellen, die auf die Bedürfnisse kleiner Bevölkerungsgruppen zugeschnitten sind und daher keine profitablen Märkte bedienen.

In die Lage therapeutischer Waisen, die derzeit so kennzeichnend für die Kinder- und Jugendpsychiatrie ist, könnten zukünftig viele weitere Patientengruppen geraten. Je größer das Verständnis der molekularen und genetischen Mechanismen wird, die psychiatrischen Erkrankungen zugrunde liegen, desto mehr setzt sich die Erkenntnis durch, dass scheinbar ähnliche pathologische Erscheinungsbilder auf ganz unterschiedliche Weise entstehen können. Demzufolge werden die Patientengruppen immer kleiner werden, für die ein bestimmter Behandlungsansatz geeignet erscheint. Dies wird zur Folge haben, dass Fragen des Schutzes spezieller Bevölkerungsgruppen, z.B. von Kindern, alten, demenzkranken oder auch geistig behinderten Menschen, immer mehr an Bedeutung gewinnen werden. Auf lange Sicht ist damit zu rechnen, dass die Entwicklung hin zu immer spezifischeren Behandlungsansätzen für verschiedene Genotypen eine ganz neue Ausrichtung der Gerechtigkeitsdebatte in Medizinrecht und Medizinethik nach sich ziehen wird.

Heutzutage zielen die meisten neuen Möglichkeiten zur Intervention am Gehirn auf Erwachsene mit schweren Erkrankungen und ungünstiger Prog-nose ab. Zukünftig könnten dagegen vermehrt neuroprotektive Verfahren zur Verfügung stehen, mit denen sich die Entwicklung von Kindern so beeinflussen ließe, dass diese gar nicht erst anfällig für psychiatrische Erkrankungen werden würden. Allerdings sind die ethischen und rechtlichen Rahmenbedingungen für Forschungsvorhaben im Bereich der Neuroprotektion noch viel zu wenig erforscht.

1.2 Neurotransplantation und Gentransfer

Das zweite Kapitel dieser Studie ist Methoden der zellulären und molekularen Intervention am Gehirn im Bereich der wiederherstellenden Neurochirurgie gewidmet. In den letzten Jahrzehnten hat das Wissen über die Funktionsweise des Gehirns auf zellulärer und molekularer Ebene dramatisch zugenommen. Darüber hinaus konnte in Tierversuchen gezeigt werden, dass es möglich ist, geschädigte Teilsysteme des Gehirns durch Zellimplantation und Gentransfer funktionell wiederherzustellen. Auf der Grundlage der Implantation von (unreifen) Nervenzellen (Neurotransplantation) und der Injektion viraler Vektoren zum Zweck des therapeutischen Gentransfers wurden in den letzten Jahrzehnten experimentelle klinische Behandlungsansätze für eine Reihe von degenerativen und traumatischen Hirnschädigungen erprobt.

Bei Verfahren der Neurotransplantation im Humanbereich werden neue Zellen als Zellsuspension oder auch Fragmente unreifen Hirngewebes implantiert. Dagegen lässt sich die Neurotransplantation nicht als Methode für den Ersatz *ausgedehnter* Hirnareale betrachten, welche aufgrund degenerativer Veränderung oder verletzungsbedingt ausgefallen sind. Das ausgereifte Gehirn ist ein morphologisch heterogenes Organ, bestehend aus komplexen Netzwerken miteinander verbundener Nervenzellen, die in Kerngebieten (Nuclei) oder Schichten angeordnet sind und über einen oder mehrere neuronale Schaltkreise ihre Funktion ausüben, indem je nach Zelltyp spezifische chemische Botenstoffe für den Signalaustausch verwendet werden (Neurotransmission). Aufgrund der Unzahl von Verknüpfungen zwischen Dendriten und Axonen stellt das Gehirn eine viel zu komplexe Struktur dar, als dass es sich einem Computer vergleichen ließe, dessen Module im Fall eines Defektes schlicht ausgetauscht werden können. Für das Einbringen neuer Nervenzellen sind Transplantate aus unreifen Neuronen erforderlich, da reife Nervenzellen sich nach einer Transplantation nicht in die neuronalen Netzwerke des Gehirns eines Erwachsenen integrieren.

Unreife Nervenzellen lassen sich entweder direkt aus abgetriebenen menschlichen Embryonen gewinnen, oder indirekt durch eine der folgenden Methoden: 1) durch die *In-vitro*-Vermehrung und/oder Ausdifferenzierung menschlicher Stamm- bzw. Keimzellen zu einem neuronalen Phänotyp; oder 2) durch die Ausdifferenzierung von Zelllinien neuronaler Vorläuferzellen.

In der Praxis beinhaltet Neurotransplantation die gezielte Injektion kleiner Mengen (µl) von Zellen oder Gewebsfragmenten in geschädigte Hirnregionen. Außer für den Ersatz verlorener oder funktionsgestörter Zellen *(cellular restoration)* lässt sich die Neurotransplantation auch für das Einbringen von Zellen mit regenerativen Eigenschaften heranziehen. Ziel ist dabei beispielsweise, den Verlust eines bestimmten Proteins zu kompensieren oder die Proteinexpression einzuleiten, um so das Überleben und die Konnektivität von Nervenzellen zu erhöhen bzw. zu steuern *(molecular restoration)*. Die therapeutische Wirkung von Verfahren der Neurotransplantation setzt niemals sofort ein, sondern entwickelt sich im Verlauf mehrerer Monate. Diese Zeitspanne benötigen die Zellen zum Heranreifen und zur Integration in neuronale Netzwerke bzw. zur Ausbildung ihres neurotrophen oder regenerativen Effekts.

Ein neues molekulares Verfahren zur Wiederherstellung des Nervensystems bedient sich einer genetischen Intervention, in deren Verlauf eine Kopie des jeweiligen therapeutischen Gens in die DNS von Hirnzellen eingefügt wird. Realisiert wird der Gentransfer gegenwärtig durch die Injektion von Virusvektoren – dabei handelt es sich um Viren, die mit molekularbiologischen Verfahren so konstruiert werden, dass sie Zellen zwar infizieren und ihnen Gene übertragen können, ohne jedoch fähig zur Vermehrung zu sein. Gentransfer und Zellimplantation lassen sich auch kombinieren, um das therapeutische Potential eines Transplantats zu verbessern.

Im klinischen Bereich ist die Parkinson-Erkrankung der Testfall für Verfahren der Neurotransplantation gewesen. Fetale dopaminerge Nervenzellen, die dem Mesencephalon abgetriebener menschlicher Föten entnommen und in das dopamin-verarmte Striatum von Patienten implantiert wurden, verringerten deren motorische Störungen. Obwohl dadurch gezeigt wurde, dass die Neurotransplantation beim Menschen im Prinzip möglich und ein im Großen und Ganzen sicheres Verfahren ist, war die therapeutische Wirksamkeit in der Praxis unterschiedlich ausgeprägt und führte nie zu einer vollständigen Beseitigung der Parkinson-Symptomatik. Neben diesen Ergebnissen beim Morbus Parkinson wird im Kapitel zu Neurotransplantation und Gentransfer auch der gegenwärtige Stand der klinischen Studien zu Chorea Huntington, Morbus Alzheimer, Multipler Sklerose, amyotropher Lateralsklerose, Epilepsie und Schlaganfall besprochen. In keinem dieser Anwendungsfälle haben die zellulären oder molekularen Interventionen am Gehirn bisher den Status allgemein anerkannter klinischer Therapien erreicht.

Sowohl bei Zell- als auch bei Gentherapien für das erkrankte oder geschädigte Gehirn handelt es sich um invasive Eingriffe in die organische Basis unserer Personalität. Im Gegensatz zur Einnahme von Medikamenten, die einfach gestoppt werden kann, sind diese invasiven Interventionen irreversibel oder allenfalls teilweise reversibel. Zudem wird es mit diesen Verfahren niemals vollständig möglich sein, den Zustand des Gehirns, wie er vor dem

Auftreten der jeweiligen Störung gewesen ist, hinsichtlich seiner Morphologie oder der Qualität und Quantität der neuronalen Verschaltungen wiederherzustellen. Es kann daher auch nie ausgeschlossen werden, dass beim Empfänger dieser Behandlungsmaßnahmen unerwünschte physiologische und psychische Nebenwirkungen auftreten, auch wenn diese sich nicht unbedingt im alltäglichen Leben bemerkbar machen müssen. Es wird gelegentlich argumentiert, Zell- oder Gentherapien mit minimalen Nebenwirkungen würden möglich werden, sobald die lokale zelluläre oder molekulare Ursache einer Hirnstörung präzise feststellbar sei. Es ist daher entscheidend, diese experimentellen Eingriffe in das Gehirn in sorgfältig strukturierten klinischen Studien zu evaluieren. Dabei sollten sowohl die Auswahl geeigneter Patienten als auch das Erfassen des Ergebnisses – die Krankheitssymptomatik und mögliche Nebenwirkungen betreffend – anhand eines standardisierten und krankheitsspezifischen Untersuchungsprotokolls erfolgen. Nur auf diese Weise lassen sich die Resultate verschiedener Arten von Interventionen hinsichtlich ihrer genuinen Wirksamkeit vergleichen, so dass die fragwürdige Kontrolle des Behandlungserfolgs durch Scheinoperationen unnötig werden könnte.

Sowohl eine Reihe internationaler Forschungsorganisationen als auch nationale Institutionen haben ethische Richtlinien zur Gewinnung und Verwendung von menschlichen Embryonalzellen für Transplantationszwecke formuliert. Wegen der unauflösbaren Kontroversen zum Thema der freiwilligen Abtreibung und, mehr noch, wegen der logistischen Herausforderung, große Mengen von Zellen „auf Lager zu haben“, sucht man jedoch nach alternativen Quellen für Nervenzellen. Das Problem ließe sich mit embryonalen Stammzellen bewältigen, die sich selbst unendlich vervielfältigen und in beliebige Arten von Körperzellen ausdifferenzieren können. Allerdings haben sich diesbezüglich erneut ethische Debatten aufgetan. Die *In-vitro*-Erzeugung und Nutzung von menschlichen Embryonen im Präimplantationsstadium ist bislang weitgehend auf Forschung im Bereich der Reproduktionsmedizin beschränkt. In manchen Ländern ist diese Möglichkeit unter strikter Kontrolle durch Aufsichtsbehörden zulässig, in anderen Ländern ist sie vollständig verboten. Manche fordern die Erlaubnis zur Nutzung der Stammzellen von Embryonen im Präimplantationsstadium, die im Rahmen der *In-vitro*-Fertilisation überzählig erzeugt werden. Prinzipiell ließe sich auf diese Weise eine unerschöpfliche Quelle an Stammzelllinien erschließen. Auch Tiere werden als alternative Quelle zur Gewinnung von Zellen für Transplantate in Erwägung gezogen. Bei Patienten mit Morbus Parkinson oder Chorea Huntington wurde der Einsatz solcher Transplantate allerdings bereits ohne therapeutischen Erfolg erprobt. Die ethischen Bedenken gegen derartige Formen der Xenotransplantation betreffen zum einen die Auswahl und das Wohlergehen der als Transplantatquellen herangezogenen Tiere. Zum anderen wird auf Seiten des Patienten auf die Gefahr der Infektion mit tierischen Krankheitserregern (Zoonosen) und das Erfordernis einer langfristigen immunsuppressiven Behandlung hingewiesen. Außerdem gibt es Bedenken bezüglich der psychologischen Akzeptanz der Xenotransplantation durch die Transplantatempfänger.

Eine weitere Möglichkeit zur Gewinnung von neuronalen Transplantaten könnte in der Kultivierung adulter somatischer Stammzellen bestehen, die in vielen Organen des Körpers vorhanden sind. Wenn man von genetisch bedingten Hirnstörungen absieht, könnte in diesem Fall der Patient als sein eigener Zellspender auftreten. Diese Art der Zelltherapie hätte den Vorteil, dass im Anschluss an die Implantation keine Abstoßungsreaktionen zu erwarten wären. Bislang ist die Fähigkeit zur Ausdifferenzierung in verschiedene Zelltypen bei im Labor kultivierten somatischen Stammzellen jedoch weit weniger ausgeprägt als bei embryonalen Stammzellen.

Bezüglich der Risiken zellulärer und molekularer therapeutischer Eingriffe in das Gehirn wird häufig darauf verwiesen, diese könnten zu einer Veränderung personaler Identität oder zu einer Übertragung von Persönlichkeitsmerkmalen führen. Allerdings lässt sich die Identität einer Person keiner bestimmten Hirnstruktur zuweisen. Aus biologischer Sicht ist sie vielmehr ein Ergebnis der Aktivität des Gehirnes, das sich mit seinen neuronalen Netzwerken in dynamischer Interaktion mit der Umgebung befindet (Plastizität). Es ist ausgeschlossen, dass die winzigen bei Transplantationen übertragenen Zellmengen zur Übertragung von Persönlichkeitsmerkmalen führen könnten. Es ist darüber hinaus unwahrscheinlich, dass sie so tiefgreifende Veränderungen des gesamten Gehirns verursachen könnten, dass ein Wechsel personaler Identität die Folge wäre. Während größere Veränderungen im kognitiven Bereich oder längerfristige psychiatrische Komplikationen ebenfalls nicht zu erwarten sind, ist das Auftreten subtiler Persönlichkeitsveränderungen hingegen durchaus möglich. Diese werden sich vielleicht nicht im Alltag zeigen, könnten aber in Situationen extremer Beanspruchung auffallen. Dennoch dürfte die Einschätzung des Verhältnisses von Nutzen und Risiken der Tendenz nach positiv ausfallen. Die Gefahr der Entwicklung von Tumoren ist ein Sicherheitsrisiko, mit dem besonders die Möglichkeit der Kultivierung von Transplantaten aus embryonalen oder somatischen Stammzellen behaftet ist. Die Grundlagenforschung bemüht sich derzeit, den Prozess der Ausdifferenzierung von Stammzellen so zu beherrschen, dass sich reine Nervenzellpopulationen ergeben. Die experimentelle Anwendung von Transplantaten, die aus Stammzellen entwickelt wurden, sollte an Menschen daher erst dann erprobt werden, wenn der Prozess ihrer Differenzierung sicher kontrolliert werden kann.

Es ist nicht unwahrscheinlich, dass die klinische Neurowissenschaft in eine Ära der experimentellen zellulären und molekularen Neurochirurgie eintritt. Neurotransplantation und Gentransfer haben das Potential, die wiederherstellende Medizin des Gehirns durch neue Ansätze zur Behandlung von Hirnstörungen und zur Prävention von degenerativen Prozessen zu revolutionieren. In jüngster Zeit wurde Gentransfer auch als mögliche zukünftige Strategie zur Behandlung von Verhaltensstörungen und psychiatrischen Erkrankungen wie Depressionen, Angststörungen, kognitiven Störungen und Schizophrenie diskutiert.

1.3 Neuroprothetik des zentralen Nervensystems

Es ist in der Medizin bereits heute durchaus üblich, direkte Verbindungen zwischen elektronischen Geräten und dem zentralen Nervensystem herzustellen. Diese Technologie enthält zugleich

- Aussichten auf zukünftige medizinische Anwendungen,
- Potential im Hinblick auf das Enhancement menschlicher Fähigkeiten,
- Raum für eine Vielzahl bloßer Spekulationen, die sich in Science-Fiction-Romanen und -Filmen niederschlagen.

Sowohl für die klare Unterscheidung dieser verschiedenen Aspekte als auch für die wissenschaftliche Analyse der gegensätzlichen Positionen in der gegenwärtigen öffentlichen Debatte über mögliche soziale Konsequenzen bietet es sich an, zum einen die Geschichte der Neuroelektronik und zum anderen die aktuellen Entwicklungen in diesem Gebiet zu hinterfragen.

Zwar ist bereits seit den Lebzeiten von Galvani und Volta im späten 18. Jahrhundert bekannt, dass Nerven sich durch elektrischen Strom erregen lassen. Doch eröffnete erst die in den sechziger Jahren des letzten Jahrhunderts entwickelte Computertechnologie die Möglichkeit zur Herstellung von miniaturisierten elektronischen Geräten, die sich im menschlichen Körper implantieren lassen, ohne dass externe Drahtverbindungen zu großem Laborgerät erforderlich sind. Naheliegenderweise wurden als erste Anwärter auf derartige Implantate in Gestalt ertaubter Menschen solche Patienten in Erwägung gezogen, die den Ausfall eines kompletten Sinneskanals zu beklagen haben. Cochlear-Implantate wandeln den durch ein Mikrophon aufgenommenen Schall in ein elektronisches Stimulationsmuster um, das über mehr als 20 Elektroden an den Hörnerv übertragen wird. Das Cochlear-Implantat ist heutzutage mit mehr als 200.000 Trägern weltweit die erfolgreichste Neuroprothese und vermittelt der Mehrheit seiner Träger sogar die Fähigkeit zur (gegenüber Normalhörenden sicherlich eingeschränkten) Kommunikation per Telefon. Tatsächlich sind die Implantate inzwischen so ausgereift, dass manche Patienten auf der einen Seite mit einem Cochlear-Implantat ausgestattet werden, auf der Gegenseite dagegen mit einem konventionellen Hörgerät, um das dort noch vorhandene Gehör zu verstärken. Insofern bei diesen Patienten ein künstlicher Sinneskanal mit einem erheblich beeinträchtigten, aber noch funktionstüchtigen physiologischen Sinneskanal auf der Gegenseite „kooperiert", bietet sich damit ein regelrechtes „Cyborg"-Szenario. Die technologische Entwicklung hat darüber hinaus ein weiteres, ähnliches Implantat hervorgebracht, welches direkt mit dem Hirnstamm verbunden ist. Der von diesen Implantaten vermittelte Höreindruck ist jedoch weit schlechter als der durch am Hörnerv ansetzende Cochlear-Implantate erzeugte.

Der komplette Verlust des Sehvermögens stellte eine weitere Herausforderung dar: Retina-Implantate können mittlerweile die gesamte Bandbreite der für Menschen sichtbaren Lichtintensität vermitteln. Gegenwärtig kann ein subretinales Implantat (40x40 Elemente auf einem 3x3mm großen Chip) theoretisch eine räumliche Auflösung von 0,6 Grad, ein Sehfeld von ungefähr 12 Grad und eine Sehschärfe von 0,1 vermitteln. Auch epiretinale Implantate für erblindete Patienten befinden sich in der klinischen Erprobung. Kortikale Sehimplantate sind inzwischen so weit entwickelt, dass die Unterscheidung der Umrisse und Lage von Gegenständen möglich erscheint, wodurch manchen blinden Patienten eine grobe Fähigkeit zur Orientierung in ihrer Umgebung zurück gegeben werden könnte. Weil mit diesen Implantaten eine Verbindung zwischen Elektronik und Kortex, also der dünnen Nervenschicht auf der Oberfläche des Gehirns, hergestellt wird, handelt es sich bei ihnen im weiteren Sinn um Mensch-Computer-Schnittstellen (*human-computer interfaces* – HCIs), nämlich um Geräte, die verloren gegangene motorische oder sensorische Funktionen wiederherstellen. Allerdings wird dieser Terminus derzeit noch ausschließlich zur Bezeichnung von neuroelektronischen Schnittstellen verwendet, die *nicht* stimulieren, sondern lediglich elektrische Hirnaktivität aufnehmen und so verarbeiten, dass vollständig gelähmte Patienten künstliche Gliedmaßen oder Kommunikationsmittel wie Computer steuern können.

Nicht-invasive Varianten von HCIs werden häufig als Hirn-Computer-Schnittstellen (*brain-computer interfaces* – BCIs) bezeichnet. Das größere Interesse haben in letzter Zeit jedoch die invasiven Hirn-Maschine-Schnittstellen (*brain-machine interfaces* – BMIs) erregt, deren Vorteil in der Möglichkeit zur Aufzeichnung elektrischer Aktivität mit hoher räumlicher und zeitlicher Auflösung liegt. Im Jahre 2005 wurde an der Duke-University einem querschnittgelähmten Patienten eine Anordnung von 96 Elektroden in diejenige Region des motorischen Kortex implantiert, die für die Kontrolle von Arm- und Handbewegungen zuständig ist. Decoder gestatten es dem Patienten, Emails zu öffnen und Geräte wie z.B. einen Fernseher zu bedienen, selbst während er sich mit jemandem unterhält. Weiterhin kann er eine Handprothese öffnen und schließen und einfache Handlungen mit einem Roboterarm ausführen.

Diese Errungenschaften dienen primär der medizinischen Hilfeleistung in Situationen, in denen alle anderen Behandlungsoptionen versagen. Selbstverständlich regen sie auch die Vorstellungskraft an und darüber hinaus wissenschaftliche Projekte, die sich dem *Enhancement* von Leistungen gesunder Menschen widmen. Da die mit der Implantation von Elektroden und dem möglichen Versagen von Geräten verbundenen Risiken immer besser beherrscht werden können, ist es mit der heutigen Technologie theoretisch möglich, zusätzliche, künstliche Gliedmaßen einzig über willkürlich beeinflussbare Hirnströme zu steuern. HCIs könnten neue nonverbale, unsichtbare Wege der Kommunikation erschließen. Durch elektrische Stimulation bestimmter Hirnregionen (oder auch mit geringeren Risiken durch die Stimulation des Vagus-Nervs) lässt sich die Stimmungslage verändern und das Selbstvertrauen steigern. Einer der Gründe, weshalb diese direkten HCIs nicht zur Verwendung bei „normalen" Menschen in Betracht gezogen werden, liegt darin, dass diese Technologien immer noch mehr oder weniger invasive Eingriffe erfordern, bei denen relativ umfangreiche Elektrodenanordnungen in das zentrale Nervensystem implantiert werden.

Wenn mit der Verbesserung von Möglichkeiten zur telemetrischen Stimulation die Notwendigkeit direkter Kontaktstellen zwischen Elektroden und Gewebe entfällt, erscheint ein Enhancement von Sinnesleistungen nicht mehr als besonders weit hergeholte Vorstellung. Manche Formen sensorischen Enhancements sind schon heute ohne jeden invasiven Eingriff möglich (beispielsweise Ultraschallhören mittels Sonar oder Infrarotsehen mit Nachtsichtgeräten). Implantate zur Erzielung des gleichen Effekts werden allenfalls dann akzeptiert werden, wenn sie vollkommen sicher sind. Dagegen könnten heute noch nicht verfügbare Implantate, die effizient und in erheblichem Umfang kognitive Fähigkeiten wie z.B. Gedächtnisleistungen verbessern würden, selbst trotz erheblicher Risiken und Nebenwirkungen auf Akzeptanz stoßen. Sollte es jemals möglich sein, menschliche kognitive Fähigkeiten durch das Anschließen eines technischen Gerätes mit sehr geringem Risiko zu erweitern (z.B. mit einem „Gedächtnis-Chip"), dann ist kaum einzusehen, warum Menschen eine solche Möglichkeit nicht würden nutzen wollen. Dies gilt insbesondere für den Fall, dass eine entsprechende elektronische Schnittstelle jederzeit abgeschaltet werden könnte.

Jeder neue Schritt in der Entwicklung elektronischer Neuroimplantate birgt die Möglichkeit des Missbrauchs in sich. Vielen wird ein Enhancement durch Herstellen einer Verbindung zwischen elektronischen Geräten und menschlichem Gehirn zumindest auf den ersten Blick moralisch fragwürdig erscheinen. Die Öffentlichkeit ist angesichts der Vielzahl von Science-Fiction-Szenarien mit Cyborgs, welche die angeblich unmittelbar bevorstehende Transformation der Menschheit in eine halb-elektronische Art vor Augen führen, zwar eher ratlos, dennoch haben diese Szenarien bereits Überreaktionen gegen jede Form wissenschaftlichen Fortschritts im Bereich der Neuroprothetik provoziert. Andere mögen dagegenhalten, diese Technologien enthielten vielmehr die Verheißung, das Leben noch lebenswerter zu machen – vorausgesetzt, dass die Gesellschaft eine Antwort auf die sozialen Herausforderungen findet, vor die uns alle neuen Methoden des Eingriffs in das Gehirn stellen.

1.4 Elektrische Hirnstimulation bei psychiatrischen Störungen

Bei der elektrischen Hirnstimulation werden Elektroden in das Gehirn implantiert, um durch hochfrequenten elektrischen Strom die Symptome von Patienten mit Bewegungsstörungen (wie z.B. beim Morbus Parkinson) oder schweren psychiatrischen Erkrankungen, die sich nicht medikamentös beherrschen lassen, zu verringern. Während früher häufig chirurgische Methoden zur lokalen Zerstörung von Nervengewebe in tief gelegenen Hirnregionen angewendet wurden, bevorzugen die meisten Neurochirurgen derzeit die elektrische Stimulation aufgrund ihrer Reversibilität und Anpassbarkeit gegenüber dieser älteren Methode.

Zwangsstörungen und schwere Depressionen sind die beiden psychiatrischen Indikationen, bei deren Behandlung sich die elektrische Hirnstimulation bislang bewährt hat. Dennoch befindet sich die Methode auch für diese Krankheitsbilder noch im Erprobungsstadium. Die wesentliche Triebfeder für die Entwicklung von Stimulationsverfahren zur Therapie von Zwangsstörungen und Depressionen liegt in der Vielzahl schwerkranker, therapierefraktärer Patienten, die dringend der Behandlung bedürfen.

Beim Verfahren der transkraniellen Magnetstimulation (TMS) werden magnetische Impulse mithilfe einer handgeführten Stimulationsspule über bestimmten Kopfregionen ausgelöst. Die Spule ist mit einem Stimulator verbunden, der die magnetischen Impulse generiert. Durch die Magnetfelder, die über die Zeit wechseln, kann in verschiedenen Strukturen des Gehirns ein elektrischer Strom erzeugt werden. Im Gegensatz zur elektrischen Hirnstimulation handelt es sich bei TMS um ein nicht-invasives Verfahren. Beide Techniken sind in der klinischen Praxis entwickelt worden. Erst im Nachhinein wurden grundlegende neurobiologische Erkenntnisse gewonnen, welche die ihnen zugrunde liegenden Wirkmechanismen zumindest teilweise klären.

Patienten mit Tiefenhirnelektroden können mit einer Handbedienung ausgestattet werden, mit deren Hilfe sie bestimmen können, wann sie stimuliert werden und wann nicht. Mit dieser Ein/Aus-Kontrolle bietet sich eine praktikable Möglichkeit, den Bedenken zu begegnen, wonach Stimulationstechniken zur Manipulation von Patienten dienen könnten. Da Patienten jedoch nicht in der Programmierung des Stimulationsgeräts geübt sind, ist es eine zweischneidige Idee, ihre Autonomie dadurch bewahren zu wollen, dass man ihnen die Einstellung der Stimulationsparameter überlässt. Die Patienten selbst sehen es nicht als ethisches Problem an, dass ein Stimulationsgerät ihre psychische Verfassung beeinflusst, so lange es ihnen nur Erleichterung verschafft. Sie vergleichen den Apparat mit anderen implantierbaren Geräten wie z.B. Schrittmachern, die bei der Behandlung von Herzerkrankungen eingesetzt werden.

Das Einsetzen eines elektrischen Hirnstimulators geschieht durch einen chirurgischen Eingriff in das Gehirn. Aufgrund der historisch negativen Besetzung des Begriffes „Psychochirurgie“ wird heutzutage meist von „Neurochirurgie für psychiatrische Störungen“ gesprochen. In Frankreich wurde diese Art von Chirurgie in den letzten Jahrzehnten gar nicht durchgeführt. Noch im Jahr 2002 hat das „Comité Consultatif National d'Ethique pour les Sciences de la Vie et de la Santé“ entschieden, das Verbot gegen chirurgische Verfahren zur Behandlung psychiatrischer Störungen aufrechtzuerhalten. Dagegen hat das Komitee wegen der Reversibilität und Anpassbarkeit der elektrischen Hirnstimulation ihrer Erprobung bei Zwangsstörungen im Rahmen eines Forschungsvorhabens zugestimmt. Eine Forschungskooperation, die sich um die Optimierung der elektrischen Hirnstimulation zur Behandlung von Patienten mit Zwangsstörung bemüht, hat selbstverpflichtende Richtlinien entwickelt, die beispielhaft zeigen sollen, wie sich die Anwendung von neurochirurgischen Verfahren in der Psychiatrie auf verantwortungsvolle Weise regeln lassen könnte. Außerdem ist es bereits gängige Praxis, Patienten mit psychiatrischen Störungen, bei denen ein neurochirurgischer Eingriff erwogen wird, durch ein beratendes, interdisziplinäres Gremium begutachten zu lassen, das in jedem einzelnen Fall über die Eignung des betreffenden Patienten für die Operation entscheidet.

Innovative Weiterentwicklungen im Bereich der Hirnstimulation werden in der Forschung unter Laborbedingungen bereits erprobt, haben aber noch nicht die Klinik erreicht. Solche Weiterentwicklungen betreffen etwa die Miniaturisierung von Elektroden und Stimulatoren, die Verwendung von Nanotechnologie, Telemedizin, Fernüberwachung und Fernbedienung. Insbesondere für den Fall einer möglichen zukünftigen Fernbedienung ist die Entwicklung spezifischer Sicherheitsauflagen erforderlich.

2 Begriffliche Klärungen

2.1 Die Relevanz verschiedener Bedenken zur personalen Integrität

Diejenigen, die schon die therapeutische Anwendung neuer Techniken zum Eingriff in das Gehirn für ethisch fragwürdig halten, begründen dies für gewöhnlich nicht mit dem Risiko psychischer Nebenwirkungen als solcher. Vielmehr stellen sie die neuen Behandlungsmethoden zumeist deswegen in Frage, weil diese im Vergleich zu etablierten Verfahren Patienten auf eine radikalere und tiefer greifende Art und Weise verändern könnten. Sehr verbreitet ist das Bedenken, die neuen Interventionstechniken könnten die personale Identität gefährden. Die Suggestivwirkung einer so monströsen Aussicht wie der, jemand werde „durch Herumbasteln an seinem Gehirn“ möglicherweise zu jemand anderem gemacht, könnte vielversprechende Forschungsbereiche in der öffentlichen Meinung in Misskredit bringen. Das wiederum könnte die künftige Entwicklung dringend benötigter neuer Behandlungsmethoden vereiteln. Bei einzelnen Patienten könnte die vage Befürchtung, nach einer therapeutischen Maßnahme nicht mehr „der zu sein, der man war", zu Vorurteilen gegenüber dem betreffenden medizinischen Verfahren führen. Aus diesen Gründen haben wir uns in der vorliegenden Studie darum bemüht, die Sorgen zu zerstreuen, neue therapeutische Möglichkeiten in Psychopharmakologie, Neurotransplantation, Neuroprothetik und elektrischer Hirnstimulation könnten die personale Identität der zu behandelnden Patienten gefährden. Weil derartige Bedenken indes schwer greifbar und präzisierbar sind, lassen sie sich auch nur schwer widerlegen. Unsere Versuche, solchen Vorbehalten gegenüber neuen Arten von Eingriffen ins Gehirn einen klaren Sinn zu geben, führten uns schließlich zu dem Ergebnis, dass sich ein echter Wechsel personaler Identität als profunde dissoziative Störung manifestieren müsste, also z.B. als retrograde Amnesie oder dissoziative Identitätsstörung. Beschreibt man freilich die Möglichkeit einer Gefährdung personaler Identität auf diese Weise, dann wird deutlich, dass es sich dabei keineswegs um eine bisher unbekannte Art psychischer Nebenwirkungen handelt, sondern um einen Effekt, der prinzipiell ebenso gut auch durch bereits klinisch etablierte neurochirurgische Eingriffe verursacht werden könnte.

Allerdings gibt es bisher keine Hinweise, dass irgendeine der in dieser Studie untersuchten Interventionsformen mit nennenswerter Wahrscheinlichkeit dissoziative Störungen verursachen oder andere schwere Nebenwirkungen auf die Psyche haben könnte, die einer Bedrohung personaler Identität gleich oder auch nur nahe kämen. Und selbst wenn ein bestimmter Typus therapeutischer Eingriffe ins Gehirn gelegentlich derartig schwere psychische Schäden nach sich zöge, so müsste dennoch von Fall zu Fall entschieden werden, ob es akzeptabel – oder womöglich sogar ratsam – wäre, einen Eingriff dieser Art trotz dieses Risikos durchzuführen. Behandlungsentscheidungen unter Risikogesichtspunkten treffen zu müssen, gehört zum allgemeinen Geschäft der Medizin. Neben der Verfügbarkeit, Effektivität und Sicherheit alternativer Therapieoptionen müssen dabei auch die mit dem Unterlassen jeglicher Behandlung für den Patienten verbundenen Gefahren berücksichtigt werden. Die schwierigen ethischen Dilemmata, die für medizinische Risiko-Nutzen-Abwägungen charakteristisch sind, treten keineswegs nur bei der Entscheidung über therapeutische Methoden der Intervention ins Gehirn auf.

➔ Eine Verengung der öffentlichen Debatte auf radikale und offenkundige psychische Veränderungen, von denen Patienten betroffen sein könnten, mag dazu führen, dass anderen Nebenwirkungen, die eigentlich größeren Anlass zur Sorge geben, nicht die gebührende Aufmerksamkeit gewidmet wird. Die Rede ist von *subtilen* Veränderungen der Psyche im Allgemeinen und der Persönlichkeit im Speziellen, die leicht unbemerkt bleiben können.

Im Abschnitt 3.1.1 werden wir konkrete Vorschläge formulieren, wie bestehende Forschungs- und Behandlungsrichtlinien fortzuschreiben wären, um dem Auftreten subtiler Formen psychischer Nebenwirkungen Rechnung zu tragen.

2.2 Grenzen des Sozialsystems Medizin: Behandlung – Enhancement – Prävention

Aus nicht-therapeutischen Anwendungen neuer Techniken zum Eingriff in das menschliche Gehirn ergeben sich neuartige soziale Herausforderungen. Das gilt insbesondere dann, wenn mit solchen Techniken Zwecke des Enhancements verfolgt werden, möglicherweise aber auch schon bei bloßer Nutzung zur Prävention. Diese Feststellung nötigt zunächst zur Klärung der Begriffe Therapie, Prävention und Enhancement sowie der Beziehungen zwischen ihnen. Wir tun dies, indem wir den „Enhancement"-Begriff zunächst in seiner umgangssprachlichen Bedeutung nehmen, um ihn anschließend als einen *prima facie* negativen Grenzbegriff in doppeltem Sinn näher zu bestimmen: erstens als etwas, das nicht als Bestandteil einer recht verstandenen Medizin betrachtet werden kann bzw. sollte, und zweitens als etwas, dass nicht zum Arsenal dessen gehört, was „Behandlung" heißt. Eine solche Analyse wirft offenkundig zwei grundlegende Fragen auf: (1) Was gehört zur wohldefinierten Sphäre der Medizin?, und (2) Was bedeutet „Behandlung"?

2.2.1 Die Legitimität genuin medizinischer Verfahren

Für die erste Frage halten wir als Prämisse fest, dass der Begriff der Medizin zumindest in einer Hinsicht normativ zu verstehen ist: Alle indizierten medizinischen Maßnahmen haben eine normative Eigenschaft gemeinsam, nämlich die, im jeweiligen Kontext legitim zu sein. Um diese Auffassung weiter zu erläutern, unterscheiden wir zwischen dem gesellschaftlichen (in irgendeiner Weise öffentlich finanzierten) Gesamtsystem Medizin einerseits und medizinischem Handeln als einer interpersonellen Praxis zwischen Individuen bzw. einem intrapersonellen Verhalten einzelner Personen zu sich selbst andererseits. Antworten auf die Frage nach angemessenen Grenzen der Medizin können ersichtlich unterschiedlich ausfallen, je nachdem, ob es um die Begrenzung des Systems der Medizin im ersteren Sinne geht (also um die Beschränkung dessen, was ein öffentliches Gesundheitssystem an Leistungen zur Verfügung stellen sollte), oder aber um die Grenzen zulässigen medizinischen Handelns im letzteren Sinn (also um die Grenzen dessen, was jemand als medizinischen Eingriff an sich selbst oder an anderen durchführen darf). Es liegt auf der Hand, dass Handlungen, die im inter- oder im intrapersonellen Verhältnis unzulässig sind, als illegitim auch aus dem Leistungskatalog eines wohlgeordneten Systems der öffentlichen Gesundheitsfürsorge ausgeschlossen werden müssen. Im umgekehrten Fall gilt dieses Entsprechungsverhältnis jedoch nicht: Viele medizinische Maßnahmen, die gegebenenfalls mit guten Gründen vom Leistungskatalog des öffentlichen Gesundheitssystems ausgeschlossen sind, also nicht zu jener Grundversorgung gehören, die ein solches System für alle Mitglieder bereitstellen sollte, können gleichwohl rechtmäßig sein, wenn sie von einem Arzt an einer anderen Person mit deren Einwilligung, oder wenn sie von einer Person an sich selbst vorgenommen werden. Als erläuterndes Beispiel mögen solche medizinische Eingriffe dienen, die allein zu kosmetischen bzw. ästhetischen Zwecken vorgenommen werden.

2.2.2 Enhancement versus Behandlung

Die Unterscheidung zwischen Heilbehandlung und Enhancement markiert eine plausible Grenze des sozialen Systems Medizin. Oder genauer: sie markiert *eine* der *beiden* plausiblen Grenzen; die andere wird durch den Begriff der Prävention gekennzeichnet (dem wir uns weiter unten zuwenden). Das begriffliche Gegensatzpaar „Heilbehandlung/Enhancement" allein besagt freilich noch nichts darüber, wo genau in jedem konkreten Einzelfall diese Grenze zu ziehen wäre. Das führt uns zur zweiten der oben formulierten Fragen. Wir schlagen vor, die relevante Grenzziehung nicht mittels einer Definition des Enhancement-Begriffs vorzunehmen, sondern umgekehrt den Begriff der Krankheit (in einem weiten, Behinderungen einschließenden Sinn) zu klären, also das konzeptuelle Gegenstück und das praktische Objekt dessen zu bestimmen, was „Heilbehandlung" heißt. (Dies genau macht „Enhancement" zum negativen Grenzbegriff im oben angedeuteten Sinn.) Der Krankheitsbegriff ist seit langem Gegenstand intensiver Debatten innerhalb der Philosophie, der Medizin und des Medizinrechts. In deren Verlauf sind zahlreiche unterschiedliche Konzeptionen entwickelt worden. Wir selbst stimmen im Wesentlichen einem Krankheitsbegriff zu, den der Philosoph Norman Daniels vorgeschlagen hat. Er bestimmt Krankheit als signifikante Abweichung von spezies-typischen Funktionsnormen physischer und/oder psychischer Systeme, Fähigkeiten und Eigenschaften des Menschen. Im Unterschied freilich zu Daniels sind wir nicht der Meinung, dass sich daraus ein rein deskriptiver oder naturalistischer Krankheitsbegriff ergibt. Denn was im Einzelfall noch innerhalb des Bereichs spezies-typischer Funktionsnormen liegt und was andererseits als hinreichend bedeutsame Abweichung von diesen zu gelten hat, ist nicht einfach eine Frage wissenschaftlich ermittelbarer Tatsachen. Vielmehr erfordern komplexe Grenzfälle unvermeidlich *Entscheidungen.* Diese enthalten stets ein irreduzibles normatives Element, das weder dem Beweis noch der Widerlegung durch die Naturwissenschaften (etwa der Biologie) zugänglich ist.

Das ist die von uns gewählte und präzisierte begriffliche Grundlage. Danach hat jeder technische Eingriff als Enhancement zu gelten, der jemandes physischen oder psychischen Zustand in mindestens einer bestimmten Hinsicht zu verbessern beabsichtigt, dabei aber nicht als Behandlung einer Krankheit (im Behinderungen einschließenden Sinne) beurteilt werden kann.

2.2.3 Der Zweck der Medizin: Krankheiten bekämpfen

Zur Bestimmung der legitimen Sphäre der Medizin als eines sozialen Systems ist die Unterscheidung zwischen Behandlung und Enhancement nicht ausreichend: sie lässt den Begriff der Prävention unberücksichtigt. Zu jedem der beiden Begriffe unserer bisherigen Dichotomie – zu „Heilbehandlung" wie zu „Enhancement" – weist der Begriff der Prävention eine gewisse Nähe auf: Einerseits sind Präventionsmaßnahmen in normativer Hinsicht offenbar ebenso *a limine* legitim wie Maßnahmen der Behandlung. Therapeutische wie präventive Maßnahmen sind gleichermaßen Mittel zur Bekämpfung von Krankheiten; daher ist es gerechtfertigt, die letzteren nicht anders als die ersteren dem Bereich legitimer Medizin zuzurechnen. Betrachtet man andererseits nur die jeweiligen äußeren Formen des medizinischen Handelns, so erscheinen bestimmte exemplarische Arten der Prävention eher als Formen eines Enhancements. Das gilt ersichtlich nicht für alle Arten der Prävention, sehr wohl aber etwa für eine so zentrale Präventionsform wie die der Impfung. Impfungen dienen der Stärkung und damit dem „Enhancement" bestimmter natürlicher Fähigkeiten des Körpers zur (potentiellen) Neutralisierung pathogener Mikroorganismen und anderer Krankheitserreger, denen der Körper künftig ausgesetzt sein könnte. Aus diesem Grund betrachten wir Prävention als ein selbständiges Konzept und erweitern die Dichotomie von Behandlung und Enhancement entsprechend zur Trichotomie „Behandlung – Prävention – Enhancement".

Für die Frage nach den sinnvollen Schranken der Medizin als soziales System entstehen daraus keine weiteren Probleme. Wie wir bereits angedeutet haben, lässt sich jeder potentiell geeignete Versuch, dem Eintreten eines Zustands mit anerkanntem Krankheitswert vorzubeugen, mit gleichem Recht dem wohldefinierten Bereich legitimer Medizin zuschlagen wie Maßnahmen zur Behandlung der betreffenden Krankheit.[305] Dies gilt ohne prinzipiellen Unterschied auch für die Prävention bzw. die Therapie psychischer Erkrankungen durch neue Methoden des Eingreifens ins Gehirn.

---

[305] Unterschiede zwischen Behandlung und Prävention gibt es freilich im Hinblick auf die Frage, ob entsprechende Maßnahmen in einem System öffentlicher Gesundheitsfürsorge nicht nur legitim, sondern möglicherweise sogar geboten (obligatorisch) sind. Das wird für Behandlungen in erheblich weiter reichendem Maße zu bejahen sein als für Vorbeugemaßnahmen. Im Ganzen geht es dabei aber vorwiegend um ein Problem der gerechten und klugen Verteilung knapper und kostspieliger Ressourcen, das uns hier nicht weiter beschäftigen soll.

2.2.4 Enhancement dient nicht dem Zweck der Medizin

Auf der Basis dieser Klärung unserer Grundbegriffe ergibt sich folgendes Postulat:

➔ „Reine" Enhancement-Maßnahmen (also solche, die nicht wenigstens auch als Beitrag zur Prävention von Krankheit/Behinderung verstanden werden können) sollten in den wohldefinierten Bereich legitimer Medizin als eines sozialen Systems nicht einbezogen werden.

Wir räumen ausdrücklich ein, dass sich aus dieser Empfehlung in bestimmten Fällen Probleme individueller Gerechtigkeit ergeben können. Doch kann keine theoretische Strategie zur Abgrenzung des Bereichs der Medizin das Auftreten derartiger Probleme vollständig vermeiden. Die von uns entwickelte und empfohlene Strategie weist diesen Problemen ihren plausibelsten begrifflichen und normativen Ort zu. All dies schließt im Übrigen nicht aus, dass ein und dieselbe medizinisch-technische Maßnahme in einem Fall als Enhancement und in einem anderen Fall als Behandlung gelten kann. Wenn zum Beispiel eine Person *A* den spezies-typischen Standard bezüglich einer bestimmten kognitiven Funktion *x* unterschreitet, ohne dabei die diagnostischen Kriterien einer geistigen Behinderung zu erfüllen, dann ist ein Eingriff, der bei dieser Person *x* verbessert, als Enhancement zu beurteilen. Dagegen lässt sich ein äußerlich exakt gleicher Eingriff bei einer Person *B*, die hinsichtlich *x* so beeinträchtigt ist, dass sie im klinischen Sinne als geistig behindert gelten kann, zutreffend als Behandlung klassifizieren. Wichtig ist schließlich das Folgende: Der Gesetzgeber, aber auch andere „Wächter" des Gesundheitswesens, wie z.B. Gerichte und Krankenversicherungen, bedürfen zur Erfüllung ihrer jeweiligen Aufgaben einer gewissen „robusten" Entscheidungsbefugnis für die Feststellung, welche konkreten medizinischen Maßnahmen in dieses System gehören und welche nicht. Solche Entscheidungen sind niemals nur dem Kriterium individueller Gerechtigkeit verpflichtet. Sie müssen stets auch dem Erfordernis genügen, innerhalb des Gesamtsystems verallgemeinerbar und damit auf das gesamte Spektrum hinreichend ähnlicher Fälle in Gegenwart und Zukunft anwendbar zu sein. Deshalb müssen sie auch den Zwängen Rechnung tragen, die aus der Knappheit kostspieliger lebensrettender Ressourcen resultieren. Zur Bewältigung dieser Aufgabe bedarf es der erwähnten robusten Entscheidungszuständigkeit. Demnach kann es durchaus vorkommen, dass eine spezielle medizinische Maßnahme in der einen Rechtsordnung als Behandlung aufgefasst wird und folglich der Sphäre legitimer Medizin zugehört, während sie in einer anderen Rechtsordnung als „Enhancement" aus diesem Bereich ausgeschlossen werden mag.

2.2.5 Selbst-Enhancement versus Enhancement anderer

Was nun die Grenzen der Medizin als einer interpersonellen bzw. intrapersonellen Praxis betrifft, so nehmen wir die Unterscheidung zwischen

Behandlung und Prävention einerseits und Enhancement andererseits nur als provisorischen Ausgangspunkt für weitergehende Analysen. Auf der einen Seite ist es offensichtlich, dass jede Maßnahme, die zutreffend als Behandlung beurteilt wird, *ipso facto* gerechtfertigt ist, wenn sie von einer Person (regelmäßig einem Arzt) an einer anderen Person (dem Patienten) als medizinische Maßnahme vorgenommen wird und die dabei üblichen Erfordernisse gewahrt sind: das Selbstbestimmungsrecht des Patienten (sein Recht auf *informed consent)* sowie die sachkundige Abwägung des beabsichtigten therapeutischen Nutzens gegenüber möglichen Nebenwirkungen. In diesem begrenzten Sinn dient unsere begriffliche Trichotomie einmal mehr als nützlicher normativer Ausgangspunkt. Doch auf der anderen Seite, und in deutlichem Gegensatz zu unseren Betrachtungen zur Medizin als sozialem System, ist keineswegs klar, dass jede körperliche oder psychische Verbesserung, die außerhalb der Sphäre von Therapie und Prävention liegt, also jedes Enhancement, allein deshalb schon den Verdacht, geschweige denn das Verdikt der Illegitimität auf sich ziehen müsste. Ganz im Gegenteil: Viele der heute verfügbaren oder für die Zukunft vorstellbaren Enhancement-Maßnahmen scheinen keine inter- oder intrapersonellen Normen, seien sie ethischer oder rechtlicher Provenienz, zu verletzen.

Gleichwohl gibt es normative Grenzen. Zu deren Klärung unterscheiden wir Fälle des Selbst-Enhancements von Fällen des Enhancements anderer. Innerhalb der ersten Kategorie differenzieren wir weiter zwischen Fällen, an denen nur eine Partei beteiligt ist, und solchen, bei denen zwei Parteien involviert sind. Die zuerst genannten betreffen Situationen, in denen eine einwilligungsfähige Person ein Verfahren des Enhancements ausschließlich an sich selbst anwendet. In Zwei-Parteien-Fällen geht es dagegen um Enhancement-Maßnahmen, die eine Person von einer anderen an sich vornehmen lässt. Im Standardfall handelt es sich dabei um einen Arzt, der ein Enhancement an einer Person mit deren aufgeklärter Einwilligung durchführt. Innerhalb dieses prinzipiellen Schemas lassen sich zahlreiche normative Probleme unterscheiden. Sie reichen von spezifischen Fragen konkreter Nebenwirkungen bis hin zu abstrakten Gerechtigkeitsfragen. Die Ergebnisse unserer systematischen Analyse dieser Probleme werden weiter unten dargestellt.

Andere normative Probleme treten auf, wenn an Stelle des Selbst-Enhancements (auch des mittelbaren mit Hilfe einer anderen Person) Fälle des genuinen Fremd-Enhancements betrachtet werden. Für diese ist eine Struktur typisch, die sie als „Drei-Parteien-Fälle" kennzeichnet: Normalerweise gibt es dabei eine Person *X*, die einen Eingriff des Enhancements bei einer anderen Person *Y* wünscht bzw. über einen solchen entscheidet, der wiederum von einer dritten Person *Z* (für gewöhnlich ein medizinischer Fachmann) ausgeführt wird. Wir analysieren die speziellen Probleme, die sich aus dieser Konstellation ergeben, anhand zweier exemplarischer Situationstypen: In Situationen des einen Typs verlangen Eltern ein Enhancement ihrer minderjährigen Kinder, in Situationen des anderen Typs geht es um Strafgefangene, die dem Staat besonderen Anlass geben, die Möglichkeit ihres mentalen Enhancements in Erwägung zu ziehen. Die Ergebnisse der Analyse dieser Situationstypen werden mit den entsprechenden Empfehlungen unter 3.3 dargelegt.

3 Normative Grundlagen

Die Bewältigung der sozialen Herausforderungen, die von den in dieser Studie untersuchten Entwicklungen ausgehen, bedarf nicht der Einführung neuartiger ethischer Grundprinzipien. Vielmehr lassen sich die meisten der hier angesprochenen normativen Probleme in angemessener Weise durch die Anwendung der bereits unter 1.1 in dieser Zusammenfassung erwähnten Prinzipien der medizinischen Ethik klären: den Prinzipien des Schädigungsverbots *(nonmaleficence)*, des Gebots zur Hilfe *(beneficence)*, der Achtung fremder Autonomie *(respect for autonomy)* sowie der Gerechtigkeit *(justice)*.[306] Diese vier Prinzipien ergeben ein geeignetes Ordnungsschema für den Rest dieser Zusammenfassung. In ihrem (und seinem) Rahmen werden wir einige handlungsorientierte Schlussfolgerungen ziehen, um auf diese Weise die interdisziplinäre Debatte voranzubringen, die öffentliche Diskussion anzuregen und politische Entscheidungsträger sowie weitere Interessengruppen bei ihren Beschlüssen zu unterstützen.

3.1 Schädigungsverbot: Das Vermeiden von Schaden bei Eingriffen in das Gehirn

Die generelle negative Pflicht, anderen keinen Schaden zuzufügen, kann als das grundlegende moralische Prinzip aller historisch bekannten Zeiten und Kulturen angesehen werden. Entsprechend stellt es auch für das Gesundheitswesen und die medizinische Forschung das wichtigste ethische Grundprinzip dar. Gelegentlich findet es seinen Ausdruck in Form der altehrwürdigen Maxime *primum non nocere*. Es besagt, dass Handlungen, die Schaden zufügen, *prima facie* falsch sind, d.h. dass sie im Allgemeinen, nämlich auf einer abstrakten normativen Ebene, einem Verbot unterliegen. Freilich können solche generell verbotenen Handlungen im Einzelfall legitim sein, wenn gewisse rechtfertigende Umstände vorliegen: In solchen Fällen muss der Schaden, der einem Menschen durch eine an ihm vorgenommene, von seiner aufgeklärten Einwilligung getragene medizinische Maßnahme entstehen

[306] In bewusster Abweichung von der Vorlage von Beauchamp und Childress (2001) beginnen wir unsere Abhandlung mit dem Prinzip des Nicht-Schadens, um dessen vorrangige Bedeutung für unsere gegenwärtigen Fragen zu unterstreichen.

kann, überwogen werden durch den vernünftigerweise zu erwartenden Nutzen der Maßnahme. Bei der Analyse solcher Güterabwägungen beschränken wir uns auf die Berücksichtigung der Interessen des betroffenen Subjekts, da wir, jedenfalls im Prinzip, utilitaristische Rechtfertigungen der Schädigung von Personen im Hinblick auf das Wohlergehen anderer ablehnen.[307]

3.1.1 Zum Umgang mit Nebenwirkungen in Forschung und medizinischer Praxis

Im Zusammenhang von Entscheidungen über die Zulässigkeit von Eingriffen in das Gehirn kommt das Prinzip des Schädigungsverbots vorwiegend bei der Beurteilung von Nebenwirkungen zum Tragen. Denn bei den intendierten Primäreffekten von zulässigen Behandlungs- bzw. Präventionsmaßnahmen handelt es sich *per definitionem* nicht um Schäden. Und aus unserer Bestimmung des Enhancement-Begriffs folgt, dass die beabsichtigte Wirkung eines auf Enhancement abzielenden Verfahrens zumindest von der Person, die sich dem Verfahren unterzieht, als Verbesserung betrachtet wird. Daher stellen auch die intendierten Primäreffekte von Enhancements grundsätzlich keine Schäden dar. (Dies gilt vorbehaltlich einiger näherer Bestimmungen, mit denen wir uns unter 3.1.3 beschäftigen werden.)

Die Überwachung subtiler psychischer Nebenwirkungen

In den Vorbemerkungen zu dieser Zusammenfassung haben wir argumentiert, dass es in erster Linie subtile psychische Nebenwirkungen sind, die guten Grund geben, innovative Methoden zum Eingriff in das zentrale Nervensystem sorgfältig zu prüfen. Wenn wir über subtilen psychischen Schaden sprechen, beziehen wir uns auf negative Nebenwirkungen, die erstens leicht übersehen werden können und die zweitens entweder die Persönlichkeit betreffen oder aber psychische Funktionen, die für Personalität selbst konstitutiv sind.[308] Auch wenn die Möglichkeit derartiger psychischer Schädigun-

---

[307] Freilich räumen auch die meisten deontologischen (und andere nicht-utilitaristische) Moralkonzeptionen zu Recht ein, dass Abwägungen zwischen Nutzen und Schaden über Personengrenzen hinweg, wenn auch nur in engen Grenzen, zulässig sein können. Damit werden (vergleichsweise schwache) Solidaritätspflichten anerkannt, die es einer Person *X* im Gefahrenfall gestatten, einer anderen Person *Y* einen geringfügigen Schaden zuzufügen, auch wenn diese für das Zustandekommen der Gefahr, die *X* droht, schlechterdings unzuständig ist, sofern der aus dieser Handlung für *X* enstehende Nutzen der Gefahrabwendung den Schaden für *Y* bei weitem überwiegt. Zwar spielt dieses Prinzip für die klinische Forschung an Nicht-Einwilligungsfähigen eine gewisse Rolle, doch können wir es an dieser Stelle getrost vernachlässigen; für das Thema dieser Studie ist es nicht von Bedeutung.

[308] Damit sind insbesondere gemeint: diskriminative Fähigkeiten (Wahrnehmen und Wiedererkennen), episodisches Gedächtnis, Lern-, Sprach- und Denkfähigkeiten, Dispositionen zur Befriedigung natürlicher Bedürfnisse und schließlich die Fähigkeiten, Zwecke verfolgen sowie Lust und Unlust empfinden zu können. Für Details vgl. Kapitel 5.3.

gen keineswegs nur bei Eingriffen in das Gehirn gegeben ist, weisen solche Interventionen wegen der Schlüsselrolle des Gehirns für die Psyche in dieser Hinsicht doch ein besonderes Risiko auf. Weiterhin ist die Annahme plausibel, dass jede Intervention in das Gehirn, die mit der *Absicht* ausgeführt wird, Einfluss auf die Psyche zu nehmen, ein zusätzliches Risiko für subtile Nebenwirkungen besagter Art birgt. Daher erscheinen uns die folgenden Forderungen angebracht:

➔ Während der Forschungsphase sollte jede neue Methode zur Intervention am Gehirn systematisch auf Nebenwirkungen geprüft werden, welche die Persönlichkeit oder psychische Funktionen, die für Personalität konstitutiv sind, betreffen.

➔ Wenn ein bestimmter Interventionstyp, der für bestimmte therapeutische oder präventive Anwendungen zugelassen ist, bekanntermaßen subtile Nebenwirkungen auf die Persönlichkeit oder auf solche psychischen Fähigkeiten haben kann, die für Personalität konstitutiv sind, dann sollte jede Person, an deren Gehirn ein Eingriff dieses Typs vorgenommen wird, im Anschluss sorgfältig auf das Auftreten solcher Nebenwirkungen hin untersucht werden, damit sie gegebenenfalls eine entsprechende Behandlung erfahren kann.

Für die meisten erst kürzlich entwickelten Methoden der Intervention am Gehirn – einschließlich der in dieser Studie untersuchten – wurden gewisse Anstrengungen unternommen, diesen Forderungen nachzukommen. Insgesamt glauben wir allerdings, dass ein Bedarf an konsequenteren Kontrollen mit verbesserten methodischen Verfahren besteht. An dieser Stelle können keine detaillierten Vorschläge für entsprechende Vorgehensweisen gemacht werden. Vielmehr soll es genügen, zum einen auf einige Aspekte hinzuweisen, die größere Aufmerksamkeit bei der Überwachung subtiler psychischer Schäden verdienen, und zum anderen einige Hindernisse zu benennen, die dem entgegenstehen.

Zunächst kann die „Subtilität“ von Nebenwirkungen auf der Ebene der Psyche darin bestehen, dass sie erst nach längerer Zeit offenbar werden. Das ist besonders einschlägig für Eingriffe während der Entwicklungsphase des Gehirns (die bei Menschen von der intrauterinen bis zur postpubertären Phase reicht), da es in diesem Zeitraum besonders schwer ist, die Nachwirkungen eines Eingriffs in dem komplexen Gefüge natürlicherweise auftretender Veränderungen zu erkennen. Würde Langzeitnebenwirkungen die ihnen gebührende Aufmerksamkeit geschenkt, könnte dies zu dem Problem führen, dass Sicherheitsprüfungen für neue Arten von Interventionen am Gehirn zeit- und kostenaufwendiger würden. Um die Entwicklungskosten für neue Interventionstypen in einem handhabbaren Rahmen zu halten, könnte man zusätzlich zu einer angemessen langen klinischen Testphase vor der Zulassung umfangreiche Kontrolluntersuchungen im Anschluss an die Markteinführung einfordern. Allerdings können einer

Implementierung dieser Überwachungsstrategie, je nach Lage der nationalen Datenschutzgesetzgebung, Zugriffsbeschränkungen auf die relevanten Daten entgegenstehen. Der vermutlich einfachste Weg zur Auflösung dieses normativen Konflikts bestünde darin, Patienten in Anbetracht ihres eigenen Interesses an Langzeit-Sicherheitsstudien die Möglichkeit zum Verzicht auf bestimmte Rechte zum Schutz einschlägiger persönlicher Daten einzuräumen.

Auch wenn wir in dieser Studie nicht auf die methodologische Debatte über Testinstrumente zur Untersuchung von Persönlichkeitsveränderungen eingehen konnten, lassen sich aus dem in Kapitel 5 entwickelten narrativen Ansatz zur Bestimmung des Persönlichkeitsbegriffs einige für diese Debatte relevante Konsequenzen ziehen. Da das *Selbstverständnis* einen wesentlichen Teil des Charakters einer Person ausmacht, muss es bei jeder umfassenden Beurteilung von Persönlichkeitsveränderungen, die aus Interventionen am Gehirn resultieren könnten, Berücksichtigung finden. Zu diesem Zweck ist es erforderlich, die Bekundungen und Erzählungen zu beachten, mit denen Personen vermitteln, wer sie sind. Allerdings lassen sich Persönlichkeitsveränderungen nicht einfach dadurch zuverlässig feststellen, dass man Patienten vor und nach einem Eingriff fragt, ob sich ihre Persönlichkeit verändert habe oder nicht. Vielmehr sollte systematisch versucht werden, Unterschiede festzustellen zwischen der Selbsteinschätzung einer Person und der Art und Weise, wie andere die Auswirkung eines Eingriffs auf ihre Persönlichkeit beschreiben. Werden derartige Unterschiede entdeckt und scheinen diese zudem für die Bewertung des Eingriffs von erheblicher Bedeutung, dann ist es ratsam, objektivere Verfahren zur Beschreibung der umstrittenen Persönlichkeitsmerkmale zu wählen, beispielsweise in Form der Bezugnahme auf Verhaltensindikatoren. Anstatt lediglich die Ausprägung einzelner Persönlichkeitseigenschaften durch Maßgrößen zu bestimmen, sollte auch ihre relative Bedeutung im ganzheitlichen Gefüge des Charakters einer Person mit beachtet werden. Dabei muss wiederum die Möglichkeit verschiedener Beurteilungen aus der Perspektive der ersten bzw. dritten Person berücksichtigt werden.

Die Subtilität von Persönlichkeitsveränderungen

Ein besonderer Grund dafür, dass in der Folge eines Eingriffs eintretende Persönlichkeitsveränderungen unbemerkt bleiben können, wenn nicht eigens nach ihnen gesucht wird, liegt in der (glücklicherweise) großen Anpassungsfähigkeit von Personen. Anstatt daher besonders ins Auge zu fallen, werden Persönlichkeitsveränderungen in vielen Fällen harmonisch in das personale Selbstverständnis eingefügt. Insbesondere das Wertesystem, das einen wichtigen Teil des Selbstverständnisses darstellt, reagiert häufig in sehr dynamischer Weise auf Persönlichkeitsveränderungen. In provokanter Form könnte man diesen weiteren Aspekt der Subtilität von Persönlichkeitsveränderungen wie folgt ansprechen: Wie auch immer sich der Charakter einer Person durch einen Eingriff in ihr Gehirn verändern mag, wird sie sich aller Voraussicht nach mit ihrer veränderten Persönlichkeit anfreunden, so dass ihr letztlich kein Schaden entsteht. – Zum einen ist jedoch ein solch „positiver" Ausgang des Anpassungsprozesses weitaus weniger sicher als es diese Aussage suggeriert, und zum anderen ist die in ihr enthaltene Schlussfolgerung schlicht und ergreifend falsch. Denn selbst wenn eine Person eine bestimmte Veränderung ihrer Persönlichkeit für sich genommen gutheißt, könnten die sich aus dieser Veränderung im Weiteren ergebenden Konsequenzen dennoch eine erhebliche Schädigung bedeuten. Wenn die betroffene Person beispielsweise ziemlich alleine dasteht mit der Wertschätzung ihrer veränderten Persönlichkeit, so dass ihr alle anderen aufgrund ihrer Veränderung den Rücken kehren, dann stellt die resultierende Isolation sicherlich einen Schaden für die Person dar. Doch selbst wenn die herbeigeführten Veränderungen soziale Billigung erfahren, muss das nicht bedeuten, dass kein Schaden entstanden ist. Man wird die Möglichkeit einer Schädigung in diesem Kontext jedoch so lange unterschätzen, wie man ausschließlich die Bewertung in Betracht zieht, die eine Person abgibt *nachdem* ihre Persönlichkeit bereits versehentlich durch einen Eingriff verändert wurde. Dem halten wir entgegen:

➔ Ob die Aussicht darauf, dass ein Eingriff in das Gehirn eine bestimmte Form von Persönlichkeitsveränderung zur möglichen Nebenwirkung hat, akzeptabel oder gar wünschenswert ist, kann ausschließlich von den betroffenen Personen selbst *vor* der Durchführung des Eingriffs entschieden werden.

Dies impliziert auch, dass es für die Frage der Klassifizierung einer Persönlichkeitsveränderung als Schaden irrelevant ist, ob *sonst irgend jemand* die Möglichkeit des Auftretens dieser Veränderung als Nebenwirkung eines Eingriffs begrüßt. Wenn nun eine Person eine mögliche Persönlichkeitsveränderung als Schaden empfindet, dann gilt im selben Sinne, dass niemand außer ihr selbst darüber befinden kann, ob dieses Risiko eines Eingriffs annehmbar ist oder nicht. Selbstverständlich ist es für Personen, die darüber nachdenken, sich einem bestimmten Eingriff zu unterziehen, von erheblichem Belang, wie vorhersehbar die genaue Art und wie wahrscheinlich das Auftreten einer möglichen Persönlichkeitsveränderung ist. In jedem Fall sollten Personen explizit darüber in Kenntnis gesetzt werden, dass Nebenwirkungen auf Ebene der Persönlichkeit mit Veränderungen ihrer Sichtweise auf die erzielten Effekte einhergehen können. Wenn ein Patient dieses Risiko zu tragen bereit ist (und der Eingriff ausgeführt wird), müssen möglicherweise resultierende Veränderungen seiner subjektiven Kriterien zur Bewertung des Interventionsergebnisses akzeptiert werden, so dass sie anschließend den nunmehr verbindlichen Maßstab zur Beurteilung des Wohlbefindens des Patienten bilden.

3.1.2 Möglichen Schaden durch sorgfältigen Studienentwurf minimieren

Die klinische Forschung wird durch Gesetze geregelt, welche das Einholen informierter Einwilligung (s. Abschnitt 3.3) und die Evaluierung durch Medizinethik-Kommissionen zur Voraussetzung für die Genehmigung von Forschungsvorhaben erklären. Dies gilt auch für die neuen Interventionsmöglichkeiten am Gehirn, die in dieser Studie besprochen wurden. Das mit ihnen verbundene besondere Risiko, subtile psychische Nebenwirkungen nach sich zu ziehen, unterstreicht jedoch das allgemeine Erfordernis zur sorgfältigen Studienplanung. Abgesehen davon, dass klinische Studien nicht durchgeführt werden sollen und sogar als unethisch gelten müssen, wenn mit ihnen grundsätzlich keine eindeutig interpretierbaren und gehaltvollen Resultate erzielt werden können, gilt außerdem, dass die Bedeutung erhobener Befunde höher einzustufen ist, wenn ein standardisiertes Protokoll für die Messung der wesentlichen Symptome von Hirnstörungen verwendet wird. Es würde die zur Sicherstellung der Bedeutsamkeit der Ergebnisse benötigte Anzahl von Patienten, die sich experimentellen Eingriffen in das zentrale Nervensystem unterziehen müssten, minimieren, wenn solche standardisierten Evaluationsprotokolle verfügbar wären. Das führt zu folgender Empfehlung:

➔ Für die Durchführung experimenteller Forschungsvorhaben an Patienten mit neurologischen und psychiatrischen Störungen sollten standardisierte krankheitsspezifische Untersuchungspläne *(core assessment protocols)* mit schematisierten Zeitvorgaben etabliert werden, um (1) die Erhebung aussagekräftiger Resultate zu gewährleisten und (2) Vergleichsmöglichkeiten zwischen verschiedenen Behandlungsansätzen zu schaffen.

Da für jede neurologische oder psychiatrische Hirnstörung ein spezifischer Untersuchungsplan benötigt wird, sind diese selbst Gegenstand der Forschung und Konsensfindung durch Wissenschaftler und Kliniker, die auf bestimmte Krankheitsbilder des Gehirns spezialisiert sind. Diese Empfehlung richtet sich daher in erster Linie an Wissenschaftler, anstatt den Gesetzgeber zum Handeln aufzurufen. Sie spricht sich jedoch für die Bildung multizentrischer Kooperationen bei klinischen Studien zu neuen Interventionsformen aus, wie dies im Bereich der Pharmakologie bereits üblich ist.

3.1.3 Mögliche Schädigungen durch Enhancement

Wie bereits erwähnt, können die beabsichtigten Primäreffekte von Enhancement-Verfahren grundsätzlich nicht als Schaden betrachtet werden. Denn um überhaupt als Enhancement gelten zu können, muss das Verfahren zumindest in den Augen derjenigen Personen, an denen es durchgeführt wird, in wenigstens einer Hinsicht eine Verbesserung verheißen – nämlich in der Hinsicht, die letztlich den Beweggrund für die Intervention liefert. Eine Verbesserung ist kein Schaden. Und da die intendierten Wirkungen nur an der Person eintreten, die um den Eingriff gebeten hat, gibt grundsätzlich nur das eigene, womöglich idiosynkratische Urteil dieser Person selber den Ausschlag in der Frage, ob diese Wirkungen als vorteilhaft, also als unschädlich, zu beurteilen sind oder nicht.[309]

Gibt es illegitime Ziele von Enhancements?

Diese rein subjektive Beurteilung eines bestimmungsgemäßen Ausgangs von Enhancements allein nach Maßgabe der individuellen Präferenzen der jeweils betroffenen Person entspricht gewiss prinzipiell grundlegenden ethischen Normen. Dies gilt in der Tat ausnahmslos, sofern nur eine Partei beteiligt ist: Was eine – jedenfalls im Ganzen – zurechnungsfähige Person ausschließlich mit sich selbst anstellt, fällt prinzipiell unter den Schutz ihrer Privatsphäre, ungeachtet eines etwa abweichenden Urteils anderer Leute über den jeweiligen Eingriff.[310] In „Zwei-Parteien-Fällen" unterliegt dieses Prinzip jedoch bestimmten Einschränkungen. Die meisten entwickelten Rechtsordnungen kennen bestimmte Grenzen der Rechtfertigung für *physische* Eingriffe, die eine Person am Körper einer anderen vornimmt, selbst wenn für diese Eingriffe eine aufgeklärte Einwilligung gegeben wurde. Diese rechtlichen Beschränkungen greifen dann, wenn der Eingriff einen gravierenden Verstoß gegen „die guten Sitten" – verstanden als fundamentale, allgemein geteilte ethische Prinzipien und Regeln – darstellt.[311] Dieses begrenzende Rechtsprinzip mag nicht nur die unmittelbaren physischen Auswirkungen eines Eingriffs in Betracht ziehen, sondern zusätzlich auch weitere, mit ihm zusammenhängende und beabsichtigte Folgen (und in einigen Rechtssystemen geschieht dies auch). Dann ließe sich der reine körperliche Eingriff nach objektiv-normativen Kriterien schon und allein deshalb als rechtswidrige Schädigung (im oben erläuterten Sinne eines „gravierenden Sittenverstoßes") beurteilen, weil die mit ihm verbundenen Sekundärfolgen als sittenwidrig zu beurteilen sind – unbeschadet des Umstands, dass die betroffene Person selbst den Eingriff als Enhancement betrachtet.

Zwei Arten von Fällen sind hier zu unterscheiden: zum einen Enhancements, die nur aufgrund ihres funktionellen Nutzens für illegitime („sittenwidrige") Ziele angestrebt werden; und zum anderen Enhancements, die als solche, nämlich als Verbesserung, nur von der sie begehrenden Person aufge-

[309] Mögliche negative Folgen der massenhaften Anwendung eines bestimmten Enhancement-Verfahrens auf die Gesellschaft sind ein anderes Thema, das hier unter der Überschrift „Gerechtigkeit" (3.4) behandelt wird.

[310] Wir lassen hier einmal spezielle Konstellationen beiseite, in denen sich aus einer besonderen moralischen Verpflichtung gegenüber anderen (z.B. der Verpflichtung einer Mutter gegenüber ihrem minderjährigen Kind) für eine Person die Pflicht ergeben mag, ihre eigene Persönlichkeit nicht auf bestimmte Weise zu verändern.

[311] Der Einfachheit halber zitieren wir hier den Wortlaut von § 228 des deutschen Strafgesetzbuches; die meisten anderen Rechtsordnungen enthalten Normen mit mehr oder weniger ähnlichen Formulierungen.

fasst werden, von jedem vernünftigen Beobachter dagegen als schwerwiegende Schädigung beurteilt würden. Zu Fällen des ersten Typs: Wenn eine Person in der Absicht, sich der Verantwortung für einen von ihr begangenen Mord zu entziehen, eine Veränderung ihrer Psyche im Sinne einer dissoziativen Störung anstrebte, die eine komplette Auslöschung der Erinnerung an dieses Verbrechen beinhaltete, so hätte sie durchaus nachvollziehbare Gründe, diese Veränderung als für sich vorteilhaft und damit als Enhancement zu betrachten. Die Rechtsordnung kann jedoch diese subjektive Definition von Enhancement sehr wohl als irrelevant verwerfen. Dann beginge der Arzt, der im Wissen um die Absichten des Mörders einen solchen Eingriff vornähme, trotz Vorliegens einer aufgeklärten Einwilligung eine rechtswidrige Körperverletzung. Weitere Beispiele für Enhancements, die in rechtswidriger (z.B. betrügerischer) Absicht erstrebt werden, sind unschwer vorstellbar und sollten als realistische zukünftige Möglichkeit ernst genommen werden.

Für die zweite Art von Fällen ist die Erfindung eines veranschaulichenden Szenarios erheblich schwieriger. Man müsste sich eine Person vorstellen, die tatsächlich den Wunsch hat, ihre kognitiven Fähigkeiten in erheblichem Maße zu beschneiden und die dies für sich selbst als Enhancement begreift. Die meisten Menschen würden ein derartiges Szenario wohl als völlig unrealistisch erachten. Doch ein wohldokumentierter analoger Fall aus dem Bereich physischer Interventionen lässt es als voreilig erscheinen, eine solche Möglichkeit *a limine* zurückzuweisen. In den vergangenen Jahren ist in verschiedenen Ländern eine beachtliche Anzahl von Fällen bekannt geworden, in welchen Chirurgen von ansonsten normalen, d.h. zurechnungsfähigen, Personen dazu gedrängt wurden, an ihnen Amputationen gesunder Gliedmaßen vorzunehmen.[312] Vergleichbare Phänomene im psychischen Bereich sind nach unserer Kenntnis bislang nicht dokumentiert. Dass sie gleichwohl auftreten könnten, sollte jedoch nicht leichfertig ausgeschlossen werden. An solche Fälle kann man im Prinzip auf zweierlei Weise herangehen: Entweder erachtet man ein derartig seltsames Verlangen oder jedenfalls das mit seinem Unerfülltbleiben verbundene Leid (das sich als regelrechte Depression manifestieren kann) als psychische Störung, so dass dann, unter bestimmten Umständen, die gewünschte, objektiv schädigende Intervention durchaus als gerechtfertigte Behandlung gelten könnte.[313] Oder man weist die Idee der Rechtfertigung eines solchen Eingriffs kategorisch mit der Begründung

[312] Fälle sogenannter „selbstgewählter Amputierter“ *(Amputees-by-choice)*, s. Bayne und Levy (2005).

[313] Selbstverständlich würde die Rechtfertigung eines so gravierenden Eingriffs ein entsprechend gravierendes Leiden des Patienten in Folge seiner Störung zur Voraussetzung haben. Aber eben dies könnte durchaus gegeben sein. In einigen der Fälle von Amputation-auf-Verlangen sollen die betroffenen Personen ernsthaft in Erwägung gezogen haben, Suizid zu begehen, falls ihnen ihr Wunsch verweigert würde.

zurück, dass es sich dabei unter allen denkbaren Umständen um einen gravierenden Sittenverstoß im oben erwähnten Sinn handelt. Gegenwärtig mag man getrost abwarten, was die weitere Debatte zu diesem Problem ergeben wird. Fälle wie die geschilderten haben sicherlich einen exotischen und futuristischen Beigeschmack und werden, wenn überhaupt, nur als seltene Ausnahmen in Erscheinung treten. Das ist jedoch kein Grund, ihre Möglichkeit zu ignorieren. Gegenwärtig bedarf es keiner neuen Rechtsnormen zur Behandlung dieser hypothetischen Szenarien. Doch in dem Maße, in welchem zukünftige Entwicklungen von Eingriffen in das Gehirn neue Möglichkeiten der Einflussnahme auf die Psyche eröffnen, sollte die Forschung in diesen Dingen ebenfalls vorangetrieben werden, um die empirische Grundlage für normative Lösungen zu schaffen, für die sich dann ein Bedarf durchaus ergeben mag.

In einem gewissen Zusammenhang mit dem obigen Problem steht die Frage, ob Techniken des mentalen Enhancements für rein militärische Zwecke entwickelt oder angewendet werden dürfen: mit dem Ziel, die kognitiven, emotionalen oder motivationalen Charakteristika von Soldaten zu verbessern, um sie zu effizienteren Kämpfern zu machen. Jede normativ beglaubigte Antwort darauf müsste freilich den Bereich der Bio- oder Neuroethik überschreiten und die Sphäre der politischen Ethik betreten, insbesondere den Bereich der Rechts- und Moralphilosophie von Krieg und Frieden. Aus nahe liegenden Gründen können wir im Zuge der Behandlung unseres Themas nicht in diese Debatte eintreten. Was sich jedoch ganz allgemein sagen lässt, ist das Folgende: Solange man (wie die Autoren dieses Buches) anerkennt, dass ein Staat einen bewaffneten Konflikt unter gewissen Umständen (gemäß den strengen Kriterien des gegenwärtigen Völkerrechts) *gerechtfertigterweise* austragen kann, lassen sich Einwände gegen mögliches Enhancement zu militärischen Zwecken jedenfalls nicht schon durch den bloßen Hinweis darauf begründen, dass es hier um militärische Zwecke geht. Eine ganz andere Frage ist es, ob das Risiko des Missbrauchs solcher Techniken in bewaffneten Konflikten oder zu völkerrechtswidrigen kriegerischen Zwecken nicht zu hoch ist, als dass sich die Mitwirkung von Wissenschaftlern an militärischen Forschungsvorhaben rechtfertigen ließe. Aber jeder Versuch einer Antwort auf diese Fragen würde die Grenzen dieser Untersuchung sprengen. Daher wollen wir es bei einer allgemeinen Mahnung zu dringender Vorsicht bei jeglichem Einsatz von Wissenschaft zur Etablierung von Techniken belassen, die der Tötung von Menschen dienen (oder die Tötung von Menschen in Kauf nehmen). Als letzte hier einschlägige Frage erwähnen wir die Besorgnis, die Verwendung solcher Techniken könnte dazu führen, dass auf Soldaten (bzw. auf Personen, die Soldaten werden möchten) offen oder versteckt Druck ausgeübt werde, in ein Enhancement einzuwilligen. Ein solcher Druck könnte eine Beschneidung ihres Rechts auf persönliche Selbstbestimmung oder sogar ein politisches Unrecht darstellen; daher werden wir uns dieses Themas (wenn auch in etwas allgemeinerer Form) in den Abschnitten zu Authentizität (3.3.2) und politischer Gerechtigkeit (3.4.2) annehmen.

Zum Umgang mit möglichen Nebenwirkungen von Enhancements

Anders als therapeutische Maßnahmen sind Eingriffe, die auf ein mentales Enhancement abzielen, nicht Gegenstand einer moralischen *prima facie*-Verpflichtung von Ärzten (beziehungsweise des Gesundheitssystems); sie können allenfalls als moralisch zulässig gelten. Aus diesem Grund gewinnen nachteilige Nebenwirkungen bei reinen Enhancements generell größeres Gewicht für den Abwägungsprozess, der im Zentrum jeder Risikobewertung steht. Daher mag ein und dasselbe negative Ergebnis als mögliche Nebenwirkung einer Behandlung akzeptabel, im Fall eines Enhancements jedoch unannehmbar sein.

Bei der Beurteilung der Risiken von Enhancements nimmt nicht nur die Bedeutung möglicher Nebenwirkungen zu; auch der Bereich der für die Bewertung relevanten Nebenwirkungen selbst erweitert sich erheblich. Auf Seiten des ausführenden Mediziners ergibt sich daraus eine doppelte Ausweitung seiner Informationspflichten: Erstens muss er sich über mögliche psychische Besonderheiten seiner Klienten gründlicher informieren, als dies im Fall therapeutischer Maßnahmen geboten wäre. Zweitens muss er seine Klienten umfassender über mögliche unerwünschte Nebenwirkungen in Kenntnis setzen, selbst wenn diese sehr subtil und entlegen erscheinen. Diese Maximen weichen natürlich nicht von den geläufigen Prinzipien der Medizinethik und des Medizinrechts ab; dennoch verdienen es die Besonderheiten, die sich bei ihrer Anwendung auf Fälle mentalen Enhancements ergeben, hervorgehoben zu werden.

Als Schlussfolgerung dieser Diskussion halten wir fest:

➔ Die bloße Tatsache, dass mentales Enhancement für Individuen, die sich ihm unterziehen, mit physischen oder psychischen Risiken verbunden sein kann, rechtfertigt es unseres Erachtens nicht, solche Maßnahmen prinzipiell ethisch zu verwerfen oder gar rechtlich zu verbieten. Im Vergleich zu therapeutischen Interventionen muss jedoch unterstrichen werden, dass bei Fällen reinen Enhancements drohende negative Nebenwirkungen gegenüber den beabsichtigten positiven Wirkungen schwerer wiegen. Ärzte, die zu bloßen Zwecken des Enhancements Eingriffe durchführen, unterstehen gegenüber ihren Klienten erweiterten Informationspflichten. Konsequenterweise sind sie auch verpflichtet, sich selbst in entsprechend umfangreicherem Maße zu informieren.

Aus verfassungsrechtlichen Gründen ist es in liberalen, demokratischen Gesellschaften nicht zulässig, das Recht paternalistisch zur öffentlichen Kontrolle individueller Präferenzen und selbstbezogener Handlungen autonomer Bürger zu instrumentalisieren. Dasselbe gilt, wenn auch nur in eingeschränktem Umfang, für säkulare Konzeptionen der Ethik, zu denen die

Autoren dieser Studie sich im Großen und Ganzen und trotz Meinungsverschiedenheiten in einzelnen Aspekten bekennen. Eine religiöse Ethik mag zu anderen Schlussfolgerungen gelangen. Wir betonen ausdrücklich unseren Respekt für solche Positionen. Allerdings möchten wir auch hervorheben, dass sie in säkularen Gesellschaften, die wegen der Vielfalt der in ihnen vorhandenen ethischen Konzeptionen im Wesentlichen nur rechtsförmig zu steuern sind, keine allgemeine Verbindlichkeit mehr beanspruchen können. *A fortiori* gilt, dass genuin religiösen Auffassungen keine prägende Rolle bei der Ausgestaltung der Rechtsordnung zukommen darf.

3.2 Hilfe leisten („Wohltun"): Die Grenzen zwischenmenschlicher Wohltätigkeit

3.2.1 Behandlung und Prävention

Das Prinzip der Hilfeleistung statuiert eine positive Verpflichtung, dem Wohlergehen anderer zu dienen. Ob die Moral generell und von jedermann verlangen kann, anderen nicht nur keinen Schaden zuzufügen, sondern ihnen auch Gutes zu tun (von speziellen Situationen und Beziehungen abgesehen, in denen fraglos jedermann zu derartigem Tun verpflichtet ist), darüber lässt sich lange streiten. Im Gesundheitswesen Tätige unterstehen jedoch ganz offensichtlich einer solchen Verpflichtung. Sie handeln als Funktionsträger eines Systems, dessen Bereitstellung als Ganzes ebenso zu den fundamentalen positiven Pflichten moderner Staaten gehört wie die rechtliche Sicherung des Zugangs zu diesem System für alle Bürger. Dabei ist es ersichtlich notwendig, die Hilfeleistungspflicht sowohl des einzelnen Mediziners als auch des gesamten öffentlichen Gesundheitswesens zu begrenzen. Innerhalb dieser Grenzen umfasst das generelle Prinzip der Hilfeleistung die zugelassenen Therapien mittels neuartiger Eingriffe in das Gehirn ganz genauso wie alle anderen Methoden zur Behandlung menschlicher Krankheiten. Ist eine Intervention ins Gehirn – egal welcher Art und welchen Umfangs – als legitime (nicht-schädigende) Behandlungsmethode anerkannt, steht sie demnach im Einklang mit den gängigen Kriterien zur Abwägung beabsichtigter Primäreffekte gegenüber absehbaren negativen Nebenwirkungen, so ist sie *per definitionem* hilfreich. (Ob die voranschreitende Ausweitung des Bereichs medizinischer Behandlungsoptionen neue und striktere Rationierungsvorschriften für neu entwickelte Methoden erfordert, ist eine andere Frage, die besser im Abschnitt zur „Gerechtigkeit" aufgehoben ist als im vorliegenden Abschnitt zum Prinzip der Hilfeleistung.)

3.2.2 Verantwortlichkeit und Haftung für Enhancement

→ Ein Enhancement gesunder Menschen gehört nicht zum genuinen Aufgabenbereich der Beschäftigten im Gesundheitswesen, deren Aufgabe vielmehr die Behandlung und vorbeugende Verhinderung von Krankheiten ist. Ausschließlich auf Enhancement abzielende Eingriffe in das Gehirn unterliegen deshalb nicht der prinzipiellen Hilfeleistungspflicht der Medizin. Dass es schwer entscheidbare Grenzfälle gibt, bleibt davon unberührt.

Wie bereits dargelegt, sollten reine Enhancement-Maßnahmen aus dem Leistungskatalog der Medizin als eines öffentlichen und öffentlich finanzierten Systems ausgeschlossen werden. Dies impliziert auch, dass sie nicht in den Bereich der individuellen ärztlichen Pflicht zur Hilfe fallen. Ärzte sind durch keine – nicht einmal durch eine *prima facie* – Pflicht zur Durchführung von Enhancement-Maßnahmen angehalten. Dies gilt für mentale nicht anders als für rein physische („kosmetische") Enhancements.

Soweit jedoch die Nebenwirkungen einer medizintechnischen Maßnahme des Enhancements, die von einer zurechnungsfähigen Person an sich selbst oder aber von einem (medizinischen oder nicht-medizinischen) Akteur an einer wirksam einwilligenden Person vorgenommen werden, selbst Krankheitswert besitzen (z.B. den einer Sucht), werden sie zum legitimen Gegenstand der Behandlung durch spezialisiertes Personal des Gesundheitswesens. Diese Behandlungen selbst fallen eindeutig unter das Prinzip der gebotenen Hilfeleistung. Da dies für ihre Ursache jedoch nicht gilt, stellt sich die Frage, ob und inwieweit die finanziellen Kosten zur Behandlung dieser Nebenwirkungen von Krankenversicherungssystemen abgedeckt werden sollen, die auf einer zwangsrechtlichen Solidarpflicht gründen, sei diese klassisch sozialversicherungsrechtlicher oder steuerrechtlicher Provenienz. Eine generelle und normativ zwingende Antwort auf diese Frage gibt es nicht. Wenn die finanziellen Mittel eines nationalen Systems der Gesundheitsfürsorge die Übernahme der Kosten für Behandlungen solcher durch Enhancement verursachter Krankheiten erlauben, mögen sie durchaus in diesem System integriert werden. Doch weder das Prinzip der Hilfeleistung noch das der Gerechtigkeit fordert eine solche Integration. Insofern unterliegt es einem weitreichenden Ermessensspielraum der jeweiligen nationalen Gesetzgebung, ob sie die Übernahme solcher Kosten dem Individuum aufbürden will, das sich einer Maßnahme des Enhancements unterzogen und das Risiko einer Folgeerkrankung bewusst auf sich genommen hat. Um Missverständnisse zu vermeiden, möchten wir hervorheben, dass dieser Ermessensspielraum sich nur auf die Kosten, nicht aber auf die Behandlung selbst bezieht. Deren Einbeziehung in ein wohlgeordnetes Gesundheitswesen wird vielmehr vom Prinzip der gebotenen Hilfeleistung gefordert. Daraus folgt, dass Personen, die die Behandlungskosten von Krankheiten nicht bezahlen können, welche in der Folge eines Enhancement-Eingriffs in ihr Gehirn entstanden sind, gleichwohl behandelt werden müssen; die anfallenden Kosten sind dann vom Sozialversicherungssystem entsprechend seiner jeweiligen rechtlichen Ausgestaltung zu tragen.

3.2.3 Öffentliche Forschungsfinanzierung

Staaten unterstehen einer positiven *prima facie*-Verpflichtung zur Förderung von Forschungsvorhaben im Dienste des medizinischen Fortschritts. Diese Pflicht unterliegt selbstverständlich einer Vielzahl von Beschränkungen, für deren konkrete Handhabung ein weitreichendes staatliches Ermessen besteht. Dieses allgemeine Prinzip der medizinischen Ethik gilt, *mutatis mutandis*, auch für die Erforschung von neuen Methoden zur Intervention am Gehirn, solange es dabei um neue Möglichkeiten der Behandlung und der Prävention geht. Auch wenn diese Art von Forschung im Prinzip keine speziellen normativen Probleme aufwirft, drängt sich die Frage auf, ob der Umfang der öffentlichen Fördermittel dem tatsächlichen klinischen Bedarf in diesem Bereich gerecht wird.

Um die Berechtigung dieser Frage einzusehen, muss man sich die weitreichenden Konsequenzen vergegenwärtigen, die Krankheiten und Verletzungen des Gehirns, psychiatrische Störungen wie Depression und Schizophrenie, die Begleiterscheinungen des Alterns sowie stressbezogene Erkrankungen für das Funktionieren von Menschen in der Gesellschaft haben. Im Jahr 2004 litten allein in der EU 127 Millionen Menschen an Hirnerkrankungen, entsprechend 27% der Gesamtbevölkerung. Ein erheblicher Anteil der gegenwärtigen Gesundheitsausgaben entfällt auf die Behandlung von Hirnstörungen. Für 2004 wurden diese Kosten auf 386 Milliarden Euro geschätzt, wobei dieser Betrag nur die finanziellen Aufwendungen für die medizinische Versorgung erfasst, während die indirekten sozialen Kosten unberücksichtigt bleiben. Auf Erkrankungen des Gehirns (neurologische, neurochirurgisch behandelbare, psychiatrische und vaskuläre) entfällt ein geschätzter Anteil von 35% der Gesamtausgaben für alle Krankheiten in Europa, und damit ein größerer Anteil als auf Krebs oder Herzversagen. Diese Zahlen[314] werden im Gefolge der wachsenden Lebenserwartung wahrscheinlich weiter ansteigen: „Der Körper überlebt das Gehirn." Verbesserungen der klinischen Methoden bei der Behandlung von Erkrankungen des Gehirns setzen Grundlagenforschung in angemessenem Umfang voraus. Mit dem wachsenden *Verständnis* des Gehirns vermehren sich auch die Möglichkeiten zur *Intervention*. Jeder Durchbruch im Bereich der Neurowissenschaft wurde durch die enge Zusammenarbeit von Grundlagenforschung und klinischer Forschung ermöglicht. Für keine der neuen Techniken zur Intervention am Gehirn wurde bislang der mögliche therapeutische Nutzen zur Behandlung der genannten Hirnstörungen voll ausgeschöpft.

Trotz der oben bezifferten Lasten für Individuum und Gesellschaft wird nur ein Bruchteil der Gesamtausgaben für Erkrankungen des Gehirns in neurowissenschaftliche Forschung investiert. Auf europäischer Ebene hat

[314] Alle Angaben wurden der Studie „The Cost of Disorders of the Brain in Europe" des European Brain Council entnommen, die in einem Themenheft des European Journal of Neurology veröffentlicht worden ist (Andlin-Sobocki et al. 2005).

das ausgelaufene fünfte Rahmenforschungsprogramm nur einen Anteil von 0.01% der geschätzten medizinischen Kosten für Hirnstörungen in Europa für die Erforschung dieser Erkrankungen zur Verfügung gestellt. Sofern nicht ausreichende Energie und finanzielle Mittel für die Hirnforschung verausgabt werden, könnte die Gesellschaft bald allen Grund dazu haben, Politik und Wissenschaft anzuklagen, weil sie keinen angemessenen Beitrag zur Besserung der Lage geleistet haben.

Die normative Situation ist vollkommen anders, wenn es um Forschungsvorhaben geht, die ausschließlich auf die Entwicklung von Interventionen am Gehirn für reine Enhancement-Zwecke abzielen. Man mag wohl daran zweifeln, dass derartige (d.h. *nur* für Enhancement einschlägige) Forschung überhaupt möglich ist oder vernünftigerweise in Erwägung gezogen werden kann. Aber wie dem auch sei – sollte eine solche Forschung möglich sein oder werden, so fällt sie jedenfalls nicht in den normativen Anwendungsbereich des Prinzips der gebotenen Hilfe. Daher fordern wir:

➔ Forschung, die ausschließlich auf die Entwicklung von Mitteln für mentales Enhancement durch Intervention am Gehirn gerichtet ist, sollte nicht mit öffentlichen Mitteln gefördert werden, die für das soziale System der Gesundheitsfürsorge bestimmt sind. Ebensowenig sollte die praktische Anwendung der Produkte dieser Forschung zur Realisierung mentalen Enhancements durch das Gesundheitssystem finanziell gefördert werden.

Dieses Prinzip betrifft jedoch nicht die Grundlagenforschung zu den Bedingungen der Wirksamkeit von Verfahren des Enhancements oder zu deren pathogenen Eigenschaften. Eine plausible Analogie aus dem Bereich des rein körperlichen Enhancements bietet sich hier zur Erläuterung an: Forschung, die auf neue Dopingmethoden im Sport ausgerichtet ist, verdient gewiss keine öffentliche Förderung, wohl aber die Grundlagenforschung zu den funktionellen und krankheitsverursachenden Mechanismen solchen Dopings. Selbstverständlich legt nichts von dem hier Gesagten ein moralisches Verdikt, geschweige denn ein gesetzliches Verbot solcher Forschung nahe. Ihre Durchführung sollte jedoch vollständig privater Initiative und Finanzierung überlassen bleiben.

3.3 Autonomie: Probleme der informierten Einwilligung und von Zwang

Bekanntlich ist Autonomie ein komplexer und facettenreicher Begriff. Wir unterscheiden grob Autonomie als Souveränität, d.h. Selbstbestimmung, von Autonomie als Authentizität, etwa im Sinne eines Im-Einklang-Stehens mit der eigenen individuellen Natur. In dieses grundlegende Schema fügen wir weitere begriffliche Unterscheidungen ein. Anschließend analysieren wir die zugehörigen Probleme erstens aus rechtlicher Perspektive, die ausschließlich für den Bereich der „Autonomie als Souveränität" einschlägig ist, und zweitens aus der Perspektive der Ethik, die sowohl Aspekte der Souveränität als auch der Authentizität umfasst. Es sollte beachtet werden, dass die letztgenannten Probleme nur im Zusammenhang mit (beabsichtigten) Enhancements auftreten. Denn was auch immer *gerechtfertigterweise* unter Therapie oder Prävention subsumierbar ist, kann jedenfalls schwerlich in den Verdacht geraten, auf „nicht-authentischen" Entscheidungen zu basieren. Bei manchen Formen von Enhancement mag sich dies dagegen durchaus anders verhalten.

3.3.1 Behandlung, Prävention und Forschung

Das Ziel, Krankheiten durch therapeutische oder präventive Interventionen am Gehirn zu bekämpfen, erzeugt mit Bezug auf die Bedingungen von Autonomie noch keine spezifischen normativen Probleme. Jedoch kommt einigen der üblichen Prinzipien, die medizinische Eingriffe generell regeln, im Hinblick auf therapeutische Eingriffe in das Gehirn eine besondere Bedeutung zu.

Die schwere Fassbarkeit psychischer Schäden als Hindernis für eine aufgeklärte Einwilligung

Die Achtung vor der Autonomie eines Patienten (bzw. einer Versuchsperson) verlangt, dass im Voraus seine aufgeklärte Einwilligung eingeholt wird. Auf Seiten des Patienten ist für die Ausübung seiner Autonomie eine ausreichende Kenntnis der Art, der Methode, des Nutzens sowie möglicher Nebenwirkungen einer geplanten medizinischen Intervention nicht nur in normativer, sondern auch in begrifflicher Hinsicht notwendig. Der Akt der Einwilligung lässt sich als Ausdruck der Selbstbestimmung einer Person nur insofern werten, als diese *weiß,* wozu sie ihre Einwilligung erteilt. Daher hat das Gebot, einem Patienten dieses Wissen zu vermitteln, indem man ihn mit allen verfügbaren Informationen versorgt, welche für seine Entscheidungsfindung relevant sein können, die gleiche zwingende, Autonomie schützende Verbindlichkeit wie die Pflicht des Arztes, kurative Interventionen ohne Einwilligung gänzlich zu unterlassen. Weder für die Zwangsbehandlung eines zurechnungsfähigen Patienten noch für ein Erschleichen seiner Einwilligung durch Zurückhalten wichtiger Informationen gibt es eine Rechtfertigung. Dies gilt selbst dann, wenn der Patient ohne Behandlung einem hohen Mortalitätsrisiko ausgesetzt ist. Wir betonen, dass die besonderen Merkmale von Eingriffen in das Gehirn keinen Grund bieten, von diesem wohlbegründeten Prinzip des Medizinrechts und der Medizinethik abzuweichen.

Eine Eigenheit möglicher Auswirkungen solcher Eingriffe liegt darin, dass sie manchmal in ihrer Tragweite und Bedeutung nur schwer greifbar sind. Das mag selbst für den behandelnden Arzt gelten, und gilt sicher in gesteigertem Maße für Patienten. Beispielsweise zeigt unsere Studie, dass es nicht immer offensichtlich ist, was das Auftreten eines Wechsels personaler Identität bedeutet. Wenn eine bestimmte Art von Intervention ins Gehirn mit dem

Risiko eines Wechsels der Identität verbunden ist, kann es schwierig zu vermitteln sein, dass diese Nebenwirkung in bestimmtem Sinn von endgültiger Natur ist. Dieses Problem mag noch durch die Tatsache erschwert werden, dass Patienten mit einem ernsthaften medizinischen Befund bereit sind, nach jedem Strohhalm zu greifen, der Erleichterung verspricht. Um den Schweregrad solcher Schäden hervorzuheben, könnte es hilfreich sein, die in Kapitel 5 eingeführte Metapher des „psychischen Todes" aufzugreifen. Allerdings kann dieser Ausdruck durchaus auch im Sinne einer irreführenden Übertreibung missverstanden werden. In unserer Besprechung dieser Problematik weisen wir darauf hin, dass selbst schwere dissoziative Störungen, die die klarste Manifestation eines Wechsels personaler Identität darstellen, anders als der Tod überwunden werden können. Auf der anderen Seite gibt es keine Garantie für eine derartige Genesung. In dieser Hinsicht könnte der Vergleich zu Zuständen des Komas dazu geeignet sein, dem Patienten nachdrücklich zu verdeutlichen, dass in einem wichtigen Sinn sein persönliches Selbst, das primär konstituiert wird durch sein gegenwärtiges subjektives Bewusstsein, nach einem Eingriff im Falle eines möglicherweise als Nebenwirkung auftretenden dissoziativen Zustands so lange nicht mehr vorhanden wäre als dieser Zustand andauert – möglicherweise also für immer.

Obwohl bloße Persönlichkeitsveränderungen einen weniger drastischen Typ psychischen Schadens darstellen, besteht die Gefahr, dass sie ebenfalls als mögliche Nebenwirkungen unterschätzt werden. Bezüglich dieser Nebenwirkungen ist von entscheidender Bedeutung, dass ihre potentiellen Erscheinungsformen so detailliert wie möglich beschrieben werden, um Personen im Prozess der Abwägung des Für und Wider einer bestimmten Intervention zu unterstützen. Allerdings ist dabei ebenso wichtig, die prinzipiellen Grenzen der Prognostizierbarkeit von Persönlichkeitsveränderungen zu vermitteln, die sich daraus ergeben, dass jede Veränderung des narrativ strukturierten Ganzen eines Selbstverständnisses eine Kette unabsehbarer Folgen nach sich ziehen kann.

Das Ausüben von Autonomie unter äußerem Zwang

Zweifel an der Möglichkeit einer wahrhaft autonomen Einwilligung können aufkommen, wenn es um die Durchführung eines therapeutischen Eingriffs am Gehirn einer (ansonsten zurechnungsfähigen) Person geht, die sich gegenwärtig in Gefängnishaft befindet oder einer anderen rechtmäßigen Form des Gewahrsams unterliegt. Zur genaueren Erläuterung: Situationen, in denen es um die Behandlung (durch Intervention am Gehirn) einer im Verlaufe einer Haftstrafe ausbrechenden Krankheit geht, stellen hier keine besonderen Probleme dar. Das schon erwähnte Verbot von Zwangsbehandlungen zurechnungsfähiger Personen trifft auf Strafgefangene ebenso wie auf alle anderen zu. Problematisch sind jedoch Situationen wie die folgende: Ein Gefangener hat (1) die volle Dauer seiner gesetzlichen Haftstrafe verbüßt, muss aber (2) in Haft, nämlich in Sicherheitsverwahrung, verbleiben, weil er (3) eine gravierende Form soziopathischer Störung aufweist, die ihn (unbehandelt) zu einer dauerhaften Gefahr für seine Mitbürger macht, die jedoch (4) durch eine neue Methode der Intervention ins Gehirn behandelt werden könnte. (Wir sind uns völlig darüber im Klaren, dass die Projektion derartiger medizinischer Möglichkeiten gegenwärtig noch von einem Hauch von Science Fiction umgeben ist; dies könnte sich jedoch in nicht allzu ferner Zukunft ändern.) Die resultierende normative Frage ist nun: Lässt die Wahlmöglichkeit, vor die man einen solchen Soziopathen stellen könnte, sich nämlich entweder dem besagten Eingriff zu unterziehen oder auf unbestimmte Zeit in Sicherheitsverwahrung zu verbleiben, genügend Spielraum für eine autonome und damit rechtswirksame Einwilligung in einen solchen Eingriff?

Die Antwort lautet „Ja". Die Autonomie und damit auch die Wirksamkeit einer gegebenen Einwilligung entfällt nicht allein schon wegen der Höhe des Drucks, unter dem sie gegeben wird. Wenn etwa dieser Druck nicht von anderen Personen ausgeübt oder kontrolliert wird, sondern natürlichen Ursprungs ist, dann mag er beliebig groß sein, groß genug sogar, jeder vernünftigen Person eine Entscheidung mit annähernd hundertprozentiger Sicherheit aufzuzwingen, ohne doch deshalb die Autonomie dieser Entscheidung auch nur im Mindesten zu berühren. Beispielhaft: Wenn ein Patient mit Nierenkrebs vor die Alternative gestellt ist, entweder in die operative Entfernung der betroffenen Niere einzuwilligen oder binnen weniger Monate zu sterben, so wird er sich höchstwahrscheinlich für den Eingriff entscheiden. Seine Einwilligung zur Operation ist zweifellos autonom (und damit wirksam), auch wenn er das übermächtige Empfinden haben mag, keine Wahl zu haben. Im Gegensatz dazu wäre die Einwilligung einer Person, die unter Morddrohungen genötigt wird, der Entnahme einer ihrer Nieren zu Transplantationszwecken zuzustimmen, *nicht* autonom und daher unwirksam. Projiziert man diese grundsätzlichen Überlegungen auf das Problem des Psychopathen in Haft, so ist zunächst zu bedenken, dass der Druck, der auf eine Person von anderen ausgeübt wird, die dazu von Rechts wegen ermächtigt oder sogar verpflichtet sind, als ein Druck angesehen werden sollte, der von den Rechtsnormen selbst ausgeht. Für die Autonomie der Rechtsunterworfenen liegt der Zwang der geltenden Rechtsordnung (als eines Teils der sozialen Umwelt) auf der gleichen Ebene des äußerlich Vorgegebenen wie die Macht, die von der kausalgesetzlichen Ordnung der natürlichen Umwelt ausgeht.[315] Daher sind Entscheidungen, die Personen unter der Zwangsgewalt rechtlicher Normen treffen, nicht weniger autonom als Entscheidungen, die unter dem Einfluss der zwingenden Kraft natürlicher Gegebenheiten gefällt werden. Dabei macht es keinen Unterschied, ob der Zwang auf der unmittelbar selbstvollstreckenden Wirkung dieser Normen auf das Subjekt der Entscheidung

[315] Wir gehen hier von dem Regelfall *legitimer* Rechtssysteme aus. Die Unterdrückungsmechanismen terroristischer oder totalitärer Regime sind ein anderer Fall; ein unter solchen Bedingungen Inhaftierter, dem ein derartiges Enhancement angesonnen würde, wäre in der Tat das Opfer einer rechtswidrigen Nötigung.

beruht, oder von Mittelsleuten ausgeübt wird, die im Rahmen ihrer rechtlichen Kompetenzen handeln. Demnach bleibt festzuhalten:

Sollte jemals ein Verfahren der Intervention am Gehirn entwickelt werden, mit dem sich schwere Psychopathie mit einem vernünftigen Verhältnis von Nutzen und Risiken behandeln ließe, dann spräche nichts dagegen, Personen in Sicherheitsverwahrung die Behandlung mit diesem Interventionsverfahren anzubieten. Dies gilt insbesondere für den Fall, dass dies für den Betroffenen die einzige Alternative dazu darstellt, für unbestimmte Zeit in Gewahrsam zu verbleiben. Der schiere Druck, dem der Häftling in dieser Wahlsituation ausgesetzt ist, verletzt weder seine Autonomie, noch beraubt er seine Entscheidung ihrer rechtlichen Gültigkeit. Wir sind der Meinung, dass der Staat unter solchen Umständen nicht nur berechtigt, sondern sogar dazu verpflichtet wäre, ein solches Angebot zu unterbreiten.

3.3.2 Enhancement und die Grenzen der Autonomie

Enhancement als möglicher „Verstoß gegen die guten Sitten"

Beim Abwägen von Fragen der Autonomie bezüglich Maßnahmen des Enhancements müssen wiederum rechtliche von rein ethischen Überlegungen getrennt werden. Was das Recht anbelangt, so verweisen wir auf unsere obigen Bemerkungen zu den Grenzen der Rechtfertigbarkeit des Zufügens körperlichen Schadens unter Einwilligung der jeweils betroffenen zurechnungsfähigen Personen. Wir haben die relevante Schwelle unter exemplarischer Anleihe bei der Formulierung des § 228 des deutschen Strafgesetzbuchs bestimmt: „Wer eine Körperverletzung mit Einwilligung der verletzten Person vornimmt, handelt nur dann rechtswidrig, wenn die Tat trotz der Einwilligung gegen die guten Sitten verstößt." Der Beschränkung dessen, was ein Arzt zu tun berechtigt ist, muss auf Seiten des Patienten ersichtlich eine Einschränkung der Freiheit des Verfügens über die eigene körperliche Unversehrtheit entsprechen. Diese Verfügungsbeschränkung bezieht sich auf die Möglichkeit, zur Vornahme medizinisch-technischer Eingriffe am eigenen Körper andere Personen wirksam zu ermächtigen. In solchen Zwei-Parteien-Fällen darf der Arzt keine Interventionen durchführen, in die der Patient wegen ihres Verstoßes „gegen die guten Sitten" nicht wirksam einwilligen kann. Dabei liegt die Schwelle für einen solchen Verstoß in Fällen reinen Enhancements gewiss deutlich niedriger als bei therapeutischen Maßnahmen.[316] Jedoch bedeutet die bloße Tatsache, dass ein zu reinen Zwecken

---

[316] Tatsächlich können Behandlungen, die im Einklang mit anerkannten medizinischen Standards stehen, diese Schwelle *niemals* übertreten; denn sie setzen neben der informierten Einwilligung des Patienten auch eine angemessene Abwägung von Risiken und Nutzen eines Eingriffs voraus. Ausschließlich Behandlungen, die mit einem grob unverhältnismäßigen Risiko behaftet sind, beträchtlichen und unwiderruflichen Schaden als Nebenwirkung zu verursachen, können trotz Vorliegen der informierten Einwilligung als hinreichender „Sittenverstoß" gewertet werden. Dies mag etwa auf die meisten Fälle der „Auf-Wunsch-Amputierten" zutreffen (s. o. Fußnote 313).

des Enhancements vorgenommener Eingriff ins Gehirn absehbar signifikante Veränderungen der psychischen Eigenschaften einer Person nach sich ziehen kann, noch nicht, dass mit einem solchen Eingriff *ipso facto* jene Schwelle überschritten wird. Daher ist auch die wirksame Einwilligung zu einem solchen Eingriff keineswegs schon *per se* ausgeschlossen.

➔ Wenn eine Intervention anstatt therapeutischen nur Zielen des Enhancements dient, dann stellt dies allein noch keinen „groben Sittenverstoß" im erläuterten Sinn dar. Zugunsten der Zulässigkeit einer Intervention zum Zweck des individuellen Enhancements fällt die individuelle Freiheit (Autonomie als Selbstbestimmung) der Person, die ein solches Enhancement wünscht, gravierend (wenn auch nicht allein entscheidend) ins Gewicht.

Dennoch kann das Gesetz der Freiheit zur Selbstverfügung legitime Grenzen setzen. Und es tut dies (1) im Hinblick auf körperliche Folgen, sofern diese schweren, unverhältnismäßigen und unwiderruflichen Schaden bedeuteten, und (2) im Hinblick auf psychische Folgen, sollten diese ihrer Art nach selbst als vergleichsweise schädlich gelten können oder wenn sie offensichtlich nur um zukünftiger betrügerischer Zwecke willen erwünscht sind.

Es muss betont werden, dass die normativen Probleme, die mit den psychischen Wirkungen von Eingriffen ins Gehirn zum Zwecke des Enhancements zusammenhängen, bislang nur ansatzweise zum Gegenstand rechtswissenschaftlicher Diskussion gemacht worden sind. Wo genau die Grenze gezogen werden sollte, die sich aus dem Kriterium der Sittenwidrigkeit ableiten lässt, ist alles andere als klar. Hier besteht noch erheblicher Diskussionsbedarf. Wovor wir gegenwärtig warnen möchten, ist der mögliche Missbrauch einer anerkannten Rechtsfigur (der Formel des „Verstoßes gegen die guten Sitten"), die zur Anwendung in anderen Zusammenhängen entwickelt wurde, zum Zwecke eines voreiligen und möglicherweise ideologischen Kampfes gegen „künstliche" Methoden der menschlichen Selbstentwicklung.

Gewiss, auf der abstrakt-semantischen Ebene jener Rechtsfigur sind die beiden oben erwähnten Grenzen der Autonomie in Zwei-Parteien-Fällen weitgehend unbestritten; und für Interventionen, die auf mentales Enhancement abzielen, gilt dies ohne jede Abstriche. Andererseits fällt es jedoch nicht leicht, diese abstrakte Figur durch halbwegs realistische Beispielfälle für unseren Zusammenhang zu illustrieren. Wir glauben, dass dies Gesetzgeber und Gerichte zur Vorsicht gegenüber übereilten rechtlichen Verdikten anhalten sollte. Denn solche Verbote haben stets ihren gesellschaftlichen Preis – und sei es „nur" der einer Einbuße an persönlicher Freiheit. Es mag andere und bessere Gründe und Wege für das Recht geben, die möglicherweise unerwünschte Entwicklung von Verfahren des mentalen Enhancements zu verhindern, als die bequeme Abkürzung über das Prinzip des „groben Sittenverstoßes" zu nehmen.

Enhancement von Kindern: Der Umfang der elterlichen Entscheidungsgewalt

Ein ganz anderes Thema sind Enhancement-Interventionen am Gehirn, die an Kindern mit „stellvertretender Einwilligung“ der Eltern vorgenommen werden. Hinsichtlich therapeutischer Maßnahmen scheinen sich bei Kindern keine besonderen normativen Probleme für Eingriffe ins Gehirn zu ergeben, die nicht auch für andere medizinische Interventionen einschlägig wären. Aber reine Enhancements stellen in der Tat eine spezifische Problematik dar. Um diese zu erhellen, heben wir eine oft übersehene Einsicht hervor, der in solchen Fällen besondere Bedeutung zukommt: „Stellvertretende Einwilligung“ darf nicht missverstanden werden als stellvertretende Ausübung der Autonomie des Kindes (oder einer anderen unmündigen Person) durch den Berechtigten. Der Begriff „Autonomie“ schließt eine solche Möglichkeit gerade aus. Was auch immer Autonomie noch sein mag, schon begrifflich bezeichnet sie ein Vermögen, das nicht vertretungsweise für einen anderen ausgeübt werden kann. Vielmehr umfasst das Elternrecht zur Erteilung oder Verweigerung „stellvertretender Einwilligungen“ für ihre Kinder zwei Funktionen, die beide nichts mit der Autonomie der Kinder zu tun haben: *Erstens* sollen Eltern die Möglichkeit haben, Kontrolle darüber auszuüben, wie mit ihrem Kind verfahren wird – eine Kontrolle, die sie ausschließlich zum Wohl des Kindes ausüben dürfen. Und *zweitens* verwirklichen sie damit ihr genuines Elternrecht auf weitgehende Bestimmung der Formen und Wege des Aufwachsens ihres Kindes – freilich erneut nur innerhalb bestimmter Grenzen, die durch die Rechte und das Wohl des Kindes gezogen werden.

Was Eingriffe in das Gehirn zum Zweck des mentalen Enhancements anbelangt, so hat dieser Doppelaspekt der elterlichen Autorität eine zweifache (und leicht paradox anmutende) Folge. Hinsichtlich der Frage, welche Art von „Geist“ oder Charakter zu besitzen im wohlverstandenen Interesse eines Menschen liegt (seinem Wohlergehen am ehesten dienlich ist), gibt es keinen objektiv begründbaren Maßstab. Daher gewährt das Recht Eltern aus gutem Grund einen umfangreichen Ermessensspielraum bei der Beeinflussung und Lenkung der seelischen Entwicklung ihrer Kinder entsprechend ihrem eigenen (elterlichen) Gutdünken. Zum Zweck der Formung von Charaktereigenschaften und der Ausbildung intellektueller Fähigkeiten ihrer Kinder haben Eltern somit eine weitreichende rechtliche Befugnis der Vermittlung, ja des Oktrois ihres eigenen Wertesystems an ihre Kinder. Sie dürfen die geistige Entwicklung eines Kindes dabei sogar in eine Richtung lenken, die vernünftige Menschen als schädlich für das Kind erachten würden. Dieser rechtliche Ermessensspielraum deckt ohne weiteres auch die Befugnis, Entscheidungen zugunsten der Förderung ganz bestimmter psychischer Merkmale zu treffen, selbst wenn dies die Entwicklung anderer Eigenschaften behindert, die allgemein als wichtig für das zukünftige Wohlergehen eines Kindes erachtet werden. Soweit es dagegen um das körperliche Wohl ihres Kindes geht, haben Eltern keinerlei Befugnis, aktuell oder potentiell schädliche Entscheidungen zu treffen. Denn in diesem Bereich gibt es relativ eindeutige, objektive Standards des Wohlergehens; sie dürfen durch elterliche Entscheidungen nicht verletzt werden. Auf der Grundlage geltender Rechtsprinzipien können physisch-invasive medizinische Maßnahmen an Kindern durch elterliche Einwilligung nur in dem Maße autorisiert werden, in dem sie zur Behandlung von Krankheiten erforderlich sind. Eltern können beispielsweise nicht wirksam in Eingriffe der kosmetischen Chirurgie an ihren Kindern einwilligen, um damit ihre eigenen ästhetischen Präferenzen zu verwirklichen. (Etwas anderes gilt selbstverständlich, wenn solche chirurgischen Maßnahmen therapeutischen Charakter haben, z.B. erhebliche körperliche Missbildungen zu beseitigen bestimmt sind.)

➔ Auch wenn Eltern also ein gesetzlich verbrieftes Recht zur Einflussnahme auf die psychischen Merkmale ihrer Kinder nach Maßgabe ihrer eigenen Wertvorstellungen (und im Modus traditioneller Erziehungsmaßnahmen) haben, endet dieses Recht stets dort, wo die körperliche Unversehrtheit des Kindes beginnt. Nach allgemeinen Rechtsprinzipien ist damit *a fortiori* ausgeschlossen, dass Eltern eine wirksame Einwilligung zu Eingriffen in das Gehirn eines Kindes zum bloßen Zwecke des Enhancements geben könnten.

Zwischen dem weiten Spielraum, mittels traditioneller Erziehungsmethoden die psychische Entwicklung sogar in schädliche Richtungen zu lenken, und dem Fehlen jeglichen Spielraums zum Herbeiführen etwaiger nützlicher Enhancements durch neuartige auf das Gehirn einwirkende Interventionsmethoden, besteht ein offensichtliches Ungleichgewicht. Und ebenso offensichtlich erzeugt dies eine gewisse normative Spannung. Auch diesem Problem haben Rechtswissenschaftler und Rechtsphilosophen sich bisher noch nicht ausreichend zugewandt.

Wir drängen darauf, eine solche Debatte in Wissenschaft und Gesellschaft zu beginnen. Erforderlich erscheint dies vor allem vor dem Hintergrund der Tatsache einer sich schnell ausbreitenden Praxis, Kindern durch die Gabe von Wirkstoffen wie z.B. Methylphenidat (das, wie mittlerweile bekannt ist, tiefgreifenden Einfluss auf Physiologie und Struktur des Gehirns ausübt) zu kognitivem Enhancement zu verhelfen. Gemessen an der oben skizzierten Rechtslage, dürfte diese gegenwärtige Praxis weitgehend illegitim sein. Wir glauben, dass sie derzeit aus zwei Gründen stillschweigend toleriert wird: (1) Weil man kollektiv die Augen vor den physischen, sprich neuronalen Effekten solcher Medikamente verschließt, und (2) wegen einer sich weitgehend unbemerkt ausbreitenden Medikalisierung von Varianten kindlichen Verhaltens, die ehedem zwar ebenfalls als unerwünscht, aber doch als (noch) normal beurteilt wurden. Dieser Prozess einer halbwegs klandestinen Ausweitung des Krankheitsbegriffs, und damit zusammenhängend des Begriffs der Therapie, auf früher als normal erachtete psychische Merkmale von Kindern ist in verschiedener Hinsicht problematisch: Begünstigt wird diese Tendenz durch die konzeptuelle Vagheit des Begriffs „psychische Krankheit"; sie übertrifft definitorische Unbestimmtheiten in der rein somatischen Sphäre bei weitem. Handelt es sich bei einem etwas zappeligen Kind um einen „minderschweren Fall" von ADHS, oder bleibt dieses Kind einfach in geringfügigem, wenngleich unerwünschtem Maße hinter elterlichen Erwartungen zurück, ohne jedoch damit das Spektrum des Normalen zu verlassen? Zu einem guten Teil spielt sich die besagte stillschweigende Medikalisierung außerhalb der normativen Kontrolle durch rechtliche Institutionen ab. Dadurch entstehen soziale Risiken, deren die Gesellschaft gewahr werden sollte. Dies soll keinesfalls bedeuten, dass alle am Gehirn ansetzenden Maßnahmen des Enhancements von Kindern gesetzlich verboten werden sollten. Es geht vielmehr (1) um Klarheit, (2) um Aufrichtigkeit, und (3) um ein vernünftiges Maß an sozialer Kontrolle über einen Prozess, der sich gegenwärtig allein auf der Basis unterschiedlicher faktischer Interessen entwickelt und sich dabei jeder Verpflichtung zur normativen Rechtfertigung entzieht. Gewiss wird es Möglichkeiten des Enhancements durch Interventionen am Gehirn geben, die trotz entsprechender Nachfrage seitens der Eltern für deren Kinder nicht akzeptabel sind. Doch ebenso sicher werden sich andere Methoden etablieren, deren Anwendung sich auf der Basis legitimer elterlicher Sorge um ihren Nachwuchs rechtfertigen lässt. Die gesamte Thematik bedarf der weiteren Klärung durch gesellschaftliche, wissenschaftliche und rechtlich-ethische Diskussion.

➔ In Anbetracht der vielen möglichen und noch unerforschten Langzeitfolgen von Maßnahmen der Einflussnahme auf das Gehirn halten wir gegenwärtig ein eher strenges Vorsichts-Prinzip für angebracht. Im Einklang mit der aktuellen Gesetzeslage sollten bei Kindern chirurgische Eingriffe am Gehirn und elektromagnetische Stimulationsverfahren des Gehirns zu reinen Enhancement-Zwecken verboten bleiben, bis ein gesellschaftlicher Konsens zu den komplexen einschlägigen normativen Fragen erreicht ist.

➔ Angesichts der Tendenz einer sich ausbreitenden Medikalisierung sollten pharmazeutische Interventionen mit möglichen Langzeitwirkungen auf das Gehirn strikteren Kontrollen unterworfen werden, und zwar nicht nur in finanzieller Hinsicht, d.h. durch Ablehnung einer Kostenübernahme seitens der Sozialversicherung, sondern auch mittels der Durchsetzung existierender Rechtsnormen zum Schutz von Kindern.

Die Authentizität betreffende Bedenken

Nach der rechtlichen Klärung wenden wir uns den ethischen Problemen und damit der zweiten abstrakten Bedeutung von Autonomie zu: der Authentizität. Hinsichtlich des Enhancements eigener psychischer Merkmale sollten zwei Fragen unterschieden werden. Die erste betrifft die *Motive* für solche

Interventionen, die zweite deren mögliches *Ergebnis*. Bei der ersten Frage geht es, grob gesagt, um das Vorliegen hinreichend authentischer Beweggründe, während die zweite problematisiert, ob eine „mental enhancte" Person noch ein hinreichend authentisches Selbst aufweist, um als wahrhaft autonom gelten zu können. Beide Fragen setzen gewisse moralische Pflichten autonomer Personen gegenüber sich selbst voraus, anhand derer jeweils das Hinreichen der Authentizität zu bemessen ist.

Wir behandeln hier nicht das generelle philosophische Problem moralischer „Pflichten gegenüber sich selbst", wie sie von Kant behauptet und seither kontrovers diskutiert worden sind. Zwar erkennen wir die Möglichkeit der Begründung solcher Pflichten auf der Basis einer säkularen Ethik grundsätzlich an. Jedoch können wir dieses Problem hier ohne Bedenken ignorieren. Denn eine moralische Pflicht dazu, das Enhancement (die Verbesserung) der eigenen mentalen Fähigkeiten zu unterlassen, gibt es ganz offensichtlich nicht. Im Gefolge Kants würden viele eher das Gegenteil behaupten, nämlich die Geltung einer moralischen Pflicht zur Entwicklung der eigenen natürlichen geistigen Anlagen. Ob man nun bloß die Erlaubnis besitzt oder sogar dazu verpflichtet ist, sich selbst zu verbessern, beide Möglichkeiten setzen die individuelle Freiheit voraus, bestimmte psychische Merkmale zur Verbesserung auszuwählen, da sich nicht alle im gleichen Maße verbessern lassen. Im Prinzip erstreckt sich diese Wahlfreiheit auch auf die Mittel und Wege der Selbstverbesserung. Das bedeutet, dass sich die grundsätzliche moralische Berechtigung zur Gestaltung des eigenen Geists nicht alleine aufgrund der Künstlichkeit oder „Unnatürlichkeit" neuer Methoden zur Intervention am Gehirn in Zweifel ziehen, geschweige denn ganz aufgeben oder gar durch eine moralische Verpflichtung zum genauen Gegenteil ersetzen lässt. Zwar könnte, wie wir bereits gesehen haben, die Anwendung von Interventionsmethoden für mentales Enhancement im Hinblick auf Risiken und Nebenwirkungen sowie mögliche unlautere Nutzungsabsichten Grund zur Sorge geben. Und in Zwei-Parteien-Fällen mögen diese Bedenken nicht nur ein moralisches, sondern auch ein rechtliches Verbot rechtfertigen. Solche Verbote dienen der Vermeidung von Schädigungen Dritter, die auf dem kollusiven Zusammenspiel zweier einverstandener Vertragspartner beruhen und auf eine Sittenwidrigkeit im oben beschriebenen Sinne hinauslaufen. Vorgänge dieser Art verletzen soziale Interessen. Ihr Verbot hat damit aber ersichtlich nicht die Bewahrung eines „natürlichen" (Enhancement-freien) psychischen *Status quo* zum Ziel.

Ein zweites Bedenken zum Thema Authentizität entstammt der Furcht, eine massenhafte Anwendung von auf das Gehirn einwirkenden mentalen Enhancements könnte alle Menschen einem subtilen oder sogar massiven Druck aussetzen, sich diesen neuen Anforderungen des sozialen Wettbewerbs zu unterwerfen. Kollektiver Druck dieser Art gäbe sicher Grund zu einer ganzen Reihe von Besorgnissen. Entsprechende Entwicklungstendenzen sollten beobachtet und im Falle ihres hinreichenden Nachweises mit

Hilfe politischer und rechtlicher Instrumente korrigiert werden. Ein derartiger sozialer Druck könnte allerdings, so unerwünscht er auch wäre, nicht die Authentizität bzw. die rechtliche Autonomie individueller Entscheidungen beeinträchtigen, mit denen ihm nachgegeben würde. Auch von anderen gesellschaftlichen Entwicklungen wie beispielsweise neuen Modetrends oder technischen Neuerungen (z.B. Telefon oder Computer) lässt sich ja nicht gut behaupten, sie minderten die Autonomie ihrer Anhänger bzw. Nutzer, wiewohl sie unbestritten großen Einfluss auf diesbezügliche individuelle Entscheidungen ausüben. Gewiss gibt es einen bedeutenden moralischen Unterschied zwischen dem sozialen Druck, der jemanden etwa zur Benutzung eines Computers veranlasst, um in seinen beruflichen Leistungen konkurrenzfähig zu bleiben, und dem Druck, der jemanden aus demselben Grund bewegen könnte, ein Enhancement der eigenen mentalen Fähigkeiten durch einen Eingriff in sein Gehirn anzustreben. Doch dieser Unterschied betrifft nicht die Autonomie oder Authentizität der Entscheidungen, die unter solchem Druck getroffen werden. Vielmehr betrifft er die Unantastbarkeit der körperlichen Sphäre, die gegen Eingriffe und externe Zwänge, die zu solchen Eingriffen drängen mögen, wesentlich intensiver geschützt ist als die Nötigungsfreiheit des eigenen Verhaltens gegen die Zwänge der sozialen Entwicklung. (Wir werden auf diesen Punkt *sub specie* „Gerechtigkeit" noch einmal zurückkommen.)

Schließlich sehen wir keinen überzeugenden Grund, daran zu zweifeln, dass eine Person mit künstlich optimierten Fähigkeiten insofern weiterhin ein authentisches Selbst hat, als ihre Entscheidungen immer noch im Einklang mit ihrer Natur stehen können. Man mag freilich skeptisch sein, was den subjektiven Wert eines solchen Enhancements für die betroffene Person selbst anbelangt. Wie in Kapitel 6 gezeigt, gilt zumindest für manche menschlichen Fertigkeiten, dass bei der Beurteilung von Ergebnissen die zu ihrer Realisierung eingesetzten Mittel durchaus eine Rolle spielen. In solchen Fällen hängt unsere Bewunderung für die Leistungen anderer Menschen anscheinend in erheblichem Maße von dem persönlichen Aufwand ab, der mit dem Erwerb der entsprechenden Fertigkeit verbunden war. Die Entwertung von athletischen Leistungen, die nachweislich durch Doping ermöglicht wurden, spricht diesbezüglich Bände. Das darf als Warnung gegen allzu flinke und einfache Abkürzungen auf dem Weg zu erstrebten Zielen verstanden werden und rechtfertigt gewiss die Mahnung, jeden Rückgriff auf künstliches mentales Enhancement genau zu erwägen und im Zweifelsfall davon Abstand zu nehmen. Die mögliche Entwertung der erzielten Ergebnisse durch die eingesetzten Mittel *kann* auf einem Mangel an Authentizität der Person beruhen, die von diesen Mitteln Gebrauch macht. Doch muss dies nicht so sein – so wenig wie irgendwelche anderen nutz- oder sinnlosen (oder gar verschlimmernden) Modifikationen der Persönlichkeit die Authentizität der betroffenen Person allein schon aufgrund ihrer bloßen Nutz- oder Sinnlosigkeit kompromittieren müssen. Ein in diesem Punkt abweichendes Urteil, das ein künstliches mentales Enhancement als Verletzung einer Pflicht gegen sich selbst beurteilte, wäre lediglich der Ausdruck einer abweichenden ethischen Auffassung. Daraus ergäbe sich jedoch – wie wir hervorheben möchten – keine hinreichende normative Grundlage für ein rechtliches Verbot. Moderne Verfassungsstaaten sind nicht berechtigt, ausschließlich *moralische* Pflichten, selbst wenn sie als solche begründet sind, in geltendes Recht umzusetzen.

3.4 Gerechtigkeit: Ungleichheit; gerechte Verteilung; politische Gerechtigkeit

„Gerechtigkeit" ist ein mindestens ebenso komplexer Begriff wie „Autonomie". Wir unterscheiden, in gängiger Weise, vier Facetten seiner Bedeutung: distributive, kommutative (ausgleichende), korrigierende und politische Gerechtigkeit. Nur die erste und die letzte Bedeutung sind von Belang für die Fragen unserer Untersuchung.

Allgemein gesprochen zielen Theorien distributiver Gerechtigkeit darauf ab, faire Verteilungsprinzipien für bestimmte Güter und Lasten zu etablieren, die sich aus den Interaktionen von Mitgliedern auf Kooperation beruhender Gesellschaften ergeben. Moral-, Rechts- und politische Philosophie haben eine Vielzahl solcher Prinzipien entwickelt und vorgeschlagen. Sie variieren in verschiedenen Hinsichten, etwa in den Fragen, welche Güter es überhaupt gerecht zu verteilen gilt (z.B. Einkommen, Möglichkeiten, Wohlbefinden) oder anhand welcher Kriterien bzw. Mechanismen die Allokation solcher Güter vorgenommen werden sollte (z.B. Gleichheit, Verdienst, Bedürftigkeit, Regeln des freien Marktes). Ungeachtet der Vielfalt von Meinungen zu all diesen Fragen herrscht Konsens darüber, dass nicht alle Gegenstände, nur weil sie einen Wert besitzen, bereits zu Gegenständen werden, deren Verteilung anhand von Gerechtigkeitsprinzipien zu regeln wäre. Ausschließlich „gesellschaftliche Grundgüter", um John Rawls' bekannten Terminus zu verwenden, sind angemessener Gegenstand distributiver Gerechtigkeit, d.h. Güter, die (1) kein Bestandteil der natürlichen Ausstattung sind, und die (2) für jedes vernünftige Mitglied einer Gesellschaft von Wert sind, welche individuellen Präferenzen und persönlichen Lebenspläne es auch ansonsten hegen mag. Medizinische Dienstleistungen zählen sicherlich zu diesen Grundgütern. Sie unterliegen der sozialen Verteilung und dienen dem Erhalt oder der Wiederherstellung der Gesundheit, welche im Sinne einer „All-Zweck-Voraussetzung" eine Ermöglichungsbedingung für beliebige Lebenspläne vernünftiger Personen darstellt. Weniger einvernehmlich bestimmbar ist hingegen, auf welches Spektrum menschlichen Befindens (von lebensbedrohlichen Zuständen bis hin zu idiosynkratischen persönlichen Präferenzen) sich die Allokation medizinischer Dienste beziehen sollte.

„Politische Gerechtigkeit" wollen wir für die Zwecke dieser Studie so verstehen, dass sie alle anderen der Medizin zukommenden Aufgaben umfasst, die tatsächlich oder potentiell die Rechte und Interessen jedes Individuums, aber auch der Gesellschaft als Ganzes berühren. Zu diesen Aufgaben gehören daher die Prüfung, die Kontrolle und erforderlichenfalls die Korrektur sozialer Entwicklungen im Bereich der Medizin.

3.4.1 Probleme der Verteilungsgerechtigkeit

Hinsichtlich der gerechten Allokation von Ressourcen ergeben sich für keine der drei genuinen Sphären der Medizin (Behandlung, Prävention und Forschung) normative Probleme, die spezifisch den Gegenstand dieser Untersuchung beträfen. Die außerordentliche Komplexität einiger der neuen Methoden zur Intervention am Gehirn könnte zu der Frage herausfordern, ob bei ihnen Kosten und Nutzen in einem vernünftigen Verhältnis zueinander stehen. Angesichts mancher Interventionsmöglichkeiten könnte zweifelhaft erscheinen, ob es klug ist, sie als medizinische Behandlungen anzuerkennen. Je weniger schwerwiegend beispielsweise die Einbuße an Funktionalität ist, die durch eine Neuroprothese wiederhergestellt werden kann, desto eher wird deren Einsatz von Krankenversicherungen und anderen Geldgebern mit Leistungen der kosmetischen Chirurgie und anderen Grenzfällen zwischen Therapie und Enhancement verglichen werden. Aber dies sind bekannte Probleme, die sich regelmäßig bei innovativen, technologisch aufwendigen und dementsprechend ungewöhnlich teuren medizinischen Mitteln stellen. Sie betreffen nicht primär Prinzipien der Gerechtigkeit, sondern vielmehr definitorische Fragen sowie Belange politischer und ökonomischer Klugheit.

Maßnahmen des Enhancements dagegen werfen tatsächlich schwierige Gerechtigkeitsfragen auf. Wir werden uns mit zwei denkbaren einschlägigen Folgen von Enhancement beschäftigen, von denen die eine die Möglichkeit einer Verschärfung von Ungleichheit, die andere die Verschwendung von Ressourcen betrifft.

Könnte Enhancement bestehende soziale Ungleichheiten verschärfen?

Die Möglichkeit einer Verschärfung von Ungleichheit in Folge einer verstärkten Nutzung von Enhancementverfahren steht im Zusammenhang mit dem von uns geforderten strikten Ausschluss solcher Maßnahmen aus öffentlich finanzierten sozialen Gesundheitssystemen. Werden nämlich die Kosten für Enhancements auch nicht *anderweitig* über öffentliche Mittel finanziert bzw. subventioniert, dann folgt, dass nur diejenigen Menschen von dem Nutzwert verbesserter psychischer Merkmale zu profitieren in der Lage sind, die sich die erforderlichen Maßnahmen aus eigenen Mitteln leisten können. Weil die meisten der betreffenden Dienstleistungen sehr kostspielig sein und bleiben dürften, werden nur Wohlhabende und deren Angehörige in den Genuss der mit ihnen verbundenen Vorteile kommen. Dies wiederum mag bestehende soziale Ungleichheiten verschärfen, da sich auf diese Weise ein ohnehin schon privilegierter Personenkreis in vielen Bereichen zusätzliche Wettbewerbsvorteile sichern könnte.

Sollte sich diese Aussicht bewahrheiten, so gäbe es sicher guten Grund zu ernsthafter Sorge um die Verteilungsgerechtigkeit. Bestimmte kognitive Fähigkeiten wie Aufmerksamkeit oder Intelligenz sind „positionierende" oder „relationale Güter" *(positional goods)* in dem Sinne, dass sie ihren Besitzern im gesellschaftlichen Wettbewerb um begehrte Stellungen und Güter gegenüber anderen Personen erhebliche Vorteile verschaffen. In dem Maße, in dem solche Fähigkeiten nach und nach ihren bisherigen Status einer unverfügbaren natürlichen „Mitgift" verlieren und zum Gegenstand gezielter Manipulation durch menschliche Intervention werden, werden auch die Mittel zu solchen Interventionen allmählich zum Gegenstand der distributiven Gerechtigkeit. Das könnte eine Wirkungsspirale in Gang setzen, nämlich diese: Wenn (1) Mittel mentalen Enhancements nur Vermögenden verfügbar sind, (2) der Gebrauch dieser Mittel wesentliche Wettbewerbsvorteile beim Vermögenserwerb verschafft, und wenn (3) eine stark ungleiche Wohlstandsverteilung mit Blick auf distributive Gerechtigkeit zur Besorgnis Anlass gibt, dann führt künstliches mentales Enhancement ganz offensichtlich zu einer Verschärfung problematischer Muster der sozialen Verteilung.

Bekanntlich ist die dritte genannte Prämisse seit jeher Gegenstand philosophischer Kontroversen. Wir können uns an dieser Stelle nicht eingehend mit dieser Debatte befassen. Der Hinweis möge genügen, dass auch in dezidiert liberalen Staaten die gesetzgebenden Instanzen zweifellos dazu berechtigt sind, soziale Entwicklungen nach Möglichkeit zu korrigieren, die zu einem dramatischen Anwachsen der Ungleichverteilung von Vermögenswerten unter ihren Bürgern führen. Das gilt insbesondere dann, wenn es nicht etwa besondere Verdienste auf Seiten der Privilegierten sind, die solche Entwicklungstendenzen antreiben. Das Prädikat „unverdient" träfe aber in hohem Maß gerade auf die relationalen Vorteile zu, die aus künstlich herbeigeführtem mentalen Enhancement resultieren würden, sollten sich die eben skizzierten sozialen Tendenzen nachhaltig durchsetzen. Dies scheint uns Grund genug für ein moralisches Warnsignal. Wir möchten daher betonen, dass mögliche Entwicklungen wie die beschriebenen von zuständigen politischen, wissenschaftlichen und gesellschaftlichen Institutionen aufmerksam verfolgt werden sollten:

➔ Sollten sich klare Anzeichen dafür ergeben, dass die wachsende Verfügbarkeit käuflicher Mittel zum mentalen Enhancement einer Entwicklung hin zu krasser Ungleichverteilung von Wohlstand und damit von sozialen Chancen Vorschub leistet, so müssen Gegenmaßnahmen ergriffen werden.

Die zu diesem Zweck ergriffenen Maßnahmen müssen selbstverständlich gängigen Kriterien der Verhältnismäßigkeit entsprechen. Dabei darf der Staat aus einem breiten Spektrum an Möglichkeiten auswählen, die von fiskalischen Maßnahmen über Restriktionen bei der Erteilung von Zulassungen für medizinische Enhancement-Verfahren bis hin zur *ultima ratio* des rechtlichen Verbots bzw. der Strafandrohung reichen. Wir möchten hervorheben, dass es kaum genügen würde, einem negativen sozialen Trend der besagten Art durch eine teilweise Umverteilung ungerecht-ungleichmäßig angehäufter Vermögenswerte im Wege des Steuerrechts entgegenzuwirken. Denn eine erhebliche Ungleichverteilung sozialer Chancen, handele es sich bei diesen nun um berufliche Stellungen oder um andere für die individuelle Lebensqualität bedeutsame Güter, bedeutet auch eine Ungleichverteilung fundamentaler Voraussetzungen für Selbstachtung. Sofern es sich hierbei, folgt man John Rawls, um das wichtigste gesellschaftliche Grundgut überhaupt handelt, lassen sich auf dessen Erwerb bezogene Ungleichheiten nicht allein auf finanziellem Wege kompensieren.

Nachdem wir all dies dargelegt haben, möchten wir gleichwohl ein doppeltes Caveat gegen ein voreiliges politisches Eingreifen zum gegenwärtigen Zeitpunkt formulieren:

(1) Ob die skizzierten negativen Entwicklungen Wirklichkeit werden ist eine empirische Frage. Sie lässt sich nicht durch bloße theoretische Spekulationen beantworten. So plausibel diese auch erscheinen mögen, müssen sie doch durch feststellbare Tatsachen belegt werden. Bis jetzt gibt es keine derartigen Belege. Selbst technologisch hoch entwickelte Gesellschaften mit einem starken Interesse an Wissenschaft und technischen Innovationen sind bisher noch recht weit entfernt von den beschriebenen nachteiligen Folgen für die Verteilungsgerechtigkeit. Selbstverständlich ist es legitim, wenn Politik mögliche unerwünschte Entwicklungen vorbeugend zu vermeiden trachtet. Das erfordert jedoch ein komplexes Abwägen zwischen protektiven und freiheitlichen Interessen. Dieser Abwägungsprozess wiederum muss auf ausreichenden Informationen über drohende Risiken basieren. Ohne das entsprechende Wissen sind sinnvolle und verhältnismäßige Gegenmaßnahmen schwer vorstellbar. Wir meinen, dass die gegenwärtig Gesetzgebern und anderen politischen Entscheidungsträgern verfügbaren Informationen noch keine vernünftige Beurteilung dieser Fragen gestatten. Da politische Hindernisse, ganz zu schweigen von gesetzlichen Verboten, stets auf Kosten der individuellen und sozialen Freiheit gehen, schlagen wir vor, dass Regierungen und Gesetzgeber ihre Politik einstweilen auf die oben empfohlenen Maßnahmen einer aufmerksamen Überwachung beschränken.

(2) Unsere Mahnung zu politischer Zurückhaltung wird durch eine weitere Überlegung gestützt. Wie bereits gesagt stellen bestimmte geistige Vermögen relationale Güter dar, die zu Wettbewerbsvorteilen in einer Vielzahl von Kontexten des sozialen Lebens verhelfen. Doch das ist noch nicht alles. Man könnte sagen, dass diese Fähigkeiten auch einen „unabhängigen" Wert haben, dass sie nämlich für sich genommen von Wert sind für das individuelle Leben und Wohlbefinden des über sie verfügenden Menschen. Wer mit besonders gut ausgebildeten kognitiven Fähigkeiten gesegnet ist, mag erfolg-

reich in Konkurrenzsituationen bestehen können. Darüber hinaus bilden diese Fähigkeiten auch die Grundlage für die Ausprägung und Befriedigung intellektueller Vorlieben, die allein dem Zweck des persönlichen Vergnügens dienen, oder begünstigen die Erfüllung individueller Neigungen zu Kunst, Literatur oder Wissenschaft, frei von ökonomischem Gewinnstreben. Die Freiheit zur Ausbildung eigener Fähigkeiten zur Ermöglichung eines erfüllteren geistigen Lebens sollte weder ignoriert noch geringgeschätzt werden. Diese Betrachtungen bekräftigen den oben unterbreiteten Vorschlag, gegenwärtig von prohibitiven Interventionen in die Entwicklung und Anwendung von am Gehirn ansetzenden Techniken mentalen Enhancements abzusehen.

Bedeutet Enhancement eine Verschwendung medizinischer Ressourcen?

Bei der befürchteten Folge der Ressourcenverschwendung durch die Verwendung medizinischer Mittel zu Zwecken bloßen Enhancements geht es um das Problem einer möglichen Vergeudung knapper medizinischer Ressourcen in Bereichen jenseits von Therapie oder Prävention. Ob sich dieser Vorwurf rechtfertigen lässt, hängt nicht von der Frage ab, wer für den Ge- bzw. Missbrauch dieser Mittel bezahlt; deshalb ist auch nicht von Belang, dass unserem oben entwickelten Argument zufolge stets der private Abnehmer des Enhancements dessen unmittelbare Kosten tragen sollte, nie dagegen das öffentlich finanzierte Gesundheitswesen. Die Kritik weist vielmehr auf eine absolute *Limitation* medizinischer Ressourcen hin. Es geht um die Tatsache, dass medizinische Mittel, einschließlich der Arbeitskraft von Spezialisten, die für einen bestimmten Zweck eingesetzt werden, notwendigerweise unverfügbar für andere mögliche Anwendungen sind. Werden sie für Zwecke des Enhancements genutzt, fehlen die eingesetzten Mittel im wesentlich wichtigeren therapeutischen Bereich, stehen also für potentiell lebensrettende oder heilende Verwendungen nicht zur Verfügung. Selbst wenn keine direkte Verbindung zwischen der Verwendung von Mitteln in einem und ihrem Fehlen in einem anderen konkreten Aufgabenbereich bestehen mag, lässt sich die unterstellte Abhängigkeit im Blick auf das Ganze des Gesundheitssystems doch kaum leugnen.

Der erhobene Vorwurf erwiese sich als berechtigt, wenn eine von zwei empirischen Voraussetzungen erfüllt ist: Erstens könnte er sich auf die Annahme stützen, dass die Gesamtheit der medizinischen Ressourcen in einer gegebenen Gesellschaft immer (oder jedenfalls normalerweise) von ihren Mitglieder vollständig nachgefragt oder in Anspruch genommen wird, so dass diese Ressourcen jederzeit in nahezu vollem Umfang genutzt werden. Ungeachtet der Knappheit medizinischer Ressourcen scheint dies allerdings keine sehr plausible Annahme zu sein. Zweitens würde der Vorwurf der Ressourcenverschwendung ebenfalls beglaubigt, wenn die massenhafte Bindung medizinischer Ressourcen durch Zwecke mentalen Enhancements tatsächlich einen zumindest spürbaren Mangel ihrer Verfügbarkeit für Behandlungsmaßnahmen nach sich zöge. Auch in diesem Fall würde die Verwendung medizinischer Mittel für reines Enhancement als gewissermaßen parasitär gegenüber ihrer primären Zweckbestimmung zu beurteilen sein, und dieser Missstand ließe sich als Verletzung von Prinzipien distributiver Gerechtigkeit kritisieren. Schließlich stellt nicht nur die Anwendung, sondern bereits die Herstellung medizinischer Mittel eine gewaltige und permanente Belastung gesellschaftlicher finanzieller Ressourcen dar.

Wir halten diesen Vorwurf bis zu einem gewissen Grad für plausibel, vorausgesetzt, dass die empirische Annahme, auf welcher er basiert, korrekt ist. Gegenwärtig ist unklar, ob dies der Fall ist oder nicht. (Mit ebenso gutem Recht könnte man den Vorwurf der Ressourcenverschwendung gegen die gegenwärtig weithin akzeptierte Praxis der kosmetischen Chirurgie erheben.) Die besagte Kritik liefert hinreichenden Grund für einen moralischen Warnhinweis, verbunden mit der Aufforderung, die soziale Entwicklung in den einschlägigen Aspekten zu beobachten. Andererseits ergibt sich jedoch auch an dieser Stelle keine hinreichende Grundlage für ein sofortiges gesetzliches Verbot möglicher Anwendungen von Interventionen am Gehirn zum Zweck mentalen Enhancements.

3.4.2 Allgemeine Probleme der politischen Gerechtigkeit

Bei der Diskussion der Authentizitätsthematik haben wir bereits auf das Risiko hingewiesen, dass sich in Folge einer verbreiteten Nutzung invasiver Methoden mentalen Enhancements diejenigen Personen wachsendem Druck ausgesetzt sehen könnten, die sich einerseits solchen Eingriffen nicht unterziehen möchten, aber andererseits die erheblichen Wettbewerbsnachteile nicht hinnehmen wollen, die aus ihrer Ablehnung resultieren könnten. Wie bereits ausgeführt, würde diese Art von sozialem Druck nicht die rechtliche Autonomie der betreffenden Personen beschneiden. Folglich bliebe auch die Gültigkeit ihrer Einwilligung zu einem invasiven Eingriff in ihr Gehirn unangetastet, sollten sie jenem Druck nachgeben. Der Staat, hier in Gestalt des Gesetzgebers, hat jedoch sicherlich das Recht und innerhalb der Grenzen seiner Entscheidungsgewalt auch *prima facie* die Pflicht zur Intervention, um seine Bürger vor der Nötigung durch solche sozialen Anforderungen abzuschirmen. Auch wiegt der soziale Druck, sich einem invasiven körperlichen Eingriff zu unterziehen, sicher erheblich schwerer als beispielsweise der auf die Mitglieder weitgehend motorisierter Gesellschaften wirkende „Zwang“ zum Erwerb eines Führerscheins und zur Nutzung eines Kraftfahrzeugs im Interesse des Erhalts der eigenen Wettbewerbsfähigkeit. Angesichts der vorrangigen Verpflichtung des Staates, Leib und Leben seiner Bürger zu schützen, gibt selbst jede nur indirekte und mittelbare Gefährdung der körperlichen Integrität Anlass zur sorgfältigen Prüfung der Frage, ob es geboten sein könnte, eine diese Gefährdung hervorbringende Entwicklung mit Hilfe rechtlicher Verbote aufzuhalten.

Erneut hängt die Plausibilität von Forderungen nach mehr oder weniger unmittelbaren Verboten an einer empirischen Frage – diesmal an der, ob der befürchtete soziale Druck hin zu mentalem Enhancement tatsächlich im Entstehen begriffen ist. Und wiederum lässt sich von heutiger Warte aus die Antwort nicht mit annähernd wünschenswerter Sicherheit vorhersehen. Dies gibt uns die Veranlassung zu einem dritten, letzten und besonders wichtigen Warnhinweis mit Blick auf die Sorge um soziale Gerechtigkeit:

➔ Die zuständigen politischen Instanzen und wissenschaftlichen Einrichtungen sollten ein besonderes Augenmerk darauf richten, ob die individuelle Freiheit, auf hirn-invasives Enhancement zu verzichten, in Gefahr geraten könnte. Sollten deutliche Anzeichen für eine solche Entwicklung erkennbar werden, scheint eine staatliche Intervention zum Schutz derjenigen Bürger geboten, die ein Enhancement ablehnen.

Solange jedoch keine Belege für diese Art von Entwicklung vorhanden sind, sollten Verbote unterbleiben. Liberale Verfassungsstaaten sind nicht berechtigt, legislative Maßnahmen gegen Bedrohungen des Gemeinwesens zu treffen, deren Auftreten noch ungewiss ist. Dies gilt insbesondere dann, wenn man den von einer Bedrohung ausgehenden unerwünschten Folgen im Fall ihres künftigen Auftretens noch immer rechtzeitig entgegentreten könnte.

Wesentliche Ergebnisse und Empfehlungen

- Die Autoren dieser Studie haben neuartige Methoden zur Intervention am Gehirn aus den Bereichen Psychopharmarkologie, Neurotransplantation, Neuroprothetik und elektrische Hirnstimulation eingehend untersucht. Sie erkennen deren Potential zu therapeutischer Hilfe für den Einzelnen und zum Nutzen für die Gesellschaft an. Da solche Eingriffe unmittelbar auf das Gehirn einwirken, muss ihre Anwendung mit besonderer Sorgfalt erfolgen, auch wenn sie ausschließlich therapeutischen Zwecken zu dienen bestimmt sind.
- Eine Verengung der öffentlichen Debatte auf radikale und offenkundige psychische Veränderungen, von denen Patienten betroffen sein könnten, mag dazu führen, dass anderen Nebenwirkungen, die eigentlich größeren Anlass zur Sorge geben, nicht die gebührende Aufmerksamkeit gewidmet wird. Die Rede ist von subtilen Veränderungen der Psyche im Allgemeinen und der Persönlichkeit im Speziellen, die leicht unbemerkt bleiben können.
- Während der Forschungsphase sollte jede neue Methode zur Intervention am Gehirn systematisch auf Nebenwirkungen geprüft werden, welche die Persönlichkeit oder psychische Funktionen, die für Personalität konstitutiv sind, betreffen.
- Wenn ein bestimmter Interventionstyp, der für bestimmte therapeutische oder präventive Anwendungen zugelassen ist, bekanntermaßen subtile Nebenwirkungen auf die Persönlichkeit oder auf solche psychischen Fähigkeiten haben kann, die für Personalität konstitutiv sind, dann sollte jede Person, an deren Gehirn ein Eingriff dieses Typs vorgenommen wird, im Anschluss sorgfältig auf das Auftreten solcher Nebenwirkungen hin untersucht werden, damit sie gegebenenfalls eine entsprechende Behandlung erfahren kann.
- Ob die Aussicht darauf, dass ein Eingriff in das Gehirn eine bestimmte Form von Persönlichkeitsveränderung zur möglichen Nebenwirkung hat, akzeptabel oder gar wünschenswert ist, kann ausschließlich von den betroffenen Personen selbst *vor* der Durchführung des Eingriffs entschieden werden.
- Für die Durchführung experimenteller Forschungsvorhaben an Patienten mit neurologischen und psychiatrischen Störungen sollten standardisierte krankheitsspezifische Untersuchungspläne *(core assessment protocols)* mit schematisierten Zeitvorgaben etabliert werden, um (1) die Erhebung aussagekräftiger Resultate zu gewährleisten und (2) Vergleichsmöglichkeiten zwischen verschiedenen Behandlungsansätzen zu schaffen.

- Wenn eine Intervention anstatt therapeutischen nur Zielen des Enhancements dient, dann stellt dies allein noch keinen „Verstoß gegen die guten Sitten“ dar. Zugunsten der Zulässigkeit einer Intervention zum Zweck des individuellen Enhancements fällt die individuelle Freiheit (Autonomie als Selbstbestimmung) der Person, die ein solches Enhancement wünscht, gravierend (wenn auch nicht allein entscheidend) ins Gewicht.
- Die bloße Tatsache, dass mentales Enhancement für Individuen, die sich ihm unterziehen, mit physischen oder psychischen Risiken verbunden sein kann, rechtfertigt es unseres Erachtens nicht, solche Maßnahmen prinzipiell ethisch zu verwerfen oder gar rechtlich zu verbieten. Im Vergleich zu therapeutischen Interventionen muss jedoch unterstrichen werden, dass bei Fällen reinen Enhancements drohende negative Nebenwirkungen gegenüber den beabsichtigten positiven Wirkungen schwerer wiegen. Ärzte, die zu bloßen Zwecken des Enhancements Eingriffe durchführen, unterstehen gegenüber ihren Klienten erweiterten Informationspflichten. Konsequenterweise sind sie auch verpflichtet, sich selbst in entsprechend umfangreicherem Maße zu informieren.
- Ein Enhancement gesunder Menschen gehört nicht zum genuinen Aufgabenbereich der Beschäftigten im Gesundheitswesen, deren Aufgabe vielmehr die Behandlung und vorbeugende Verhinderung von Krankheiten ist. Ausschließlich auf Enhancement abzielende Eingriffe in das Gehirn unterliegen deshalb nicht der prinzipiellen Hilfeleistungspflicht der Medizin. Dass es schwer entscheidbare Grenzfälle gibt, bleibt davon unberührt.
- „Reine“ Enhancement-Maßnahmen (also solche, die nicht wenigstens auch als Beitrag zur Prävention von Krankheit/Behinderung verstanden werden können) sollten in den wohldefinierten Bereich legitimer Medizin als eines sozialen Systems nicht einbezogen werden.
- Forschung, die ausschließlich auf die Entwicklung von Mitteln für mentales Enhancement durch Intervention am Gehirn gerichtet ist, sollte nicht mit öffentlichen Mitteln gefördert werden, die für das soziale System der Gesundheitsfürsorge bestimmt sind. Ebensowenig sollte die praktische Anwendung der Produkte dieser Forschung zur Realisierung mentalen Enhancements durch das Gesundheitssystem finanziell gefördert werden.
- Auch wenn Eltern ein gesetzlich verbrieftes Recht zur Einflussnahme auf die psychischen Merkmale ihrer Kinder nach Maßgabe ihrer eigenen Wertvorstellungen (und im Modus traditioneller Erziehungsmaßnahmen) haben, endet dieses Recht stets dort, wo die körperliche Unversehrtheit des Kindes beginnt. Nach allgemei-

nen Rechtsprinzipien ist damit *a fortiori* ausgeschlossen, dass Eltern eine wirksame Einwilligung zu Eingriffen in das Gehirn eines Kindes zum bloßen Zwecke des Enhancements geben könnten.

- In Anbetracht der vielen möglichen und noch unerforschten Langzeitfolgen von Maßnahmen der Einflussnahme auf das Gehirn halten wir gegenwärtig ein eher strenges Vorsichts-Prinzip für angebracht. Im Einklang mit der aktuellen Gesetzeslage sollten bei Kindern chirurgische Eingriffe am Gehirn und elektromagnetische Stimulationsverfahren des Gehirns zu reinen Enhancement-Zwecken verboten bleiben, bis ein gesellschaftlicher Konsens zu den komplexen einschlägigen normativen Fragen erreicht ist.
- Angesichts der Tendenz einer sich ausbreitenden Medikalisierung sollten pharmazeutische Interventionen mit möglichen Langzeitwirkungen auf das Gehirn strikteren Kontrollen unterworfen werden, und zwar nicht nur in finanzieller Hinsicht, d.h. durch Ablehnung einer Kostenübernahme seitens der Sozialversicherung, sondern auch mittels der Durchsetzung existierender Rechtsnormen zum Schutz von Kindern.
- Sollte jemals ein Verfahren der Intervention am Gehirn entwickelt werden, mit dem sich schwere Psychopathie mit einem vernünftigen Verhältnis von Nutzen und Risiken behandeln ließe, dann spräche nichts dagegen, Personen in Sicherheitsverwahrung die Behandlung mit diesem Interventionsverfahren anzubieten. Dies gilt insbesondere für den Fall, dass dies für den Betroffenen die einzige Alternative dazu darstellt, für unbestimmte Zeit in Gewahrsam zu verbleiben. Der schiere Druck, dem der Häftling in dieser Wahlsituation ausgesetzt ist, verletzt weder seine Autonomie, noch beraubt er seine Entscheidung ihrer rechtlichen Gültigkeit. Wir sind der Meinung, dass der Staat unter solchen Umständen nicht nur berechtigt, sondern sogar dazu verpflichtet wäre, ein solches Angebot zu unterbreiten.
- Sollten sich klare Anzeichen dafür ergeben, dass die wachsende Verfügbarkeit käuflicher Mittel zum mentalen Enhancement einer Entwicklung hin zu krasser Ungleichverteilung von Wohlstand und damit von sozialen Chancen Vorschub leistet, so müssen Gegenmaßnahmen ergriffen werden.
- Die zuständigen politischen Instanzen und wissenschaftlichen Einrichtungen sollten ein besonderes Augenmerk darauf richten, ob die individuelle Freiheit, auf hirn-invasives Enhancement zu verzichten, in Gefahr geraten könnte. Sollten deutliche Anzeichen für eine solche Entwicklung erkennbar werden, scheint eine staatliche Intervention zum Schutz derjenigen Bürger geboten, die ein Enhancement ablehnen.

List of Abbreviations

AACAP	American Academy of Child and Adolescent Psychiatry
AADC	L-amino acid decarboxylase
AAV	adeno-associated viral
ABI	auditory brainstem implant
AD	Alzheimer's disease
ADHD	attention deficit hyperactivity disorder
AIDS	acquired immuno-deficiency syndrome
ALS	amyotrophic lateral sclerosis
APA	American Psychiatric Association
BCI	brain-computer interface
BDNF	brain-derived neurotrophic factor
BIID	body integrity identity disorder
BMI	brain-machine interface
BNST	bed nucleus of the stria terminalis
CAP	core assessment protocol
CAPIT	Core Assessment Program for Intracerebral Transplantations
CAPIT-HD	Core Assessment Program for Intracerebral Transplantation in Huntington's Disease
CAPSIT-PD	Core Assessment Program for Surgical Interventional Therapies in Parkinson's Disease
CAPTN	Child and Adolescent Psychiatry Trials Network
CATIE study	Clinical Antipsychotic Trials of Intervention Effectiveness study
CBT	cognitive behaviour therapy
CDRS-R	Children's Depression Rating Scale, Revised
CHMP	Committee for Medicinal Products for Human Use
CI	cochlear implant
CM	centrum medianum-parafascicular nucleus
CMV	cytomegalovirus
CNS	central nervous system
CNTF	ciliary neurotrophic factor
CPU	central processing unit

CT	computerised tomography
DARPA	Defence Advanced Research Projects Agency
DAT	dopamine transporter
DBS	deep brain stimulation
DEA	US American Drug Enforcement Administration
DID	dissociative identity disorder
DNA	deoxyribonucleic acid
DSM III/IV	Diagnostic and Statistical Manual of Mental Disorders 3rd/4th edition, published by the American Psychiatric Association
EBS	electrical brain stimulation
EBV	Epstein-Barr virus
EC	European Commission
ECC	embryonic carcinoma cell
ECT	electroconvulsive therapy
EEG	electro-encephalogram
EGC	embryonic germ cell
EGE	European Group on Ethics in Science and New Technologies
EMEA	European Medicines Agency
ESC	embryonic stem cell
EUDRACT	European Clinical Trials Data Base
FDA	U.S. Food and Drug Administration
FDAMA	Food and Drug Administration Modernisation Act
FES	functional electrical stimulation
GABA	gamma amino butyric acid
GAD	glutamic acid decarboxylase
GAF-Scale	Global Assessment of Functioning Scale
GDNF	glia cell-derived neurotrophic factor
GLP	good laboratory practice
GPi	global pallidus
HCFA	Health Care Financing Administration
HCHP	Harvard Community Health Plan
HCI	human-computer interface
HD	Huntington's disease
HIV	human immunodeficiency virus
HSVtk gene	herpes simplex virus thymidine kinase gene
HTLV	human T-cell leukemia virus
ICD-10	International Classification of Diseases and Related Health Problems 10th edition, published by the World Health Organisation (WHO)

ICM	inner cell mass
IQ	intelligence quotient
IVF	in vitro fertilisation
LBS	Layton BioScience Inc.
LGL	lateral geniculate ganglion
LV	lentiviral
MAOI	monoamine oxidase inhibitor
MDD	major depressive disorder
MemCrit	memory criterion (for personal identity)
MEMS	micro-electro-mechanical systems
MHRA	Modern Humanities Research Association
MIG-HD	Multicentric Intracerebral Grafting in Huntington's Disease
MMT	multimodal treatment study
MPH	Methylphenidate
MRI	magnetic resonance imaging
MS	multiple sclerosis
MSA	multiple system atrophy
MTA	Multimodal Treatment Study of Children with ADHD
NAcc	nucleus accumbens
NECTAR	Network of European CNS Transplantation and Restoration
NGF	nerve growth factor
NIMH	National Institute of Mental Health
NMP	neuromotor prosthesis
NPY	neuropeptide Y
NT-3	neurotrophin-3
NTS	nucleus tractus solitarius
OCD	obsessive compulsive disorder
OLG	Oberlandesgericht (Higher Regional Court)
PD	Parkinson's disease
PERV	porcine endogenous retrovirus
PET	positron emission tomography
PI-Crit	criterion for personal identity
PNS	peripheral nervous system
POMS	Profile of Mood States
PPN	pedunculo-pontine nucleus
PRN	pro re nata (=according to need)
p-trait	personality trait
PTSD	posttraumatic stress disorder

PVS	persistent vegetative state
RNA	ribonucleic acid
RNAi	RNA interference
rTMS	repetitive Transcranial Magnetic Stimulation
SCHIP	(U.S.) State Children's Health Insurance Program
SCNT	somatic cell nuclear transfer
siRNA	small interfering RNA
SSC	somatic stem cell
SSRI	selective serotonin reuptake inhibitor
STN	subthalamic nucleus
SUDS	Subjective Units of Distress Scale
TADS	Treatment for Adolescents with Depression Study
TAU	treatment as usual
TCAs	tricyclic antidepressants
TMS	transcranial magnetic stimulation
UPDRS	Unified Parkinson's Disease Rating Scale
Vim	ventral intermediate nucleus of the thalamus
VNS	vagal nerve stimulation
VZV	varicella-zoster virus
WPA	World Psychiatric Association
YBOCS	Yale-Brown Obsessive-Compulsive Scale

Glossary[317]

AFFECTIVE DISORDERS: see MOOD DISORDERS

ALZHEIMER'S DISEASE (AD):
AD is a neurodegenerative disease characterised by progressive cognitive deterioration together with declining activities of daily living and neuropsychiatric symptoms or behavioural changes. It is the most common type of dementia. The pathological process consists of neuronal loss and atrophy, typically observed as the deposition of amyloid plaques and neurofibrillary tangles. Although susceptibility genes have been identified the ultimate cause of the disease is unknown (cf. Section 2.4.3).

AMNESIA:
Refers to different types of memory disorders. Individuals suffering from anterograde amnesia (ICD-10: R41.1) are severely impaired in their ability to form new lasting memories. While their short-term memory is usually intact, they forget everything they experience shortly afterwards. In contrast, people with retrograde amnesia (ICD-10: R41.2) are unable to recall events which occurred before onset of amnesia. A third type of memory disorder is so-called dissociative amnesia (ICD-10: F44.0) which is characterised by an inability to recall certain EPISODIC or autobiographic memories usually related to traumatic or stressful events. Depending on whether the memory loss is either quite generalised or rather confined to a certain period of time, different subtypes of dissociative amnesia can be distinguished.

AMYOTROPHIC LATERAL SCLEROSIS (ALS):
ALS is a progressive fatal neurodegenerative disease caused by the gradual degeneration of motoneurons which control voluntary muscle movement. The disease does not necessarily debilitate the patient's mental functioning. ALS most commonly strikes people between 40 and 60 years of age. Currently the disease cannot be cured (cf. Section 2.4.4).

---

[317] The glossary contains only a small selection of technical terms from neurophysiology and -anatomy. For a succinct introduction into structure and functioning of the nervous system see Section 2.2.

Anterograde amnesia: see AMNESIA

Antipsychotic drugs: see NEUROLEPTICS

Anxiolytics:
Drugs for the treatment of anxiety disorders. Anxiolytics are generally divided into two groups of medication, benzodiazepines and non-benzodiazepines (cf. Section 1.1.3).

Attention deficit hyperactivity disorder (ADHD):
The term ADHD is not included in the ICD-10 but is comparable to the so-called "hyperkinetic disorders" which are represented in its various forms (either single or in combination with other disorders) in the F9x chapter of the ICD-10. The diagnosis of a hyperkinetic disorder requires severe symptoms of inattention (for example concentration problems), hyperactivity (for example extensive restlessness) and impulsivity (for example an inability to wait) for at least six months which are present in two separate contexts (e.g. at school and at home). Symptoms need to be present before the age of six (cf. Section 1.4.2.2).

Autistic disorders:
Can be found in the subchapter F84.x of the ICD-10 (pervasive developmental disorders). Patients with autistic disorders present with an impairment of social interaction and communication and with stereotypical, repeated patterns of interests and activities. The child's behaviour does not suit its age. Patients show an inability to get into social contact with others and have no real interest to participate in group activities. The patients seem to lack empathy or the ability to perceive moods or responses of others. They routinely engage in unusual patterns of behaviour and resist or have significant difficulty with new experiences or transitions. Often the acquisition and proper use of language is impaired as well.

Bipolar disorders (ICD-10: F31.x):
Characterised by alternating episodes of depression and elevated (hypomanic or manic) mood. A minimum of two episodes of changing mood is required for bipolar disorders to be diagnosed. The different subgroups are divided according to the affective state and to whether or not psychotic symptoms are present.

BORDERLINE PERSONALITY DISORDER:

Defined as a subtype of the emotionally unstable **PERSONALITY DISORDERS** in the ICD-10 (F60.31). Patients with this disorder tend to act impulsively, without giving a thought on possible consequences. Symptoms include instability of self perceptions and goals, a tendency to engage in intensive yet unstable relationships, a fear of abandonment and repeated **SELF-INJURIOUS** threats or actions combined with a steady feeling of emptiness.

BRADYKINESIA: see **PARKINSON'S DISEASE**

CHOLESTEATOMA:

A type of cyst located in the middle ear mostly developing as a consequence of repeated ear infections.

CONDUCT DISORDERS:

"Characterised by a repetitive and persistent pattern of dissocial, aggressive or defiant conduct. Such behaviours should amount to major violations of age-appropriate social expectations" (ICD-10: F91.x). Typical examples include fire setting, truancy, fighting, stealing, repeated lying, unusual temper tantrums, etc. Conduct disorders can be combined with hyperkinetic disorders.

CORE ASSESSMENT PROTOCOL:

Basic and standardised evaluation protocol allowing to establish or follow in time the clinical success of a new treatment for a disease against other available treatments in an unbiased and quantitative manner. A core assessment protocol is disease-specific and also allows pre-/post-treatment comparisons. When employed in clinical research it can reduce the number of patients subjected to experimental treatments and it can improve the comparison and evaluation of new treatment approaches (cf. Section 2.6.2).

CYSTIC MYELOPATHY (ALSO CALLED "SYRINGOMYELIA"):

Refers to the development of a cyst filled with cerebrospinal fluid within the spinal cord. Cystic myelopathy is an infrequent, but potentially devastating, complication following traumatic spinal cord injury.

DEMENTIA:

A chronic and often progressive decline and loss of cognitive functions, including memory, thought, orientation, interpretation, calculation, learning, speech and judgement. Often concomitant decline of emotional control, social behaviour or motivation can be found. Dementia can be found in

ALZHEIMER'S DISEASE, cerebrovascular disorders and other disorders affecting the brain, as well as with HIV infections and PARKINSON'S DISEASE. Intellectual performance and cognitive functioning decrease over time thus leading to a reduced ability to live everyday life.

DEPRESSIVE DISORDERS:
Belong to the subgroup of affective disorders in the ICD-10. Depressive episodes could be classified as either mild, moderate or severe according to the ability of the depressed individual to participate in everyday life. Symptoms include: depressed mood, diminished interest or pleasure in most activities, loss of weight or appetite, fatigue or loss of energy and sleep disorders. Depressive episodes which are followed by manic episodes constitute the subclass of so-called BIPOLAR DISORDERS.

DISSOCIATIVE AMNESIA: see AMNESIA

DISSOCIATIVE IDENTITY DISORDER (DID):
(DSM IV: 300.14; classified as "multiple personality disorder" under ICD-10: F44.8) An individual with DID apparently exhibits different personalities ("alters") which seem to take turns controlling the individual's behaviour. When under the control of one alter, the person is often unable to remember events that occurred while other alters were in control.

DYSKINESIA:
Difficulty or distortion in performing voluntary movements; see also TARDIVE DYSKINESIA.

DYSTHYMIA:
Chronically depressed state of mind, less severe than in major depression.

EPISODIC MEMORY:
The recollection of events of one's own life.

EXTRA-PYRAMIDAL SIDE EFFECTS:
Physical symptoms, including TARDIVE DYSKINESIA, tremor, slurred speech, restlessness, muscular spasms and rigidity, which primarily occur in reaction to NEUROLEPTICS.

Gene transfer/therapy:

The insertion of genes into an individual's cells or tissues to treat diseases, in particular hereditary diseases. The technology is still in its infancy, but gene transfer by means of genetically modified viruses unable to reproduce as a virus and used as transport medium for a therapeutic gene (viral vector-mediated gene transfer) has been used with some success. However, gene transfer so far has certainly not been established as gene therapy (cf. Section 2.3.4).

Glial cells:

Second main type of cell in the central nervous system next to neurons. Glial cells surround neurons holding them in place and insulating them from one another. Furthermore, they supply neurons with nutrients and oxygen. In recent years more and more functions of glial cells have been recognised, for instance, they also participate in signal transmission in the central nervous system.

Huntington's disease (HD):

A rare inherited neurological disorder caused by a trinucleotide repeat expansion in the huntingtin gene. This expansion produces mutant huntingtin protein causing neuronal cell death especially in the striatal areas of the brain, thus leading to abnormal body movements (chorea) and a lack of coordination, but also affecting mental abilities and aspects of personality. The symptoms become noticeable in a person's forties, but can occur at any age depending on the length of the trinucleotide repeat. Being a genetic disorder, there is currently no cure (cf. Section 2.4.2).

Mania (ICD-10: F30.x):

An affective disorder associated with inadequate elevated mood, increased speech and energy, decreased need for sleep, hyperactivity, feeling of "racing thoughts", behavioural dyscontrol, reckless, daredevil behaviour without loosing thoughts about possible risks, and increased libido. Delusions and hallucinations can be present but are not necessary for diagnosis. Sometimes manic episodes can be found as an interlude of depression. This is called a BIPOLAR DISORDER.

Mastectomy:

The surgical removal of one or two breasts, partially or completely.

Mental enhancement:

Summarises the enhancement of cognitive capacities ("cognitive enhancement"), emotional ("mood enhancement"), motivational states and processes, and of "autonomic states", i.e. mental states emerging from autonomic functions of the CNS and, like these functions themselves, not subject to volitional control, such as dreaming, proprioceptive awareness, or sexual arousal.

Micro-electro-mechanical systems (MEMS):
Integrated systems of mechanical elements, sensors, actuators, and electronics on a common substrate (e.g. silicon) built through microfabrication technology.

Mood (affective) disorders:
This category of ICD-10 (F3x) comprises manic episodes, hypomania (elated and irritable mood below the threshold to mania), BIPOLAR DISORDER, DEPRESSIVE DISORDERS, cyclothymia (continued mood fluctuations) and DYSTHYMIA. The core symptoms are changes of mood and affect to either a depressed form or – on the other side of the scale – a lifted, even manic state of mind. Disorders are classified according to their severity and the presence or absence of psychotic symptoms. Symptoms typical for a depressed state of mind are e.g.: loss of interest, decreased mood, sleep irregularities, fatigue or feelings of diminished energy, whereas concomitant symptoms of a manic state include: increased talkativeness, delusional thinking, flight of ideas, increased activity, restlessness, decreased need to sleep, reckless behaviour or unnecessary expenses.

Multiple personality disorder: see DISSOCIATIVE IDENTITY DISORDER

Multiple sclerosis (MS):
A chronic inflammatory disease of the central nervous system (CNS) resulting in focal loss of myelin and therefore loss of neuronal activity. MS can cause a variety of symptoms, including changes in sensation, visual problems, muscle weakness, depression, difficulties with coordination and speech, severe fatigue, short term memory loss, problems with balance, overheating and pain. MS causes impaired mobility and disability in more severe cases. MS may take several different forms, with new symptoms occurring either in discrete attacks or slowly accruing over time. Between attacks, symptoms may resolve completely, but permanent neurological problems often persist. The exact cause of MS remains unknown and the disease has no cure. MS primarily affects adults, its age of onset typically is between 20 and 40 years (cf. Section 2.4.5).

Narcolepsy:
A disorder causing the patient to spontaneously and unwillingly fall asleep. The disorder often starts in late adolescence or young adulthood and leads to uncontrollable sleep attacks. Narcolepsy seems to be caused either through a

genetic defect leading to a diminished production of the protein Orexin or an increased level of acetylcholine and dopamine (both of them are neurotransmitters helping to send information over the synaptic cleft thus connecting neuronal cells) within the brain.

Neural grafting:
Neurotransplantation of undifferentiated or immature neural cells.

Neural prosthetics:
Summarises technologies aimed at the restitution or bridging of lost or disturbed neural function (e.g. sensory or motor deficits). Central neural prostheses are electronic devices that connect to the brain for the purpose of stimulation or detection of brain activity.

Neuroenhancement: see **mental enhancement**

Neurosis:
The term dates back to the beginning of modern psychotherapy and can be found in the ICD-10 within different contexts as it is used in defining **obsessive compulsive disorder** (anankastic neurosis, F42), **post traumatic stress disorder** (traumatic neurosis, F43.1), **dysthymia** (neurotic depression, F34.1), hypochondriacal disorder (hypochondriacal neurosis, F45.2) and "other specified neurotic disorders" (e.g.: psychasthenic neurosis, F48.8).

Neuroleptics:
A class of drugs predominantly used to treat psychosis (hence these drugs are also referred to as "antipsychotics"). Older agents like chlorpromazine are called "traditional" or "typical" neuroleptics. During the 1990s a new generation of antipsychotic drugs were developed commonly referred to as "atypical" neuroleptics (cf. Section 1.1.3).

Neuromodulation:
Refers to technologies aimed at influencing erroneous function in neural networks by means of electrical stimulation.

Neuroteratology, functional/behavioural:
Functional neuroteratology, also called behavioural teratology, is a field of research focussing on the subtle changes in functional aspects of the brain in relation to abnormal events during prenatal and postnatal brain development. It does not describe the gross anatomical changes known as teratology, but the often hidden cellular and molecular changes in the brain caused by

environmental factors, food and drug intake or severe burdens in young life that only show up in later life as minor or more significant and cumbersome behavioural and mental incapacities. Subtle changes as found in functional neuroteratological studies with laboratory animals (controlled influences in early life and tests in adulthood) could be indicative of and are sometimes proven to underlie differences in physical and mental capacities and personality traits of human beings.

Neurotransplantation:

Implantation of cells into the central nervous system. These cells can be either immature neurons or cells which can differentiate into neurons after implantation and thus replace lost or dysfunctional neurons (neural grafting) or GLIAL CELLS or non-neural cells to support functional repair of the central nervous system. Neurotransplantation is seen as a promising technique for the treatment of various neurodegenerative disorders.

Nootropic substance:

Any natural or synthetic substance improving human cognitive abilities. The term covers medications for the treatment of cognitive impairment as well as agents by which an enhancement of normal cognitive abilities may be achieved.

Obsessive compulsive disorder (OCD; ICD-10: F42.x):

The patients suffer from recurrent and persistent obsessional thoughts (often in a stereotyped form) and/or feel driven to repeatedly perform compulsive acts. OCD is closely linked to anxiety disorders insofar patients consider their behaviour necessary to ward off harm to themselves or others. If they try to resist their obsessional thoughts and rituals the related anxiety usually increases.

Off-label use:

The use of an approved medication outside the terms of its product license („label"), e.g. in a non-approved age group or indication.

Orphan drugs:

Medications for the treatment of rare diseases.

Parkinson's disease (PD):

A progressive degenerative disease of the central nervous system, primarily affecting dopaminergic neurons in the brain's substantia nigra. The cardinal symptoms of PD are tremor in hands, arms, legs, jaw, and face; rigidity or stiffness of the limbs and trunk; BRADYKINESIA (slowness of movement) or akinesia (inability to initiate movement); postural instability or impaired balance and coordination. The most widely used form of treatment is levodopa (L-dopa) helping to compensate for the depletion of dopamine. However, prolonged use of levodopa may give rise to TARDIVE DYSKINESIA. (Cf. Section 2.4.1)

PERSISTENT VEGETATIVE STATE (PVS):

A state of unconsciousness not as profound as coma. Unlike in coma, patients in PVS may open and move their eyes and sometimes show a sleep-wake cycle. Although they exhibit some spontaneous movements they are considered "awake but not aware" because of their unresponsiveness to most external stimuli.

PERSONALITY DISORDERS (ICD-10: F6x):

The behaviour of patients with personality disorders deviates extremely or significantly from the way in which the average individual in a given culture perceives, thinks, feels and, particularly, relates to others. These patterns of behaviour have to be stable over the years (often with an onset in childhood or adolescence) and concern a variety of behavioural and psychological functions of the person affected. Because of the requirement of long-term stability it is considered inappropriate to diagnose a personality disorders before the age of 16 or 17. ICD-10 differentiates the following types of personality disorders: paranoid, schizoid, dissocial, emotionally unstable, histrionic, anankastic, anxious, dependent, combined and further specific and unspecified personality disorders.

PHARMACODYNAMICS:

The study of the time course and mechanisms of drug action and of the relationship between drug concentration and physiological effect.

PHARMACOKINETICS:

Uses mathematical models to describe and predict the time course of drug absorption, distribution, metabolism and excretion, these being the processes that determine the concentrations in various body tissues after drug administration.

POST-TRAUMATIC STRESS DISORDER (PTSD; ICD-10: F43.1):

Describes a delayed or protracted response to an overwhelming stressful situation (such as natural disasters, war, accident, torture and rape). Typical symptoms include so-called "flashback" memories, a feeling of numbness and emotional dullness, anhedonia and the avoidance of situations which are connected with the trauma. Sometimes panic attacks and massive anxiety can be triggered via the memory of the traumatic situation.

Psychosis/psychotic states:
Can be found in different subgroups of the ICD-10 (particularly in the F0x, F2x and F3x group). During psychotic states of mind the perception of reality is impaired (often accompanied by delusions and hallucinations).

(Psycho)stimulants:
A broad category of substances inducing heightened alertness, increased vigilance and – depending on their effectiveness – a sense of well-being and euphoria. Some of these substances are prescribed for medical conditions (e.g. Methylphenidate), others are manufactured for illicit substance abuse (e.g. cocaine), and others again can be found in over-the-counter decongestants, herbal extracts, caffeinated beverages, and cigarettes (cf. Section 1.4.3.1).

Psychotropic substance:
Any natural or synthetic substance which has an effect on cognitive, emotional and motivational states or processes including, e.g., antidepressive agents, hallucinogens, and tranquilising agents.

Retrograde amnesia: see Amnesia

Schizoaffective disorders (ICD-10: F25x):
Episodic disorders where both schizophrenic and affective symptoms can be present at the same time. Criteria for affective disorders are combined with schizophrenia-like symptoms such as delusions, auditory hallucinations, speech disorders, catatonic symptoms (motor irregularities) and thought disorders. Affective symptoms can be either depressive or manic or sometimes even combined.

Schizophrenia (ICD-10: F2x):
Goes along with thought disturbances, delusions and affective impairment without intellectual disabilities. Symptoms include: delusions, hallucinations, so-called "negative symptoms" (such as affective flattening, alogia or avolition), formal thought disorder, feelings of thought control from outside and behavioural changes of the person often leading to social withdrawal. Symptoms have to be present for at least one month. Often a prodromal phase can be seen in adolescents before the onset of schizophrenic symptoms. A prodromal phase can be accompanied by diminished interest, absence from work, social withdrawal and dysphoria to an extent atypical for the person affected. Several forms of schizophrenia can be differentiated including: paranoid schizophrenia, hebephrenic schizophrenia, catatonic schizophrenia, schizophrenia simplex and undifferentiated schizophrenia.

SELF-INJURIOUS BEHAVIOUR:
Defined by Favazza (1998) as "deliberate, nonsuicidal destruction of one's own body tissue." Favazza differentiated between major self-mutilation such as "eye enucleation and castration, commonly associated with psychosis and intoxication", stereotypic self-mutilation which includes "such acts as head banging and self-biting most often accompanying TOURETTE'S SYNDROME and severe mental retardation" and superficial/moderate self-mutilation for which "compulsive acts such as trichotillomania [repeated urge to pull out scalp and body hair] and skin picking and such episodic acts as skin cutting and burning" are typical.

SHAM SURGERY:
In order to control for placebo effects of surgical interventions participants of clinical trials are put in a position where they cannot tell whether they received the surgical treatment in question or not. In the case of neurosurgical procedures this may include giving general anaesthesia to participants and drilling a hole in the outer layer of the skull (cf. Section 2.6.1).

SMART PILL: see NOOTROPIC SUBSTANCE

STEM CELLS:
Primal cells with the ability to renew themselves through cell division and differentiate into a wide range of specialised cell types. Three broad categories of mammalian stem cells exist: embryonic stem cells, derived from blastocysts as pre-implantation embryos, somatic (adult) stem cells, which are found in matured tissues, and cord blood stem cells. As stem cells can be readily grown under laboratory conditions and transformed into specialised cells with characteristics consistent with cells of various tissues including nervous tissue, their use in medical therapies has been proposed and is currently being explored.

STIMULANTS: see PSYCHOSTIMULANTS

TARDIVE DYSKINESIA (TD):
A possible side effect associated with the prolonged use of NEUROLEPTIC medication. The expression "tardive" indicates that the DYSKINESIAS can continue even after the drugs are no longer taken. TD originates from a dopamine (a neurotransmitter) blockade within the basal ganglia – a region of the brain responsible for motor control. TD can lead to irregular movements of tongue, mouth or body. So far there seems to be no pharmaceutical substance to effectively combat TD.

Torsades de pointes dysrhythmia:
A special pattern of cardiac dysrhythmia.

Tourette's syndrome (ICD-10: F95.2):
Describes a combination of vocal and multiple motor tics starting before the age of 18. Before onset of vocal tics there is often a history of motor tics. The tics may consist of vocalisations and gestures which are of an obscene nature.

Xenotransplantation:
The transplantation of living cells, tissues or organs (xenografts) from one species to another, in particular from animals (e.g. pigs) to human beings.

References

Abbott A (2002) Brain implants show promise against obsessive disorder. Nature 419 (Oct 17):685

Abbott A (2005) Deep in thought. Nature 436(July 7):18–19

Abe K (2000) Therapeutic potential of neurotrophic factors and neural stem cells against ischemic brain injury. J Cereb Blood Flow Metab 20:1393–1408

Abelson J, Curtis G, Sagher O, Albucher R, Harrigan M, Taylor S, Martis B, Giordani B (2005) Deep brain stimulation for refractory obsessive-compulsive disorder. Biol Psychiatry 57:510–516

Adams F, Aizawa K (2001) The bounds of cognition. Philosophical Psychology 14:43–64

Advisory Group on the Ethics of Transplantation (1996) Animal Tissues into Humans. Her Majesty's Stationary Office, Norwich

Aebischer P, Schluep M, Deglon N, Joseph JM, Hirt L, Heyd B, Goddard M, Hammang JP, Zurn AD, Kato AC, Regli F, Baetge EE (1996) Intrathecal delivery of CNTF using encapsulated genetically modified xenogeneic cells in amyotrophic lateral sclerosis patients. Nat Med 2:696–699

Agar N (2004) Liberal Eugenics. Blackwell, Oxford

Alataris K, Berger, TW, Marmarelis VZ (2000) A novel network for nonlinear modeling of neural systems with arbitrary point-process inputs. Neural Netw 13(2):255–266

Albin RL (2002) Sham surgery controls: Intracerebral grafting of fetal tissue for Parkinson's disease and proposed criteria for use of sham surgery controls. J Med Ethics 28:322–325

Alexy R (1983) Theorie der juristischen Argumentation. Suhrkamp, Frankfurt

Allen DB, Fost NC (1990) Growth hormone therapy for short stature: Panacea or Pandora's box? Journal of Pediatrics 117:16–21

Altmann J (2004) Military uses of nanotechnology: Perspectives and concerns. Security Dialogue 35(1):61–79

Aman MG, Marks RE, Turbott SH, Wilsher CP, Merry SN (1991) Methylphenidate and thioridazine in the treatment of intellectually subaverage children: Effects on cognitive-motor performance. J Am Acad Child Adolesc Psychiatry 30(5):816–24

Amitai Y, Frischer H (2006) Excess fatality from desipramine in children and adolescents. Journal of the American Academy of Child & Adolescent Psychiatry 45(1):54–60

Anderson D, Ahmed A (2003) Treatment of patients with intractable obsessive-compulsive disorder with anterior capsular stimulation. J Neurosurg 98:1104–1108

Anderson KD, Panayotatos N, Corcoran TL, Lindsay RM, Wiegand SJ (1996) Ciliary neurotrophic factor protects striatal output neurons in an animal model of Huntington disease. Proc Natl Acad Sci USA 93:7346–7351

Andlin-Sobocki P, Jönsson B, Wittchen H-U, Olesen J (eds) (2005) Cost of disorders of the brain in Europe. Eur J Neurology 12 (suppl. 1)

Angell M (2004) The Truth About the Drug Companies. Random House, New York

Angold A, Erkanli A, Egger HL, Costello EJ (2000) Stimulant treatment for children: A community perspective. Journal of the American Academy of Child and Adolescent Psychiatry 39(8):975–984

Antoinette T, Iyengar S, Puig-Antich J (1990) Is locked seclusion necessary for children under the age of 14? Am J Psychiatry 147:1283–1289

Aouizerate B, Cuny E, Martin-Guehl C, Guehl D, Amieva H, Benazzouz A, Fabrigoule C, Allard M, Rougier A, Bioulac B, Tignol J, Burbaud P (2004) Deep brain stimulation of the ventral caudate nucleus in the treatment of obsessive-compulsive disorder and major depression. J Neurosurg 101:682–686

Archer DR, Cuddon PA, Lipsitz D, Duncan LD (1997) Myelination of the canine central nervous system by glial cell transplantation: a model for repair of human myelin disease. Nature Med 1:54–59

Arendash GW, Gorski RA (1982) Enhancement of sexual behavior in female rats by neonatal transplantation of brain tissue from males. Science 217:1276–1278

Ariès P (1960) L'Enfant et la Vie Familiale sous l'Ancien Régime. Paris, Plon

Aristoteles (1951) Die Nikomachische Ethik. Gigon O (ed) Artemis, Zürich

Arjona V, Minguez-Castellanos A, Montoro RJ, Ortega A, Escamilla F, Toledo-Aral JJ, Pardal R, Mendez-Ferrer S, Martin JM, Perez M, Katati MJ, Valencia E, Garcia T, Lopez-Barneo J (2003) Autotransplantation of human carotid body cell aggregates for treatment of Parkinson's disease. Neurosurgery 53:321–328

Armenteros JL, Whitaker AH, Welikson M, Stedge DJ, Gorman J (1997) Risperidone in adolescents with schizophrenia: an open pilot study. J Am Acad Child Adolesc Psychiatry 36(5):694–700

Armstrong RJ, Svendsen CN (2000) Neural stem cells: from cell biology to cell replacement. Cell Transplant 9:139–152

Asano T, Sasaki K, Kitano Y, Terao K, Hanazono Y (2006) In vivo tumor formation from primate embryonic stem cells. Methods Mol Biol 329:459–67

Austin JK, McNelis AM, Shore CP, Dunn DW, Musick B (2002) A feasibility study of a family seizure management program: "Be Seizure Smart". J Neurosci Nurs 34(1):30–37

Avigen Announces Encouraging Early Data from Parkinson's Disease Clinical Trial (2005) http://www.avigen.com/non_financial_release/2005/2005_Avigen_EarlyData_PDClinicalTrial_071805.htm

Bach FH, Fishman JA, Daniels N, Proimos J, Anderson B, Carpenter CB, Forrow L, Robson SC, Fineberg HV (1998) Uncertainty in xenotransplantation: individual benefit versus collective risk. Nature Med 4:141–144

Bachelin C, Lachapelle F, Girard C, Moissonnier P, Serguera-Lagache C, Mallet J, Fontaine D, Chojnowski A, Le Guern E, Nait-Oumesmar B, Baron-Van Evercooren A (2005) Efficient myelin repair in the macaque spinal cord by autologous grafts of Schwann cells. Brain 128:540–549

Bachoud-Lévi AC, Déglon N, Nguyen JP, Bloch J, Bourdet C, Winkel L, Rémy P, Goddard M, Lefaucheur JP, Brugières P, Baudic S, Cesaro P, Peschanski M, Aebischer P (2000a) Neuroprotective gene therapy for Huntington's disease using a polymer encapsulated BHK cell line engineered to secrete human CNTF. Hum Gene Ther 11:1723–1729

Bachoud-Lévi AC, Gaura V, Brugières P, Lefaucheur P, Boissé MF, Maison P, Baudic S, Ribeiro MJ, Bourdet C, Remy P, Cesaro P, Hantraye P, Peschanski M (2006) Effect of foetal neural transplants in patients with Huntington's disease 6 years after surgery: a long-term follow-up study. Lancet Neurol 5:303–309

Bachoud-Lévi AC, Hantraye P, Peschanski M (2002) Fetal neural grafts for Huntington's disease: a prospective view. Mov Disord 17:439–444

Bachoud-Lévi AC, Remy P, Nguyen JP, Brugieres P, Lefaucheur JP, Bourdet C, Baudic S, Gaura V, Maison P, Haddad B, Boisse MF, Grandmougin T, Jeny R, Bartolomeo P, Dalla Barba G, Degos JD, Lisovoski F, Ergis AM, Pailhous E, Cesaro P, Hantraye P, Peschanski M (2000b) Motor and cognitive improvements in patients with Huntington's disease after neural transplantation. Lancet 356:1975–1979

Backlund E-O, Granber P-O, Hamberger B, Sedvall G, Seiger A, Olson L (1985) Transplantation of adrenal medullary tissue to striatum in parkinsonism: first clincal trials. J Neurosurg 62:169–173

Bailey P, Bremer F (1938) A sensory cortical representation of the vagus nerve. Neurophysiology pp 405–412

Bakay RAE, Barrow DL, Fiandaca MS, Iuvone PM, Schiff A, Collins DC (1987) Biochemical and behavioral correction of MPTP Parkinson-like syndrome by fetal cell transplantation. Am NY Acad Sci 495:623–640

Bankiewicz KS, Eberling JL, Kohutnicka M, Jagust W, Pivirotto P, Bringas J, Cunningham J, Budinger TF, Harvey-White J (2000) Convection-enhanced delivery of AAV vector in parkinsonian monkeys: in vivo detection of gene expression and restoration of dopaminergic function using pro-drug approach. Exp Neurol 164:2–14

Bankiewicz KS, Forsayeth J, Eberling JL, Sanchez-Pernaute R, Pivirotto P, Bringas J, Herscovitch P, Carson RE, Eckelman W, Reutter B, Cunningham J (2006) Long-term clinical improvement in MPTP-lesioned primates after gene therapy with AAV-hAADC. Mol Ther Jul 6

Bankiewicz KS, Kao H, Bernal J, Pierce GF, Johnson KW (2005) AAV2-mediated gene delivery to monkey putamen: evaluation of an infusion device and delivery parameters. Exp Neurol 194:476–83

Bankiewicz KS, Plunkett RJ, Jacobowitz DM, Porrino L, Di Porzio U, London WT, Kopin IJ, Oldfield EH (1990) The effect of fetal mesencephalon implants on primate MPTP-induced parkinsonism: histochemical and behavioral studies. J Neurosurg 72:231–244

Barch DM (2004) Pharmacological manipulation of human working memory. Psychopharmacology 174:126–135

Barker RA, Kendall AL, Widner H (2000) Neural tissue xenotransplantation: what is needed prior to clinical trials in Parkinson's disease? Neural Tissue Xenografting Project. Cell Transplant 9:235–246

Barkley RA, Fischer M, Smallish L, Fletcher K (2003) Does the treatment of attention-deficit/hyperactivity disorder with stimulants contribute to drug use/abuse? A 13-year prospective study. Pediatrics 111:97–109

Barnett SR, dosReis S, Riddle MA, The Maryland Youth Practice Improvement Committee for Mental Health (2002) Improving the management of acute aggression in state residential and inpatient psychiatric facilities for Youths. J Am Acad Child Adolesc Psychiatry 41:897–905

Baron-Cohen S (1997) Mindblindness: an essay on autism and theory of mind. MIT-Press, Cambridge Mass

Baron U, Bujard H (2000) Tet repressor-based system for regulated gene expression in eukaryotic cells: principles and advances. Methods Enzymol 327:401–421

Barondes SH (2003) Better than Prozac. Creating the Next Generation of Psychiatric Drugs. Oxford University Press, Oxford New York

Battaglia J, Moss S, Rush J, Kang J, Mendoza R, Leedom L, Dubin W, McGlynn C, Goodman L (1997) Haloperidol, lorazepam, or both for psychotic agitation? A multicenter, prospective, double-blind, emergency department study. Am J Emerg Med 15:335–340

Battmer RD, Dillier N, Lai WK, Weber BP, Brown C, Gantz BJ, Roland JT, Cohen NJ, Shapiro W, Pesch J, Killian MJ, Lenarz T (2004) Evaluation of the neural response telemetry (NRT) capabilities of the nucleus research platform 8: initial results from the NRT trial Int J Audiol 43 suppl 1:10–5, 10–15

Bayne T, Levy N (2005) Amputees by choice: body integrity identity disorder and the ethics of amputation. Journal of Applied Philosophy 22(1):75–86

Beauchamp TL, Childress J (2001) Principles of Biomedical Ethics. 5th edn, Oxford University Press, Oxford New York

Beadle EA, McKinley DJ, Nikolopoulos TP, Brough J, O'Donoghue GM, Archbold SM (2005a) Long-term functional outcomes and academic-occupational status in implanted children after 10 to 14 years of cochlear implant use. Otol Neurotol 26(6):1152–1160

Beadle, EA, McKinley DJ, Nikolopoulos TP, Brough J, O'Donoghue GM, Archbold SM (2005b) Long-term functional outcomes and academic-occupational status in implanted children after 10 to 14 years of cochlear implant use. Otol Neurotol 26(6):1152–1160

Belkadi AM, Gény C, Naimi S, Jeny R, Peschanski M, Riche D (1997) Maturation of fetal human neural xenografts in the adult rat brain. Exp Neurol 144:369–380

Belzen van MJ, Heutink P (2006) Genetic analysis of psychiatric disorders in humans. Genes, Brain and Behavior 5(suppl. 2):25–33, 260–269

Ben Menachem E (2002) Vagus-nerve stimulation for the treatment of epilepsy. Lancet Neurol 1(8):477–482

Ben Menachem E, French A (2005) VNS Therapy versus the latest antiepileptic drug. Epileptic Disord 7 suppl 1:22–26

Benabid AL (2003) Deep brain stimulation for Parkinson's disease. Curr Opin Neurobiol 13:696–706

Benabid AL, Pollak P, Gervason CL, Hoffmann D, Gao DM, Hommel M, Perret JE, De Rougemont J (1991) Long term suppression of tremor by chronic stimulation of the ventral intermediate nucleus thalamic nucleus. Lancet 337:403–406

Benabid AL, Wallace B, Mitrofanis J, Xia R, Piallat B, Chabardes S, Berger F (2005) A putative generalized model of the effects and mechanism of action of high frequency electrical stimulation of the central nervous system. Acta Neurol Belg 105:149–157

Bender L, Cottington F (1942) the use of amphetamine sulfate (benzedrine) in child psychiatry. Am J Psychiatry 99:116–121

Beracochea D, Celerier A, Peres M, Pierard C (2003) Enhancement of learning processes following an acute modafinil injection in mice. Pharmacol Biochem Behav 76(3–4):473–9

Berger TW, Ahuja A, Courellis SH, Deadwyler SA, Erinjippurath G, Gerhardt GA, Gholmieh G, Granacki JJ, Hampson R, Hsaio MC, LaCoss J, Marmarelis VZ, Nasiatka P, Srinivasan V, Song D, Tanguay AR, Wills J (2005) Restoring lost cognitive function. IEEE Eng Med Biol Mag 24(5):30–44

Bernal JD (1929) The World, the Flesh and the Devil. K. Paul Trench & Trubner, London

Berthoud HR, Neuhuber WL (2000) Functional and chemical anatomy of the afferent vagal system. Auton Neurosci 85(1–3):1–17

Beynon AJ, Snik AF, van den Broek P (2003) Comparison of different speech coding strategies using a disability-based inventory and speech perception tests in quiet and in noise. Otol Neurotol 24(3):392–396

Biederman J, Faraone SV (2005) Attention-deficit hyperactivity disorder. Lancet 366:237–248

Biederman J, Wilens T, Mick E, Spencer T, Faraone S (1999) Pharmacotherapy of attention-deficit/hyperactivity disorder. Lancet 366:237–248

Bieniek SA, Ownby RL, Penalver A, Dominguez RA (1998) A double-blind study of lorazepam versus the combination of haloperidol and lorazepam in managing agitation. Pharmaotherapy 18:57–62

Birbaumer N, Kubler A, Ghanayim N, Hinterberger T, Perelmouter J, Kaiser J, Iversen I, Kotchoubey B, Neumann N, Flor H (2000) The thought translation device (TTD) for completely paralyzed patients. IEEE Trans Rehabil Eng 8(2):190–193

Bird ED, Coyle JT (1986) Huntington's disease. In: Herman S, Bachelard HS, Lunt GG, Marsden CD (eds) Clinical Neurochemistry. Academic Press Inc, London, pp 1–57

Björklund A (1992) Dopaminergic transplants in experimental parkinsonism: cellular mechanisms of graft-induced functional recovery. Curr Opin Neurobiol 2:683–689

Björklund A (2005) Cell therapy for Parkinson's disease: problems and prospects. Novartis Found Symp 265:174–86

Björklund A, Stenevi U (1979) Reconstruction of the nigrostriatal dopamine pathway by intracerebral nigral transplants. Brain Res 177:555–560

Bjornson CR, Rietze RL, Reynolds BA, Magli MC, Vescovi AL (1999) Turning brain into blood: a hematopoietic fate adopted by adult neural stem cells in vivo. Science 283:534–537

Bleuler E (1916) Lehrbuch der Psychiatrie. Springer, Berlin

Bloch J, Bachoud-Lévi AC, Deglon N, Lefaucheur JP, Winkel L, Palfi S, Nguyen JP, Bourdet C, Gaura V, Remy P, Brugieres P, Boisse MF, Baudic S, Cesaro P, Hantraye P, Aebischer P, Peschanski M (2004) Neuroprotective gene therapy for Huntington's disease, using polymer-encapsulated cells engineered to secrete human ciliary neurotrophic factor: results of a phase I study. Hum Gene Ther 15:968–975

BMA British Medical Association (1988) BMA guidelines on the use of fetal tissue. Lancet 1:1119

Boer GJ (1994) Ethical guidelines for the use of human embryonic or fetal tissue for experimental and clinical neurotransplantation and research. Journal of Neurology 242:1–13

Boer GJ (1996) The self-restraining ethical guidelines of NECTAR for the clinical neurotransplantation investigations. In: Hubig C, Poser H (eds) Cognitio Humana – Dynamik des Wissens und der Werte. Universität Leipzig, Leipzig, pp 1420–1427

Boer GJ (1999) Ethical issues in neurografting of human embryonic cells. Theor Med Bioeth 20:461–475

Boer GJ, Widner H (2002) Clinical neurotransplantation: core assessment protocol rather than sham surgery as control. Brain Res Bull 58:547–553

Boer GJ (2006) Restorative therapies for Parkinson's disease: ethical issues. In: Brundin P, Olanow CW (eds) Restorative Therapies for Parkinson's Disease. Springer, New York, pp 12–49

Boorse C (1975) On the distinction between disease and illness. Philosophy and Public Affairs 5(1):49–68

Boorse C (1977) Health as a theoretical concept. Philosophy of Science 44(4):542–573

Boorse C (1997) A rebuttal on health. In: Humber JM, Almeder RF (eds) What is Disease? Humana Press, Totowa, NJ, pp 1–134

Bopp J, Burtchaell JT (1988) Report of the Human Fetal Tissue Research Panel, vol 1. US Government Printing Office, Washington

Borlongan CV, Saporta S, Poulos SG, Othberg A, Sanberg PR (1998) Viability and survival of hNT neurons determine degree of functional recovery in grafted ischemic rats. NeuroReport 9:2837–2842

Borlongan CV, Skinner SJ, Geaney M, Vasconcellos AV, Elliott RB, Emerich DF (2004) Intracerebral transplantation of porcine choroid plexus provides structural and functional neuroprotection in a rodent model of stroke. Stroke 35:2206–2210

Bosco E, D'Agosta L, Mancini P, Traisci G, D'Elia C, Filipo R (2005) Speech perception results in children implanted with Clarion devices: Hi-resolution and standard resolution modes. Acta Otolaryngol 125(2):148–158

Bothe HW, Engel M (1998) Neurobionik. Umschau, Frankfurt am Main

Bradley C (1937) The behaviour of children receiving benzedrine. American Journal of Psychiatry 94:577–585

Bradley C, Bowen M (1940) School performance of children receiving amphetamine (benzedrine) sulfate. Am J Orthopsychiatry 10:782–788

Bradley C, Bowen M (1941) Amphetamine (benzedrine) therapy of children's behavior disorders. Am J Orthopsychiatry 11:92–103
Bradley C, Green E (1940) Psychometric performance of children receiving amphetamine (benzedrine) sulfate. Am J Psychiatry 97:388–394
Brazelton TR, Rossi FM, Keshet GI, Blau HM (2000) From marrow to brain: expression of neuronal phenotypes in adult mice. Science 290:1775–1779
Brent DA (2004) Antidepressants and pediatric depression – the risk of doing nothing. The New England Journal of Medcine 351(16):1598–1601
Brindley GS, Lewin WS (1968) The sensations produced by electrical stimulation of the visual cortex. J Physiol 196(2):479–93
Brock DW (2003) Genetic Engineering. In: Frey RG, Wellman CH (eds) A Companion to Applied Ethics. Blackwell, Oxford, pp 356–368
Brundin P, Dunnett S, Björklund A, Nikkhah G (2001) Transplanted dopaminergic neurons: more or less? Nat Med 7:512–513
Brundin P, Karlsson J, Emgård M, Kaminski Schierle GS, Hansson O, Petersen A, Castilho RF (2000) Improving the survival of grafted dopaminergic neurons: a review over current approaches. Cell Transplant 9:179–195
Buchanan A, Brock DW, Daniels N, Wikler D (2000) From Chance to Choice. Genetics & Justice. Cambrige University Press, Cambridge
Buckley PF (2001) Broad therapeutic use of atypical antipsychotic medications. Biol Psychiatry 50:912–924
Burke J, Loeber R, Birmaher B (2002) Practice parameter for the use of stimulant medications in the treatment of children, adolescents and adults. Journal of the American Academy of Child & Adolescent Psychiatry 41(2):26–49
Buss S (2002) Personal Autonomy. In: Stanford Encyclopedia of Philosophy. http://plato.stanford.edu/contents.html
Butcher J (2003) Cognitive enhancement raises ethical concerns. The Lancet 362:132–133
Butler D (1998) Last chance to stop and think on risks of xenotransplants. Nature 391:320–324
Caldwell JJ, Caldwell J, Smythe NR, Hall K (2000) A double-blind, placebo-controlled investigation of the efficacy of modafinil for sustaining the alertness and performance of aviators: a helicopter simulator study. Psychopharmacology 150:272–282
Calmels MN, Saliba I, Wanna G, Cochard N, Fillaux J, Deguine O, Fraysse B (2004) Speech perception and speech intelligibility in children after cochlear implantation. Int J Pediatr Otorhinolaryngol 68(3):347–351
Campbell M, Rapoport JL, Simpson GM (1999) Antipsychotics in children and adolescents. J Am Acad Child Adolesc Psychiatry 38:537–545
Canterbury R (2003) Deep brain stimulation for obsessive-compulsive disorder, Editorial. J Neurosurg 98:941–942
Caplan AL, Engelhardt T Jr, McCartney JJ (eds) (1981) Concepts of Health and Disease. Interdisciplinary Perspectives. Reading
Carlezon WA Jr, Konradi C (2004) Understanding the neurobiological consequences of early exposure to psychotropic drugs: linking behavior with molecules. Neuropharmacology 47:47–60
Carmena JM, Lebedev MA, Crist RE, O'Doherty JE, Santucci DM, Dimitrov DF, Patil PG, Henriquez CS, Nicolelis MA (2003) Learning to control a brain-machine interface for reaching and grasping by primates. PLoS Biol 1(2):E42
Carpenter LL, Friehs GM, Price LH (2003) Cervical vagus nerve stimulation for treatment-resistant depression. Neurosurg Clin N Am 14(2):275–282
Carpenter RH (2002) Reaching out: Cortical Mechanisms of Directed Action. Curr Biol 12(15):R517–R519

Cattaneo L, Voss M, Brochier T, Prabhu G, Wolpert DM, Lemon RN (2005) A cortico-cortical mechanism mediating object-driven grasp in humans. Proc Natl Acad Sci USA 102(3):898–903

Cedarbaum JM, Chapman C, Charatan M, Stambler N, Andrews L, Zhan C, Radka S, Morrisey D, Lakings D, Brooks BR (1995) The pharmacokinetics of subcutaneously administered recombinant human ciliary neurotrophic factor (rHCNTF) in patients with amyotrophic lateral sclerosis: Relation to parameters of the acute-phase response. Clin Neuropharmacol 18:500–514

Challas G, Brauer W (1963) Tourette's disease: relief of symptoms with R 1625. Am J Psychiatry 120:283–284

Chapel J, Brown N, Jenkins R (1964) Tourette's disease: symptomatic relief with haloperidol. Am J Psychiatry 121:608–610

Chapin JK, Moxon KA, Markowitz RS, Nicolelis MA (1999) Real-time control of a robot arm using simultaneously recorded neurons in the motor cortex. Nat Neurosci 2(7):664–670

Chatterjee A (2004) Cosmetic neurology. The controversy over enhancing movement, mentation, and mood. Neurology 63:968–974

Chauvet GA, Berger TW (2002) Hierarchical model of the population dynamics of hippocampal dentate granule cells. Hippocampus 12(5):698–712

Chen R, Han DD, Gu HH (2005) A triple mutation in the second transmembrane domain of mouse dopamine transporter markedly decreases sensitivity to cocaine and methylphenidate. J Neurochem 94:352–359

Cheng H, Liao KK, Liao SF, Chuang TY, Shih YH (2004) Spinal cord repair with acidic fibroblast growth factor as a treatment for a patient with chronic paraplegia. Spine 29:E 284–288

Chilcoat HD, Breslau N (1999) Pathways from ADHD to early drug use. Journal of the American Academy of Child and Adolescent Psychiatry 38(11):1347–1354

Chow AY, Chow VY (1997) Subretinal electrical stimulation of the rabbit retina. Neurosci Lett 225(1):13–6

Chow, AY, Chow VY, Packo, KH, Pollack JS, Peyman GA, Schuchard R (2004) The artificial silicon retina microchip for the treatment of vision loss from retinitis pigmentosa. Arch Ophthalmol 122(4):460–469

Chow AY, Pardue MT, Chow VY, Peyman GA, Liang C, Perlman JI, Peachey NS (2001) Implantation of silicon chip microphotodiode arrays into the cat subretinal space. IEEE Trans Neural Syst Rehabil Eng 9(1):86–95

Christman J (ed) (1989) The Inner Citadel: Essays on Individual Autonomy. Oxford University Press, New York

Chu K, Kim M, Jung KH, Jeon D, Lee ST, Kim J, Jeong SW, Kim SU, Lee SK, Shin HS, Roh JK (2004) Human neural stem cell transplantation reduces spontaneous recurrent seizures following pilocarpine-induced status epilepticus in adult rats. Brain Res 1023:213–221

Cibelli JB, Kiessling AA, Cunniff K, Richards C, Lanza RP, West MD (2001) Somatic cell nucleus transfer in humans: pronuclear and early embryonic development. J Regen Med 2:25–31

Clark A (2005) Intrinsic content, active memory and the extended mind. Analysis 65:1–11

Clark A, Chalmers D (1998) The extended mind. Analysis 58:7–19

Clark GM, Tong YC, Martin LF (1981) A multiple channel cochlear implant: an evaluation using open-set CID sentences. Laryngoscope 91:628–634

Clark PA (2002) Placebo surgery for Parkinson's disease: do the benefits outweigh the risks? J Law Med Ethics 30:58–68

CNESVS (National Consultative Ethics Committee for Life Sciences and Health) (1984) Recommendation on the Use of Embryo Tissue as well as Tissue of Dead Foetuses for Therapeutic, Diagnostic and Scientific Purposes. Le Comité, Paris

CNESVS (National Consultative Ethics Committee for Life Sciences and Health) (1990) Statement on Intracerebral Graft of Mesencephalic Tissue of Human Embryo Origin in Patients with Parkinsonism for Therapeutic Experimentation. Le Comité, Paris

Cochlear Corp (2005) New developments in Cohlea Implant technology. Healthy Aims Dissemination Day, Freiburg, 1.12.2005

Coffman KL, Sher L, Hoffman A, Rojter S, Folk P, Cramer DV, Vierling J, Villamel F, Podesta L, Demetriou A, Makowka L (1998) Survey results of transplant patient's attitudes on xenografting. Psychosometics 39:379–383

Colaizzi J (2005) Seclusion & restraint. A historical perspective. Journal of Psychosocial Nursing 43:31–37

Cole J (1995) Pride and a Daily Marathon. MIT Press, Cambridge, Mass

Colletti V, Carner M, Miorelli V, Colletti L, Guida M, Fiorino F (2004) Auditory brainstem implant in posttraumatic cochlear nerve avulsion. Audiol Neurootol 9(4):247–255

Colletti, V, Carner M, Miorelli V, Guida M, Colletti L, Fiorino F (2005) Auditory brainstem implant (ABI): new frontiers in adults and children. Otolaryngol Head Neck Surg 133(1):126–138

Colletti V, Fiorino F, Carner M, Sacchetto L, Miorelli V, Orsi A (2002) Auditory brainstem implantation: the University of Verona experience. Otolaryngol Head Neck Surg 127(1):84–96

Colletti V, Fiorino F, Sacchetto L, Miorelli V, Carner M (2001) Hearing habilitation with auditory brainstem implantation in two children with cochlear nerve aplasia. Int J Pediatr Otorhinolaryngol 20; 60(2):99–111

Colletti V, Shannon RV (2005) Open set speech perception with auditory brainstem implant? Laryngoscope 115(11):1974-1978

Comité Consultatif National d'Ethique pour les sciences de la vie et de la santé (2002) La neurochirurgie fonctionelle d'affections psychiatriques sévères. Avis N 71, 25 avril 2002

Cooper P (2005) Education in the age of Ritalin. In: Rees D, Rose S (eds) The New Brain Sciences. Perils and Prospects. Cambridge University Press, Cambridge, pp 249–262

Copray S, Balasubramaniyan V, Levenga J, de Bruijn J, Liem R, Boddeke E (2006) Olig2 overexpression induces the in-vitro differentiation of neural stem cells into mature oligodendrocytes. Stem Cells 24:1001–1010

Cosgrove R (2004) Deep brain stimulation and psychosurgery, Editorial. J Neurosurg 101:574–576

Cosyns P, Caemaert J, Haaijman W, van Veelen C, Gybels J, van Manen J, Ceha J (1994) Functional stereotactic neurosurgery for psychiatric disorders: An experience in Belgium and The Netherlands. Adv Tech Stand Neurosurg 21:239–279

Cosyns P, Gabriëls L, Nuttin B (2003) Deep brain stimulation in treatment-refractory obsessive-compulsive disorder. Verh K Acad Geneeskd Belg 65(6):385–399; Discussion 399–400

Council of Europe (1997) Convention for the Protection of Human Rights and Dignity of the Human Being with Regard to the Application of Biology and Medicine. European Treaty Series 164

CPMP Working Party on Efficacy of Medicinal Products (1990) EEC Note for guidance: Good clinical practice for trials on medicinal products in the European Community. Pharmacol Toxicol 67:361–72

Craelius W (2002) The bionic man: restoring mobility. Science 295(5557):1018–1021

Croonenberghs J, Fegert JM, Findling RL, De Smedt G, Van Dongen S (2005) Risperidone in children with behavior disorders and subaverage intelligence: A 1-year, open-label study of 504 patients. J Am Acad Child Adolesc Psychiatry1:64–72

Crouch RA (1997) Letting the deaf be deaf. Reconsidering the use of cochlear implants in prelingually deaf children. Hastings Cent Rep 27(4):14–21
Crumley FE (1990) Chemical restraint? J Am Acad Child Adolesc Psychiatry 29:982
Cutts KK, Jasper HH (1939) Effect of benzedrine sulphate and phenobarbital on behavior problem children with abnormal electroencephalograms. Arch Neurol Psychiatr 41:1138
Daar AS (1997) Ethics of xenotransplantation: animal issues, consent, and the likely transformation of transplant ethics. World J Surg 21:975–982
Daar AS (1998) Analysis of factors for the prediction of the response to xenotransplantation. Ann NY Acad. Sci 862:222–233
Daniels N (1985) Just Health Care. Cambridge University Press, New York
Daniels N (1996) Justice and Justification. Reflective Equilibrium in Theory and Practice. Cambridge University Press, Cambridge
Daniels N (2000) Normal functioning and the treament-enhancement distinction. Camb Q Healthc Ethics 9:309–322
Daniels N, Sabin JE (1996) Determining "medical necessity" in mental health practice. In: Daniels N, Justice and Justification. Reflective Equilibrium in Theory and Practice. Cambridge University Press, Cambridge, pp 232–256
Danto AC (1981) The Transfiguration of the Commonplace. Harvard University Press, Cambridge, Mass
Danto AC (1985) Narration and Knowledge. Columbia University Press, New York
Das GD, Altman J (1971) Transplanted precursors of nerve cells: their fate in the cerebellum of young rats. Science 173:637–638
Das S, Buchman CA (2005) Bilateral cochlear implantation: current concepts. Curr Opin Otolaryngol Head Neck Surg, 13(5):290–293
Date I, Shingo T, Ohmoto T, Emerich DF (1997) Long-term enhanced chromaffin cell survival and behavioral recovery in hemiparkinsonian rats with co-grafted polymer-encapsulated human NGF-secreting cells. Exp Neurol 147:10–17
Davis KL Charney D, Coyle JT, Nemeroff C (eds) (2002) Neuropsychopharmacology: The Fifth Generation of Progress. Lippincott Williams & Wilkins, New York
Deacon T, Dinsmore J, Costantini LC, Ratliff J, Isacson O (1998) Blastula-stage stem cells can differentiate into dopaminergic and serotonergic neurons after transplantation. Exp Neurol 149:28–41
Defer GL, Geny C, Ricolfi F, Fenelon G, Monfort JC, Remy P, Villafane G, Jeny R, Samson Y, Keravel Y, Gaston A, Degos JD, Peschanski M, Cesaro P, Nguyen JP (1996) Long-term outcome of unilaterally transplanted Parkinsonian patients. I. clinical approach. Brain 119:41–50
Defer GL, Widner H, Marie RM, Remy P, Levivier M (1999) Core assessement program for surgical interventional therapies in Parkinsons' disease (CAPSIT-PD). Movement Disorder 14:572–584
DeGiorgio CM, Schachter SC, Handforth A, Salinsky M, Thompson J, Uthman B, Reed R, Collins S, Tecoma E, Morris GL, Vaughn B, Naritoku DK, Henry T, Labar D, Gilmartin R, Labiner D, Osorio I, Ristanovic R, Jones J, Murphy J, Ney G, Wheless J, Lewis P, Heck C (2000) Prospective long-term study of vagus nerve stimulation for the treatment of refractory seizures. Epilepsia 41(9):1195–1200
DeGranpere R (1999) Ritalin Nation. Norton, New York
DeGrazia D (2005) Human Identity and Bioethics. Cambridge University Press, Cambridge
Dekkers WJM, Boer GJ (2001) Sham surgery in patients with Parkinson's disease: is it morally acceptable? J Med Ethics 27:151–156
De la Fuente-Fernandez R, Ruth TJ, Sossi V, Schulzer M, Calne DB, Stoessel AJ (2001) Expectation and dopamine release: mechanism of the placebo effect in Parkinson's disease. Science 293:1164–1166
Delay J, Deniker P (1955) Neuroleptic effects of chlorpromazine in therapeutics of neuropsychiatry. Int Rec Med Gen Pract Clin 168:318–26

Delgado JM (1952) Responses evoked in waking cat by electrical stimulation of motor cortex. Am J Physiol 171(2):436–446
Delgado JM (1967) Aggression and defense under cerebral radio control. UCLA Forum Med Sci 7:171–193
Delgado JM (1969) Physical control of the mind. Harper & Row, New York
Delgado JM, Anand BK (1953) Increase of food intake induced by electrical stimulation of the lateral hypothalamus. Am J Physiol 172(1):162–168
Delgado JM, Delgado-Garcia JM, Grau C (1976) Mobility controlled by feedback cerebral stimulation in monkeys. Physiol Behav 16(1):43–49
Delgado JM, Hamlin H, Chapman WP (1952) Technique of intracranial electrode implacement for recording and stimulation and its possible therapeutic value in psychotic patients. Confin Neurol 12(5–6):315–319
Delgado JM, Hamlin H, Koskoff YD (1955) Electrical activity after stimulation and electrocoagulation of the human frontal lobe. Yale J Biol Med 28(3–4):233–244
Delgado JM, Lipponen V, Weiss G, Del Pozo F, Monteagudo JL, McMahon R (1975) Two-way transdermal communication with the brain. Am Psychol 30(3):265–273
Delgado JM, Rosvold HE, Looney E (1956) Evoking conditioned fear by electrical stimulation of subcortical structures in the monkey brain. J Comp Physiol Psychol 49(4):373–380
Dell P, Olson R (1951) Projections 'secondaires' mesencephaliques, diencephaliques et amygdaliennes des afferences viscerales vagales. C R Soc Biol 145:1088–1091
DeMause L (ed) (1974) The history of childhood. New York, Harper Torchbook
Dennett D (1992) The self as a center of narrtaive gravity. In: Kessel F, Cole P, Johnson D (eds) Self and Consciousness: Multiple Perspectives. Erlbaum, Hillsdale
Department of Health and Human Services. Health Care Financing Administration (1999) 42 CFR part 482, Medicare and Medicaid programs; hospital condition of participation: patients′ rights; interim final rule with comment
Deutsch A (1949) The mentally ill in America: a history of their care and treatment form colonial times. Columbia University, New York
Devinsky O (1999) Patients with refractory seizures. N Engl J Med 340:1565–1570
De Wert G (2002) The use of human embryonic stem cells for research: an ethical evaluation. Prog Brain Res 138:405–470
De Wert G, Berghmans RL, Boer GJ, Andersen S, Brambati B, Carvalho AS, Dierickx K, Elliston S, Nunez P, Osswald W, Vicari M (2002) Ethical guidance on human embryonic and fetal tissue transplantation: a European overview. Med Health Care Philos 5:79–90
Diederich NJ, Goetz CG (2000) Neuropsychological and behavioral aspects of transplants in Parkinson's disease and Huntington's disease. Brain Cogn 42:294–306
Diller LH (1998) Running on Ritalin: A Physician Reflects on Children, Society and Performance on a Pill. Bantam Books, New York
Djourno A, Eyries C (1957) Prothèse auditive par excitation électrique à distance du nerf sensoriel à l'aide d'un bobinage inclus à demeure. Presse Méd 35:1417–1423
Dobelle WH (2000) Artificial vision for the blind by connecting a television camera to the visual cortex. Asaio J 46(1):3–9
Dobelle WH, Mladejovsky MG (1974) Phosphenes produced by electrical stimulation of human occipital cortex, and their application to the development of a prosthesis for the blind. J Physiol 243(2):553–76
Donoghue JP (2002) Connecting cortex to machines; recent advances in brain interfaces. Nature Neuroscience Suppl 5:1085–1088
Dorfman DH, Kastner B (2004) The use of restraint for pediatric patients in emergency departments. Pediatric Emergency Care 20:151–156
Dougherty DD, Bonab AA, Spencer TJ, Rauch SL, Madras BK, Fischman AJ (1999) Dopamine transporter density in patients with attention deficit hyperactivity disorder. Lancet 354:2132–2133

Doyle JH, Doyle JB, Turnbull FM Jr (1964) Electrical stimulation of the eighth cranial nerve. Arch Otolaryngol 80:388–391

Dulcan M (1997) Practice parameters for the assessment and treatment of children, adolescents, and adults with attention-deficit/hyperactivity disorder. American Academy of Child and Adolescent Psychiatry. J Am Acad Child Adolesc Psychiatry 36(10 Supp):85–121

Dunnett SB, Björklund A, Lindvall O (2001) Cell therapy in Parkinson's disease – stop or go? Nat Rev Neurosci 2:365–369

Dunnett SB, Isacson O, Sirinathsinghji DJS, Clark DJ, Björklund A (1988) Striatal grafts in rats with unilateral neostriatal lesions. III. Recovery from dopamine-dependent motor asymmetry and deficits in skilled paw reaching. Neuroscience 24:813–820

Dunning JJ (2006) Genetic manipulation of learning and memory. In: Kaplitt MG, During M (eds) Gene therapy in the central nervous system, from bench to bedside. Academic Press, Amsterdam, pp 167–179

Dunning JJ, White DJ, Wallwork J (1994) The rationale for xenotransplantation as a solution to the donor organ shortage. Pathol Biol 42:231–235

DuPaul GJ, Barkley RA, McMurray MB (1994) Response of children with ADHD to methylphenidate: interaction with internalizing symptoms. J Am Acad Child Adolesc Psychiatry 33:894–903

During MJ, Kaplitt MG, Stern MB, Eidelberg D (2001) Subthalamic GAD gene transfer in Parkinson disease patients who are candidates for deep brain stimulation. Hum Gene Ther 12:1589–1591

During MJ, Samulski RJ, Elsworth JD, Kaplitt MG, Leone P, Xiao X, Li J, Freese A, Taylor JR, Roth RH, Sladek JR, O'Malley KL, Redmond DE (1998) In vivo expression of therapeutic human genes for dopamine production in the caudates of MPTP-treated monkeys using an AAV vector. Gene Ther 5:820–827

Durston S, Tottenham NT, Thomas KM (2003) Differential patterns of striatal activation in young children with and without ADHD. Biol Psychiatry 53:871–878

Dutch Health Council (2002) Stem cells for tissue repair. 09E, The Hague, The Netherlands

Dworkin G (1971) Paternalism. In: Wasserstrom RA (1971) Morality and the Law. Wadsworth, Belmont, pp 108–122

EC Directive of the European Parliament and Council (2003) Setting Standards of Quality and Safety for the Donation, Procurement, Testing, Processing, Storage and Distribution of Human Tissues and Cells. 2002/0128 (COD), adopted A5–0387, Brussels

Eckmiller R (1997) Learning retina implants with epiretinal contacts. Ophthalmic Res 29(5):281–289

Edgerton BJ, House WF, Hitselberger W (1982) Hearing by cochlear nucleus stimulation in humans. Ann Otol Rhinol Laryngol suppl 91 (2 Pt 3):117–124

Elger G, Hoppe C, Falkai P, Rush A J, Elger CE (2000) Vagus nerve stimulation is associated with mood improvements in epilepsy patients. Epilepsy Res 42 (2–3):203–210

Elliger T (1991) Methylphenidat – aktuelle Verordnungszahlen. Z Kinder- und Jugendpsychiat 19:268–270

Elliott C, Chambers T (2004) Prozac as a Way of Life. University North Carolina Press, Chapel Hill London

Elliott R, Sahakian BJ, Matthews K, Bannerjea A, Rimmer J, Robbins TW (1997) Effects of methylphenidateon spatial working memory and planning in healthy young adults. Psychopharmacology 131:196–206

Emerich DF, Lindner MD, Winn SR, Chen EY, Frydel BR, Kordower JH (1996) Implants of encapsulated human CNTF-producing fibroblasts prevent behavioral deficits and striatal degeneration in a rodent model of Huntington's disease. J Neurosci 16:5168–5181

Emerich DF, Winn SR, Hantraye PM, Peschanski M, Chen EY, McDermott P, Baetge EE, Kordower JH (1997) Encapsulated CNTF-producing cells protect monkeys in a model of Huntington's disease. Nature 386:395–398

Endres M, Namura S, Shiiza Sasamata M, Waeber C, Zhang I, Gomes Isla T, Hyman BT, Moskowitz MA (1998) Attenuation of delayed neuronal death after mild focal ischemia in mice by inhibition of the caspase family. J Cereb Blood Flow Metab 18:238–247

Engelhardt T (1996) The Foundations of Bioethics (2nd ed) Oxford University Press, Oxford New York

Englert H (2006) Hört, hört! Gehirn&Geist 7–8:63–70

Entorf H, Fegert JM, Kölch M (2004) Children in need of medical innovation. In: Discussion Paper No. 04-49, ZEW Zentrum für Europäische Wirtschaftsforschung GmbH, p 28

Eriksdotter Jonhagen M, Nordberg A, Amberla K, Backman L, Ebendal T, Meyerson B, Olson L, Seiger, Shigeta M, Theodorsson E, Viitanen M, Winblad B, Wahlund LO (1998) Intracerebro-ventricular infusion of nerve growth factor in three patients with Alzheimer's disease. Dement Geriatr Cogn Disord 9:246–257

Eysenck HJ (1965) Persönlichkeitstheorie und psychodiagnostische Tests. Diagnostica 11:3–27

Fabiani GE, McFarland DJ, Wolpaw JR, Pfurtscheller G (2004) Conversion of EEG activity into cursor movement by a brain-computer interface (BCI). IEEE Trans Neural Syst Rehabil Eng 12(3):331–338

Falci S, Holtz A, Akesson E, Azizi M, Ertzgaard P, Hultling C, Kjaeldgaard A, Levi R, Ringden O, Westgren M, Lammertse D, Seiger A (1997) Obliteration of a post-traumatic spinal cord cyst with solid human embryonic spinal cord grafts: first clinical attempt. J Neurotrauma 14:875–884

Falkner F, Tanner JM (eds) (1978) Human growth 1, Principles and Prenatal Growth. Baillière Tindall, London

Farah MJ (2002) Emerging ethical issues in neuroscience. Nature Neuroscience 5:1123–1129

Farah MJ (2005) Neuroethics: The practical and the philosophical. Trends in Cognitive Sciences 9:34–40

Farah MJ, Illes J, Cook-Deegan R, Gardner H, Kandel E, King P, Parens E, Sahakian B, Wolpe PR (2004) Neurocognitive enhancement: what can we do and what should we do? Nat Rev Neurosci 5(5):421–425

Fassas A, Passweg JR, Anagnostopoulos A, Kazis A, Kozak T, Havrdova E, Carreras E, Graus F, Kashyap A, Openshaw H, Schipperus M, Deconinck E, Mancardi G, Marmont A, Hansz J, Rabusin M, Zuazu Nagore FJ, Besalduch J, Dentamaro T, Fouillard L, Hertenstein B, La Nasa G, Musso M, Papineschi F, Rowe JM, Saccardi R, Steck A, Kappos L, Gratwohl A, Tyndall A, Samijn J (2002) Autoimmune disease working Party of the EBMT (European group for blood and marrow transplantation). Hematopoietic stem cell transplantation for multiple sclerosis. A retrospective multicenter study. J Neurol 249:1088–1097

Favazza AR (1998) The coming of age of self-mutilation. The Journal of Nervous and Mental Disease 186(5):259–268w

Fegert JM (1999) Eugenik und die Phantasie vom Designerkind aus kinder-, jugendpsychiatrischer und psychotherapeutischer Sicht. In: Byrd BS, Hruschke J, Joerden JC (eds) Annual Review of Law and Ethics. Jahrbuch für Recht und Ethik. Duncker & Humblot, Berlin, pp 239–255

Fegert JM (2001) Methylphenidat und kein Ende? Ist die medikamentöse Behandlung des hyperkinetischen Syndroms tatsächlich ein Thema für Suchtmediziner? Suchtmedizin in Forschung und Praxis 3:185–186

Fegert JM (2002) Psychopharmakotherapie – Happy Pills oder chemische Zwangsjacke? In: Knopp M-L, Ott G (eds) Total durchgeknallt. Hilfen für Kinder und Jugendliche in psychischen Krisen. Psychiatrie-Verlag, Bonn, pp 184–190

Fegert JM (2003) Ethical and legal problems in treating schizophrenic patients with neuroleptics during childhood and adolescence. Child Adolesc Psychophamacol 8:5

Fegert JM (2004a) Depressionsbehandlung mit SSRI in der Kinder- und Jugendpsychiatrie – Ein Forschungs- oder ein Informationsdebakel? Nervenheilkunde 23:60–64

Fegert JM (2004b) Förderung der seelischen Gesundheit und Prävention im Kindes- und Jugendalter. In: Aktion Psychisch Kranke, Schmidt-Zadel R, Kunze H, Peukert R (eds) Prävention bei psychischen Erkrankungen. Neue Wege in Praxis und Gesetzgebung. Psychiatrie-Verlag, Bonn, pp 91–124

Fegert JM, Glaeske G, Janhsen K, Ludolph A, Ronge C (2002) Arzneimittel-Versorgung von Kindern mit hyperkinetischen Störungen anhand von Leistungsdaten der GKV. In: Projektbericht Kooperationsprojekt Universität Bremen, Zentrum für Public Health – Universitätsklinikum Ulm, Klinik für Kinder- und Jugendpsychiatrie/Psychotherapie

Fegert JM, Häßler F, Rothärmel S (1999) Atypische Neuroleptika in der Jugendpsychiatrie. Schattauer Verlag, Stuttgart New York

Fegert JM, Herpertz-Dahlmann B (2004) Editorial. Zum Einsatz von selektiven Serotoninwiederaufnahmehemmern (SSRI) bei depressiven Kindern und Jugendlichen. Zeitschrift für Kinder- und Jugendpsychiatrie und Psychotherapie 32(2):74–75

Fegert JM, Herpertz-Dahlmann B (2005) Serotoninwiederaufnahme-Hemmer im Kindes- und Jugendalter. Warnhinweise der Behörden, Analyseergebnisse und Empfehlungen. Der Nervenarzt, online first

Fegert JM, Jahnsen K, de Jong-van den Berg LTW, Zito JM (2004) SSRI Use in Children and Adolescents in Europe and the United States: Cause of Concern? IACAPAP, Berlin

Fegert JM, Kölch M, Zito JM, Glaeske G, Janhsen K (2006) Antidepressant use in children and adolescents in Germany. Journal of Child and Adolescent Psychopharmacology 16(1/2):197–206

Fegert JM, Wolfslast G (2006) Wissenschaftlicher Ergebnisbericht des Projektes Patientenaufklärung, Informationsbedürfnis und Informationspraxis in der Kinder und Jugendpsychiatrie und Psychotherapie. Vandenhoek & Rupprecht, Göttingen

Feigin A, Kaplitt M, During M, Strybing, K, Cox M, Dhawan V, Eidelberg D (2005) Gene Therapy for Parkinson's disease with AAV-GAD. An open-label, dose escalation, safety-tolerability trial 1. Mov Disorders 20:1236

Feinberg J (1986) Harm to Self. The Moral Limits of the Criminal Law. Vol. III. Oxford University Press, New York

Feinberg J (1992) The child's right to an open future. In: Feinberg J, Freedom and Fulfillment. Chapter 3, Princeton University Press, Princeton, pp 76–97

Felten DL (1994) Cell transplantation and research design. Science 263:1546

Fernandez E, Alfaro A, Tormos JM, Climent R, Martinez M, Vilanova H, Walsh V, Pascual-Leone A (2002) Mapping of the human visual cortex using image-guided transcranial magnetic stimulation. Brain Res Protoc 10(2):115–124

Fernandez E, Ferrandez J, Ammermuller J, Normann RA (2000) Population coding in spike trains of simultaneously recorded retinal ganglion cells. Brain Res 887(1):222–229

Fernandez E, Pelayo F, Romero S, Bongard M, Marin C, Alfaro A, Merabet L (2005) Development of a cortical visual neuroprosthesis for the blind: the relevance of neuroplasticity. J Neural Eng 2(4):R1–R12

Feron F, Perry C, Cochrane J, Licina P, Nowitzke A, Urquhart S, Geraghty T, Mackay-Sim A (2005) Autologous olfactory ensheathing cell transplantation in human spinal cord injury. Brain 128:2951–2960

Ferraro L, Fuxe K, Tanganelli S, Tomasini MC, Rambert FA, Antonelli T (2002) Differential enhancement of dialysate serotonin levels in distinct brain regions of the awake rat by modafinil: possible relevance for wakefulness and depression. J Neurosci Res 68(1):107–12

Feucht M, Laube T, Bornfeld N, Walter P, Velikay-Parel M, Hornig R, Richard G (2005) Development of an epiretinal prosthesis for stimulation of the human retina. Ophthalmologe 102(7):688–691

Fields D (2005) Erasing memories. Scientific American Mind 16:28–35

FIGO (2003) Research on pre-embryos. In: Recommendations on Ethical Issues in Obstetrics and Gynecology by the FIGO Committee for the Ethical Aspects of Human Reproduction and Women's Health, pp 22–23

Findling RL (2004) The Relevance of Pharmacokinetic Studies of Antidepressants. IACAPAP Meeting, Berlin

Findling RL, Fegert JM, De Smedt G (2001) Interim Results from a Multicenter Study of the Long-Term Safety and Efficacy of Risperidone in Children and Adolescents with Severe Disruptive Behaviors and Subaverage IQ. APA Institute on Psychiatric Services, October 10–14, 2001, Orlando, Florida

Fine A (1986) Transplantation in the central nervous system. Sci Am 255:42–52

Fink JS, Schumacher JM, Ellias SL, Palmer EP, Saint-Hilaire M, Shannon K, Penn R, Starr P, VanHorne C, Kott HS, Dempsey PK, Fischman AJ, Raineri R, Manhart C, Dinsmore J, Isacson O (2000) Porcine xenografts in Parkinson's disease and Huntington's disease patients: preliminary results. Cell Transplant 9:273–278

Fish B (1960a) Drug therapy in child psychiatry: pharmacological aspects. Compr Psychiatry 1:212–227

Fish B (1960b) Drug therapy in child psychiatry: psychological aspects. Compr Psychiatry 1:55–61

Flax JD, Aurora S, Yang C, Simonin C, Wills AM, Billinghurst LL, Jendoubi M, Sidman RL, Wolfe JH, Kim SU, Snyder EY (1998) Engraftable human neural stem cells respond to developmental cues, replace neurons and express foreign genes. Nature Biotech 16:1033–1039

Fogassi L, Luppino G (2005) Motor functions of the parietal lobe. Curr Opin Neurobiol 15(6):626–631

Fontaine D, Mattei V, Borg M, van Langsdorff D, Magnie MN, Chanalet S, Robert P, Paquis P (2004) Effect of subthalamic nucleus stimulation on obsessive-compulsive disorder in a patient with Parkinson's disease. J Neurosurg 100:1084–1086

Ford, NM (2002) The Prenatal Person: Ethics from Conception to Birth. Blackwell, Oxford

Fost N (1986) Drugs in sports: A sceptical view. Hastings Center Report 4:5–10

Foster D (2003) Oral presentation. In: Transcripts of Council Discussions of the President's Council on Bioethics. Friday Jan 17th, 2003. Session 6: Neuropsychopharmacology and Public Policy, available at http://bioethics.gov/transcripts/jan03/ session6.html (accessed on November 28th, 2006)

Frank S, Kieburtz K, Holloway R, Kim S (2005) What is the risk of sham surgery in Parkinson disease clinical trials? A review of published reports. Neurology 65:1101–1103

Franke R, Hart D (2006) Die Leistungspflicht der gesetzlichen Krankenversicherung für Heilversuche. Medizinrecht 2006:131–138

Frankfurt HG (1999) Necessity, Volition, and Love. Cambridge University Press, Cambridge

Franklin RJ, Gilson JM, Franceschini IA, Barnett SC (1996) Schwann cell-like myelination following transplantation of an olfactory bulb-ensheathing cell line into areas of demyelination in the adult CNS. Glia 1996(17):217–224

Franz K (1996) Betrachtungen zu Personalität und Gehirn unter dem Blickwinkel der Möglichkeit von Hirngewebetransplantationen. In: Hubig C, Poser H (eds) Cognitio Humana – Dynamik des Wissens und der Werte. Universität Leipzig, Leipzig, pp 1428–1434

Freed CR, Breeze RE, Rosenberg NL, Schneck SA, Kriek E, Qi JX, Lone T, Zhang YB, Snyder JA, Wells TH (1992) Survival of implanted fetal dopamine cells and neurologic improvement 12 to 46 months after transplantation for Parkinson's disease. New Engl J Med 237:1549–1555

Freed CR, Greene PE, Breeze RE, Tsai WY, DuMouchel W, Kao R, Dillon S, Winfield H, Culver S, Trojanowski JQ, Eidelberg D, Fahn S (2001) Transplantation of embryonic dopamine neurons for severe Parkinson's disease. New Engl J Med 344:710–719

Freed CR, Leehey MA, Zawada M, Bjugstad K, Thompson L, Breeze RE (2003) Do patients with Parkinson's disease benefit from embryonic dopamine cell transplantation? J Neurol 250, suppl 3:III 44–46

Freedman AM, Effron AS, Bender L (1955) Pharmacotherapy in children with psychiatric illness. J Nerv Ment Dis 122:479–86

Freedman C (1998) Aspirin for the mind? Some ethical worries about psychopharmacology. In Parens E (ed) Enhancing Human Traits: Ethical and Social Implications. Georgetown University Press, Washington, DC:135–150

Freedman R (2005) The choice of antipsychotic drugs for schizophrenia. New England Journal of Medicine 353:1286–1288

Freeman TB, Vawter D, Goetz CG, Leaverton PE, Cicchetti F, Hauser RA, Deacon TW, Li XJ, Hersch SM, Nauert GM, Sanberg PR, Kordower JH, Saporta S, Isacson O (2000) Transplanted fetal striatum in Huntington's disease: phenotypic development and lack of pathology. Proc Natl Acad Sci USA 97:13877–13882

Freeman TB, Vawter DE, Leaverton PE, Godbold JH, Hauser RA, Goetz CG, Olanow CW (1999) Use of placebo surgery in controlled trials of a cellular-based therapy for Parkinson's disease. New Engl J Med 341:988–991

Freeman TB, Vawter D, Goetz CG, Leaverton PE, Hauser RA, Sanberg PR, Godbold JH, Olanow CW (1997) Towards the use of surgical placebo-controlled trials. Transplant Proceed 29:1925

Freeman TB, Willing A, Zigova T, Sanberg PR, Hauser RA (2001) Neural transplantation in Parkinson's disease. Adv Neurol 86:435–445

Freeman WJ (2000) Neural transplantation, an introduction. The MIT Press, Cambridge, MA London

Freese A (1999) Restorative gene therapy approaches to Parkinson's disease. Med Clin North Am 83:537–548

Friehs GM, Zerris VA, Ojakangas CL, Fellows MR, Donoghue JP (2004) Brain-machine and brain-computer interfaces. Stroke 35(11 suppl 1):2702–2705

Frodl EM, Duan WM, Sauer H, Kupsch A, Brundin P (1994) Human embryonic dopamine neurons xenografted to the rat: effects of cryopreservation and varying regional source of donor cells on transplant survival, morphology and function. Brain Res 647:286–298

Frommer EA (1967) Treatment of childhood depression with antidepressant drugs. BMJ 1:729–732

Frommer EA (1972) Indications for antidepressant treatment with special reference to depressed preschool children. In: Annell AL (ed) Depressive States in childhood and Adolescence. John Wiley & Sons, New York, pp 449–454

Fukuyama F (2002) Our Posthuman Future: Consequences of the Biotechnology Revolution. Farar, Straus & Giroux, New York

Fulford B (2001) What is (mental) disease? An open letter to Christopher Boorse. Journal of Medical Ethics 27:80–85

Gabriëls L (2004) Doctoral Thesis: Electrical brain stimulation in treatment refractory obsessive compulsive disorder

Gabriëls L, Cosyns P, Nuttin B, Demeulemeester H, Gybels J (2003) Deep brain stimulation for treatment-refractory obsessive-compulsive disorder: psychopathological and neuropsychological outcome in 3 cases. Acta Psychiatr Scand 107:275–282

Gage FH, Björklund A, Stenevi U, Dunnett SB, Kelly PAT (1984) Intra-hippocampal septal grafts ameliorate learning impairments in aged rats. Science 225:533–536

Gage FH, Wolff JA, Rosenberg MB, Xu L, Yee JK, Shults C, Friedmann T (1987) Grafting genetically modified cells to the brain: possibilities for the future. Neuroscience 23:795–807

Gaines RA (2003) The value of deaf culture: should states have the right to mandate placement of cochlear implants? Curr Surg 60(6):600–601

Galert T (2005) Vom Schmerz der Tiere. Grundlagenprobleme der Erforschung tierischen Bewußtseins. Mentis, Paderborn

Galpern WR, Burns LH, Deacon TW, Dinsmore J, Isacson O (1996) Xenotransplantation of porcine fetal ventral meencephalon in a rat model of Parkinson's disease: functional recovery and graft morphology. Exp Neurol 140:1–13

Gansbacher B (2003) European Society of Gene Therapy. Report of a second serious adverse event in a clinical trial of gene therapy for X-linked severe combined immune deficiency (X-SCID). Position of the European Society of Gene Therapy (ESGT) J Gene Med 5:261–262

Gareth Jones D (1991) Fetal neural transplantation: placing the ethical debate within the context of society's use of human material. Bioethics 5:23–43

Garland B (ed) (2004) Neuroscience and the law. Brain, mind, and the scales of justice. Dana Press, New York

Gaura V, Bachoud-Lévi AC, Ribeiro MJ, Nguyen JP, Frouin V, Baudic S, Brugieres P, Mangin JF, Boisse MF, Palfi S, Cesaro P, Samson Y, Hantraye P, Peschanski M, Remy P (2004) Striatal neural grafting improves cortical metabolism in Huntington's disease patients. Brain 127:65–72

Gazzaniga MS (2005) The Ethical Brain. Dana Press, New York

George MS, Rush AJ, Marangell LB, Sackeim HA, Brannan SK, Davis SM, Howland R, Kling MA, Moreno F, Rittberg B, Dunner D, Schwartz T, Carpenter L, Burke M, Ninan P, Goodnick P (2005) A one-year comparison of vagus nerve stimulation with treatment as usual for treatment-resistant depression. Biol Psychiatry 58(5):364–373

George MS, Sackeim HA, Rush AJ, Marangell LB, Nahas Z, Husain MM, Lisanby S, Burt T, Goldman J, Ballenger JC (2000) Vagus nerve stimulation: a new tool for brain research and therapy. Biol Psychiatry 47(4):287–295

Gerlach M, Baving L, Fegert JM (2006) Therapie mit Lithiumsalzen in der Kinder- und Jugendpsychiatrie. Klinische Wirksamkeit und praktische Empfehlungen. Zeitschrift der Kinder- und Jugendpsychiatrie und Psychotherapie 34(3):181–189

Gernert M, Thompson KW, Löscher W, Tobin AJ (2002) Genetically engineered GABA-producing cells demonstrate anticonvulsant effects and long-term transgene expression when transplanted into the central piriform cortex of rats. Exp Neurol 176:183–192

Gethmann CF, Gerok W, Helmchen H, Henke K-D, Mittelstraß J, Schmidt-Aßmann E, Stock G, Taupitz J, Thiele F (2005) Gesundheit nach Maß. Akademie-Verlag, Berlin

Gharabaghi A, Hellwig D, Rosahl SK, Shahidi R, Schrader C, Freund HJ, Samii M (2005) Volumetric image guidance for motor cortex stimulation: integration of three-dimensional cortical anatomy and functional imaging. Neurosurgery 57 (1 suppl):114–120

Gholmieh G, Courellis S, Dimoka A, Wills JD, LaCoss J, Granacki JJ, Marmarelis V, Berger T (2004) An algorithm for real-time extraction of population EPSP and population spike amplitudes from hippocampal field potential recordings. J Neurosci Methods 136(2):111–121

Gholmieh G, Courellis S, Marmarelis V, Berger T (2002) An efficient method for studying short-term plasticity with random impulse train stimuli. J Neurosci Methods 121(2): 111–127
Gholmieh G, Soussou W, Courellis S, Marmarelis V, Berger T, Baudry M (2001) A biosensor for detecting changes in cognitive processing based on nonlinear systems analysis. Biosens Bioelectron 16(7–8):491–501
Gillberg C (2000) Typical neuroleptics in child and adolescent psychiatry. European Child & Adolescent Psychiatry 9:I/2–I/8
Glannon W (2006a) Psychopharmacology and memory. Journal of Medical Ethics 32:74–78
Glannon W (2006b) Neuroethics. Bioethics 20:37–52
Glover J (1988) I: The Philosophy and Psychology of Personal Identity. Penguin, London
Goetz CG, Janko K, Blasucci L, Jaglin JA (2003) Impact of placebo assignment in clinical trials of Parkinson's disease. Mov Disord 18:1146–1149
Goodman S (2002) France wires up to treat obsessive disorder. Nature 417(June 13):677
Graimann B, Huggins JE, Levine SP, Pfurtscheller G (2004) Toward a direct brain interface based on human subdural recordings and wavelet-packet analysis. IEEE Trans Biomed Eng 51(6):954–962
Green TA, Nestler EJ (2006) Psychiatric applications of viral vectors. In: Kaplitt MG, During MJ (eds) Gene therapy in the central nervous system, from bench to bedside. Academic Press, Amsterdam, pp 181–193
Greenhill LL, MTA Cooperative Group (1999) Chronic stimulant treatment effects of weight acquisition rates of ADHD children. Boca Raton, Florida, New Clinical Drug Evaluation Unit Program Conference Proceeding 39:26–27
Greenhill LL, Waslick B (2004) Selective Serotonin Reuptake inhibitors for the treatment of depression in 4.100 Children and Adolescents. IACAPAP, Berlin
Groevich SJ, Findling RL, Rowane WA, Friedman L, Schulz SC (1996) Risperidone in the treatment of children and adolescents with schizophrenia: A retrospective study. J Child Adolesc Psychopharmacol 6(4):251–257
Groves DA, Brown VJ (2005) Vagal nerve stimulation: a review of its applications and potential mechanisms that mediate its clinical effects. Neurosci Biobehav Rev 29(3):493–500
Grumet AE, Wyatt JL Jr, Rizzo JF (2000) Multi-electrode stimulation and recording in the isolated retina. J Neurosci Methods 101(1): 31–42
Guilford JP (1959) Personality. McGraw Hill, New York
Guttinger M, Fedele D, Koch P, Padrun V, Pralong WF, Brustle O, Boison D (2005a) Suppression of kindled seizures by paracrine adenosine release from stem cell-derived brain implants. Epilepsia 46:1162–1169
Guttinger M, Padrun V, Pralong WF, Boison D (2005b) Seizure suppression and lack of adenosine A1 receptor desensitization after focal long-term delivery of adenosine by encapsulated myoblasts. Exp Neurol 193:53–64
Gybels J, Cosyns P, Nuttin B (2002) La psychochirurgie en Belgique. Les Cahiers du Comité Consultatif National d'Ethique pour les Sciences de la Vie et de la Santé (la France) 32:18–21
Haberman RP, Samulski RJ, McCown TJ (2003) Attenuation of seizures and neuronal death by adeno-associated virus vector galanin expression and secretion. Nat Med 9:1076–1080
Habermas J (2001) Die Zukunft der menschlichen Natur. Suhrkamp, Frankfurt a.M.
Häßler F, Fegert JM (1999) Psychopharmakotherapie des selbstverletzenden Verhaltens bei Menschen mit geistiger Behinderung. Nervenarzt, 70:1025–1028
Hagell P, Piccini P, Björklund A, Brundin P, Rehncrona S, Widner H, Crabb L, Pavese N, Oertel WH, Quinn N, Brooks DJ, Lindvall O (2002) Dyskinesias following neural transplantation in Parkinson's disease. Nat Neurosci 5:627–628

Hahn T, Wolff SN, Czuczman M, Fisher RI, Lazarus HM, Vose J, Warren L, Watt R, McCarthy PL Jr, ASBMT Expert Panel (2001) The role of cytotoxic therapy with hematopoietic stem cell transplantation in the therapy of diffuse large cell B-cell non-Hodgkin's lymphoma: an evidence-based review. Biol Blood Marrow Transplant 7:308–331

Hall W (2004) Feeling better than well'. EMBO reports 5(12):1105–1109

Hansen JE (2002) Embryonic stem cell production through therapeutic cloning has fewer ethical problems than stem cell harvest from surplus IVF embryos. J Med Ethics 28:86–88

Hansson SO (2005) Implant ethics. J Med Ethics 31(9):519–525

Hantraye P, Riche D, Maziere M, Isacson O (1990) An experimental primate model for Huntington's disease: anatomical and behavioural studies of unilateral excitotoxic lesions of the caudate-putamen in the baboon. Exp Neurol 108:91–104

Harden CL (2002) The co-morbidity of depression and epilepsy: epidemiology, etiology, and treatment. Neurology 59(6 suppl 4):48–55

Harden CL, Pulver MC, Ravdin LD, Nikolov B, Halper JP, Labar DR (2000) A pilot study of mood in epilepsy patients treated with vagus nerve stimulation. Epilepsy Behav 1(2):93–99

Harris J (1998) Clones, Genes, and Immortality. Ethics and the Genetic Revolution. Oxford University Press, Oxford

Hartmann D (1998) Philosophische Grundlagen der Psychologie. Wiss Buchges, Darmstadt

Hartmann D (2000) Willensfreiheit und die Autonomie der Kulturwissenschaften. In: Handlung, Kultur, Interpretation 1:66–103, revised reprint in e-journal Philosophie der Psychologie 1 (2005), http://www.jp.philo.at/texte/HartmannD1.pdf

Hartmann D (2003) On Inferring. An Enquiry into Relevance and Validity. Mentis, Paderborn

Hartmann D, Budagian V, Bulanova E, Orinska Z, Duitman E, Brandt K, Ludwig A, Lemke G, Saftig P, Bulfone-Paus S (2005) Soluble Axl is generated by ADAM10-dependent cleavage and associates with Gas6 in mouse serum. Mol Cell Biol 25:9324–9339

Hauser RA, Freeman TB, Snow BJ, Nauert M, Gauger L, Kordower J, Olanow CW (1999) Long-term evaluation of bilateral fetal nigral transplantation in Parkinson's disease. Arch Neurol 56:179–187

Hauser RA, Furtado S, Cimino CR, Delgado H, Eichler S, Schwartz S, Scott D, Nauert GM, Soety E, Sossi V, Holt DA, Sanberg PR, Stoessl AJ, Freeman TB (2002) Bilateral human fetal striatal transplantation in Huntington's disease. Neurology 58:687–695

Healy D (2004) Let Them Eat Prozac. University Press, New York

Hechtman L, Abikoff H, Klein RG, Greenfield B, Etcovitch J, Cousins L, Fleiss K, Weiss M, Pollack S (2005) Children with ADHD treated with long-term methylphenidate and multimodal psychosocial treatment: Impact on parental practices. Journal of the American Academy of Child & Adolescent Psychiatry 43(7):830–838

Helms J, Muller J, Schon F (2004) Bilateral cochlear implantation, experiences and perspectives. Otolaryngol Pol 58(1):51–52

Heneine W, Tibell A, Switzer WM, Sandstrom P, Rosales GV, Mathews A, Korsgren O, Chapman LE, Folks TM, Groth CG (1998) No evidence of infection with porcine endogenous retrovirus in recipients of porcine islet-cell xenografts. Lancet 352:695–699

Henry TR (2002) Therapeutic mechanisms of vagus nerve stimulation. Neurology 59(6 suppl 4):3–14

HER (European Commission Working Group on Human Embryos and Research) (1994) Second Report, EC Directorate General XII, Science Research and Development, Brussels

Hermens WT, Verhaagen J (1998) Viral vectors, tools for gene transfer in the nervous system. Prog Neurobiol 55:399–432

Hermelin B, Pring L, Buhler M, Wolff S, Heaton P (1999) A visually impaired savant artist: Interacting perceptual and memory representations. Journal of Child Psychology and Psychiatry and Allied Disciplines 40:1129–1139

Hermerén G, Alivizatos N C, de Beaufort I, Capurro R, Englert Y, Labrusse-Riou C, McLaren A, Nielsen L, Puigdomenech-Rosell P, Rodota S, Virt G, Whittacker P (2005) Ethical Aspects of ICT Implants in the human body. Opinion No. 20 of the European Group on Ethics (EGE) in Science and New Technologies to the European Commission

Heuyer G, Gerard G, Galibert J (1953) Traitement de l'excitation psychomotrice chez l'enfant. Arch Franç Pediatr 9:961–963

Hildt E (1996) Hirngewebetransplantation und personale Identität. In: Hubig C, Poser H (eds) Cognitio Humana – Dynamik des Wissens und der Werte. Universität Leipzig, Leipzig, pp 1435–1442

Hildt E (1999a) Ethical aspects of neural tissue transplantation. In: Croatian Medical Journal 40/3, online at http://www.cmj.hr/1999/40/3/10411958.htm

Hildt E (1999b) Hängt die Identität des Menschen von der Identität des Gehirns ab? Zur Problematik von Hirngewebetransplantationen. In: Engels E-M (ed) Biologie und Ethik. Reclam, Stuttgart, pp 257–282

Hochberg LR, Serruya MD, Friehs GM, Mukand JA, Saleh M, Caplan AH, Branner A, Chen D, Penn RD, Donoghue JP (2006) Neuronal ensemble control of prosthetic devices by a human with tetraplegia. Nature 442(7099):164–171

Hoffer BJ, Olson L (1991) Ethical issues in brain-cell transplantation. TINS 14:384–388

Hoffmann H, Dehm J (2005) Neuroprothetik. VDE Initiative Mikromedizin, Frankfurt a.M.

Hofmann B (2001) Complexity of the concept of disease as shown through rival theoretical frameworks. Theoretical Medicine 22:211–236

Holt RF, Kirk KI, Eisenberg LS, Martinez AS, Campbell W (2005) Spoken word recognition development in children with residual hearing using cochlear implants and hearing AIDS in opposite ears. Ear Hear 26(4 suppl):82–91

Hoppe C, Helmstaedter C, Scherrmann J, Elger CE (2001) Self-reported mood changes following 6 months of vagus nerve stimulation in epilepsy patients. Epilepsy Behav 2(4):335–342

House WF, Urban J (1973) Long term results of electrode implantation and electronic stimulation of the cochlea in man. Ann Otol Rhinol Laryngol 82:504–517

Huang H (2005) Basic and clinical researches of olfactory ensheating cells for spinal cord injury. First International Spinal Cord Injury Treeatments and Trials Symposium, Hong Kong, China, 17–20 December

Huang H, Wang H, Gu Z, Li Y, Chen L, Song Y, Hao W, Zhang J, Zhang F (2004) Preliminary Report of Olfactory Ensheathing Cell Transplantatin for Amyotrophic Lateral Sclerosis (ALS). 56th Annual Meeting of American Academy Neurological Surgeons, San Francisco, CA, May 3

Huber A, Padrun V, Deglon N, Aebischer P, Mohler H, Boison D (2001) Grafts of adenosine-releasing cells suppress seizures in kindling epilepsy. Proc Natl Acad Sci USA 98:7611–7616

Huffaker TK, Boss BD, Morgan AS, Neff NT, Strecker RE, Spence MS, Miao R (1989) Xenografting of fetal pig ventral mesencephalon corrects motor asymmetry in the rat model of Parkinson's disease. Exp Brain Res 77:329–336

Hughes J (2004) Citizen Cyborg. Westview Press, Cambridge, MA

Humayun MS (2001) Intraocular retinal prosthesis. Trans Am Ophthalmol Soc 99:271–300

Humayun MS, de Juan E Jr, Dagnelie G, Greenberg RJ, Propst RH, Phillips DH (1996) Visual perception elicited by electrical stimulation of retina in blind humans. Arch Ophthalmol 114(1):40–6

Humayun MS, Freda R, Fine I, Roy A, Fujii G, Greenberg RJ, Little J, Mech B, Weiland JD, de Juan E (2005) Implanted Intraocular Retinal Prosthesis in Six Blind Subjects. Submitted to ARVO (The Association for Research in Vision and Ophthalmology)

Humayun MS, Weiland JD, Fujii GY, Greenberg R, Williamson R, Little J, Mech B, Cimmarusti V, Van Boemel G, Dagnelie G, de Juan E (2003) Visual perception in a blind subject with a chronic microelectronic retinal prosthesis. Vision Res 43(24):2573–2581

Humber JM, Almeder RF (eds) (1997) What is Disease? Humana Press, Totowa NJ

Hume D (2000) Treatise of Human Nature. Ed by Norton DF, Norton MJ. Oxford University Press, Oxford

Husserl E (1900) Logische Untersuchungen. Erster Teil: Prolegomena zur reinen Logik. Niemeyer, Halle a. d. S.

Husserl E (1901) Logische Untersuchungen. Zweiter Teil: Untersuchungen zur Phänomenologie und Theorie der Erkenntnis. Niemeyer, Halle a. d. S.

Husserl E (1913) Ideen zu einer reinen Phänomenologie und phänomenologischen Philosophie. In: Jahrbuch für Philosophie und phänomenologische Forschung 1:1–323

Hwang WS, Ryu YJ, Park JH, Park ES, Lee EG, Koo JM, Jeon HY, Lee BC, Kang SK, Kim SJ, Ahn C, Hwang JH, Park KY, Cibelli JB, Moon SY (2004) Evidence of a pluripotent human embryonic stem cell line derived from a cloned blastocyst. Science 303:1669–1674

Hyman S (2002) Ethical issues in pharmacology: Research and practice. In: Marcus SJ (ed) Neuroethics. Mapping the Field. Dana Press, New York, pp 135–143

Hyde M, Power D (2006) Some ethical dimensions of cochlear implantation for deaf children and their families. J Deaf Stud Deaf Educ 11(1):102–111

Iatrou M, Berger TW, Marmarelis VZ (1999) Application of a novel modeling method to the nonstationary properties of potentiation in the rabbit hippocampus. Ann Biomed Eng 27(5):581–591

Illg A, von der Haar-Heise S, Goldring JE, Lenarz T (1999) Speech perception results for children implanted with the CLARION cochlear implant at the Medical University of Hannover. Ann Otol Rhinol Laryngol suppl 177:93–98

Ingvar M, Ambros-Ingerson J, Davis M, Granger R, Kessler M, Rogers G, Schehr RS and Lynch G (1997) Enhancement by an Ampakine of Memory Encoding in Humans. Experimental Neurology 146:553–559

Isacson, O, Björklund, L, Pernaute RS (2001) Parkinson's disease: interpretations of transplantation study are erroneous. Nat Neurosci 4:553

Isacson O, Breakefield XO (1997) Benefits of hosting animal cells in the human brain. Nature Med 3:964–969

Isacson O, Deacon T (1997) Neural transplantation studies reveal the brain's capacity for continuous reconstruction. TINS 20:477–482

Isacson O, Deacon TW, Pakzaban P, Galpern WR, Dinsmore J, Burns LH (1995) Transplanted xenogeneic neural cells in neurodegenerative disease models exhibit remarkable axonal target specificity and distinct growth patterns of glial and axonal fibres. Nature Med 11:1189–1194

Itakura T, Uematsu Y, Nakao N, Nakai E, Nakai K (1997) Transplantation of autologous sympathetic ganglion into the brain with Parkinson's disease. Long-term follow-up of 35 cases. Stereotact Funct Neurosurg 69:112–115

James C, Albegger K, Battmer R, Burdo S, Deggouj N, Deguine O, Dillier N, Gersdorff M, Laszig RR, Sterkers O, Von Wallenberg E, Weber B, Fraysse B (2005) Preservation of residual hearing with cochlear implantation: how and why. Acta Otolaryngol 125(5):481–491

Jelden E (1996) Personale Identität: Prozeß statt Status. In: Hubig C, Poser H (eds) Cognitio Humana – Dynamik des Wissens und der Werte. Universität Leipzig, Leipzig, pp 144–1450

Jiang Q, Zhang ZG, Ding GL, Zhang L, Ewing JR, Wang L, Zhang R, Li L, Lu M, Meng H, Arbab AS, Hu J, Li QJ, Pourabdollah Nejad DS, Athiraman H, Chopp M (2005) Investigation of neural progenitor cell induced angiogenesis after embolic stroke in rat using MRI. Neuroimage 28:698–707

Jobson KO, Potter WZ (1995) International psychopharmacology algorithm project report. Introduction. Psychopharmacology Bulletin 31:457–507

Johnson AG (1994) Surgery as placebo. The Lancet 344:1140–1142

Johnson WE (1924) Logic, Part III. Cambridge UP, Cambridge

Jones R, Morris K, Nutt D (2005) Cognition Enhancers. Foresight Brain Science, Addiction and Drugs Project. University of Bristol, Bristol

Juengst ET (1998) What does enhancement mean? In Parens E (ed) Enhancing Human Traits: Ethical and Social Implications. Georgetown University Press, Washington, DC:29–47

Kant I (1903/11) Grundlegung zur Metaphysik der Sitten. Akademie-Ausgabe vol IV. Georg Reimer, Berlin, pp 385462

Kant I (1904/11) Kritik der reinen Vernunft. Akademie Ausgabe vol III. Georg Reimer, Berlin

Kant I (1907/14) Die Metaphysik der Sitten. Akademie-Ausgabe vol VI. Georg Reimer, Berlin, pp 203491

Kant I (1907/17) Anthropologie in pragmatischer Hinsicht. Akademie-Ausgabe vol VII. Georg Reimer, Berlin, pp 117–335

Kaplitt MG, During MJ (2006) Gene therapy in the central nervous system, from bench to bedside. Academic Press, Amsterdam

Kazdin AE (1984) Acceptability of aversive procedures and medications as treatment alternatives for deviant child behaviour. J Abnorm Child Psychol 12:289–301

Keller MB, Ryan ND, Strober M, Klein RG, Kutcher SP, Birmaher B, Hagino OR, Koplewicz H, Carlson GA, Clarke GN, Emslie GJ, Feinberg D, Geller B, Kusumakar V, Papatheodorou G, Sack WH, Sweeney M, Wagner KD, Weller EB, Winters NC, Oakes R, McCafferty JP (2001) Efficacy of paroxetine in the treatment of adolescent major depression: a randomized, controlled trial. J Am Acad Child Adolesc Psychiatry 40:762–772

Kelly S, Bliss TM, Shah AK, Sun GH, Ma M, Foo WC, Masel J, Yenari MA, Weissman IL, Uchida N, Palmer T, Steinberg GK (2004) Transplanted human fetal neural stem cells survive, migrate, and differentiate in ischemic rat cerebral cortex. Proc Natl Acad Sci USA 101:11839–11844

Kendall AL, Rayment FD, Torres EM, Baker HF, Ridley RM, Dunnett SB (1998) Functional integration of striatal allografts in a primate model of Huntington's disease. Nat Med 4:727–729

Kenny DA (1979) Correlation and Causality. Wiley, New York

Kersting W (2002) Kritik der Gleichheit. Velbrück, Weilerswist

Khushf G (1997) Why bioethics needs the philosophy of medicine: Some implications of reflections on concepts of health and disease. Theoretical Medicine 18:145–163

Kim SYH, Holloway RG, Frank S, Beck CA, Zimmerman C, Wilson R, Kieburtz K (2006) Volunteering for early phase gene transfer research in Parkinson disease. Neurology 66:1010–1015

Kiss JG, Toth F, Nagy AL, Jarabin J, Szamoskozi A, Torkos A, Jori J, Czigner J (2003) Neural response telemetry in cochlear implant users. Int Tinnitus J 9(1):59–60

Klosterkötter J, Hellmich M, Steinmeyer EM, Schultze-Lutter F (2001) Diagnosing schizophrenia in the initial prodromal phase. Arch Gen Psychiatry 58:158–164

Knutson B, Wolkowitz OM, Cole SW, Chan T, Moore EA, Johnson RC, Terpstra J, Turner RA, Reus VI (1998) Selective alteration of personality and social behavior by serotonergic intervention. Am J Psychiatry 155:373–379

Kocsis JD, Akiyama Y, Lankford KL, Radtke C (2002) Cell transplantation of peripheral-myelin-forming cells to repair the injured spinal cord. J Rehab Res Develop 39:287–298

Kölch M, Bücheler R, Gleiter CHH, Fegert JM (2004) Is St. John's Wort an Evidence Based Treatment-Alternative for Depressed Minors? Facts and prescribing trends in Germany. IACAPAP, Berlin

Koelega HS (1993) Stimulant drugs and vigilance performance: a review. Psychopharmacology 111:1–16

Kohama I, Lankford KL, Preiningerova J, White FA, Vollmer TL, Kocsis JD (2001) Transplantation of cryopreserved adult human Schwann cells enhances axonal conduction in demyelinated spinal cord. J Neurosci 21:944–950

Kondziolka D, Steinberg GK, Wechsler L, Meltzer CC, Elder E, Gebel J, Decesare S, Jovin T, Zafonte R, Lebowitz J, Flickinger JC, Tong D, Marks MP, Jamieson C, Luu D, Bell-Stephens T, Teraoka J (2005) Neurotransplantation for patients with subcortical motor stroke: a phase 2 randomized trial. J Neurosurg 103:6–8

Kondziolka D, Wechsler L, Goldstein S, Meltzer C, Thulborn KR, Gebel J, Jannetta P, DeCesare S, Elder EM, McGrogan M, Reitman MA, Bynum L (2000) Transplantation of cultured human neuronal cells for patients with stroke. Neurology 55:565–569

Kopell BH, Rezai AR (2003) Psychiatric neurosurgery: A historical perspective. Neurosurg Clin North Am 14(2):181–197

Kopyov OV, Jacques S, Lieberman A, Durna CM, Eagle KS (1998) Safety of intrastriatal neurotransplantation for Huntington's disease patients. Exp Neurol 149:97–108

Kordower JH, Bloch J, Ma SY, Chu Y, Palfi S, Roitberg BZ, Emborg M, Hantraye P, Deglon N, Aebischer P (1999) Lentiviral gene transfer to the nonhuman primate brain. Exp Neurol 160:1–16

Kordower JH, Emborg ME, Bloch J, Ma SY, Chu Y, Leventhal L, McBride J, Chen EY, Palfi S, Roitberg BZ, Brown WD, Holden JE, Pyzalski R, Taylor MD, Carvey P, Ling Z, Trono D, Hantraye P, Deglon N, Aebischer P (2000) Neurodegeneration prevented by lentiviral vector delivery of GDNF in primate models of Parkinson's disease. Science 290:767–773

Kordower JH, Freeman TB, Chen EY, Mufson EJ, Sanberg PR, Hauser RA, Snow B, Olanow CW (1998) Fetal nigral grafts survive and mediate clinical benefit in a patient with Parkinson's disease. Mov Disord 13:383–393

Kowatch RA, Suppes T, Carmody TJ, Bucci JP, Hume JH, Kromelis M, Emslie GJ, Weinberg WA, Rush AJ (2000) Effect size of lithium, divalproex sodium, and carbamazepine in children and adolescents with bipolar disorder. J Am Acad Child Adolesc Psychiatry 39:713–720

Kraemer HC (2004) Statistics and clinical trial design in psychopharmacology. In: Machin D, Day S, Green S, Everitt B, George S (eds) Textbook of Clinal Trials. Ch 10, John Wiley & Sons, pp 173–183

Kraepelin E (1899) Psychiatry: A Textbook for Students and Physicians. Jacques M Quen (ed) 2 vols, 1st English edn, transl of German 6th rev edn (1883) Resources in Medical History (1990) Science History Publications, Canton, MA

Kraft IA, Ardali C, Duffy JH, Hart JT, Pearce P (1965) A clinical study of chloridazepoxide used in psychiatric disorders of children. Int J Neuropsychiatry 1(5):433–7

Kramer PD (1993) Listening to Prozac: A Psychiatrist Explores Antidepressant Drugs and the Remaking of the Self. Viking, New York

Krakowski AJ (1965) Amitriptyline in treatment of hyperkinetic children: A double blind study. Psychosomatics 6:355–60

Krause KH, Dresel SH, Krause J, Kung HF, Tatsch K (2000) Increased striatal dopamine transporter in adult patients with attention hyperactive disorder: effects of methylphenidate as measured by single photon emission computed tomography. Neuroscience Letters 285:107–110

Krishnamoorthy J, King BH (1998) Open-label olanzapine treatment in five preadolescent children. J Child Adolesc Psychopharmacol 8(2):107–113

Kubler A, Neumann N, Kaiser J, Kotchoubey B, Hinterberger T, Birbaumer NP (2001) Brain-computer communication: self-regulation of slow cortical potentials for verbal communication. Arch Phys Med Rehabil 82(11):1533–1539

Kuchta J, Otto SR, Shannon RV, Hitselberger WE, Brackmann DE (2004) The multichannel auditory brainstem implant: how many electrodes make sense?

Kuhn R (1957) Über die Behandlung depressiver Zustände mit einem Iminobenzylderivat. Schweizer Med Wschr 87:1135–1140

Kumra S, Jacobsen LK, Lenane M (1998) Childhood-onset schizophrenia: an open label study of olanzapine in adolescents. J Am Acad Child Adolesc Psychiatry 37(4):377–385

Kurzweil R (1992) The Age of Intelligent Machines. MIT Press, Boston

Kurzweil R (2000) The Age of Spiritual Machines. Penguin, New York

Kurzweil R (2006) The Singularity Is Near. When Humans Transcend Biology. Penguin Group, London

Kutnick P, Kington A (2005) Children's friendships and learning in school: Cognitive enhancement through social interaction? British Journal of Educational Psychology 75:521–538

Kramer P (1993) Listening to Prozac. Penguin Books, New York

Krupa DJ, Wiest MC, Shuler MG, Laubach M, Nicolelis MA (2004) Layer-specific somatosensory cortical activation during active tactile discrimination. Science 304(5679):1989–1992

Lad SP, Neet KE, Mufson EJ (2003) Nerve growth factor: structure, function and therapeutic implications for Alzheimer's disease. Curr Drug Targets CNS Neurol Disord 2:315–334

Lakatos A, Smith PM, Barnett SC, Franklin RJ (2003) Meningeal cells enhance limited CNS remyelination by transplanted olfactory ensheathing cells. Brain 126:598–609

Lambert NM, Hartsough CS (1998) Prospective study of tobacco smoking and substance dependencies among samples of ADHD and non-ADHD participants. J Learn Disabil 31:533–544

Lane H, Bahan B (1998) Ethics of cochlear implantation in young children: a review and reply from a Deaf-World perspective. Otolaryngol Head Neck Surg 119(4):297–313

Lane H, Grodin M (1997) Ethical issues in cochlear implant surgery: an exploration into disease, disability, and the best interests of the child. Kennedy Inst Ethics J 7(3):231–251

Langston JW, Widner H, Goetz CG, Brooks D, Fahn S, Freeman T, Watts R (1992) Core assessment program for intracerebral transplantation (CAPIT). Mov Disord 7:2–13

Larsson LC, Widner H (2000) Neural tissue xenografting. Scand J Immunol 52:249–256

Laszig R (2000) Cochlear implants in children (soft surgery). Adv Otorhinolaryngol 57:87–9, 87–89

Laszig R, Aschendorff A, Schipper J, Klenzner T (2004a) Current developments in cochlear implantation. HNO 52(4):357–362

Laszig R, Aschendorff A, Stecker M, Muller-Deile J, Maune S, Dillier N, Weber B, Hey M, Begall K, Lenarz T, Battmer RD, Bohm M, Steffens T, Strutz J, Linder T, Probst R, Allum J, Westhofen M, Doering W (2004b) Benefits of bilateral electrical stimulation with the nucleus cochlear implant in adults: 6-month postoperative results. Otol Neurotol 25(6):958–968

Laszig R, Marangos N, Sollmann P, Ramsden R, Fraysse B, Lenarz T, Rask-Andersen H, Bredberg G, Sterkers O, Manrique M, Nevison B (1997) Initial results from the clinical trial of the nucleus 21-channel auditory brain stem implant. Am J Otol 18(6 suppl):160

Lau B, Stanley GB, Dan Y (2002) Computational subunits of visual cortical neurons revealed by artificial neural networks. Proc Natl Acad Sci USA 99(13):8974–8979

Lecic-Tosevski D, Christodoulou N, Herrman H et al. (2003) Consensus Statement on Psychiatric Prevention. WPA, The section's Newsletter 6:6–8

LeFever, GB, Dawson, KV, Morrow, AL (1999) The extent of drug therapy for attention deficit-hyperactivity disorder among children in public schools. American Journal of Public Health 89(9):1359–1364

Le HN, Frim DM (2002) Gene therapy for Parkinson's disease. Expert Opin Biol Ther 2:151–161

Leibniz GW (1983) Discourse de Métaphysique. Lestienne H (ed). Vrin, Paris

Lenarz T (2005) Auditory Brainstem Implant. ESBS Meeting Fulda

Lenckner T (1989) Einwilligung. In: Eser A, Luterotti Mv, Sporken P (eds) Lexikon Medizin, Ethik, Recht. Herder, Freiburg Basel Wien, pp 271–279

Lesinski-Schiedat A, Illg A, Warnecke A, Heermann R, Bertram B, Lenarz T (2006) Paediatric cochlear implantation in the first year of life Preliminary results. HNO 54(7):565–572

Leuthardt EC, Schalk G, Wolpaw JR, Ojemann JG, Moran DW (2004) A brain-computer interface using electrocorticographic signals in humans. J Neural Eng 1(2):63–71

Levin FR, Kleber HD (1995) Attention-deficit hyperactivity disorder and substance abuse: relationships and implications for tretatment. Harv Rev Psychiatry 2:246–58

Levine SP, Huggins JE, BeMent SL, Kushwaha RK, Schuh LA, Rohde MM, Passaro EA, Ross DA, Elisevich KV, Smith BJ (2000) A direct brain interface based on event-related potentials. IEEE Trans Rehabil Eng 8(2):180–185

Levivier M, Dethy S, Rodesch F, Peschanski M, Vandesteene A, David P, Wikler D, Goldman S, Claes T, Biver F, Liesnard C, Goldmanb M, Hildebrand J, Brotchi J (1997) Intracerebral transplantation of fetal ventral mesencephalon for patients with advanced Parkinson's disease. Methodology and 6-month to 1-year follow-up in 3 patients. Stereotact Funct Neurosurg 69:99–111

Lewis D (1983) Philosophical Papers, vol 1. Oxford University Press, Oxford

Liebermann JA, March JS (2005) Book reviews. Journal of the American Academy of Child and Adolescent Psychiatry 9:957–958

Lieberman JA, Stroup TS, McEvoy JP, Swartz MS, Rosenheck RA, Perkins DO, Keefe RSE, Davis SM, Davis CE, Lebowitz BD, Severe J, Hsiao JK (2005) Effectiveness of antipsychotic drugs in patients with schizophrenia (CATIE-study). New England Journal of Medicine 353:1209–1223

Lindsay R (2005) Enhancement and Justice: Problems in Determining the Requirements of Justice in a Genetically Transformed Society. Kennedy Insitute of Ethics Journal 15(1):3–38

Lindvall O (1997) Neural transplantation: a hope for patients with Parkinson's disease. NeuroReport 8:14

Lindvall O (1999) Cerebral implantation in movement disorders: state of the art. Mov Disord 14:201–205

Lindvall O, Brundin P, Widner H, Rehncrona S, Gustavii B, Frackowiak R, Leenders KL, Sawle G, Rothwell JC, Marsden CD, Björklund A (1990) Grafts of fetal dopamine neurons survive and improve motor function on Parkinson's disease. Science 247:574–577

Lindvall O, Rehncrona S, Brundin P, Gutavii B, Åstedt B, Widner H, Lindholm T, Björklund A, Leenders KL, Rothwell JC (1989) Human fetal dopamine neurons grafted to the striatum in two patients with severe Parkinson's disease: a detailed account of methodology and a 6 months follow-up. Arch Neurol 46:615–631

Lindvall O, Widner H, Rehncrona S, Brundin P, Odin P, Gustavii B, Frackowiak R, Leenders KL, Sawle G, Rothwell JC, Björklund A, Marsden CD (1992) Transplantation of fetal dopamine neurons in Parkinson's disease: one-year clinical and neurophysiological observations in two patients with putaminal implants. Ann Neurol 31:155–165

Lin EJ, Richichi C, Young D, Baer K, Vezzani A, During MJ (2003) Recombinant AAV-mediated expression of galanin in rat hippocampus suppresses seizure development. Eur J Neurosci 18:2087–2092

Linke DB (1993) Hirnverpflanzung. Die erste Unsterblichkeit auf Erden. Rowohlt, Reinbek

Lippitz B, Mindus P, Meyerson B, Kihlström L, Linquist C (1999) Lesion topography and outcome after thermocapsulotomy or gamma knife capsulotomy for obsessive-compulsive disorder: relevance of the right hemisphere. Neurosurgery 44(3):452–460

Locke J (1975) An Essay Concerning Human Understanding. Nidditch PH (ed) Clarendon, Oxford

Löscher W, Ebert U, Lehmann H, Rosenthal C, Nikkhah G (1998) Seizure suppression in kindling epilepsy by grafts of fetal GABAergic neurons in rat substantia nigra. J Neurosci Res 2:196–209

London AJ, Kadane JB (2002) Placebos that harm: sham surgery controls in clinical trials. Stat Meth Med Res 11:413–427

López-Lozano JJ, Bravo G, Brera B, Millan I, Dargallo J, Salmeán J, Uria J, Insausti J (1997) Long-term improvement in patients with severe Parkinson's disease after implantation of fetal ventral mesencephalic tissue in a cavity of the caudate nucleus: 5-year follow up in 10 patients. J Neurosurg 86:931

Lorenz K (1969) Die Begründung des principium identitatis indiscernibilium. In: Müller K, Totok W (eds) Studia Leibnitiana Supplementa, Vol III: Akten des internationalen Leibniz-Kongresses Hannover, 14.–19. Nov 1966, Band III: Erkenntnislehre, Logik, Sprachphilosophie, Editionsberichte. Franz Steiner Verlag, Wiesbaden

Lucas AP, Lockett HJ, Grimm F (1965) Amitriptylin in Childhood depression. Dis Nerv Sys 28:105–113

Luntz M, Shpak T, Weiss H (2005) Binaural-bimodal hearing: concomitant use of a unilateral cochlear implant and a contralateral hearing aid. Acta Otolaryngol 125(8):863–869

MacIntyre A (^{2}1985) After Virtue. A Study in Moral Theory. Duckworth, London

Macklin R (1999) The ethical problems with sham surgery in clinical research. New Engl J Med 341:992–996

Maclean PD (2006) The triune brain in evolution: role in paleocerebral functions. Plenum Press, New York

Madrazo I, Drucker-Colin R, Diaz V, Martinez-Mata J, Torres C, Becerril JJ (1987) Open microsurgical autograft of adrenal medulla to the right caudate nucleus in two patients with intractable Parkinson's disease. New Engl J Med 316:831–834

Madrazo I, Franco-Bourland R, Aguilera M, Ostrosky-Solis F, Cuevas C, Castregon H, Velazquez D, Grijalva E, Guizar-Sahagun G, Magallon E, Madrazo M (1991) Fetal ventral mesencephalon brain homotransplantation in Parkinson's disease; the Mexican experience. Restor Neurol 4:123–130

Madrazo I, Franco-Bourland RE, Castrejon H, Cuevas C, Ostrosky-Solis F (1995) Fetal striatal homotransplantation for Huntington's disease: first two case reports. Neurol Res 17:312–315

Maguire GQ, McGee EM (1999) Implantable brain chips? Time for debate. Hastings Cent Rep 29(1):7–13

Maitra A, Arking DE, Shivapurkar N, Ikeda M, Stastny V, Kassauei K, Sui G, Cutler DJ, Liu Y, Brimble SN, Noaksson K, Hyllner J, Schulz TC, Zeng X, Freed WJ, Crook J, Abraham S, Colman A, Sartipy P, Matsui S, Carpenter M, Gazdar AF, Rao M, Chakravarti A (2005) Genomic alterations in cultured human embryonic stem cells. Nat Genet 37:1099–1103

Mallet L, Mesnage V, Houeto J, Pelissolo A, Yelnik J, Behar C, Gargiulo M, Welter M, Bonnet A, Pillon B, Cornu P, Dormont D, Pidoux B, Allilaire J, Agid Y (2002) Compulsions, Parkinson's disease and stimulation. Lancet 360:1302–1304

Mandoki M (1997) Olanzapine in the treatment of early onset schizophrenia in children and adolescents. Biol Psychiatry Abstracts 41:22

Manrique M, Huarte A, Morera C, Caballe L, Ramos A, Castillo C, Garcia-Ibanez L, Estrada E, Juan E (2005) Speech perception with the ACE and the SPEAK speech coding strategies for children implanted with the Nucleus(R) cochlear implant. Int J Pediatr Otorhinolaryngol 69(12):1667–1674

March J (2005) Let them eat Prozac: The unhealthy relationship between the pharmaceutical industry and depression. Journal of the American Academy of Child & Adolescent Psychiatry 44(9):955–958

March JS, Silva SG, Compton S, Ginger A, DeVeaugh-Geiss J Califf R, Krishnan KR (2004) The child and adolescent psychiatry trials network (CAPTN). Journal of the American Academy of Child and Adolescent Psychiatry 43:515–518

March JS, Silva SG, Compton S, Shapiro M, Califf R, Krishnan KR (2005) The case for practical clinical trials in psychiatry. American Journal of Psychiatry 162:836–846

Marcus SJ (ed) (2002) Neuroethics. Mapping the field. Dana Press, New York

Maries E, Kordower JH, Chu Y, Collier TJ, Sortwell CE, Olaru E, Shannon K, Steece-Collier K (2006) Focal not widespread grafts induce novel dyskinetic behavior in parkinsonian rats. Neurobiol Dis 21:165–80

Marshall AH, Fanning N, Symons S, Shipp D, Chen JM, Nedzelski JM (2005) Cochlear implantation in Cochlear Otosclerosis. Laryngoscope 115(10):1728–1733

Masters KJ, Bellonci C, Bernet W, Arnold V, Beitchman J, Benson RS, Bukstein O, Kinlan J, McClellan J, Rue D, Shaw JA, Stock S (2002) Practice parameter for the prevention and management of aggressive behavior in child and adolescent psychiatric institutions, with special reference to seclusion and restraint. J Am Acad Child Adolesc Psychiatry 41(2 suppl):4S–25S

Mattay VS, Callicott, Bertolino A, Heaton I, Frank JA, Coppola R, Berman KF, Goldberg TE, Weinberger DR (2000) Effects of Dextroamphetamine on cognitive performance and cortical activation. NeuroImage 12:268–275

Matthies C, Thomas S, Moshrefi M, Lesinski-Schiedat A, Frohne C, Battmer R-D, Lenarz T, Samii M (2000) Auditory brainstem implants: current neurosurgical experiences and perspective. J Laryngol Otol 114(suppl 27):32–37

Matthiesen L (2002) Survey on Opinions from National Committees or Similar Bodies, Public Debate and National Legislation in Relation to Human Embryonic Stem Cell Research and Use, vol 1–2. EC Research Directorate-General, Brussels

Mayberg H, Lozano A, Voon V, McNeely H, Seminowicz D, Hamani C, Schwalb J, Kennedy S (2005) Deep brain stimulation for treatment-resistant depression. Neuron 45:651–660

Mazzone P, Lozano A, Stanzione P, Galati S, Scarnati E, Peppe A, Stefani A (2005) Implantation of human pedunculopontine nucleus: a safe and clinically relevant target in Parkinson's disease. Neuroreport 16(17):1877–1881

McCabe SE, Knight JR, Teter CJ, Wechsler H (2005) Non-medical use of prescription stimulants among US college students: prevalence and correlates for a national survey. Addiction 99:96–106
McConville B, Arvanitis L, Thyrum P, Smith K (1999) Pharmacokinetics, tolerability, and clinical effectiveness of quetiapine in adolescents with selected psychotic disorders. EurNeuropsychopharmacol 9, suppl 5:267
McCreery DB, Shannon RV, Moore JK, Chatterjee M (1998) Accessing the tonotopic organization of the ventral cochlear nucleus by intranuclear microstimulation. IEEE Trans Rehabil Eng 6(4):391–399
McCreery DB, Yuen TG, Bullara LA (2000) Chronic microstimulation in the feline ventral cochlear nucleus: physiologic and histologic effects. Hear Res 149(1–2):223–238
McCullagh PM (1987) The Foetus as Transplant Donor. Scientific, Social and Ethical Perspectives. Wiley, Chichester
McDermott HJ (2004) Music perception with cochlear implants: a review. Trends Amplif 8(2):49–82
McGorry PD (2000a) The nature of schizophrenia: signposts to prevention. Australian and New Zealand Journal of Psychiatry, suppl 34:14–21
McGorry PD (2000b) Evaluating the importance of reducing the duration of untreated psychosis. Australian and New Zealand Journal of Psychiatry, suppl 34:5145–5149
McKenzie JL, Waid MC, Shi R, Webster TJ (2004) Decreased functions of astrocytes on carbon nanofiber materials. Biomaterials 25(7–8):1309–1317
McKibben B (2003) Enough. Staying Human in an Engineered Age. Times Books, New York
McLaren A (1996) Research on embryos in vitro, the various types of research. Third Symposium on Bioethics 'Medically assisted procreation and the protection of the human embryo'. CDBI/SPK 22, Council of Europe, Strasbourg December 15–18
McLaren A (2001) Ethical and social considerations of stem cell research. Nature 414:129–131
McLean REG (1960) Imipramine hydrochloride (Tofranil) and enuresis. Am J Psychiatry 117:551
McRae C, Cherin E, Diem G, Vo AH, Ellgring JH, Russell D, Fahn S, Freed C (2003) Does personality change as a result of fetal tissue transplantation in the brain? J Neurol 250:282–286
Measham TJ (1995) The acute management of aggressive behaviour in hospitalized children and adolescents. Can J Psychiatry 40:330–336
Mehlman MJ (2003) Wondergenes: Genentic Enhancement and the Future of Society. Indiana University Press, Indianapolis
Mehlman MJ (2004) Cognition-Enhancing Drugs. The Milbank Memorial Quarterly 82:483–506
Mehlman MJ (2005) Genetic enhancement: Plan now to act later. Kennedy Institute of Ethics Journal 15(1):77–72
Mehta V, Spears J, Mendez I (1997) Neural transplantation in Parkinson's disease. Can J Neurol Sci 24:292–301
Mehta MA, Owen AM, Sahakian BJ, Mavaddat N, Pickard JD, Robbins TW (2000) Methylphenidate enhances working memory by modulating discrete frontal and parital lobe regions in the human brain. The Journal of Neuroscience 20:RC65:1–6
Mehring C, Rickert J, Vaadia E, Cardosa d O, Aertsen A, Rotter S (2003) Inference of hand movements from local field potentials in monkey motor cortex. Nat Neurosci 6(12):1253–1254
Meltzer CC, Kondziolka D, Villemagne VL, Wechsler L, Goldstein S, Thulborn KR, Gebel J, Elder EM, DeCesare S, Jacobs A (2001) Serial [18F] fluorodeoxyglucose positron emission tomography after human neuronal implantation for stroke. Neurosurgery 49:586–591

Mendez I, Dagher A, Hong M, Gaudet P, Weerasinghe S, McAlister V, King D, Desrosiers J, Darvesh S, Acorn T, Robertson H (2002) Simultaneous intrastriatal and intranigral fetal dopaminergic grafts in patients with Parkinson disease: a pilot study. Report of three cases. J Neurosurg 96:589–596

Mendez I, Sanchez-Pernaute R, Cooper O, Vinuela A, Ferrari D, Björklund L, Dagher A, Isacson O (2005) Cell type analysis of functional fetal dopamine cell suspension transplants in the striatum and substantia nigra of patients with Parkinson's disease. Brain 128:1498–510

Merkel R (2005) Interim Report of the "Enquete Commission on Ethics and Law of Modern Medicine" of the German Parliament – dissenting opinion. In: Deutscher Bundestag (2005) Drucksache 15/5050 (03/17/2005):78–87

Merkel R (2006) Commentary on §§ 218–219b. In: Kindhäuser U, Neumann U, Paeffgen H-U (eds) Nomos Kommentar zum Strafgesetzbuch. Vol. II. Nomos Verlag, Baden-Baden

Merzenich MM, Schindler RA, Sooy FA (1974) Introduction. In: Merzenich MM, Schindler RA, Sooy FA, Proceedings of the First International Conference on Electrical Stimulation of the Acoustic Nerve as a Treatment for Profound Sensorineural Deafness in Man. San Francisco, pp 1–3

Metzinger T (1996) Hirnforschung, Neurotechnologie, Bewußtseinskultur. Medizinethische, anthropologische und sozialphilosophische Fragen der Zukunft. In: Hubig C, Poser H (eds) Cognitio Humana – Dynamik des Wissens und der Werte. Universität Leipzig, Leipzig, pp 1467–1474

Meyerson BA (1998) Neurosurgical treatment of neutral disorders: Introduction and indications. In: Gildenberg PH, Tasker RR (eds) Textbook of Stereotactic and Functional Neurosurgery. McGraw-Hill, New York, pp 1955–1964

Mezey E, Chandross KJ, Harta G, Maki RA, McKercher SR (2000) Turning blood into brain: cells bearing neuronal antigens generated in vivo from bone marrow. Science 290:1779–1782

Michelson RP (1971) The results of electrical stimulation of the cochlea in human sensory deafness. Ann Otol Rhinol Laryngol 80:914–919

Michelson RP, Schindler RA (1981) Multichannel cochlear implant: preliminary results in man. Laryngoscope 91:38–42

Miller DE (1985) The management of misbehavior by seclusion. Milieu Ther 4:13–18

Miller RG, Petajan JH, Bryan WW, Armon C, Barohn RJ, Goodpasture JC, Hoagland RJ, Parry GJ, Ross MA, Stromatt SC (1996) A placebo-controlled trial of recombinant human ciliary neurotrophic (rhCNTF) factor in amyotrophic lateral sclerosis. rhCNTF ALS Study Group. Ann Neurol 39:256–260

Millon T (2004) Masters of the Mind. Exploring the Story of Mental Illness from Ancient Times to the New Millennium. Wiley & Sons, Hoboken, NJ

Missa J-N (1998) Psychosurgery and physical brain manipulation. In: Encyclopedia of Applied Ethics, vol 3. Academic Press, pp 735–744

Mittoux V, Joseph JM, Conde F, Palfi S, Dautry C, Poyot T, Bloch J, Deglon N, Ouary S, Nimchinsky EA, Brouillet E, Hof PR, Peschanski M, Aebischer P, Hantraye P (2000) Restoration of cognitive and motor functions by ciliary neurotrophic factor in a primate model of Huntington's disease. Hum Gene Ther 11:1177–1187

Mittoux V, Ouary S, Monville C, Lisovoski F, Poyot T, Conde F, Escartin C, Robichon R, Brouillet E, Peschanski M, Hantraye P (2002) Corticostriatopallidal neuroprotection by adenovirus-mediated ciliary neurotrophic factor gene transfer in a rat model of progressive striatal degeneration. J Neurosci 22:4478–4486

Möller HJ (2004) SSRI zu Recht unter Anklage. Psychopharmakotherapie 3:69–70

Molina B, Pelham W, Roth J (1999) Stimulant Medication and Substance Use by Adolescents with a Childhood History of ADHD (poster). Presented at the biennial meeting of the International Society for Research in Child and Adolescent Psychopathology, June 17–20, Barcelona

Molitch M, Eccles AK (1937) The effect of benzedrine sulfate on the intelligence scores of children. Am J Psychiatry 94:587–590

Molitch M, Sullivan JP (1937) The effect of benzedrine sulfate on children taking the New Stanford Achievement Test. Am J Orthopsychiatry 7:519–522

Moreno J (2006) Mind Wars: Brain Research and National Defense. University of Chicago Press, Chicago

Morgan JP (1982) The first reported case of electrical stimulation of the human brain. J Hist Med Allied Sci 37(1):51–64

Morris GL 3rd, Mueller WM (1999) Long-term treatment with vagus nerve stimulation in patients with refractory epilepsy. The vagus nerve stimulation study group E01-E05. Neurology 53(8):1731–1735

Morris K (2002) Remote possibility of sensory prostheses. Lancet Neurol 1(2):79

Muller J, Helms J (2005) Cochlear implantation maintaining remaining deep tone hearing. HNO 53(9):753–755

Muller J, Schon F, Helms J (2002) Speech understanding in quiet and noise in bilateral users of the MED-EL COMBI 40/40+ cochlear implant system. Ear Hear 23(3):198–206

Murphy FA (1996) The public health risk of animal organ and tissue transplantation into humans. Science 273:746–747

Nahas Z, Marangell LB, Husain MM, Rush AJ, Sackeim HA, Lisanby SH, Martinez JM, George MS (2005) Two-year outcome of vagus nerve stimulation (VNS) for treatment of major depressive episodes. J Clin Psychiatry 66(9):1097–1104

Nakao N, Kakishita K, Uematsu Y, Yoshimasu T, Bessho T, Nakai K, Naito Y, Itakura T (2001) Enhancement of the response to levodopa therapy after intrastriatal transplantation of autologous sympathetic neurons in patients with Parkinson disease. J Neurosurg 95:275–284

Nasto B (1997) Xenotransplant firms get xenophobic. Nature Biotech 15:1239

Nemeroff CB, Mayberg HS, Krahl SE, McNamara J, Frazer A, Henry TR, George MS, Charney DS, Brannan SK (2006) VNS therapy in treatment-resistant depression: Clinical evidence and putative neurobiological mechanisms. Neuropsychopharmacology 31(7):1345–1355

Netto CA, Hodges H, Sinden JD, LePeillet E, Kershaw T, Sowinski P, Meldrum BS, Gray JA (1993) Foetal grafts from hippocampal regio superior alleviate ischaemic-induced behavioural deficits. Behav Brain Res 58:107–112

Neuper C, Muller GR, Kubler A, Birbaumer N, Pfurtscheller G (2003) Clinical application of an EEG-based brain-computer interface: a case study in a patient with severe motor impairment. Clin Neurophysiol 114(3):399–409

Newmann TB (2004) A black-box warning for antidepressants in children? The New England Journal of Medicine 351(16):1595–1598

Nicholls JG (2001) From neurons to brain. Sinauer Ass, Sunderland, Mass

Nicolelis MA (2001) Actions from thoughts. Nature 409(6818):403–407

Nicolelis MA (2002) The amazing adventures of robotrat. Trends Cogn Sci 6(11):449–450

Nicolelis MA (2003) Brain-machine interfaces to restore motor function and probe neural circuits. Nat Rev Neurosci 4(5):417–422

Nicolelis MA, Chapin JK (2002) Controlling robots with the mind. Sci Am 287(4):46–53

Nikolopoulos TP, Archbold SM, O'Donoghue GM (1999) The development of auditory perception in children following cochlear implantation. Int J Pediatr Otorhinolaryngol 49 suppl 1:189–191

Nishino H, Borlongan CV (2000) Restoration of function by neural transplantation in the ischemic brain. Prog Brain Res 127:461–476

Noe F, Nissinen J, Filippi F, During MJ, Pitkänen A, Vezzani A (2005) rAAV-mediated neuropeptide gene expression in the hippocampus of chronically epileptic rats reduces spontaneous seizures ensuing after electrically-induced status epilepticus. 59th Annual Meeting American Epilepsy Society, Washington, DC, abstract 2.O85

Noggle R (2002) Special agents: Children's autonomy and parental authority. In: Archard D, MacLeod CM (eds) The Moral and Political Status of Children. Oxford University Press, Oxford New York, 97–117

Noonan HW (²2003) Personal Identity. Routledge, Oxford

Normann RA, Maynard EM, Rousche PJ, Warren DJ (1999) A neural interface for a cortical vision prosthesis. Vision Res 39(15):2577–2587

Normann RA, Warren DJ, Ammermuller J, Fernandez E, Guillory S (2001) High-resolution spatio-temporal mapping of visual pathways using multi-electrode arrays. Vision Res 41(10-11):1261–75

Normile D, Vogel G, Couzin J (2006) Cloning. South Korean team's remaining human stem cell claim demolished. Science 311:156–157

Northoff G (1995) Ethische Probleme bei Hirngewebstransplantationen. Eine aktuelle Übersicht. Ethik in der Medizin 7:87–98

Northoff G (1996a) Personale Identität und Erste-Person-Perspektive bei Erkrankungen des Gehirns: Theoretische und empirische Implikationen. In: Hubig C, Poser H (eds) Cognitio Humana – Dynamik des Wissens und der Werte. Universität Leipzig, Leipzig, pp 1451–1458

Northoff G (1996b) Do brain tissue transplants alter personal identity? Inadequacies of some "standard" arguments. Journal of Medical Ethics 22:174–180

Northoff G (2001) Personale Identität und operative Eingriffe in das Gehirn. Mentis, Paderborn

Nozick R (1974) Anarchy, State, and Utopia. Basic Books, New York

Nozick R (1981) Philosophical Explanations. Harvard University Press, Cambridge, Mass

Nuffield Council on Bioethics (1996) Animal-to-Human Transplants. London

Nuffield Council on Bioethics (2000) Stem Cell Therapy: The Ethical Issues. Dorchester

Nunes R (2001) Ethical dimension of paediatric cochlear implantation. Theor Med Bioeth 22(4):337–349

Nuttin B, Cosyns P, Demeulemeester H, Gybels J, Meyerson B (1999) Electrical stimulation in anterior limbs of internal capsules in patients with obsessive-compulsive disorder. Lancet 354:1526

Nuttin B, Gabriëls L, Cosyns P, Gybels J (2000) Electrical stimulation of the brain for psychiatric disorders. Central Nervous System Spectrums 5(11):35–39

Nuttin B, Gybels J, Cosyns P, Gabriels L, Meyerson B, Andréewitch S, Rasmussen S, Greenberg B, Friehs G, Rezai A, Montgomery E, Malone D, Fins J (2002) Deep brain stimulation for psychiatric disorders. Neurosurgery 51:519

Nuttin B, van Kuyck K (2002) Diepe hersenstimulatie voor psychiatrische aandoeningen, de stand van zaken. Nederlands Tijdschrift voor Neurologie 5:373–376

Nuttin B, Gabriëls L, van Kuyck K, Cosyns P (2003a) Electrical stimulation of the anterior limbs of the internal capsules in patients with severe obsessive-compulsive disorder: anecdotal reports. Neurosurgery Clinics of North America 14:267–274

Nuttin B, Gabriëls L, Cosyns P, Meyerson B, Andréewitch S, Sunaert S, Maes A, Dupont P, Gybels J, Gielen F, Demeulemeester H (2003b) Long-term electrical capsular stimulation in patients with obsessive-compulsive disorder. Neurosurgery 52:1263–1274

Nuttin B, Gybels J, Cosyns P, Gabriëls L, Meyerson B, Andreewitch S, Rasmussen S, Greenberg B, Friehs G, Rezai A, Montgomery E, Malone D, Fins J (2003c) Deep brain stimulation for psychiatric disorders. Letter to the editor, Neurosurgical Clinics of North America 14:XV–XVI

Nylund D (2000) Treating Huckleberry Finn. Jossey-Bass, San Francisco, p 27

Oduncu FS (2003) Stem cell research in Germany: ethics of healing vs. human dignity. Med Health Care Philos 6:5–16

Ohl FW, Deliano M, Scheich H, Freeman WJ (2003a) Analysis of evoked and emergent patterns of stimulus-related auditory cortical activity. Rev Neurosci 14(1-2):35–42

Ohl FW, Deliano M, Scheich H, Freeman WJ (2003b) Early and late patterns of stimulus-related activity in auditory cortex of trained animals. Biol Cybern 88(5):374–379

Ohl FW, Scheich H, Freeman WJ (2000) Topographic analysis of epidural pure-tone-evoked potentials in gerbil auditory cortex. J Neurophysiol 83(5):3123–3132

Ohl FW, Scheich H, Freeman WJ (2001) Change in pattern of ongoing cortical activity with auditory category learning. Nature 412(6848):733–736

Okun M, Bowers D, Springer U, Shapira N, Malone D, Rezai A, Nuttin B, Heilman K, Morecraft R, Rasmussen S, Greenberg B, Foote K, Goodman W (2004) What's in a "smile?" Intraoperative observations of contralateral smiles induced by deep brain stimulation, Neurocase 10(4):271–279

Olanow CW (2005) Double-blind, placebo-controlled trials for surgical interventions in Parkinson disease. Arch Neurol 62:1343–1344

Olanow CW, Goetz CG, Kordower JH, Stoessl AJ, Sossi V, Brin MF, Shannon KM, Nauert GM, Perl DP, Godbold J, Freeman TB (2003) A double-blind controlled trial of bilateral fetal nigral transplantation in Parkinson's disease. Ann Neurol 54:403–414

Olanow CW, Kordower JH Freeman TB (1996) Fetal nigral transplantation as a therapy for Parkinson's disease. TINS 19:102–109

Olds J (1956) A preliminary mapping of electrical reinforcing effects in the rat brain. J Comp Physiol Psychol 49(3):281–285

Olds J (1958) Self-stimulation of the brain; its use to study local effects of hunger, sex, and drugs. Science 127(3294):315–324

Olds J, Olds ME (1958) Positive reinforcement produced by stimulating hypothalamus with iproniazid and other compounds. Science 127(3307):1175–1176

Olds J (1963) Self-stimulation experiments. Science 140:218–220

Olfson M, Marcus SC, Greenberg T (2003) Relationship between antidepressant medication treatment and suicide in adolescents. Archives of General Psychiatry 60:978–982

O'Rahilly R, Müller F (1987) Developmental Stages in Human Embryos. Carnegie Institution of Washington, Washington

Oshana MAL (2005) Autonomy and self-identity. In: Anderson J, Christman J (eds) Autonomy and the Challenges to Liberalism: New Essays. Cambridge University Press, New York, pp 77–97

Ostroff JM, David EA, Shipp DB, Chen JM, Nedzelski JM (2003) Evaluation of the high-resolution speech coding strategy for the Clarion CII cochlear implant system. J Otolaryngol 32(2):81–86

Otto SR, Brackmann DE, Hitselberger WE, Shannon RV, Kuchta J (2002) Multichannel auditory brainstem implant: update on performance in 61 patients. J Neurosurg 96(6):1063–1071

Otto SR, Brackmann DE, Staller S, Menapace CM (1997) The multichannel auditory brainstem implant: 6-month coinvestigator results. Adv Otorhinolaryngol 52:1–7

Outka G (2002) The ethics of human stem cell research. Kennedy Inst Ethics J 12:175–213

Palacios R, Golunski E, Samaridis J (1995) In vitro generation of hematopoietic stem cells from an embryonic stem cell line. Proc Natl Acad Sci USA 92:7530–7534

Palfi S, Conde F, Riche D, Brouillet E, Dautry C, Mittoux V, Chibois A, Peschanski M, Hantraye P (1998) Fetal striatal allografts reverse cognitive deficits in a primate model of Huntington disease. Nat Med 4:963–966

Paratore S, Alessi E, Coffa S, Torrisi A, Mastrobuono F, Cavallaro S (2006) Early genomics of learning and memory: a review. Genes, Brain and Behavior 5:209–221

Parens E (1995a) The goodness of fragility: On the prospect of genetic technologies aimed at the enhancement of human capacities. Kennedy Inst Ethics J 5:141–153

Parens E (1995b) What research? Which embryos? Hastings Cent Rep 25(1):36

Parens E (ed) (1998) Enhancing Human Traits: Ethical and Social Implications. Georgetown University Press, Washington, DC

Parens E (2002) How far will the term enhancement get us as we grapple with new ways to shape ourselves? In: Neuroethics. Mapping the Field. Marcus SJ (ed) pp 152–158

Parfit D (1984) Reasons and Persons. Oxford University Press, Oxford

Paternite CE, Loney J, Salisbury H, Whaley MA (1999) Childhood inattention-overactivity, aggression and stimulant medication history as predictors for young adult outcomes. J Child Adolesc Psychopharmacol 9(3):169–184

Patience C, Patton GS, Tacheuchi Y, Weiss RA, McClure MO, Rydberg L, Breimer ME (1998) No evidence of pig DNA or retroviral infection in patients with short-term extracorporeal connection to pig kidneys. Lancet 352:699–701

Patience C, Takeuchi Y, Weiss RA (1997) Infection of human cells by an endogenous retrovirus of pigs. Nature Med 3:282–286

Peel Report, Department of Health and Social Security (1972) The Use of Fetuses and Fetal Material for Research, Report of the Advisory Group. Her Majesty's Stationary Office, London

Penfield W (1950a) Observations on the anatomy of memory. Folia Psychiatr Neurol Neurochir Neerl 53(2):349–351

Penfield W (1950b) The supplementary motor area in the cerebral cortex of man. Arch Psychiatr Nervenkr Z Gesamte Neurol Psychiatr 185(6–7):670–674

Perlow MJ, Freed WJ, Hoffer BJ, Seiger A, Olson L, Wyatt RJ (1979) Brain grafts reduce motor disabilities produced by destruction of nigrostriatal dopamine system. Science 204:643–647

Persson J, Bringlöv E, Nilsson LG, Nyberg L (2004) The memory-enhancing effects of Ginseng and Gingko biloba in healthy volunteers. Psychopharmacology 172:430–434

Pesaran B, Pezaris JS, Sahani M, Mitra PP, Andersen RA (2002) Temporal structure in neuronal activity during working memory in macaque parietal cortex. Nat Neurosci 5(8):805–811

Peschanski M, Césaro P, Hantraye P (1995) Rationale for intrastriatal grafting of striatal neuroblasts in patients with Huntington's disease. Neuroscience 68:273–285

Peschanski M, Césaro P, Hantraye P (1996) What is needed versus what would be interesting to know before undertaking neural transplantation in patients with Huntington's disease. Neuroscience 71:899–900

Peschanski M, Defer GL, Dethy S, Hantraye PM, Levivier M, Nguyen JP, Cesaro P (1999) The need for phase III studies in experimental surgical treatments of Parkinson's disease. Adv Neurol 80:651–653

Peschanski M, Defer GL, N'Guyen JP, Ricolfi F, Monfort JC, Remy P, Geny C, Samson Y, Hantraye P, Jeny R (1994) Bilateral motor improvement and alteration of L-dopa effect in two patients with Parkinson's disease following intrastriatal transplantation of foetal ventral mesencephalon. Brain 117:487499

Peschanski M, Dunnett SB (2002) Cell therapy for Huntington's disease, the next step forward. Lancet Neurology 1:81

Pezet S, McMahon SB (2006) Neurotrophins: mediators and modulators of pain. Annu Rev Neurosci 29:507–38

Pfingst BE (2001) Auditory prostheses. In: Chapin JK, Moxon KA (eds) Neural Prostheses for Restoration of Sensory and Motor Function. CRC Press, London, pp 3–45

Pfurtscheller G, Muller GR, Pfurtscheller J, Gerner HJ, Rupp R (2003a) 'Thought'-control of functional electrical stimulation to restore hand grasp in a patient with tetraplegia. Neurosci Lett 351(1):33–36

Pfurtscheller G, Neuper C, Muller GR, Obermaier B, Krausz G, Schlogl A, Scherer R, Graimann B, Keinrath C, Skliris D, Wortz M, Supp G, Schrank C (2003b) Graz-BCI: state of the art and clinical applications. IEEE Trans Neural Syst Rehabil Eng 11(2):177–180

Philpott LM, Kopyov OV, Lee AJ, Jacques S, Duma CM, Caine S, Yang M, Eagle KS (1997) Neuropsychological functioning following fetal striatal transplantation in Huntington's chorea: three case presentations. Cell Transplant 6:203–212

Philipps LJ, Yung AR, McGorry PD (2000) Identification of young people at risk of psychosis: validation of personal assessment and crisis evaluation clinic intake criteria. Aust N Z J Psychiatry 34 Suppl:164–9

Piccini P, Brooks DJ, Björklund A, Gunn RN, Grasby PM, Rimoldi O, Brundin P, Hagell P, Rehncrona S, Widner H, Lindvall O (1999) Dopaminergic release from nigral transplants visualized in vivo in a Parkinson's patient. Nat Neurosci 2:1137–1140

Plaha P, Gill S (2005) Bilateral deep brain stimulation of the pedunculopontine nucleus for Parkinson's disease. Neuroreport 16 (17):1883–1887

Pluchino S, Martino G (2005) The therapeutic use of stem cells for myelin repair in autoimmune demyelinating disorders. J Neurol Sci 233:117–119

Pluchino S, Quattrini A, Brambilla E, Gritti A, Salani G, Dina G, Galli R, Del Carro U, Amadio S, Bergami A, Furlan R, Comi G, Vescovi AL, Martino G (2003) Injection of adult neurospheres induces recovery in a chronic model of multiple sclerosis. Nature 422:688–694

Pogge T (1994) John Rawls. Beck, München

Polgar S, Morris ME, Reilly S, Bilney B, Sanberg PR (2003) Reconstructive neurosurgery for Parkinson's disease: a systematic review and preliminary meta-analysis. Brain Res Bull 60:1–24

Poliakov GI (1972) Neuron Structure of the Brain. Harvard University Press, Cambridge, Mass

Polkinghorne J (1989) Review of the Guidance on the Research Use of Fetuses and Fetal Material (Cm.762). Her Majesty's Stationery Office, London

Postman N (1982) The Disappearance of Childhood. Delacorte Press, New York

Poussaint AF, Ditman KS (1965) A clinical trial of protriptyline in childhood enuresis. Psychosomatics 6:413–6

President's Council on Bioethics (PCB) (2003) Beyond Therapy: Biotechnology and the Pursuit of Happiness. A report of The President's Council on Bioethics. US Government Printing Office, Washington DC

Pulsinelli WA, Jacewicz M, Levy DE, Petito CK, Plum F (1997) Ischemic brain injury and the therapeutic window. Ann NY Acad Sci 835:187–193

Quante M (1996) Hirngewebetransplantation und die Identität der Person: ein spezifisch ethisches Problem. In: Hubig C, Poser H (eds) Cognitio Humana – Dynamik des Wissens und der Werte. Universität Leipzig, Leipzig, pp 1459–1466

Quante M (2002) Personales Leben und menschlicher Tod. Personale Identität als Prinzip der biomedizinischen Ethik. Suhrkamp, Frankfurt a.M.

Quaranta N, Bartoli R, Priore AL, Fernandez-Vega S, Giagnotti F, Quaranta A (2005) Cochlear implantation in otosclerosis. Otol Neurotol 26(5):983–987

Quinn N, Brown R, Craufurd D, Goldman S, Hodges J, Kieburtz K, Lindvall O, MacMillan J, Roos R (CAPIT-HD committee) (1996) Core assessment programme for intracerebral transplantation in Huntington's disease (CAPIT-HD). Mov Disord 11:143–150

Quintana H, Keshavan M (1995) Case study: risperidone in children and adolescents with schizophrenia. J Am Acad Child Adolesc Psychiatry 34(10):1292–1296

Rabinovich SS, Seledtsov VI, Banul NV, Poveshchenko OV, Senyukov VV, Astrakov SV, Samarin DM, Taraban VY (2005) Cell therapy of brain stroke. Bull Exp Biol Med 139:126–128

Raeymaekers P, Rondia K, Slob M (ed) (2004) Connecting brains and society. The present and future of brain science: What is possible, what is desirable? King Baudouin Foundation, Rathenau Institute

Ralph MR, Foster RG, Davis FC, Menaker M (1990) Transplanted suprachiasmatic nucleus determines circadian period. Science 247:975–978

Rapoport JL (1965) Childhood behavior and learning problems treated with imipramine. Int J Neuropsychiatry 1:635–642

Rapoport JL, Buchsbaum MS, Zahn TP, Weingartner H, Ludolw E, Mikkelsen EJ (1978) Dextroamphetamine: Cognitive and behavioral effects in normal prepubertal boys. Science:560–562

Rapoport JL (1980) Dextroemphetamine: Its cognitive and behavioral effects in normal and hyperactive boys and normal men. Archives of General Psychiatry 37:933–943

Rappley MD, Gardiner JC, Jetton JR, Houang RT (1995) The use of methylphenidate in Michigan. Arch Pediatr Adolesc Med 149:675–679

Rauschecker JP, Shannon RV (2002) Sending sound to the brain. Science 295:1025–1029

Rawls J (1971) A Theory of Justice. Harvard University Press, Cambridge

Rawls J (1993) Political Liberalism. Columbia University Press, New York

Rawls J (2001) Justice as Fairness. A Restatement. Harvard University Press, Cambridge

Raymon HK, Thode S, Gage FH (1997) Application of ex vivo gene therapy in the treatment of Parkinson's disease. Exp Neurol 144:82–91

Reid T (1983) Essays on the intellectual powers of man. In: Hamilton W (ed) The Works of Thomas Reid. Reprinted. Olms, Hildesheim

Reinisch JM, Sanders SA (1982) Early barbiturate exposure: the brain, sexually dimorphic behavior and learning. Neurosci Biobehav Rev 6:311–319

Reinisch JM, Sanders SA, Mortensen EL, Rubin DB (1995) In utero exposure to phenobarbital and intelligence deficits in adult men. JAMA 274:1518–1525

Richichi C, Lin EJ, Stefanin D, Colella D, Ravizza T, Grignaschi G, Veglianese P, Sperk G, During MJ, Vezzani A (2004) Anticonvulsant and antiepileptogenic effects mediated by adeno-associated virus vector neuropeptide Y expression in the rat hippocampus. J Neurosci 24:3051–3059

Riordan CE (1999) Statement of the American Psychiatric Association to the Senate Finance Committee: Hearing on Seclusion and Restraint of Psychiatric Patients. http://www.psych.org/pub_pol_adv/sec_res_rior_test.cfm

Rita P (2004) Tactile sensory substitution studies. Ann NY Acad Sci 1013:83–91

Rizzo JF 3rd, Wyatt J, Humayun M, de Juan E, Liu W, Chow A, Eckmiller R, Zrenner E, Yagi T, Abrams G (2001) Retinal prosthesis: an encouraging first decade with major challenges ahead. Ophthalmology 108(1):13–14

Robertson JA (1988) Rights, symbolism and public policy in fetal tissue transplants. Hastings Center Report 6

Rohwedel J, Guan K, Zuschratter W, Jin S, Ahnert-Hilger G, Furst D, Fassler R, Wobus AM (1998) Loss of beta1 integrin function results in a retardation of myogenic, but an acceleration of neuronal, differentiation of embryonic stem cells in vitro. Dev Biol 201:167–184

Rorty AO, Wong D (1990) Aspects of identity and agency. In: Rorty A, Flanagan O (eds) Identity, Character, and Morality: Essays in Moral Psychology. MIT Press, Cambridge

Rosahl SK (2006) Implantierbarer Blutdruckmodulator. DP 10 2005 044 560.8-54. Deutsches Patentamt

Rosahl SK, Lenarz T, Matthies C, Samii M, Sollmann WP, Laszig R (2004) Hirnstammimplantate zur Wiederherstellung des Hörvermögens. Dt Ärzteblatt 101(4):180–188

Rosahl SK, Mark G, Herzog M, Pantazis C, Gharabaghi F, Matthies C, Brinker T, Samii M (2001) Far-field responses to stimulation of the cochlear nucleus with microsurgically placed penetrating and surface electrodes in the cat. J Neurosurg 95:845–852

Rosenfeld JV (2002) James IV Lecture. Epilepsy surgery, hypothalamic hamartomas and the quest for a cure. J R Coll Surg Edinb 47:653–659

Roskies A (2002) Neuroethics for the new millenium. Neuron 35:21–23

Rosser AE, Barker RA, Harrower T, Watts C, Farrington M, Ho AK, Burnstein RM, Menon DK, Gillard JH, Pickard J, Dunnett SB (2002) NEST-UK. Unilateral transplantation of human primary fetal tissue in four patients with Huntington's disease: NEST-UK safety report ISRCTN no 36485475. J Neurol Neurosurg Psychiatr 73:678–685, 95:275–84

Rothärmel S (1999) Die Einwilligungsfähigkeit – ein janusköpfiges Institut. In: Fegert JM, Häßler F, Rothärmel S (eds) Atypische Neuroleptika in der Jugendpsychiatrie. Schattauer, Stuttgart

Rothärmel S, Dippold I, Wiethoff K, Wolfslast G, Fegert JM (2005) Patientenaufklärung, Informationsbedürfnis und Informationspraxis in der Kinder- und Jugendpsychiatrie. Vandenhoeck & Rupprecht, Göttingen

Roughley N (2005) Was heisst „menschliche Natur"? Begriffliche Differenzierungen und normative Ansatzpunkte. In: Bayertz K (ed) Die menschliche Natur: Welchen und wieviel Wert hat sie? Mentis, Paderborn:133-156.

Roybon L, Christophersen NS, Brundin P, Li J-Y (2004) Stem cell therapy for Parkinson's disease: where do we stand? Cell Tissue Res 318:261–273

Rubinstein JT (2004) How cochlear implants encode speech. Curr Opin Otolaryngol Head Neck Surg 12(5):444–448

Rush AJ, George MS, Sackeim HA, Marangell LB, Husain MM, Giller C, Nahas Z, Haines S, Simpson RK Jr, Goodman R (2000) Vagus nerve stimulation (VNS) for treatment-resistant depressions: a multicenter study. Biol Psychiatry 47(4):276–286

Rush AJ, Marangell LB, Sackeim HA, George MS, Brannan SK, Davis SM, Howland R, Kling MA, Rittberg BR, Burke WJ, Rapaport MH, Zajecka J, Nierenberg AA, Husain MM, Ginsberg D, Cooke RG (2005a) Vagus nerve stimulation for treatment-resistant depression: a randomized, controlled acute phase trial. Biol Psychiatry 58(5):347–354

Rush AJ, Sackeim HA, Marangell LB, George MS, Brannan SK, Davis SM, Lavori P, Howland R, Kling MA, Rittberg B, Carpenter L, Ninan P, Moreno F, Schwartz T, Conway C, Burke M, Barry JJ (2005b) Effects of 12 months of vagus nerve stimulation in treatment-resistant depression: a naturalistic study. Biol Psychiatry 58(5):355–363

Rutecki P (1990) Anatomical, physiological, and theoretical basis for the antiepileptic effect of vagus nerve stimulation. Epilepsia 31 suppl 2:1–6

Sacks O (1985) The Man who Mistook His Wife for a Hat. And Other Clinical Tales. Touchstone, New York

Safer D, Zito J, Fine E (1996) Increased methylphenidate usage for attention deficit hyperactivity disorder in the 1990s. Pediatrics 98:1084–1088

Safer D, Zito J (2006) Treatment-emergent adverse events from selective serotonin reuptake inhibitors by age group: Children versus adolescents. J Child Adolesc Psychopharmacol 16(1-2):159–169
Sagot Y, Tan SA, Baetge E, Schmalbruch H, Kato AC, Aebischer P (1995) Polymer encapsulated cell lines genetically engineered to release ciliary neurotrophic factor can slow down progressive motor neuronopathy in the mouse. Eur J Neurosci 7:1313–1322
Salinsky MC, Uthman BM, Ristanovic RK, Wernicke JF, Tarver, WB (1996) Vagus nerve stimulation for the treatment of medically intractable seizures. Results of a 1-year open-extension trial. Vagus nerve stimulation study group. Arch Neurol 53(11):1176–1180
Sampaio E, Maris S, Rita P (2001) Brain plasticity: 'visual' acuity of blind persons via the tongue. Brain Res 908(2):204–207
Sanberg PR, Borlongan CV, Othberg AI, Saporta S, Freeman TB, Cameron DF (1997) Testis-derived Sertoli cells have a trophic effect on dopamine neurons and alleviate hemiparkinsonism in rats. Nat Med 3:1129–1132
Sanftner LM, Sommer JM, Suzuki BM, Smith PH, Vijay S, Vargas JA, Forsayeth JR, Cunningham J, Bankiewicz KS, Kao H, Bernal J, Pierce GF, Johnson KW (2005) AAV2-mediated gene delivery to monkey putamen: evaluation of an infusion device and delivery parameters. Exp Neurol 194:476–483
Santhanam G, Ryu SI, Yu BM, Afshar A, Shenoy KV (2006) A high-performance brain-computer interface. Nature 442(7099):95–198
Sass KJ, Buchanan CP, Westerveld M, Marek KL, Farhi A, Robbins RJ, Naftolin F, Vollmer TL, Leranth C, Roth RH, Price RH, Bunney BS, Elsworth JD, Hoffer PB, Redmond E, Spencer DD (1995) General cognitive ability following unilateral and bilateral fetal ventral mesencephalic tissue transplantation for treatment of Parkinson's disease. Arch Neurol 52:680–686
Savitz SI, Dinsmore J, Wu J, Henderson GV, Stieg P, Caplan LR (2005) Neurotransplantation of fetal porcine cells in patients with basal ganglia infarcts: A preliminary safety and feasibility study. Cerebrovasc Dis 20:101–107
Schellinger PD, Orberk E, Hacke W (1997) Antithrombotic therapy after cerebral ischemia. Fortschr Neurol Psychiatr 65:425–434
Schindler RA (1999) Personal reflections on cochlear implants. Ann Otol Rhinol Laryngol 177(suppl):4–7
Schläpfer TE, Kosel M, Fisch H (2006) Repetitive transcranial magnetic stimulation (rTMS) in depression. Poiesis and Praxis 4:111–127
Schmidt EM, Bak MJ, Hambrecht FT, Kufta CV, O'Rourke, DK, Vallabhanath P (1996) Feasibility of a visual prosthesis for the blind based on intracortical microstimulation of the visual cortex. Brain 119(2):507–22
Schmidt K, Solanto MV, Sanchez-Kappraff M, Vargas P, Wein S (1984) The effect of stimulant medication on academic performance, in the context of multimodal treatment, in attention deficit disorders with hyperactivity: two case reports. J Clin Psychopharmacol 4(2):100–3
Schneider PJ (1824) Entwurf zu einer Heilmittellehre gegen psychische Krankheiten. Laupp, Tübingen
Schorr M, Zhou L, Schwechheimer K (1996) Expression of ciliary neurotrophic factor is maintained in spinal motor neurons of amyotrophic lateral sclerosis. J Neurol Sci 140:117–122
Schulze H, Hess A, Ohl FW, Scheich H (2002) Superposition of horseshoe-like periodicity and linear tonotopic maps in auditory cortex of the Mongolian gerbil. Eur J Neurosci 15(6):1077–1084
Schwabe U, Paffrath D (2005) Arzneiverordnungs-Report 2005. Aktuelle Daten, Kosten; Trends und Kommentare. Heidelberg, Springer
Schwartz AB (2004) Cortical neural prosthetics. Annu Rev Neurosci 27:487–507

Scothorne RJ (1968) Early development. In: Passmore R, Robson JS (eds) A Companion to Medical Studies, vol 1. Blackwell Scientific Publications, Oxford, chapter 18
Segev R (2005) Well-being and fairness in the distribution of scarce health ressources. Journal of Medicine and Philosophy 30:231–260
Selgelid MJ (2003) Ethics and eugenic enhancement. Poiesis and Praxis 1:239–261
Serruya MD, Hatsopoulos NG, Paninski L, Fellows MR, Donoghue JP (2002) Instant neural control of a movement signal. Nature 416(6877):141–142
Shamblott MJ, Axelman J, Littlefield JW, Blumenthal PD, Huggins GR, Cui Y, Cheng L, Gearhart JD (2001) Human embryonic germ cell derivatives express a broad range of developmentally distinct markers and proliferate extensively in vitro. Proc Natl Acad Sci USA 98:113–118
Shannon KM, Kordower JH (1996) Neural transplantation for Huntington's disease: experimental rationale and recommendations for clinical trials. Cell Transplant 5:339–352
Shannon RV (1989) Threshold functions for electrical stimulation of the human cochlear nucleus. Hear Res 40(1–2):173–7
Shannon RV, Otto SR (1990) Psychophysical measures from electrical stimulation of the human cochlear nucleus. Hear Res 47(1–2):159–68
Shaw K, Turner J, Del Mar C (2001) Tryptophan and 5-Hydroxytryptophan for Depression. Cochrane Database of Systematic Reviews, Issue 1. Art. No.: CD003198. DOI: 10.1002/14651858.CD003198
Shen Y, Muramatsu SI, Ikeguchi K, Fujimoto KI, Fan DS, Ogawa M, Mizukami H, Urabe M, Kume A, Nagatsu I, Urano F, Suzuki T, Ichinose H, Nagatsu T, Monahan J, Nakano I, Ozawa K (2000) Triple transduction with adeno-associated virus vectors expressing tyrosine hydroxylase, aromatic-L-amino-acid decarboxylase, and GTP cyclohydrolase I for gene therapy of Parkinson's disease. Hum Gene Ther 11:1509–1519
Shoemaker S (1970) Persons and their pasts. In: American Philosophical Quarterly 7:269–85
Shoemaker S, Swinburne R (1984) Personal Identity. Blackwell, Oxford
Siep L (2002) Moral und Gattungsethik. Deutsche Zeitschrift für Philosophie 50:111–120
Simmons FB (1966) Electrical stimulation of the auditory nerve in man. Arch Otolaryngol 84:2–54
Simon RL (1984) Good competition and drug-enhanced performance. Journal of the Philosophy of Sport XI:6–13
Simon RL (1995) Good competition and drug enhanced performance. In: Morgan WJ, Meier KV (eds) Philosophic Inquiry in Sport, 2nd edn. Human Kinetics Publishers, Champaign, Illinois
Singer P (1990) Embryo Experimentation. Ethical, legal and social issues. Cambridge University Press, Cambridge
Skinner MW, Arndt PL, Staller SJ (2002a) Nucleus 24 advanced encoder conversion study: performance versus preference. Ear Hear 23(suppl 1):2–17
Skinner MW, Holden, LK, Whitford, LA, Plant KL, Psarros C, Holden TA (2002b) Speech recognition with the nucleus 24 SPEAK, ACE, and CIS speech coding strategies in newly implanted adults. Ear Hear 23(3):207–223
Sladek JR, Shoulson I (1988) Neural transplantation: a call for patience rather than patients. Science 240:1386–1388
Solanto MV (1998) Neuropsychopharmacological mechanism of stimulant drug action in attention-deficit-hyperactivity disorder. A review and integration. Behav Brain Res 94:127–152
Solanto MV (2002) Dopamine dysfunction in AD/HD: integrating clinical and basic neuroscience research. Behav Brain Res 130:65–71

Solomon PR, Adams F, Silver A, Zimmer J, DeVeaux R (2002) Gingko for memory enhancement. JAMA 288:835–840
Sorrentino A (2004) Chemical restraints for the agitated, violent, or psychotic pediatric patient in the emergency department: controversies and recommendations. Curr Opin Pediatr 16:201–205
Spaemann R (1996) Personen: Versuche über den Unterschied zwischen 'etwas' und 'jemand'. Klett-Cotta, Stuttgart
Spanaki MV, Allen LS, Mueller WM, Morris GL 3rd (2004) Vagus nerve stimulation therapy: 5-year or greater outcome at a university-based epilepsy center. Seizure 13(8):587–590
Spencer T, Beiderman J, Wilens T, Harding M, O'Donnell D, Griffin S (1996) Pharmacotherapy of attention-deficit hyperactivity disorder across the life cycle. Journal of the American Academy of Child and Adolescent Psychiatry 35(4):409–432
Stahl SM (2000) Essential Psychopharmacology. Neuroscientific Basis and Practical Applications, 2nd edn. Cambridge University Press, Cambridge
Stanley GB, Li FF, Dan Y (1999) Reconstruction of natural scenes from ensemble responses in the lateral geniculate nucleus. J Neurosci 19(18):8036–8042
Stark A (2006) The Limits of Medicine. Cambridge University Press, Cambridge
Stempsey WE (2000) A pathological view of disease. Theoretical Medicine 21:321–330
Steven SS, Jones RC (1939) The mechanisms of hearing by electrical stimulation. J Acoust Soc Am 10:261–269
Sternbach RA (1968) Pain. A Psychophysiological Analysis. Academic Press, New York
Stieglitz T (2006) Neuro-technical interfaces to the central nervous system. Poiesis and Praxis 4:95–109
Stilley CS, Ryan CM, Kondziolka D, Bender A, DeCesare S, Wechsler L (2004) Changes in cognitive function after neuronal cell transplantation for basal ganglia stroke. Neurology 63:1320–1322
Stoye JP, Le Tissier P, Takeuchi Y, Patience C, Weiss RA (1998) Endogenous retrovirus: a potential problem for xenotransplantation? Ann NY Acad Sci 862:67–74
Strawson G (2004) Against narrativity. Ratio 17/4:428–452
Strawson PF (1959) Individuals. An Essay in Descriptive Metaphysics. Methuen, London
Strawson PF (1966) The Bounds of Sense. An Essay on Kant's 'Critique of Pure Reason.' Methuen, London
Sturm V, Lenartz D, Koulousakis A, Treuer H, Herholz K, Klein J, Klosterkötter J (2003) The nucleus accumbens: a target for deep brain stimulation in obsessive-compulsive and anxiety-disorders. Journal of Chemical Neuroanatomy 26:293–299
Sturma D (1997) Philosophie der Person. Die Selbstverhältnisse von Subjektivität und Moralität. Schöningh, Paderborn
Swaab DF, Boer K (2001) Functional teratogenic effects of chemicals on the developing brain. In: Levene MI, Chervenak FA, Whittle MJ (eds) Fetal and neonatal neurology and neurosurgery. Chirchill Livingstone, London, chapter 15, pp 251–265
Swaab D, Goren L, Hofmann M (1992) The human hypothalamus in relation to gender and sexual orientation. Progress in Brain Research 93:205–219
Swanson J (1993) Effect of stimulant medication on hyperactive children: A review of review. Exceptional Child 60:154–162
TADS-Study-Group (2004) The treatment for adolescents with depression study (TADS): Short-Term Effectiveness and Safetys Outcomes. JAMA 7:807–820
Tan SA, Deglon N, Zurn AD, Baetge EE, Bamber B, Kato AC, Aebischer P (1996) Rescue of motoneurons from axotomy-induced cell death by polymer encapsulated cells genetically engineered to release CNTF. Cell Transplant 5:577–587

Tang Y-P, Shimizu E, Dube GR, Rampon C, Kerchner GA, Zhuo M, Liu G, Tsien JZ (1999) Genetic enhancement of learning and memory in mice. Nature 401:63–69
Talwar SK, Xu S, Hawley, ES, Weiss SA, Moxon KA, Chapin JK (2002) Rat navigation guided by remote control. Nature 417(6884):37–38
Tasker RR, Siqueira J, Hawrrylyshyn P, Organ LW (1983) What happened to VIM thalamotomy for Parkinson's disease. Appl Neurophysiol 46:68–83
Taylor C (1989) Sources of the Self. The Making of the Modern Identity. Cambridge University Press, Cambridge
Taylor DM, Tillery SI, Schwartz AB (2002) Direct cortical control of 3D neuroprosthetic devices. Science 296(5574):1829–1832
Taylor DM, Tillery SI, Schwartz AB (2003) Information conveyed through brain-control: cursor versus robot. IEEE Trans. Neural Syst Rehabil Eng 11(2):195–199
Tenenbaum L, Lehtonenm E, Monahanm PE (2003) Evaluation of risks related to the use of adeno-associated virus-based vectors. Curr Gene Ther 3:545–565
Theodore WH, Fisher RS (2004) Brain Stimulation for Epilepsy. The Lancet – Neurology (2):111–118
The President's Council on Bioethics (2003) Beyond Therapy. Biotechnology and the Pursuit of Happiness. Washington D.C.
The President's Council on Bioethics, Transcripts of Council Sessions (cited by the exact date). Available at http://bioethicsprint.bioethics.gov/transcripts
Thompson KW (2005) Genetically engineered cells with regulatable GABA production can affect afterdischarges and behavioral seizures after transplantation into the dentate gyrus. Neuroscience 133:1029–1037
Thompson KW, Suchomelova LM (2004) Transplants of cells engineered to produce GABA suppress spontaneous seizures. Epilepsia 45:4–12
Thompson WG (1980) Succesful brain grafting. NY Med J 15:701
Thomson JA, Itskovitz-Eldor J, Shapiro SS, Waknitz MA, Swiergiel JJ, Marshall VS, Jones JM (1998) Embryonic stem cell lines derived from human blastocysts. Science 282:1145–1147
Toma JG, Akhavan M, Fernandes KJ, Barnabe Heider F, Sadikot A, Kaplan DR, Miller FD (2001) Isolation of multipotent adult stem cells from the dermis of mammalian skin. Nat Cell Biol 3:778–784
Toren P, Laor N, Weizman A (1998) Use of atypical neuroleptics in child and adolescent psychiatry. Journal of Clinical Psychiatry 59 (12):644–656
Totoiu MO, Nistor GI, Lane TE, Keirstead HS (2004) Remyelination, axonal sparing, and locomotor recovery following transplantation of glial-committed progenitor cells into the MHV model of multiple sclerosis. Exp Neurol 187:254–265
Treffert DA (2006) Extraordinary People: Understanding Savant Syndrome. Backinprint.com
Tremblay JP, Malouin F, Roy R, Huard J, Bouchard JP, Satoh A, Richards CL (1993) Results of a triple blind clinical study of myoblast transplantations without immunosuppressive treatment in young boys with Duchenne muscular dystrophy. Cell Transplant 2:99–11
Trinh JV, Nehrenberg DL, Jacobsen JP, Caron MG, Wetsel WC (2003) Differential psychostimulant-induced activation of neural circuits in dopamine transporter knockout an wild type mice. Neuroscience 118:297–310
Tse WS, Bond AJ (2001) Serotonergic involvement in the psycho-social dimension of personality. Journal of Psychopharmacology 15:195–198
Turner DC, Robbins TW, Clark L, Aron AR, Dowson J, Sahakian BJ (2003) Cognitive enhancing effects of modafinil in healthy volunteers. Psychopharmacology 165:260–269
Turner DC, Clark L, Dowson J, Robbins TW, Sahakian BJ (2004) Modafinil improves cognition and response inhibition in adult attention-deficit/hyperactivity disorder. Biol Psychiatry 55(10):1031–40

Turrone P, Kapur S, Seeman MV, Flint AJ (2002) Elevation of prolactin levels by atypical antipsychotics. Am J of Psychiatry 159:133–135

Tuszynski MH (2002) Growth factor gene therapy for neurodegenerative disorders. Lancet Neurology 1:51–57

Tuszynski MH, Blesch A (2004) Nerve growth factor: from animal models of cholinergic neuronal degeneration to gene therapy in Alzheimer's disease. Prog Brain Res 146:441–449

Tuszynski MH, Smith DE, Roberts J, McKay H, Mufson E (1998) Targeted intraparenchymal delivery of human NGF by gene transfer to the primate basal forebrain for 3 months does not accelerate beta-amyloid plaque deposition. Exp Neurol 154:573–582

Tuszynski MH, Thal L, Pay M, Salmon DP, U HS, Bakay R, Patel P, Blesch A, Vahlsing HL, Ho G, Tong G, Potkin SG, Fallon J, Hansen L, Mufson EJ, Kordower JH, Gall C, Conner J (2005) A phase 1 clinical trial of nerve growth factor gene therapy for Alzheimer disease. Nat Med 11:551–555

Tyler M, Danilov Y, Bach YR (2003) Closing an open-loop control system: vestibular substitution through the tongue. J Integr Neurosci 2(2):159–164

United Nations (1948) Universal Declaration of Human Rights. Yearbook of the United Nations 1948–49. Dept of Public Information, United Nations, New York

Uthman BM, Wilder BJ, Penry JK, Dean C, Ramsay RE, Reid SA, Hammond EJ, Tarver WB, Wernicke JF (1993) Treatment of epilepsy by stimulation of the vagus nerve. Neurology 43(7):1338–1345

Vendrame M, Gemma C, de Mesquita D, Collier L, Bickford PC, Sanberg CD, Sanberg PR, Pennypacker KR, Willing AE (2005) Anti-inflammatory effects of human cord blood cells in a rat model of stroke. Stem Cells Dev 14:595–604

Veraart C, Raftopoulos C, Mortimer JT, Delbeke J, Pins D, Michaux G, Vanlierde A, Parrini S, Wanet-Defalque MC (1998) Visual sensations produced by optic nerve stimulation using an implanted self-sizing spiral cuff electrode. Brain Res 813(1):181–186

Vitiello B, Hill JL, Elia J, Cunningham E, McLeer SV, Behar D (1991) PRN medications in child psychiatric patients: A pilot placebo-controlled study. J Clin Psychiatry 52:499–501

Vitiello B, Heiligenstein JH, Riddle MA, Greenhill LL, Fegert JM (2004) The interface between publicly-funded and industry-funded research in paediatric psychopharmacology: Opportunities for integration and collaboration. Biological Psychiatry 56:3–9

Vitiello B, Jensen PS, Hoagwood K (1999) Integrating science and ethics in child and adolescent psychiatry research. Biol Psychiatry 46:1044–1049

Vogel G (2001) Parkinson's research, fetal cell transplant trial draws fire. Science 291:2060–20611

Volkow ND, Wang GJ, Fowler JS, Ding YS (2005) Imaging the effects of methylphenidate on brain dopamine: new model on its therapeutic actions for attention-deficit/hyperactivity disorder. Biol Psychiatry 57:1410–1415

Volkow ND, Wang GJ, Fowler JS, Telang F, Maynard L, Logan J, Gatley SJ, Pappas N, Wong C, Vaska P, Zhu W, Swanson JM (2004) Evidence that methylphenidate enhances the saliency of a mathematical task by increasing dopamine in the human brain. Am J Psychiatry Jul 161(7):1173–80

Volta A (1800) On the electricity excited by mere contact of conducting substances of different kinds. Trans R Soc Phil 90:403–431

Wachbroit R (2001) Health and Disease, Concepts of. In: Chadwick R (ed) The Concise Encyclopedia of the Ethics of New Technologies. San Diego, Academic Press, pp 229–233

Wagner KD, Ambrosini P, Rynn M, Wohlberg C, Yang R, Greenbaum MS, Childress A, Donnelly C, Deas D (2003) Efficacy of sertraline in the treatment of children and adolescents with major depressive disorder. J of the American Academy 290:1033

Walsh JK, Randazzo AC, Stone KL, Schweitzer PK (2004) Modafinil improves alertness, vigilance, and executive function during simulated night shifts. Sleep 27(3):434–9 Walters L (1988) Ethical issues in fetal research: a look back and a look forward. Clin Res 36:209–214

Waltzman SB, Roland JT Jr (2005) Cochlear implantation in children younger than 12 months. Pediatrics 116(4):e487–e493

Warner R (2004) Prävention in der Psychiatrie – was wirkt? In: Schmidt-Zadel R, Kunze H, Peukert R (eds) AktionPsychischKranke, Prävention bei psychischen Erkrankungen. Neue Wege in Praxis und Gesetzgebung. Psychiatrie-Verlag, Bonn, pp 62–90

Warren DJ, Normann RA (2003) Visual neuroprothesis. Handbook of neuroprosthetic methods. Finn WE, LoPresti PG (eds) CRC Press, London, pp 261–307

Warren DJ, Normann RA (2005) Functional reorganization of primary visual cortex induced by electrical stimulation in the cat. Vision Re 45(5):551–565

Warren MA (1975) On the moral and legal status of abortion. In: Wasserstrom R (ed) Today's Moral Problems. New York: McMillan, New York, pp 120–13636

Warwick K (2002) Thought to computer communication. Stud Health Technol Inform 80:61–68

Warwick K (2005) Future of computer implant technology and intelligent human-machine systems. Stud Health Technol Inform 118:125–131

Warwick K, Gasson M, Hutt B, Goodhew I, Kyberd P, Andrews B, Teddy P, Shad A (2003) The application of implant technology for cybernetic systems. Arch Neurol 60(10):1369–1373

Watts RI, Freeman TB, Hauser RA, Bakay RA, Ellias SA, Stoessel AJ, Eidelberg D, Fink JS (2001) A double blind randomized, controlled, multicenter clinical trialtrial of the safety and eficacy of stereotaxic intrastriatl implantation of fetal porcine ventral mesencephalic tissue (Neurocell™-PD) vs. imitation surgery in patients with Parkinson's disease. Parkinsonism Relat Disord 7:87

Webster JT (2004) Nano-biotechnology: carbon nanofibres as improved neural and orthopaedic implants. Nanotechnology 15:48–54

Weiland JD, Humayun MS (2003) Past, present, and future of artificial vision. Artif Organs 27(11):961–962

Weiland JD, Liu W, Humayun MS (2005) Retinal prosthesis. Annu Rev Biomed Eng 7:361–401

Weiskrantz L (ed) (1988) Thought without Language. Clarendon Press, Oxford

Weiss G, Hechtman LT (1993) Hyperactive Children Grown up: ADHD in Children, Adolescents, and Adults. 2nd ed. Guilford Press, New York

Weiss RA (1998) Transgenic pigs and virus adaptation. Nature 391:327–328

Wesensten N, Belenky G, Kautz MA, Thorne DR, Reichardt RM, Balkin TJ (2001) Maintaining alertness and performance during sleep deprivation: Modafinil versus caffeine. Psychopharmacology 159:238247

Wesnes KA, Ward T, McGinty A, Petrini O (2000) The memory enhancing effect of a Gingko biloba/Panax ginseng combination in healthy middle-aged volunteers. Psychopharmacology 152:353–361

Wever EG, Bray CW (1930) The nature of the acoustic response: the relation between sound frequency and frequency of impulses in the auditory nerve. J Exp Psychol 13:373–387

Whittington CJ, Kendall T, Fonagy P, Contrell D, Cotgrove A, Boddington E (2004) Selective serotonin reuptake inhibitors in childhood depression; systematic review of published versus unpublished data. Lancet 363:1341

Wictorin K (1992) Anatomy and connectivity of intrastriatal striatal transplants. Prog Neurobiol 38:611–639
Widner H (1994) NIH neural transplantation funding. Science 263:737
Widner H, Defer GL (1999) Dyskinesias Assessment: From CAPIT to CAPSIT. Movem Disord 14, suppl 1:60–66
Widner H, Tetrud J, Rehncrona S, Snow B, Brundin P, Gustavii B, Björklund A, Lindvall O, Langston JW (1992) Bilateral fetal mesencephalic grafting in two patients with Parkinsonism induced by 1-methyl-4-phenyl-1,2,3,6-tetrahydropyridine (MPTP). N Engl J Med 327:1556–1563
Wiggins D (1967) Identity and Spatio-Temporal Continuity. Blackwell, Oxford
Williams B (1973) The self and the future. In: Williams B (ed) Problems of the Self. Cambridge University Press, Cambridge
Wilmut I, Schnieke AE, McWhir J, Kind AJ, Campbell KH (1997) Viable offspring derived from fetal and adult mammalian cells. Nature 385:810–813
Wittgenstein L (2001) Philosophical investigations: The German text, with a revised English translation. Blackwell, Oxford
Wolf E, Zakhartchenko V, Brem G (1998) Nuclear transfer in mammals: recent developments and future perspectives. J Biotechnol 65:99–110
Woodworth T (2000) Statement before the Committee on Education and the Workforce: Subcommittee on Early Childhood, Youth and Families. May 16, 2000, available at http://www.usdoj.gov/dea/pubs/cngrtest/ct051600.htm
World Medical Association Declaration of Helsinki (2000) Ethical: Ethical principles for medical research involving human subjects. JAMA 284:3043–3045
World Psychiatric Association (WPA) (2003) Consenus statement on psychiatric prevention. WPA Sections Newsletter 2:6
Word CO, Zanna MP, Cooper J (1974) The nonverbal mediation of self-fulfilling prophecies in interracial interaction. Journal of Experimental Social Psychology 10:109–120
Worrell G, Wharen R, Goodman R, Bergey G, Murro A, Bergen D, Smith M, Vossler D, Morrell M (2005) Safety and evidence for efficacy of an implantable responsive neurostimulator (RNS™) for the treatment of medically intractable partial onset epilepsy in adults. Abstract presented at the Annual Meeting of the American Epilepsy Society (AES), Dec 2005
Wundt W (1903) Grundzüge der physiologischen Psychologie, vol 3. Barth, Leipzig
Wynn R (1996) Polar day and polar night: Month of year and time of day and the use of physical and pharmacological restraint in a North Norwegian university psychiatric hospital. Arct Med Res 55:174181
Wynn R (2002) Medicate, restrain or seclude? Strategies for dealing with violent and threatening behaviour in a Norwegian university psychiatric hospital. Scand J Caring Sci 16:287291
Xu S, Talwar SK, Hawley ES, Li L, Chapin JK (2004) A multi-channel telemetry system for brain microstimulation in freely roaming animals. J Neurosci Methods 133(1–2):57–63
Yesavage JA, Mumenthaler MS, Taylor JL, Friedman L, O'Hara R, Sheikh J, Tinklenberg J, Whitehouse PJ (2002) Donezipil and flight simulator performance: Effects on retention of complex skills. Neurology 59:123125
Yung, AR, McGorry PD (1996) The prodromal phase of first-episode psychosis: past and current conceptualizations. Schizophrenia Bulletin 22:353–370
Zabara J (1985a) Time course of seizure control to brief, repetitive stimuli. Epilepsia 26:518
Zabara J (1985b) Peripheral control of hypersynchronous discharge in epilepsy. Electroencephalogr Clin Neurophysiol 61:S162
Zaghloul KA, Boahen K (2004a) Optic nerve signals in a neuromorphic chip I: Outer and inner retina models. IEEE Trans Biomed Eng 51(4):657–666

Zaghloul KA, Boahen K (2004b) Optic nerve signals in a neuromorphic chip II: Testing and results. IEEE Trans Biomed Eng 51(4):667–675

Zhao LR, Duan WM, Reyes M, Keene CD, Verfaillie CM, Low WC (2002) Human bone marrow stem cells exhibit neural phenotypes and ameliorate neurological deficits after grafting into the ischemic brain of rats. Exp Neurol 174(1):11–20

Zimmerman DW (1998) Temporary intrinsics and presentism. In: Zimmerman DW, Inwagen P (eds) Metaphysics: The Big Questions. Blackwell, Cambridge, Mass

Zimmermann M (1982) Electrical stimulation of the human brain. Hum Neurobiol 1(4):227–229

Zito JM, Derivan AT, Greenhill LL (2004) Making Research Data Available: An Ethical Imperative Demonstrated by the SSRI Debacle. Journal of the American Academy of Child and Adolescent Psychiatry 43(5):512–514

Zito JM, Safer DJ (2005) Recent child pharmacoepidemiological findings. Journal of Child and Adolescent Psychopharmacology 15:5–9

Zito JM, Safer DJ, dosReis S, Gardner JF, Boles M, Lynch F (2000) Trends in the prescribing of psychotropic medications to preschoolers. JAMA 283:1025–1030

Zito JM, Safer DJ, dosReis S, Gardner JF, Magder L, Soeken K, Boles M, Lynch F, Riddle MA (2003) Psychotropic practice patterns for youth: A 10-year perspective. Arch Pediatr Adolesc Med 157(1):17–25

Zito JM, Safer DJ, dosReis S, Magder LS, Gardner JF, Zarin DA (1999) Psychotherapeutic medication patterns for youths with attention-deficit/hyperactivity disorder. Arch Pediatr Adolesc Med 153:1257–1263

Zöllner F, Keidel WD (1963) Gehörvermittlung durch elektrische Erregung des Nervus acusticus. Arch klin exp Ohr Nas Kehlk Heilk 181:216–223

Zrenner E (2002) Will retinal implants restore vision? Science 295(5557):1022–1025

Zrenner E, Miliczek KD, Gabel VP, Graf HG, Guenther E, Haemmerle H, Hoefflinger B, Kohler K, Nisch W, Schubert M, Stett A, Weiss S (1997) The development of subretinal microphotodiodes for replacement of degenerated photoreceptors. Ophthalmic Res 29(5):269–280

Zurn AD, Henry H, Schluep M, Aubert V, Winkel L, Eilers B, Bachmann C, Aebischer P (2000) Evaluation of an intrathecal immune response in amyotrophic lateral sclerosis patients implanted with encapsulated genetically engineered xenogeneic cells. Cell Transplant 9(4):471–484

Zurn AD, Tseng J, Aebischer P (1996) Treatment of Parkinson's disease. Symptomatic cell therapies: cells as biological minipumps. Eur Neurol 36:105–108

Further volumes of the series Ethics of Science and Technology Assessment (*Wissenschaftsethik und Technikfolgenbeurteilung*):

Vol. 1: A. Grunwald (Hrsg.) Rationale Technikfolgenbeurteilung. Konzeption und methodische Grundlagen, 1998

Vol. 2: A. Grunwald, S. Saupe (Hrsg.) Ethik in der Technikgestaltung. Praktische Relevanz und Legitimation, 1999

Vol. 3: H. Harig, C. J. Langenbach (Hrsg.) Neue Materialien für innovative Produkte. Entwicklungstrends und gesellschaftliche Relevanz, 1999

Vol. 4: J. Grin, A. Grunwald (eds) Vision Assessment. Shaping Technology for 21st Century Society, 1999

Vol. 5: C. Streffer et al., Umweltstandards. Kombinierte Expositionen und ihre Auswirkungen auf den Menschen und seine natürliche Umwelt, 2000

Vol. 6: K.-M. Nigge, Life Cycle Assessment of Natural Gas Vehicles. Development and Application of Site-Dependent Impact Indicators, 2000

Vol. 7: C. R. Bartram et al., Humangenetische Diagnostik. Wissenschaftliche Grundlagen und gesellschaftliche Konsequenzen, 2000

Vol. 8: J. P. Beckmann et al., Xenotransplantation von Zellen, Geweben oder Organen. Wissenschaftliche Grundlagen und ethisch-rechtliche Implikationen, 2000

Vol. 9: G. Banse, C. J. Langenbach, P. Machleidt (eds) Towards the Information Society. The Case of Central and Eastern European Countries, 2000

Vol. 10: P. Janich, M. Gutmann, K. Prieß (Hrsg.) Biodiversität. Wissenschaftliche Grundlagen und gesellschaftliche Relevanz, 2001

Vol. 11: M. Decker (ed) Interdisciplinarity in Technology Assessment. Implementation and its Chances and Limits, 2001

Vol. 12: C. J. Langenbach, O. Ulrich (Hrsg.) Elektronische Signaturen. Kulturelle Rahmenbedingungen einer technischen Entwicklung, 2002

Vol. 13: F. Breyer, H. Kliemt, F. Thiele (eds) Rationing in Medicine. Ethical, Legal and Practical Aspects, 2002

Vol. 14: T. Christaller et al. (Hrsg.) Robotik. Perspektiven für menschliches Handeln in der zukünftigen Gesellschaft, 2001

Vol. 15: A. Grunwald, M. Gutmann, E. Neumann-Held (eds) On Human Nature. Anthropological, Biological, and Philosophical Foundations, 2002

Vol. 16: M. Schröder et al. (Hrsg.) Klimavorhersage und Klimavorsorge, 2002

Vol. 17: C. F. Gethmann, S. Lingner (Hrsg.): Integrative Modellierung zum Globalen Wandel, 2002

Vol. 18: U. Steger et al., Nachhaltige Entwicklung und Innovation im Energiebereich, 2002

Vol. 19: E. Ehlers, C. F. Gethmann (ed) Environmental Across Cultures, 2003

Vol. 20: R. Chadwick et al., Functional Foods, 2003

Vol. 21: D. Solter et al., Embryo Research in Pluralistic Europe, 2003

Vol. 22: M. Decker, M. Ladikas (eds) Bridges between Science, Society and Policy. Technology Assessment – Methods and Impacts, 2004

Vol. 23: C. Streffer et al., Low Dose Exposures in the Environment. Dose-Effect Relations and Risk-Evaluation, 2004

Vol. 24: F. Thiele, R. A. Ashcroft, Bioethics in a Small World, 2004

Vol. 25: H.-R. Duncker, K. Prieß (eds) On the Uniqueness of Humankind, 2005

Vol. 26: B. v. Maydell, K. Borchardt, K.-D. Henke, R. Leitner, R. Muffels, M. Quante, P.-L. Rauhala, G. Verschraegen, M. Zukowski, Enabling Social Europe, 2006

Vol. 27: G. Schmid, H. Brune, H. Ernst, A. Grunwald, W. Grünwald, H. Hofmann, H. Krug, P. Janich, M. Mayor, W. Rathgeber, U. Simon, V. Vogel, D. Wyrwa, Nanotechnology. Assessment and Perspectives, 2006

Vol. 28: M. Kloepfer, B. Griefahn, A. M. Kaniowski, G. Klepper, S. Lingner, G. Steineach, H. B. Weyer, P. Wysk, Leben mit Lärm? Risikobeurteilung und Regulation des Umgebungslärms im Verkehrsbereich, 2006

Vol. 29: R. Merkel, G. Boer, J. Fegert, T. Galert, D. Hartmann, B. Nuttin, S. Rosahl: Intervening in the Brain. Changing Psyche and Society, 2007

Also the following studies were published by Springer:

Environmental Standards. Combined Exposures and Their Effect on Human Beings and Their Environment, 2003, Translation Vol. 5

Sustainable Development and Innovation in the Energy Sector, 2005, Translation Vol. 18

F. Breyer, W. van den Daele, M. Engelhard, G. Gubernatis, H. Kliemt, C. Kopetzki, H. J. Schlitt, J. Taupitz, Organmangel. Ist der Tod auf der Warteliste unvermeidbar? 2006